CONTEMPORARY IMPLANT DENTISTRY

Contemporary Implant Dentistry

CARL E. MISCH, D.D.S., M.D.S.

*Director, Oral Implantology Center
  and Oral Implant Fellowship Program
Associate Professor
Department of Prosthodontics
University of Pittsburgh
Pittsburgh, Pennsylvania*

*Associate Professor and Director
University-Hospital Residency Programs
Loma Linda University
School of Dentistry
Loma Linda, California*

*Adjunct Associate Professor
Biomedical Engineering
University of Alabama at Birmingham
Birmingham, Alabama*

*Director
Misch Implant Institute
Dearborn, Michigan*

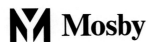 Mosby

St. Louis Baltimore Boston Chicago London Philadelphia Sydney Toronto

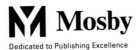

Mosby

Dedicated to Publishing Excellence

Sponsoring Editor: Robert W. Reinhardt
Developmental Editor: Carolyn Malik
Assistant Editor: Anne Gunter
Assistant Managing Editor, Text and Reference: George Mary Gardner
Production Manager: Nancy C. Baker
Proofroom Manager: Barbara M. Kelly

Mosby–Year Book, Inc.
11830 Westline Industrial Drive
St. Louis, MO 63146

1 2 3 4 5 6 7 8 9 0 GW/MV 97 96 95 94 93

Library of Congress Cataloging-in-Publication Data
   Contemporary implant dentistry / [edited by] Carl E. Misch.
       p.   cm.
   Includes bibliographical references and index.
   ISBN 0-8016-6073-4
   1. Implant dentures.   I. Misch, Carl E.
      [DNLM: 1. Dental Implantation. 2. Dental Implants. WU 640 C761
   1993]
   RK667.I45C66   1993   92-48360
   617.6'92 – dc20   CIP
   DNLM/DLC
   for Library of Congress

To my children,
Paula, Carl, Lara, David, and Jonathan.
I love them all dearly.

Contributors

Daniel E. Becker, D.D.S.
Professor, Allied Health Sciences
Sinclair Community College
Associate Director of Education
General Practice Residency
Miami Valley Hospital
Dayton, Ohio

Martha Warren Bidez, Ph.D.
Assistant Professor
Mechanical Engineering/Biomedical Engineering
University of Alabama at Birmingham
Birmingham, Alabama

Philip J. Boyne, D.M.D., D.Sc.
Department of Oral and Maxillofacial Surgery
Loma Linda University Medical Center
Loma Linda, California

Naphthali Brezniak, M.D., D.M.D., M.S.D.
Israeli Armed Services
Tel Aviv, Israel

Francine Dietsh, D.C.D., M.D.S.
Clinical Assistant Professor
Department of Prosthodontics
University of Pittsburgh
School of Dental Medicine
Pittsburgh, Pennsylvania

Lawrence P. Garetto, Ph.D.
Department of Orthodontics
Indiana University School of Dentistry
Indianapolis, Indiana

Robert A. James,
Loma Linda School of Dentistry
Loma Linda, California

Jack E. Lemons, Ph.D.
Professor and Chairman
Department of Biomaterials
University of Alabama at Birmingham
Birmingham, Alabama

Ralph V. McKinney, Jr., D.D.S., Ph.D.
(deceased)
Professor and Chairman
Department of Oral Pathology
Medical College of Georgia
Augusta, Georgia

Roland M. Meffert, D.D.S.
University of Texas Health Science Center
San Antonio, Texas

Carl E. Misch, D.D.S., M.D.S.
Director, Oral Implantology Center and Oral
  Implant Fellowship Program
Associate Professor
Department of Prosthodontics
University of Pittsburgh
Pittsburgh, Pennsylvania

Associate Professor and Director
University-Hospital Residency Programs
Loma Linda University
School of Dentistry
Loma Linda, California

Adjunct Associate Professor
Biomedical Engineering
University of Alabama at Birmingham
Birmingham, Alabama

Director
Misch Implant Institute
Dearborn, Michigan

Paul A. Moore, D.M.D., Ph.D.
Professor, Pharmacology/Physiology
Co-Director, Clinical Pharmacology
Dental Therapeutics Program
University of Pittsburgh
School of Dental Medicine
Pittsburgh, Pennsylvania

Ralph W. Phillips, D.Sc. (deceased)
Formerly, Research Professor of Dental Materials
Indiana University School of Dentistry
Indianapolis, Indiana

W. Eugene Roberts, D.D.S., Ph.D.
Professor and Chairman
Department of Orthodontics
Indiana University School of Dentistry
Indianapolis, Indiana

Mohamed Sharawy, Ph.D.
Professor and Chairman
Department of Oral Biology/Anatomy
Medical College of Georgia
Augusta, Georgia

George C. Sotereanos, D.M.D.
Director of Graduate Training in Maxillofacial
  Surgery
Presbyterian-University Hospital
Pittsburgh, Pennsylvania

Foreword

The ultimate expression of love is to give one's life for another. For many years Dr. Carl E. Misch has been sacrificing his personal life for his professional colleagues and for the organized evolution of the field of implant dentistry. *Contemporary Implant Dentistry* is the most recent manifestation of his tendency to teach, to give of himself, to enrich the lives of others.

When asked what I am most proud of in my own professional life relating to implant dentistry, I always readily answer, to have had Carl Misch as one of my students, and then to have had him become one of my teachers, and to have had him as a constant strong right arm in the worldwide development of the International Congress of Oral Implantologists and its agenda of recognition for implant dentistry.

Dr. Misch's considerable surgical skills are the result of committing long hours to the surgical method of training (something I first learned from my father), that is, interest, study, observation, assisting, being assisted, and finally mastery. Dr. Misch has continued to explore, refine, and validate new implant surgical techniques and to devise many innovative applications for standard concepts and share them unselfishly with his students and colleagues. Dr. Misch's prosthodontic skills are the result of several years of advanced private restorative practice as well as postgraduate training and teaching at the University of Pittsburgh.

Dr. Misch has served on numerous committees of many implant organizations, in many offices, and as their president; he has published extensively; he is a constant member of the international lecture circuit on implant dentistry; and he has held or holds numerous hospital and faculty appointments. He has participated in and been a key player at numerous consensus conferences: with the National Institutes of Health, for undergraduate and general practice residencies in the United States, and for predoctoral training in Europe. In addition, Dr. Misch has developed a postgraduate implant dentistry curriculum, which enjoys wide acceptance. He has been co-editor, then editor, of the *International Journal of Oral Implantology*. Further, for many years he has directed the Misch Implant Institute, dedicated to teaching routine as well as multidisciplinary implant procedures to students from around the world. Dr. Misch has shown true leadership in the field of implant dentistry, basing his teaching on extensive clinical experience and sound academic training.

All of these activities and many others I could mention have given Dr. Misch a unique insight into the science and clinical practice that has become implant dentistry in what I call its postmodern era.

Contemporary Implant Dentistry, however, reflects far more than the surgical-prosthodontic and teaching skills of one person. It organizes the totality, the "gestalt," of what a practitioner should understand and master to achieve an elegant level of clinical implant practice. Many internationally respected contributors have helped Dr. Misch achieve this goal.

Contemporary Implant Dentistry is for all members of the treatment team. It will give the reader organization and direction, medical and dental evaluation principles, language for communicating unique implant dentistry classifications, architectural and bioengineering concepts, surgical principles, alternative treatment planning, pharmacologic therapeutics, and methods for treating complications.

This is a book to be read and reread by the serious student and practitioner of implant dentistry. It projects tremendous energy, thoroughness, and commitment. It is very much Dr. Carl E. Misch.

With much personal admiration and affection.

Kenneth W.M. Judy, D.D.S., F.A.C.D., F.I.C.D.
Associate Professor
Department of Prosthodontics
University of Pittsburgh School of Dental Medicine
Pittsburgh, Pennsylvania

Preface

Organized dentistry in the early 1900s vehemently opposed fixed partial dentures. In 1911 Hunter[1] blamed the "mausoleum of gold over a mass of sepsis" for complicating anemia, gastritis, kidney disease, and lesions of the cord. Gillet in 1914 stated that the day of fixed bridgework had passed and that the next decade would see the end of its use.[2] The reformation of fixed partial dentures occurred when anatomic form, occlusion, and physiologic principles were introduced. Twenty years ago, the mere mention of the word "implant" was controversial. Organized dentistry was cautious in accepting the dental implant concept. Patients readily believed that an artificial replacement was more logical and desirable than using removable prostheses. Pioneers with vision, but all too often willing to use human experimentation, met the organized profession's skepticism. Once long-term clinical data based on sound research and scientific principles were developed, implant dentistry rapidly became an accepted alternative to removable prostheses. Today the widespread acceptance of this field is evident in almost every specialty and general practice. However, several controversial issues still remain.

The use of one implant design for all patient prosthodontic and anatomic conditions is ongoing. Forty-five years ago, when Dahl introduced the subperiosteal implant, it was popularly believed that subperiosteal implants were the most predictable treatment modality for edentulous arches. This same generalization was replaced by the root form and pin implants 25 years ago. This oversimplification then shifted to support the blade implant developed by Linkow. At one time the blade implant was the most widely used implant in the world, for both the completely and partially edentulous arch. The mandibular staple implant became the only implant system in widespread use by oral surgeons in the mid- to late 1970s, and was also touted as the only successful implant system of the time.

The latest belief of the monoimplant philosophy is the root form "osseointegrated fixture." Although this implant type has been in use for more than 25 years, not until the mid-1980s was this system introduced in North America to restore the partially or completely edentulous jaw. The newest trend of this one-implant design concept favors hydroxyapatite coating on implants.

The quest for the perfect implant will continue. However, no one implant system can accommodate all anatomic and prosthodontic conditions. The dental implant should be designed to support the indicated prosthesis, using the most predictable method for the individual patient condition. There are a myriad of patient conditions and a number of different prosthodontic requirements, and no one system can be complete or ideal for all.

Regardless of past experience in dentistry, implantology uses several unique methods and concepts not present in any existing specialty. Yet the most frequent method of training is unsupervised self-education while performing patient treatment. To seduce the practitioner, manufacturers give the impression that little skill is required and that all jaws are predictably restorable at minimal risk.

Implant dentistry developed in an era when implant education was minimal and for the most part was kept outside of the dental schools and specialty training. Malpractice litigation was rare, and few doctors were involved in treatment. Today, nine of 10 implant dentists have less than 5 years experience. The rapid assimilation of present implant dentists and the increased acceptance by the profession and patients require stricter guidelines for education and practice, especially for the teachers of implant dentistry. Implant dentistry is here to stay. A minority of practitioners will take the time and effort to learn all aspects of this rapidly growing and evolving field. The majority of practitioners can provide various aspects of treatment. Ideally, these services should be learned in a supervised hands-on program rather than self-taught in a private practice. Implant education must meet the challenge of this field and help direct the future.

The literature provided by implant companies has given the profession the luring image that implant therapy is almost 100 percent predictable. Each manufacturer, not to be outperformed, has spent millions of dollars to promote to the lay public and the profession that implants are more predictable than teeth. Teaching centers have even extracted teeth in 40-year-old patients rather than perform periodontal therapy, alleging that implants are more reliable.

The anatomy and health of the patient are always primary determinants of the outcome of the surgical procedure. When establishing a treatment plan and evaluating its prognosis, the restoring dentist must take into account a myriad of elements in dealing with the overall health of the stomatognathic system. As an implant is introduced into the treatment modality, all of the stomatognathic system has an effect on the eventual outcome.

Certainly implant dentistry represents a viable alternative for many patients in need of a removable prosthesis. But is it not a guaranteed result, without complications. It is not fair to our profession or to our patients to lump all patient conditions in a success report. Customized treatment and management of complications should be discussed with the patient based on past experience of treatment with similar or like conditions. Hence the patient with advanced atrophy who wants a fixed prosthesis cannot be compared with the patient who is satisfied with an overdenture and has abundant bone. More than 50 dental criteria influence treatment planning and its prognosis.

Not all patients need or can afford implant therapy. Removable partial and complete dentures still have indications, based on anatomic condition, health, and the patient's desires and economic priorities. For partially edentulous patients, traditional fixed prostheses are indicated whenever possible. Implant dentistry does not replace these established criteria, but only modifies the boundaries. No advanced restorative practice will not use implantology. However, it is as important to know when not to incorporate an implant in the treatment plan as it is the opposite.

Contemporary Implant Dentistry addresses the science and discipline of oral implantology. In the past, manufacturers have been the major educators in this aspect of dentistry. As a result, most all treatment is rendered with the same implant design, surgical protocol, and prosthetic approach. In contrast, this book attempts to blend the knowledge of biomaterials, biomechanics, and anatomy within the disciplines of multimodal surgery and prosthodontics. The reasons for specific clinical decisions are not based on a specific implant design but on concepts that are consistent for any design.

The first section of this book concentrates on the diagnosis and treatment plan for both the partial and completely edentulous jaw. These chapters blend together to teach undergraduate dental students the benefits and indications of implant dentistry. In addition these chapters serve as a foundation for successful planning of even the most advanced implant treatment. As a result, the experienced implant dentist will benefit from the organized approach of patient evaluation and case presentation.

The second section of the book provides the foundation sciences for oral implantology. These chapters benefit graduate students of periodontics, oral surgery, and prosthodontics. In addition, the more serious practitioner providing implant treatment will benefit, because this section provides the key to the more advanced concepts presented later in the book.

The third section presents the surgical aspects of oral implantology. The thought processes of clinical decisions are presented to enable practitioners to determine not only the ideal anatomic conditions but also to use more advanced treatments. Although these chapters are most beneficial to the surgeons of implant treatment, it is important for the astute restoring dentists to understand and appreciate surgical concerns.

The last section of this book addresses the restoration aspects of implant treatment. Because more than half of general dentists currently use implants, these chapters are designed for prosthodontic residents and restoring dentists. The advanced implant surgeons will also appreciate these chapters, to enhance their knowledge of the surgical interrelationships of treatment.

Contemporary Implant Dentistry is designed to present the thinking processes of oral implantology. The reasons certain procedures are performed over other options are addressed throughout the text. Oral Implantology has grown from the manufacturer driven treatment to the science and discipline of advanced surgical and restoring concepts. Every surgical decision affects the prosthesis. The prosthesis design and treatment affects the surgical approach. Complications most often require a combination of surgery and prosthetic considerations. Many procedures are unique solely to the discipline of oral implantology. *Contemporary Implant Dentistry* focuses on these unique aspects.

Carl E. Misch, D.D.S., M.D.S.

REFERENCES

1. Hunter W: The role of sepsis and antisepsis in medicine. *Dental Briefs* 16:852, 1911.
2. Bush AJ: Proposed classification of fixed bridge work and law governing its application. *J Natl Dent Assoc* 2:221–225, 1915.

Acknowledgments

This book is written primarily by one author. This permits consistency of thought and treatment throughout the chapters. Additional authors were asked to contribute based on past personal working relationships and undeniable leadership positions in their fields. These people often led me through the confusion of my learning curve in implant dentistry. Many, especially Bob James, Jack Lemons, and Martha Bidez, have become close personal friends, and I am especially grateful for their constant needed support. Ralph McKinney and Ralph Phillips died before this book was published. Their contributions are especially appreciated, and represent the continued commitment (in a long list) they gave to the profession and to their friends. I wish to publicly thank all participating authors for their contributions to this text and their dedication to implant dentistry.

Two individuals contributed to this book more than they know. Most responsible for the text as written is Dr. Francine Dietsh. She evaluated and edited every sentence, illustration, and photograph. She contributed often to the literature reviews and references, and helped me keep publisher deadlines. She was secretary, consultant, editor, and support during the entire project. Thank you.

Craig Misch has played many roles in my life, from 12 years younger brother, associate in my private practice, fellow in the Pittsburgh Implant Program, and now a faculty member of the Implant Graduate Program at Pittsburgh. He is my right hand. He also contributed greatly to the generic language of implant components (in some cases completely modifying my proposed terms) and also to the medication portion of the subantral grafting procedure. Thank you for your continued support.

I'd also like to acknowledge my original mentors, Ken Judy, Hilt Tatum, and Leonard Linkow. I spent hundreds of hours with these men, and their mark will forever influence my thought processes.

Ken Judy was my first mentor in oral implantology. The science and discipline of the field and its interconnection with the traditional interfacing disciplines was always understood by Ken, and taught to me in my early years of exposure. Ken Judy is still my role model for the vision of implant dentistry. In addition, he is my closest friend. Ken has always been there when I needed support, guidance, and understanding.

O. Hilt Tatum developed the concepts of autogenous and alloplastic bone augmentation specific for implant dentistry. He also developed bone manipulation and spreading procedures, along with a specific implant design for this purpose. Sinus elevation and subantral augmentation and associated implants also were first presented by Tatum. In addition, root form, plate form, and ramus frame implants were modified in surgery and design using bone biomechanic principles specific to oral implantology. Hilt allowed me to learn and participate in his teaching program on a regular basis. His appreciation for bone biomechanics and his dedication to teaching implantology influenced me for life. The influence of these advanced techniques permits implantology to treat a much broader range of patients in physical need and has dramatically extended predictable aspects of the field.

Leonard Linkow has been called the father of implant dentistry. Many other practitioners before, and during his contributions, have also influenced this field, but he has lectured more often, given more uncompensated time, and for more years than anyone else I know in this discipline. He sacrificed his personal life until implant dentistry became his life. During his recovery from bypass surgery I was honored to maintain his practice for several months. On his return I remained until his practice returned back to normal. As a result, I learned firsthand that he is most giving to his family, friends, and colleagues. Implant dentistry would not exist as it is today if Leonard Linkow were not such a hardworking and giving person.

Therefore this book is dedicated to three men who did not directly contribute to the text. However, their vision, techniques, and leadership influenced every thought presented.

Carl E. Misch, D.D.S., M.D.S.

Contents

Part I

DIAGNOSIS AND TREATMENT PLANNING

Chapter 1

Rationale for Implants

Carl E. Misch

The goal of modern dentistry is restore normal contour, function, comfort, esthetics, speech, and health, regardless of the atrophy, disease, or injury of the stomatognathic system.[1] However, the more teeth a patient is missing, the more arduous this goal becomes with traditional dentistry. As a result of research, advances in implant designs, materials, and techniques have led to predictable success in their application, and several types of implants are now available for use in rehabilitation of different clinical problems.

The overall number of dental implants used in the United States increased an estimated fourfold from 1983 to 1987. During the same period the number of practitioners who perform implant therapy increased 10-fold (Fig 1–1). Over 300,000 dental implants are expected to be inserted in the United States in the year 1992.[2] Approximately 20% of dentists currently provide dental implant treatment on a routine basis in their practices, and almost half of general dentists currently use implants for supporting fixed and removable prostheses.

EFFECT OF AGING POPULATION

In the past, geriatric dentistry meant inexpensive treatment emphasizing nonsurgical approaches. Today dental services for elderly patients are becoming increasingly important to both the public and the profession, because of the increasing age of our society.

In 1980, 30% of the U.S. population was older than 45 years, 21% was older than 50, and 11% was over 65. The over-65 age group is projected to increase to more than 20% of the population within the next 50 years (Fig 1–2). Life span has increased significantly past the age of retirement: in 1965 the average life span was 65 years; in 1990 it was 78 years.[3] Social pleasures, including dining and dating, continue throughout advanced life. Treatment alternatives, which include methods to obtain fixed prostheses with implant support, should be presented to almost any patient. Only when all treatment options are discussed can a person's needs and desires for implant dentistry be appreciated.

The increased need for implant-related services results from the combined effect of a number of factors, including (1) age-related loss of teeth, (2) anatomic condition of edentulous ridges, (3) psychological needs of the patient, (4) decreased performance of removable prostheses, (5) predictable long-term results of implant-supported prostheses, and (6) increased awareness of the benefits of implants by the profession and the public.

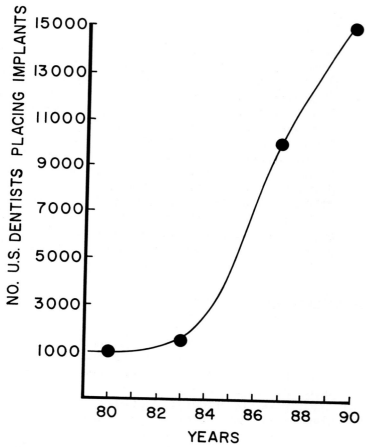

FIG 1–1.
Tenfold rise in number of U.S. dentists inserting dental implants from 1983 to 1987. Therefore, nine of 10 dentists placing implants had less than 4 years experience.

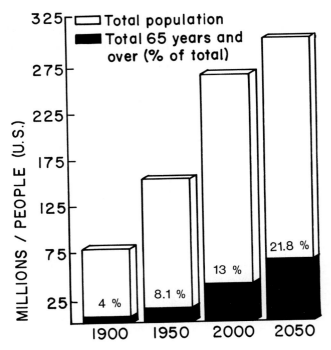

FIG 1–2.
Population older than 65 years old as a percentage of U.S. population. The lifespan of the elderly has increased to almost 80 years, and 42% of this age group have no teeth.

TOOTH LOSS RELATED TO AGE

Dental services for elderly patients represent a growing demand for the public and the dental profession. This is evident from the 1985–1986 National Survey of Oral Health in U.S. Employed Adults and Seniors, conducted by the National Institute of Dental Research (NIDR).[4] This cross-sectional study reflected the oral health of 135 million adults.

The survey revealed that Americans now can expect to retain their natural teeth longer than in the past. The present elderly population is benefiting from today's advanced knowledge and restorative techniques. In the NIDR national survey, prevalence of total edentulism of a single arch, usually the maxilla, was slight in the 30- to 34-year-old age group, but increased at around age 50 years, then began to remain constant at approximately 10%. Approximately 8 million persons have edentulism in one arch. Fifteen percent of seniors (persons over age 65) are edentulous in one arch only. The prevalence of edentulism in one arch does not change dramatically with advanced age.

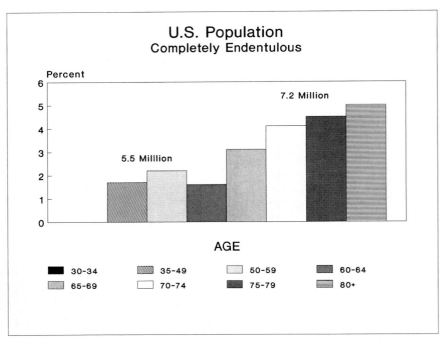

FIG 1–3.
U.S. population completely edentulous ranges from 5% to 42% after age 40 years. More than 12.5 million persons have no teeth.

Total edentulism has been noted in 5% of employed adults 40 to 44 years old, gradually increasing to almost 42% in seniors. However, these percentages are deceiving because there are more people below the age of 65 years. Before age 65 years, 5.5 million persons have lost all of their teeth, and in the 65 to 80+ years age group 7.2 million are completely edentulous (Fig 1–3). As expected, the older the person the more likely he or she is to be missing teeth. At younger ages a greater percentage of women lose their teeth, but by age 55 years men have a higher percentage of total edentulism.

These reported percentages represent over 20 million people, or about 15% of the entire U.S. adult population, who are completely edentulous in one or two arches. To place these numbers in perspective, 20 million people represent approximately two thirds of the U.S. black population or 80% of the entire population of Canada. Hence, complete edentulism remains a significant concern, and these patients often require implant dentistry to solve several related problems.

The prevalence of partial edentulism also is of interest to implant dentistry, because implants often are used in these patients. In employed adults aged 18 to 34 years the average number of missing teeth is fewer than two of 28 teeth. However, this number rapidly increases to an average of 10 teeth missing in adults

55 to 64 years old. Seniors over 65 years have lost on average 17.9 teeth, with older seniors having lost three more teeth than the younger seniors. Statistics for partial edentulism are similar for both men and women. The greatest transition from an intact dental arch to a partially edentulous condition occurs in the 35- to 54-year-old group.

Free-end edentulism is of particular concern, because in these patients teeth often are restored with removable prostheses. This condition is rarely found in persons younger than 25 years. Mandibular free-end edentulism is greater than its maxillary counterpart in all age groups. Unilateral free-end edentulism is more common than bilateral in both maxillary and mandibular arches in the younger age groups (25 to 44 years). About 13.5 million persons in these younger age groups have free-end edentulism in any arch.

In 45- to 54-year-old patients mandibular free-end edentulism also is more prevalent than in the maxillary arch, 31.3% and 13.6%, respectively. Approximately 9.9 million persons in the 45- to 54-year-old group have at least one free-end quadrant, and almost half of these have bilateral partial edentulism.

More than 40 million people in the United States have posterior edentulism

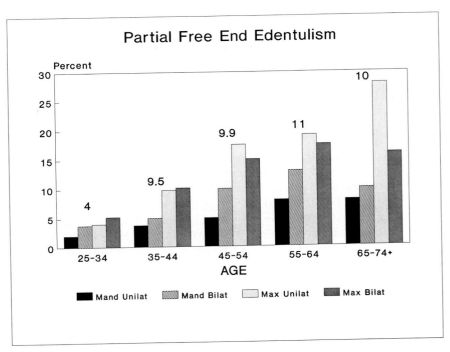

FIG 1–4.
Involvement of the mandibular arch *(Mand)* and maxillary arch *(Max)* in cases of posterior endentulism in the U.S. population, by age group. This common condition can be treated with implants and fixed prostheses.

in at least one quadrant. The pattern of posterior edentulism evolves in the 55-to 64-year-old group, where 35% of mandibular arches show free-end edentulism, compared with 18% of maxillary arches. As a result, approximately 11 million persons in this age group are potential candidates for implants. An additional 10 million show partial free-end edentulism at age 65 or older (Fig 1–4).

The number of potential patients in the United States with at least one quadrant of posterior missing teeth is more than 40 million, or twice as many as the completely edentulous population. This means almost 30% of the adult population may be candidates for a removable prosthesis. Desire for additional stability or the elimination of a removable prosthesis are the most common indications for dental implants.

The actual number of persons represented by these percentages, and their life expectancy must be addressed. A 65-year-old person can expect to live 16.7 more years, and one 80 years old can expect to live 8 more years.[3] This shift in average age to age groups who show more evidence of missing teeth guarantees that implant dentistry will continue to be needed in the future.

ALVEOLAR BONE RESORPTION

The concepts of basal bone and alveolar bone are fundamental to understanding the many concepts of implant dentistry. Basal bone forms the dental skeletal structure, contains most of the muscle attachments, and begins to form in the fetus before teeth develop. Alveolar bone first appears when Hertwig's root sheath of the tooth bud evolves.[5] The relationship between the tooth and the alveolar process continues throughout life. Wolff's law states that bone remodels in relationship to the forces applied. Bone needs stimulation to maintain its form and density. Roberts et al.[6] report that a 4% strain to the skeletal system maintains bone and helps balance the resorption and formation phenomena. The teeth transmit compressive and tensile forces to the surrounding bone. These forces may be measured as a piezoelectric effect in the imperfect crystals of durapatite that compose the inorganic portion of bone.[7] When a tooth is lost, the lack of stimulation results in a decrease in trabeculae in the area and loss of bone width, then height.[8] In a longitudinal, 25-year study of edentulous patients, lateral cephalograms demonstrated continued bone loss during this time span; a fourfold greater loss was observed in the mandible.[9]

ANATOMIC CONSEQUENCES OF EDENTULISM

The loss of teeth results in resorption of the surrounding alveolar bone and leads to atrophic edentulous ridges. This condition is associated with clinical anatomic problems (Table 1–1), which often impair the predictable results of traditional therapy. The loss of bone first results in decreased bone width. The remaining narrow residual ridge causes discomfort when the thin overlying tissues are loaded with a soft tissue–borne prosthesis. The continued atrophy of the mandible also may result in prominent mylohyoid and internal oblique ridges covered by thin, movable, unattached mucosa. The residual alveolar process continues to resorb, and the superior genial tubercles eventually become the most superior aspect of the anterior mandibular ridge. There is little to prevent the prosthesis from moving forward against the lower lip during function or speech. This condition is further compromised by the vertical movement of the distal aspect of the prosthesis during contraction of the mylohyoid and buccinator muscles, and the anterior incline of the atrophic mandible compared with that of the maxilla.

As bone loses width, then height, then width and height again, the attached gingiva gradually decreases. A very thin or absent attached tissue usually lies over the advanced atrophic mandible. The gingiva is prone to abrasions from the mobile prosthesis, and also is associated with unfavorable high muscle attachment and hypermobile tissue.

The thickness of the mucosa on the atrophic ridge depends on systemic disease or medications. Conditions such as hypertension, diabetes, anemia, and nutritional disorders all have a deleterious effect on the tissue support of removable prostheses. These disorders result in a decreased oxygen tension to the basal cells of the epithelium. Surface cell loss occurs at the same rate, but the cell formation at the basal layer is slowed. As a result, thickness of the surface tissues gradually decreases.

TABLE 1–1.

Anatomic Problems Associated With Edentulism

- Decreased width of supporting bone
- Decreased height of supporting bone
- Prominent mylohyoid and internal oblique ridges
- Progressive decrease in attached mucosa
- Prominent superior genial tubercles
- Forward movement of prosthesis from anatomic inclination
- Elevation of prosthesis with contraction; mylohyoid and buccinator muscles serving as posterior support
- Thinning of mucosa, with sensitivity to abrasion
- Loss of basal bone
- Paresthesis from dehiscient mandibular canal
- Increase in size of tongue
- More active role of tongue in mastication
- Decrease of neuromuscular control with aging
- Effect of bone loss on esthetic appearance of face

Loss of bone in the mandible is not limited to alveolar bone; portions of the basal bone also may be resorbed (Fig 1–5). The contents of the mandibular canal and/or mental foramen may become dehiscent and serve as part of the support area of the prosthesis. As a result, acute pain and/or transient to permanent paresthesia of the areas supplied by the mandibular nerve is possible.

The tongue of the patient with completely edentulous atrophic ridges usually enlarges to accommodate the increase in space formerly occupied by teeth. At the same time, the patient learns to use the tongue to limit the movements of the prostheses, and the tongue learns to take a more active role in the mastication and the digestive processes.

The decrease in neuromuscular control often associated with aging further leads to problems with traditional prosthodontics. The ability to wear a denture successfully may be largely a learned, skilled performance. The aged patient who recently becomes edentulous may lack the motor skills needed to accommodate to the new conditions.

Similar conditions exist in the partially edentulous patient who is wearing a removable soft tissue–borne prosthesis. The natural abutment teeth, which act as direct and indirect support, are submitted to additional lateral forces. These teeth also may be compromised by a deficient periodontal support. The net result is an

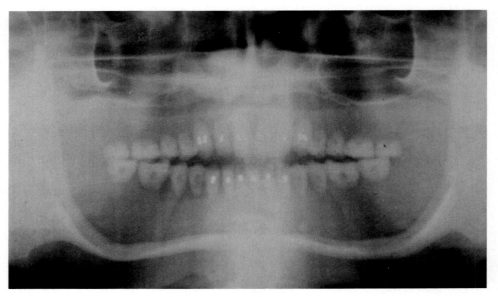

FIG 1–5.
Panoramic radiograph demonstrates advanced atrophy. Total alveolar bone and majority of basal bone have resorbed. Complications of maxillary/mandibular atrophy include paresthesia, masticatory dysfunction, speech impairment, and even pathologic fracture of the mandible.

increase in mobility of the natural teeth and removable restoration, which encourages complications.

ESTHETIC COMPLICATIONS DUE TO BONE LOSS

The facial changes that naturally occur in relation to the aging process can be accelerated and potentiated by the loss of teeth. Loss of alveolar bone can cause:

1. Prognathic appearance
2. Decrease in horizontal labial angle
3. Thinning of the lips (especially the maxilla)
4. Deepening of the nasolabial groove
5. Increased depth of associated vertical lines
6. Increase in columella-philtral angle
7. Ptosis of the muscles ("jowls" and/or "witch's chin")

A decrease in facial height from a collapsed vertical dimension results in several facial changes. The loss of labiomental angle and deepening of vertical lines in the area create a harsh appearance. As the vertical dimension progressively decreases, the occlusion evolves toward a skeletal class III malocclusion. As a result the chin rotates forward, giving a prognathic appearance, and there is a decrease in the horizontal labial angle at the corner of the lips. The patient appears unhappy when the mouth is at rest.

A thinning of the maxillary lip results from the poor lip support provided by the prosthesis and its retruded position related to the loss of crestal bone width. Women often use one of two techniques to hide this cosmetically undesirable effect: either no lipstick and little make-up, so that little attention is brought to this area of the face, or lipstick applied over the vermilion border to give the appearance of fuller lips.

Deepening of the nasolabial groove and increase in the depth of other vertical lines in the upper lip also are related to bone loss. This usually is accompanied by an increase in the columella-philtrum angle.[10] This can make the nose appear larger than if the lip had more support. Men often grow a moustache to minimize this effect. The maxillary lip looks longer, and less anterior teeth show when the lip is at rest. This has a tendency to "age" the smile, because the younger the patient the more the teeth show in relation to the upper lip at rest or when smiling.

The attachments of the masseter, mentalis, and buccinator muscles to the body and symphysis of the mandible also are affected by atrophia. The tissue sags, producing "jowls" or "witch's chin." This effect is additive because the muscles lose tone with the loss of teeth and decrease in activity.

FUNCTION AND PERFORMANCE OF REMOVABLE PROSTHESES

The difference in maximum occlusal forces recorded in a person with natural teeth and one who is completely edentulous is dramatic. In the first molar region the average force has been measured at 150 to 250 psi.[11] A patient who grinds or clenches the teeth may exert a force that approaches 1,000 psi. The maximum occlusal force in the edentulous patient is reduced to less than 50 psi. The longer the patient is edentulous the less force he or she usually is able to generate.[12]

Masticatory efficiency also is decreased with tooth loss. Ninety percent of the food chewed with natural teeth fits through a no. 12 sieve; this can be reduced to 58% in the patient wearing complete dentures.[13] The 10-fold decrease in force and the 30% decrease in efficiency affects the patient's ability to chew. Twenty-nine percent of persons with dentures are able to eat only soft or mashed foods[14]; 50% avoid many foods; and 17% claim they eat more efficiently without the prosthesis.[15]

PSYCHOLOGICAL ASPECTS OF TOOTH LOSS

The psychological effects of total edentulism are complex and varied, and range from very minimal to a state of neuroticism. A past dental health survey indicates that only 80% of the edentulous population is able to wear both removable prostheses all of the time.[16] Some patients wear only one prosthesis, usually the maxillary; others are able to wear their dentures only for short periods. In addition, approximately 7% of denture wearers are not able to wear them at all, and become dental cripples or "oral invalids." They rarely leave their home environment, and on the rare occasion when they feel forced to venture out, the thought of meeting and talking to people while not wearing teeth is unsettling.

A study of 104 completely edentulous patients seeking treatment was performed by Misch and Misch, who also compared maxillary and mandibular dentures.[15] In this study 88% of the patients claimed difficulty with speech, with one-fourth having very difficult problems. Movement of the mandibular denture was listed by 62.5% of these patients, although the maxillary prosthesis "stayed in place" most of the time at almost the same percentage. Mandibular discomfort was listed with equal frequency as movement (63.5%), and 16.5% stated they never wear the denture. In comparison, the maxillary denture was uncomfortable half as often (32.6%), and only 0.9% were seldom able to wear the denture. Function was the fourth problem reported. Half of the patients avoided many foods, and 17% claimed they were able to masticate more effectively without the prosthesis.

These patients were further divided into those accepting implant treatment (78%) and those not accepting treatment. Mandibular stability was reported unsatisfactory by 88% of patients accepting treatment, compared with 65% of patients not accepting treatment. Three fourths of patients accepting treatment stated that they were unhappy with their ability to eat and chew; half of the patients not accepting treatment reported the same complaint. Speech (94% vs. 91%) and discomfort (87% vs. 81%) were not statistically significant between the two groups.

Eighty percent of the patients treated with implant-supported prostheses judged their overall psychological health as improved compared with their state while wearing traditional, removable prosthodontic devices, and perceived the implant-supported prosthesis as an integral part of their body.[17] These findings were not reported in the patients with removable prostheses.

The psychological need of the edentulous patient is expressed in many forms. For example, in the United States more than $143 million is spent each year on denture adhesives, representing 45 million units sold. The patient is willing to accept the unpleasant taste, need for recurrent application, inconsistent denture fit, embarrassing circumstances, and continued expense for the sole benefit of increased retention of the prosthesis. Clearly, the lack of retention and psychological risk of embarrassment in the denture wearer with removable prostheses is a concern the dental profession must address.

ADVANTAGES OF IMPLANT-SUPPORTED PROSTHESES

The use of dental implants to provide support for prostheses offers a multitude of advantages compared with the use of removable soft tissue–borne restorations:

1. Maintained bone
2. Teeth positioned for esthetics
3. Maintained vertical dimension
4. Proper occlusion
5. Direct occlusal loads
6. Improved success rates
7. Increased occlusal force
8. Improved masticatory performance
9. Increased stability and retention
10. Improved phonetics
11. Improved proprioception
12. Reduced palate or flanges

A primary factor is the maintenance of alveolar bone. The dental implant placed into the bone serves not only as an anchor for the prosthetic device but also as one of the better preventive maintenance procedures in dentistry. Stress and strain may be applied to the bone surrounding the implant. As a result, the decrease in trabeculation of bone that occurs after tooth extraction is reversed. There is an increase in bone trabeculae and density when the dental implant is inserted and functioning. Hence, even grafts of iliac bone to the mandible, which usually resorb within 5 years, are instead stimulated and remain in place to support the implant. An endosteal implant can maintain bone width and height as long as the implant remains healthy. As with a tooth, peri-implant bone loss may be measured in tenths of a millimeter, and may represent more than a 20-fold decrease in lost structure compared with the resorption occurring with removable prostheses.

With an implant the teeth may be positioned to enhance esthetics and phonetics rather than in the "neutral zones" dictated by traditional denture techniques to improve the stability of a prosthesis. Independent tooth replacement may not require additional natural teeth as abutments, which may result in increased risk of complications and poorer esthetics.

The features of the inferior third of the face are closely related to the supporting skeleton. With prosthodontic treatment the vertical dimension may be similar to that with natural teeth. In addition, the implant-supported prosthesis allows an anterior cantilever of teeth for ideal facial contour and appearance in all facial planes. The facial profile may be enhanced for the long term, rather than deteriorating over the years.

Occlusion is difficult to establish and stabilize with a completely soft tissue–supported prosthesis. The mandibular prosthesis may move as much as 10 mm or more during function.[18, 19] Proper occlusal contacts occur by chance under these conditions, not by design. On the other hand, an implant-supported restoration is stable. The patient can consistently return to centric relation occlusion rather than adopt variable positions as dictated by the prosthesis instability.

With an implant-supported prosthesis the direction of the occlusal loads are controlled by the implant dentist. Horizontal forces accelerate bone loss, decrease prosthesis stability, and increase soft tissue abrasions. Therefore a decrease in horizontal forces improves the local parameters and helps to manage the underlying soft and hard tissue.

The success rate for implant prostheses is highly variable, depending on a host of factors that are different for each patient. However, compared with traditional methods of tooth replacement, the implant prosthesis offers increased longevity, improved function, bone preservation, and better psychological results. Ten-year survival surveys of fixed prostheses on natural teeth indicate decay as the most frequent reason for replacement, and survival rates are approximately 75%.[20] A major advantage is that the implant prosthesis cannot decay in the area of the implants. The implant and related prosthesis can attain a 10-year survival of greater than 95%.

The maximum occlusal force of a traditional denture ranges from 5 to 50 lb. Patients with an implant-supported fixed prosthesis may increase their maximal bite force by 85% within 2 months of completion of treatment. After 3 years the mean force may reach 300%, compared with pretreatment values. As a result, an implant prosthesis may illustrate a force similar to that of fixed restoration of natural teeth. Chewing efficiency with an implant prosthesis is greatly improved compared with that of soft tissue–borne restoration. The masticatory performance of dentures, overdentures, and natural dentition were evaluated. The traditional denture showed a 30% decrease in function, and the overdenture only 10%, compared with natural teeth. It is assumed that rigid, implant-supported bridges function similarly to natural teeth.[14]

The stability and retention of an implant-supported prosthesis are greatly improved over soft tissue–borne dentures. Mechanical means of implant retention are superior to the soft tissue retention provided by dentures and adhesives and cause fewer associated problems. The stability of the final prosthesis is variable, depending on the amount of implant support provided; yet all options demonstrate improvement.

Phonetics may be impaired by the instability of a conventional denture. The buccinator and mylohyoid muscles may flex and propel the posterior portion of the denture upward, causing clicking, regardless of the vertical dimension. As a result, a patient in whom the vertical dimension already has collapsed 10 to 20 mm may still produce clicking sounds during speech. The tongue of the denture wearer often is flattened in the posterior areas to hold the denture in position. The anterior mandibular muscles of facial expression may be tightened to prevent the mandibular prosthesis from sliding forward. The implant prosthesis is stable and retentive and does not require these manipulations.

Proprioception is awareness of a structure in time and place. The receptors in the periodontal membrane of the natural tooth help determine its occlusal position. Although endosteal implants do not have a periodontal membrane, they provide greater occlusal awareness than complete dentures. Patients with natural teeth can perceive a difference of 20 μm between the teeth, compared with 50 μm in those with rigid implant bridges, and 100 μm in those with complete dentures (either one or two).[21] As a result of improved occlusal awareness, the patient functions in a more consistent range of occlusion.

The implant restoration may have reduced flanges and/or palates. This is of benefit especially to the recent denture wearer, who often reports discomfort with the bulk of the restoration. The extended soft tissue coverage also affects the taste of food, and the soft tissue may be tender in the extended regions.

SUMMARY

The goal of modern dentistry is to return patients to oral health in a predictable fashion. The partial and complete edentulous patient may be unable to recover normal function, esthetics, comfort, or speech with traditional removable prosthesis.

The patient's function when wearing a denture may be reduced to 60% that formerly experienced with natural dentition; however, an implant prosthesis may return the function to near normal limits. The esthetics of the edentulous patient are also affected as a result of bone atrophy. Continued resorption leads to irreversible facial changes. An implant stimulates the bone and maintains its dimension in a manner similar to healthy natural teeth. As a result, the facial features are not compromised by lack of support. In addition, implant-supported restorations are positioned in relation to esthetics, function, and speech, not in "neutral zones" of soft tissue support.

The soft tissues of the edentulous patients are tender from the effects of thinning mucosa, decreased salivary flow, and unstable or unretentive prostheses. The implant-retained restoration does not require soft tissue support, and improves oral comfort.

Speech and function are compromised with prostheses, which may move 10 mm from the supporting structures during use. The tongue and perioral musculature may be compromised to limit the movement of the mandibular prosthesis. The implant abutment prosthesis is stable and retentive without the efforts of the musculature.

Implant prostheses often offer a more predictable treatment course than traditional restorations. Thus the profession and the public are becoming increasingly aware of this dental discipline. Between 1983 and 1987 there was a 10-fold increase in the number of dentists placing implants and a fourfold increase in the number of implants inserted. Manufacturers' sales have increased from a few million dollars to more than $20 million during this period. Almost every professional journal and lay publication now carries advertisements for implants. Implant dentistry finally has been accepted by organized dentistry. All U.S. dental schools now teach some awareness of implant dentistry. The current trend to expand the use of implant dentistry will continue until every restorative practice uses this modality for abutment support of both fixed and removable prostheses.

REFERENCES

1. Tatum OH: *The Omni implant system*, Alabama Implant Congress, Birmingham, Ala, May 1988.

2. National Institutes of Health Consensus Development Conference Statement on dental implants, *J Dent Educ* 52:686–691, 1988.
3. Dychtwald K: *Age wave: the challenges and opportunities of an aging America,* New York, St Martin's Press, 1988.
4. Meskin LH, Brown LJ: Prevalence and patterns of tooth loss in the U.S. employed adult and senior populations, *J Dent Educ* 52:686–691, 1988.
5. Freeman E, TenCate AR: Development of the periodontium: an electron microscopic study, *J Periodontol* 42:387–395, 1971.
6. Roberts WE et al: Bone physiology and metabolism, *Can Dent Assoc J* 15:54–61, 1987.
7. Basset CAL: Biologic significance of piezoelectricity, *Calcif Tissue Res* 1:252–272, 1968.
8. Pietrokovski J: The bony residual ridge in man, *J Prosthet Dent* 34:456–462, 1975.
9. Tallgren A: The reduction in face height of edentulous and partially edentulous subjects during long-term denture wear: a longitudinal roentgenographic cephalometric study, *Acta Odontol Scand* 24:195–239, 1966.
10. Hickey JC, Zarb GA, Bolender CL, editors: *Boucher's prosthodontic treatment for edentulous patients,* ed 9, St Louis, CV Mosby, 1985, pp 22–23.
11. Howell AW, Manley RS: An electronic strain gauge for measuring oral forces, *J Dent Res* 27:705, 1948.
12. Carr A, Laney WR: Maximum occlusal force levels in patients with osseointegrated oral implant prostheses and patients with complete dentures, *Int J Oral Maxillofac Implants* 2:101–110, 1987.
13. Rissin L et al: Clinical comparison of masticatory performance and electromyographic activity of patients with complete dentures, overdentures and natural teeth, *J Prosthet Dent* 39:508–511, 1978.
14. Carlsson GE, Haraldson T: Functional response tissue integrated prostheses. In Branemark PI, Zarb GA, Albrektsson T, editors. Chicago, Quintessence, 1985.
15. Misch LS, Misch CE: Denture satisfaction: a patient's perspective, *Int J Oral Implant* 7:43–48, 1991.
16. *Oral health of U.S. adult national findings,* U.S. Department of Health and Human Services, NIH Publ No. (87):28–68, 1987.
17. Blomberg S: Physiological response in tissue integrated prostheses: osteointegration in clinical dentistry. In Branemark PI, Zarb GA, Albrektsson T, editors. Chicago, Quintessence, 1985, pp 165–174.
18. Sheppard IM: Denture base dislodgement during mastication. *J Prosthet Dent* 13:462–468, 1963.
19. Smith D: The mobility of artificial dentures during communication. *J Prosthet Dent* 13:834–856, 1963.
20. Walton JN, Gardner FM, Agar JR: A survey of crown and fixed partial denture failures: length of service and reasons for replacement, *J Prosthet Dent*
21. Lundquist S, Haraldson T: Occlusal perception of thickness in patients with bridges on osteointegrated oral implants, *Scand J Dent Res* 92:88, 1984.

Chapter 2

Implant Terminology

Carl E. Misch

The use of dental implants in the treatment of complete and partial edentulism has become an integral treatment modality in restorative dentistry.[1-4] This is reflected in the 10-fold increase in the number of dentists who have become involved in implant dentistry between 1983 and 1987.[5] A survey published in 1990 indicated that more than 90% of oral and maxillofacial surgeons, periodontists, and prosthodontists and more than 50% of general dentists had attended a professional development course on implants during the preceding 3 years.[6] The 1988 National Institutes of Health consensus panel on dental implants recognized that restorative procedures utilizing implants differ from those of traditional dentistry, and stressed the necessity for advanced education.[1] Most practitioners have been taught the use of a specific implant system by that system's manufacturer, rather than the theory and comprehensive practice of implant dentistry. But with the ever increasing number of manufacturers entering the field, the trade names of their implant components (often unique to a particular system) have proliferated to the point of creating confusion, and several terms or abbreviations now exist that describe similar basic components.

In the team approach to implant treatment the referral base often requires that the practitioner be knowledgeable regarding many implant systems. A comparison of different endosteal implant systems reveals that no one system is best applied to all patient conditions or desires.[7-9] With the required knowledge of multiple systems and the lack of uniformity in component names, communication is hampered between manufacturers, dentists, laboratory technicians, students, and researchers. In addition, the incorporation of implant dentistry into the curriculum of most predoctoral and postdoctoral programs further emphasizes the need for standardization in implant dentistry.[10] There is a prosthetic commonality among most of the endosteal root form implant systems. This chapter provides a generic terminology that attempts to blend the continuity and familiarity of many implant systems with established definitions from the glossaries of the *Journal of Prosthetic Dentistry* and the American Academy of Implant Dentistry. [11, 12]

Oral implantology (implant dentistry) is the science and discipline concerned with the diagnosis, design, insertion, restoration, and/or management of alloplastic or autogenous oral structures to restore the loss of contour, comfort, function, esthetics, speech, and/or health of the partially or completely edentulous patient. *Implant prosthodontics* is the branch of implant dentistry concerning the restorative phase following implant placement and the overall treatment plan component before the placement of dental implants.

The prefix *allo* means other[13]; thus allografts are a category of materials that are not obtained directly from the patient. Allogenic describes materials that have an organic component, and include bone or soft tissue obtained from animals or cadavers. An alloplastic material is a relatively inert synthetic biomaterial. It is generally a metal *or* ceramic, or occasionally a polymeric material. An *oral* or *dental implant* is a biologic or alloplastic biomaterial surgically inserted into soft or hard tissues of the mouth for functional or cosmetic purposes.[13] Three categories of oral implants are discussed: endosteal, subperiosteal, and bone substitutes.

Alveolar bone has been defined as the bone of the maxilla or mandible that surrounds and supports the teeth. Once the tooth is removed, the remaining bone is termed the *residual ridge*.[11] However, the alveolar bone includes areas of bone far inferior to the roots, especially in the anterior maxilla and mandible. The term *alveolar bone* in this text includes (1) all the bone that develops as a result of tooth formation, (2) the residual ridge that is adequate or augmented for endosteal implants, and (3) the supporting surrounding bone of endosteal implants.

Osteointegration denotes at least some direct contact of living bone with the surface of an implant at the light microscopic level of magnification. The percentage of direct bone-implant contact is variable. *Rigid fixation* defines an implant with no observed mobility with 1- to 500-g force applied in a vertical or horizontal direction.

ENDOSTEAL IMPLANTS

An *endosteal implant* is an alloplastic material surgically inserted into a residual bony ridge, primarily to serve as a prosthodontic foundation.[12] The prefix *endo* means "within," and *osteal* means "bone".[13] The major subcategories of endosteal implants covered in this text are root form and plate form implants.

Root form implants are designed to use a vertical column of bone. They can be smooth, threaded, perforated, solid, hollow, or vented; can be coated or textured; and are available in submergible or nonsubmergible forms in a variety of biocompatible materials. [5, 12] There are two primary types, based on design. *Cylinder* (or *press-fit*) root form implants depend on microscopic retention and/or bonding to the bone, and usually are pushed or tapped into a prepared bone

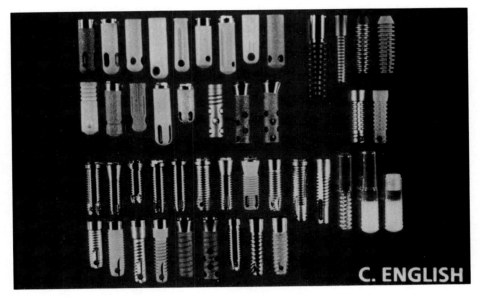

FIG 2–1.
More than 45 different implant body designs are sold in the United States. The term *root form* is the general descriptor for an implant body that uses a vertical column of bone. Many categories have been developed. This text refers to three types of root form body designs: screw, cylinder, and combination.

site. *Screw* root forms are threaded into a bone site and have obvious macroscopic retentive elements for initial bone fixation. *Combination root forms* are common, and have features of both the cylinder and screw root form. Root forms also have been described by their means of insertion, healing, surgical requirements, surface characteristics, and interface. [8, 9, 13] Although many names have been applied, the 1988 National Institutes of Health consensus statement on dental implants and the American Academy of Implant Dentistry recognize the term root form. [5, 12] (Fig 2–1).

The second major category of endosteal implants is the *plate form implant*.[12] Usually this form uses a horizontal dimension of bone, and is flat and narrow in the faciolingual dimension. This design is often called a *blade-vent implant*. The *neck* of the implant connects the implant body and permucosal abutment.

GENERIC TERMINOLOGY

A generic language for endosteal implants, both root forms and plate forms, has been developed by Misch and Misch.[14] The generic language for endosteal root form components is presented in an order similar to the method of insertion

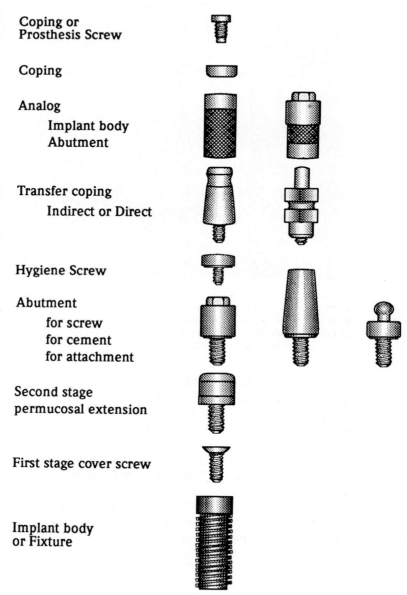

Coping or Prosthesis Screw

Coping

Analog
    Implant body
    Abutment

Transfer coping
    Indirect or Direct

Hygiene Screw

Abutment
    for screw
    for cement
    for attachment

Second stage permucosal extension

First stage cover screw

Implant body or Fixture

FIG 2–2.
Schematic of generic implant components and terminology developed by C.E. Misch and C.M. Misch.

and restoration (Fig 2–2). In formulating the terminology the five most commonly used systems in the United States were referenced, [1, 3, 4, 15, 16] with no specific implant as a model (Table 2–1).

The *body* is that portion of the implant designed to be surgically placed into the bone. It may extend slightly above the crest of the residual ridge. At the time of insertion, or first-stage surgery,[12] a *first-stage cover* is placed into the top of the implant to prevent bone, soft tissue, or debris from invading the abutment connection area during healing. If the first-stage cover is screwed into place, the term *cover screw* may be used.

After a prescribed healing period sufficient to allow a supporting interface to develop, second-stage surgery is performed to uncover or expose the implant and attach the transepithelial portion or abutment. [11, 12] This transepithelial portion is termed a *second-stage permucosal extension,* because it extends the implant above the soft tissue and results in the development of a permucosal seal around the implant. McKinney et al.[16] discussed the terminology used to describe the soft tissue interface surrounding dental implants, and suggested permucosal rather than transepithelial as a correct term.[16] Because of the lack of uniformity among the systems examined in the naming of this component, the word *extension* was selected because it is most descriptive (Fig 2–3).

The *abutment* is the portion of the implant that serves to support and/or retain a prosthesis[11] or implant superstructure. A *superstructure* is defined as a metal framework that fits the implant abutment (or abutments) and provides retention for the prosthesis,[12] such as cast bar retaining an overdenture with attachments. Three main categories of implant abutments are described according to the method by which the prosthesis or superstructure is retained to the abutment: an *abutment for screw* uses a screw to retain the prosthesis or superstructure; an *abutment for cement* uses dental cement to retain the prosthesis or superstructure; an *abutment for attachment* uses an attachment device to retain a removable prosthesis. Many manufacturers classify the abutments as fixed whenever cement retains the prostheses, and as removable when they are screw-retained. [1, 4, 15, 16] This is not accurately descriptive, because a fixed prosthesis is a restoration that is not removable by the patient[11] and may be cement-retained or screw-retained. By describing the abutment by the method of retention of the superstructure, a metal framework connected to the abutments by screws may retain a removable prosthesis with clip attachments, but the implant abutment still would be classified as an abutment for screw. The abutment may be screwed or cemented into the implant body, but this aspect is not delineated within the terminology. Each of the three types of abutments may be further classified into *straight* or *angled abutments,* describing the axial relationship between the implant body and the abutment. Many straight abutments for cemented prostheses are tapered, but the degree of taper does not change the relationship of the abutment to the implant body. An abutment for screw uses a *hygiene cover screw* placed over the

TABLE 2–1.

Manufacturer Terminology for Component Parts of Five Dental Implant Systems

Generic Term	Nobelpharma (Göteberg, Sweden)	Steri-Oss (Anaheim, Calif)	Interpore Int. (Irvine, Calif.)	Core-Vent Corp. (Encino, Calif)	Calcitek (Carlsbad, Calif)
Implant body or fixture	Branemark fixture	Steri-Oss implant	IMZ implant	Screw-Vent implant	Integral implant
First stage cover	Cover screw	Healing screw	Healing screw	Cover screw	Healing screw
Second stage permucosal extension	None	Temporary healing abutment	Second phase sealing screw, transmucosal implant extension	Healing collar	Temporary gingival cuff
Straight abutment for screw	Abutment	PME, tissue, and telescoping abutments	Abutment, complete, intramobile element	Straight or tapered insert	Abutment for removable prosthetics
Straight abutment for cement	CeraOne abutment	Threaded abutment	None	Coping	Abutment for fixed (cemented) prosthetics
Angled abutment for screw	Angled abutment	None	None	Castable coping with flat top or tapered housing	Plastic castable abutment
Angled abutment for cement	None	15° and 20° cement or screw in abutments	None	Castable coping	Preangled abutment, fixed prosthetics
Abutment for attachment	Abutment for ball attachment	Ball attachment	None	Ball screw, magnet screw	Ball overdenture, zest or magnetic attachments
Hygiene screw	Healing cap	Healing cap	Sealing cap	Hygiene insert	Comfort cap
Indirect transfer coping	Tapered impression coping	Thread timed transfer pin, impression pin	Impression post, tapered impression coping	Hexlock transfer, screw transfer	Impression post
Direct transfer coping	Impression coping	Impression coping	Square impression coping	Hexlock transfer	Transfer coping
Implant body or abutment analog	Fixture or abutment replica	Implant or abutment analog	Abutment replica, laboratory IME	Transfer and hex analogs	Implant body lab or abutment analog, transfer pin
Prefabricated coping	Gold cylinder	Bridge or bar coping alloy	Gold coping or cylinder	Titanium sheath	Gold coping
Castable coping	Plastic burnout pattern	Bridge or bar and telescoping copings	Castable coping	Plastic sheath	Waxing sleeve telescopic coping
Coping or prosthesis screw	Gold screw	Coping screw	Coping screw	Fixation screw	Coping screw

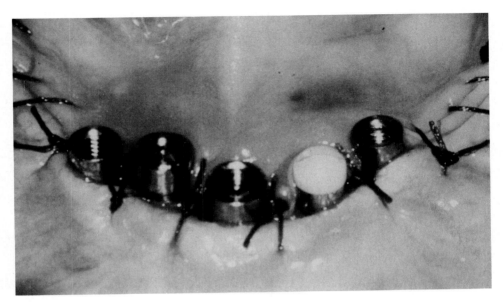

FIG 2–3.
Five second-stage permucosal extensions supplied by different implant manufacturers: *(left to right)* Steri-Oss, Core-Vent, Nobelpharma, Interpore IMZ, and Steri-Oss.

abutment between prosthetic appointments to prevent debris and calculus from entering the internally threaded portion of the abutment.

An impression is necessary to transfer the exact position and design of the implant body or abutment to a master cast. A transfer coping is used to position a die in an impression.[12] Most implant manufacturers use the terms transfer and coping to describe the component used in the final impression. Therefore a *transfer coping* is used to position an analog in an impression, and is defined by the portion of the implant it transfers to the master cast, either the *implant body coping* or *abutment transfer coping.*

Two basic techniques are used to make a master impression, and each uses a different transfer coping, based on the transfer technique performed in the mouth or on a master cast.[18] An *indirect transfer coping* utilizes an impression material requiring elastic properties.[19] The indirect transfer coping is screwed into the abutment or implant body and remains in place when the set impression is removed from the mouth. The indirect transfer is parallel sided or slightly tapered to allow ease in removal of the impression, and often has flat sides or smooth undercuts to facilitate reorientation in the impression. A *direct transfer coping* usually consists of a hollow transfer component, often square, and a long screw to secure it to the abutment or implant body. After the impression material is set the direct transfer coping screw is unthreaded to allow removal of the impression

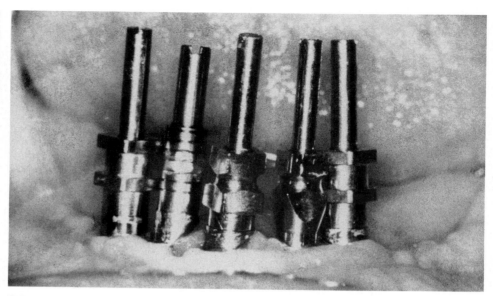

FIG 2–4.
Direct transfer copings of *(left to right)* Steri-Oss, Core-Vent, Nobelpharma, Interpore IMZ, and Steri-Oss.

from the mouth. The direct transfer coping takes advantage of impression materials having rigid properties[19] or eliminates the error of permanent deformation because it remains within the impression on its removal (Fig 2–4).

An analog is something that is analogous or similar to something else.[11] An *implant analog* is used in the fabrication of the master cast to replicate the retentive portion of the implant body or abutment. After the master impression is secured the corresponding analog (implant body, abutment for screw, or other portion) is attached to the transfer coping and the assembly is poured in stone to fabricate the master cast.

A *coping* is a thin covering,[11] usually designed to fit the implant abutment and serve as the connection between the abutment and the prosthesis or superstructure. A *prefabricated coping* usually is a metal component machined precisely to fit the abutment. A *castable coping* usually is a plastic pattern cast into the metal superstructure or prosthesis. A screw-retained prosthesis or superstructure is secured to the implant body or abutment with a *coping screw* (see Table 2–1).

SUMMARY

Independent of each other, manufacturers have developed terminology to describe the components used in implant dentistry. These terms or abbreviations often lack continuity among systems, and often do not adequately describe their use. As a result, difficulty arises in sharing concepts or techniques within the profession. Effective communication between implant surgeons, restoring dentists, laboratory technicians, faculty, and students necessitates a common language. The terminology proposed in this chapter permits the use of generic terms to broadly describe implant prosthetic components.

REFERENCES

1. Adell R et al: A 15-year study of osseointegrated implants in the treatment of the edentulous jaw, *Int J Oral Surg* 10:387–416, 1981.
2. van Steeberghe D et al: The applicability of osseointegrated oral implants in the rehabilitation of partial edentulism: a prospective multi-center study on 558 fixtures, *Int J Oral Maxillofac Implant* 3: 272, 1990.
3. Krisch A, Ackerman KL: The IMZ osteointegrated implant system, *Dent Clin North Am* 33:733–791, 1989.
4. Misch CE: The Core-Vent implant system. In *Endosteal dental implants,* St Louis, 1991, Mosby-Year Book, pp 315–330.
5. National Institutes of Health Consensus Development Conference statement on dental implants, *J Dent Educ* 52:824–827, 1988.
6. Schnitman PA: Education in implant dentistry, *J Am Dent Assoc* 121:330–332, 1990.
7. English CE: Cylindrical implants, *J Calif Dent Assoc* 16:17–20, 834–838, 1988.
8. Balkin BE: Implant dentistry: historical overview with current perspective, *J Dent Educ* 52:683–685, 1988.
9. Christensen GE, Christensen RP: *Clin Res Assoc Newslett* 13:1–4, 1989.
10. Misch CE: Dental education—meeting the demands of implant dentistry, *J Am Dent Assoc* 121:334–338, 1990.
11. Glossary of prosthodontic terms, *J Prosthet Dent* 58:717–761, 1987.
12. Glossary of implant terms, *J Oral Implant* 16:57–63, 1990.
13. Joblonsky S, editor: *Illustrated dictionary of dentistry,* Philadelphia, 1982, WB Saunders.
14. Misch CE, Misch CM: Generic terminology for root form implant prosthodontics, *J Prosthet Dent* (in press).
15. Finger IM, Guerra LR: Integral implant-prosthodontic considerations, *Dent Clin North Am* 33:793–819, 1989.
16. Hahn JA: The Steri-Oss implant system, In *Endosteal dental implants,* St Louis, 1991, Mosby-Year Book, pp 349–361.
17. McKinney RV Jr, Steflik DE, Koth DL: Per, peri, or trans? A concept for improved dental implant terminology, *J Prosthet Dent* 52:267–269, 1984.
18. Zarb GA, Jansson T: Laboratory procedures and protocol. In Branemark P-I, Zarb GA, Albrektsson T, editors: *Tissue-integrated prostheses: osseointegration in clinical dentistry,* Chicago, 1985, Quintessence, pp 292–294.
19. Phillips RW: *Skinner's science of dental materials,* ed 9, Philadelphia, 1991, WB Saunders, p 93.

Chapter 3

Implant Success or Failure: Clinical Assessment

Carl E. Misch

The answer to the question of what constitutes success in implant dentistry remains complex. There is no unanimous definition of clinical success for implants or teeth. Teeth and implants do not permit a strict diagnosis of total health or failure. A tooth with periodontal pocket depths of 5 mm may need therapy but is still within a range of "success." Failure is often easier to describe; but if a dental unit does not qualify as failure, it does not necessarily qualify as a success.

Dental implants do not decay and do not have dental pulps that may give indications of symptoms or disease; thus periodontal indices are often used for evaluation of implant success. However, classification of periodontal disease and the terms used to describe these dental conditions become controversial when applied to implants. As the causative factors, pathogenesis, and host factors become better understood, the descriptions of the tooth- or implant-related diseases evolve. The comparison between peri-implant tissue and natural teeth are discussed in Chapters 18 and 33 of this book.

NATURAL TOOTH CONDITIONS

The American Academy of Periodontology has defined five periodontal case types for diagnosis and treatment (Table 3–1).[1] These categories of disease do not indicate success or failure, but a range of health to disease.

Ideal clinical conditions for natural teeth include many factors, several of which apply to dental implants:

1. Absence of pain
2. Less than 0.1 mm initial horizontal mobility under lateral forces less than 100 g

TABLE 3–1.

Classification of Periodontitis*

Type	Terminology	Description
I	Gingitivitis	Inflammation of the gingiva characterized clinically by changes in color, gingival form, position, surface appearance, and appearance and presence of bleeding and/or exudate.
II	Slight periodontitis	Progression of gingival inflammation into deeper periodontal structures and alveolar bone crest, with slight bone loss. Usual periodontal probing depth is 3 to 4 mm, with slight loss of connective tissue attachment and slight loss of alveolar bone.
III	Moderate periodontitis	More advanced stage of type II, increased destruction of the periodontal structures, and noticeable loss of bone support possibly accompanied by an increase in tooth mobility. There may be furcation involvement in multirooted teeth.
IV	Advanced periodontitis	Further progression of periodontitis, with major loss of alveolar bone support, usually accompanied by increased tooth mobility. Furcation involvement in multirooted teeth is likely.
V	Refractory progressive periodontitis	Includes several unclassified types of periodontitis characterized either by rapid bone and attachment loss or by slow but continuous bone and attachment loss. The condition is resistant to normal therapy, and usually associated with gingival inflammation and continued pocket formation.

*After Council on Dental Care Programs, *J Am Dent Assoc* 17:371–373, 1988.

3. Less than 0.15 mm secondary mobility with lateral forces of 500 g
4. Absence of observed vertical mobility
5. Optimal probing depths of less than 2.5 mm
6. Radiographic crestal bone height 1.5 to 2.0 mm within the cemento-enamel junction
7. Intact lamina dura
8. Papilla bleeding index of grade 0 to 1 with no exudate
9. Absence of recession and furcation involvement on multirooted teeth

LITERATURE REVIEW

Several factors have been suggested for the evaluation of implant success. The most common clinical criterion reported is whether the implant is physically "in the mouth" or removed. Proponents state that this method provides the clearest presentation of the data. Critics of this criterion believe that implants which should be removed because of pain or disease may still be maintained as abutments and reported as success.

The Harvard Consensus Development Conference on dental implants in 1978 listed several conditions for implant success,[2] including that the implant type or system should succeed "75% for 5 years." This criterion is no longer acceptable for many reasons. Implant options offer greater benefit than 5 years at 75%. Implant survival today should be based on 10 or more years with higher rates. If one fourth of all cases resulted in retreatment, the cost to provide these procedures would be unrealistic for most patients.

Clinical reports of 35 published articles reviewing success from 1977 to 1989 report a wide range of criteria.[3] All of these studies reported survival rates, with a majority reporting on mobility as well as a radiographic assessment. The Loe and Silness gingival index and plaque index were also stated in about one third of the papers. The subjective criteria of discomfort was mentioned in three reports, whereas patient satisfaction was included in eight publications. The criteria described in this chapter will include:

1. Pain
2. Rigid fixation
3. Probing depth
4. Bone loss
5. Bleeding index
6. Peri-implant disease
7. Percussion
8. Radiographic evaluation

Pain

Absence of pain under vertical or horizontal forces is a primary implant criterion of evaluation. Usually (but not always) pain does not occur unless the implant is mobile. The presence of pain almost always requires removal of the implant, even in the absence of mobility. The condition rarely improves.

A natural tooth becomes hyperemic and cold temperature–sensitive as a first indicator of a problem; this warning sign does not exist with an implant. A tooth with a more serious condition becomes sensitive to heat and tender to palpation, indicating pulpitis. The implant is almost never temperature sensitive, but may become tender to percussion. Tenderness signifies a more advanced stage of complication for an implant than for a tooth, because it usually implies stress beyond physiologic limits rather than conditions that can be treated with endodontic therapy. Implant tenderness may have a successful treatment. Because this condition is usually related to excess force in amount and/or duration, treatment consists of the elimination of as much stress on the prosthesis as possible for 2 or more weeks. A major advantage of implant overdentures is that the restoration may be removed during sleep, at times when parafunction may occur, or when any tenderness develops. The occlusion and parafunctional habits should especially be addressed with implant sensitivity. The prosthesis most often should be modified, or additional implants should be placed to dissipate the forces.

Rigid Fixation

All implant abutment supports discussed in this book aim at rigid fixation as the clinical goal. Rigid fixation indicates an absence of clinical mobility of an implant under 1 to 500 g vertical or horizontal forces. It does not guarantee a direct bone-implant interface. However, when clinically observed, rigid fixation usually means that at least a portion of the implant is in direct contact with bone, although the percentage of bone contact cannot be indicated. Steflik and associates found that a lack of clinical mobility did not correlate with the presence or absence of fibrous connective tissue around an implant body.[4]

Implants with less than 0.5 mm horizontal movement may return to rigid fixation and zero mobility. This condition is unlikely, but has been observed by the author on occasion. A tooth with primary occlusal trauma shows an increase in mobility and periodontal ligament space, illustrated by a thickening in the lamina dura on radiographic study. Once the cause of trauma is eliminated, the tooth may return to zero clinical mobility and a normal radiographic appearance. This condition is not as predictable around an implant. However, the chances improve if no mobility was noted initially. If the prosthesis has already been delivered to the patient, little is lost if most forces are removed from the implant for approximately 2 months before final evaluation. A horizontally mobile implant prior to placement into function has much less chance of improving, and removal is indicated. Vertical mobility of an implant warrants removal. An implant with greater than 1 mm horizontal mobility or any vertical mobility should not remain in function, to avoid continued bone loss and a future compromised implant site. The Periotest is a computer-mechanical device that measures the damping effect against objects. A soft surface or mobile object will give higher recordings than a hard and/or rigid object. The recordings range from negative to positive numbers. Teeth with clinical zero mobility have typical ranges around 5. A nonmobile implant most often ranges from −6 to 0. This device may be used to evaluate slight changes in implant rigid fixation or note prostheses that become partially retained (Fig 3–1).

Probing Depths

Stable rigid fixated implants have reported pocket depths of 2 to 6 mm.[6] Partially edentulous patients have consistently greater probing depths around implants than around teeth.[6] A probing depth less than 3 mm is a criterion of health for a natural tooth but provides less diagnostic information for an implant, especially in the maxilla where the increased thickness of the soft tissue is variable before implant placement. A tissue thickness of 5 mm results with an initial 5-mm

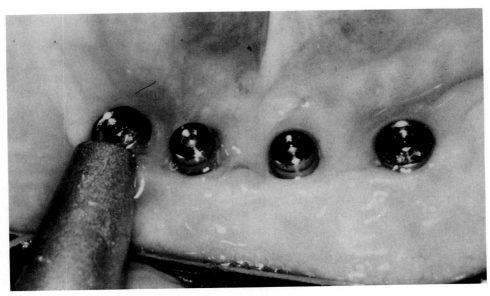

FIG 3–1.
Periotest (Siemens) may be used to evaluate implant rigid fixation or prostheses that become partially retained.

implant sulcus, unless gingiplasty is performed. However, implant sulcus depths of 6 mm or more provide an environment favorable to gram-negative microorganisms and gingival inflammation, which favors loss of bone.[7] There is a direct relationship between probing depth and oxygen tension and the effect of the latter on subgingival microflora. Therefore, the tissue thickness and implant sulcus depth should be reduced to an ideal 3 mm or less sulcular depth when esthetics are not a primary concern. Gingivoplasty to reduce pocket depth may be performed at the initial surgery, the uncovery surgery after initial healing, or before the final prosthetic impression. However, thinning the flap at initial surgery may permit greater loading of the implant body from an overlying soft tissue–borne restoration.

An increasing probing depth is more of a diagnostic criterion because it usually signifies bone loss, except in case of gingival hyperplasia or hypertrophy. The location of the probe tip subgingivally depends on the pressure used, the presence of inflammation, and the angle at which the probe is introduced next to the junctional epithelium or crest of the bone. A heavy pressure will reach the crestal bone or beyond. A positive correlation has been demonstrated between pocket depth, gingivitis, and higher plaque distribution. However, this observation was not correlated with accelerated marginal bone loss, microflora, or histologic changes indicative of periodontitis. The benefit of probing the implant sulcus is challenged in the literature because of lack of sound scientific criteria.[8] There is potential damage to the fragile attachment[9] or marring of the implant surface.[10]

A primary factor in the accuracy of probing depth is the angle at which the probe is introduced into the sulcus. Because an implant is only 4 mm in diameter, a fixed prosthesis is often contoured so that parallel probing access is not possible along the abutment. Plate form implants have undercut regions, especially on the buccal and lingual of the abutment. The probe cannot enter the region of the implant neck with any diagnostic certainty.

In spite of all the limitations, the author believes that charting the attachment level in implant permucosal areas does aid the clinician in monitoring these regions. Probing using fixed reference points on the abutment allows evaluation of crestal bone loss, especially during the first critical year of stress accommodation of the bone. Changes in crestal bone levels warrant close evaluation and early treatment. Occlusal adjustments, patient education to reduce stress on the implant system, use of parafunctional appliances, and other stress-reducing methods are required when crestal bone loss is noted.

Probing also will reveal tissue consistency, bleeding, and exudate. Care should be taken not to inoculate the implant sulcus with bacteria from a diseased periodontal site. Plastic probes are available to prevent scratching of the implant surface. Despite the uncertain meaning of pocket depth, it is an easy and quick method for assessing potential deleterious changes in the peri-implant environment and should be performed every 3 to 4 months for 1 year after the procedure. After this time, if crestal bone levels are stable, probing may be restricted to suspicious regions where bone loss is radiographically observed.

Bone Loss

The level of the crestal bone around an endosteal implant should be compared to the initial placement position of the implant. An implant originally placed 2 mm above the bone and another countersunk 2 mm below the bone cannot use the same implant reference point for judging bone loss. The probing depth may evaluate bone loss more accurately than radiographs. All sides of the implant may be evaluated. The probe is more likely to reach the crestal bone with an implant than around a tooth, because a weak hemidesmosome loose attachment is present between the implant and soft tissue above the bone.[11]

Under ideal conditions, a tooth or implant should lose minimum bone. However, it is not possible to determine precisely how much bone loss indicates success or failure. An 18-mm-high root form placed in very soft density D-4 narrow crestal bone may lose 5 mm of bone before the bone density improves and long-term stability occurs, yet the implant may still be considered successful. On the other hand, a 7-mm-high root form may be placed in dense bone and lose the same 5 mm of bone support and indicate failure. In general, if more than one third of the implant height has lost crestal bony contact, the implant is at significant risk, regardless of the original amount of implant-bone contact.

The initial bone loss around an implant during the first few years is almost always a result of excessive stress at the crestal implant–bone interface. Stress factors such as occlusal forces, cantilever length, and especially parafunction should be evaluated and reduced when initial bone loss is observed.

Bleeding Index

A bleeding index is an indicator of sulcus health. Implant success is not so related to gingival health as in the natural tooth. The inflammation may be limited to above the bone, because there is less fibrous tissue between the implant and bone interface. The most common sulcus bleeding gingival index used for implants is the Loe and Silness gingival index (GI). The GI scores the gingival inflammation on the facial, lingual, and mesial surface of all implants. The distal surface may be added if the implants are more than 2 mm apart. Easily ulcerated sulcular epithelium, reflecting inflammation, and poor oral hygiene are primary causes of bleeding on probing. Bleeding can be provoked by undue force of the probe. When the sulcus depth is less than 5 mm and the bleeding index increases, chlorhexidine often is indicated, along with other professional and home care methods. Bleeding on probing with sulcus depths in excess of 5 to 6 mm is more common and usually requires reentry surgery. Radiographic bone loss and increased pocket depth have been correlated with bleeding.[12] During first year clinical examinations of the peri-implant gingival tissues, bleeding on probing, and poor color, form, and consistency should be recorded, even if removal of the restoration is needed. After 1 year of stable probing depths, the examination may be restricted to spot checks at maintenance appointments. Removal of the prosthesis for evaluation is not indicated unless changing conditions warrant. Repeated removal of the prosthesis will wear the attachment system and cause more frequent partially retained restorations over the long-term.

Peri-Implant Disease

Gingivitis is a pathologic process involving the region of the soft tissue above the crest of bone. It can be (1) plaque associated, (2) acute necrotizing, (3) ulcerative, (4) hormonal, (5) drug-induced, or (6) spontaneously occurring. These categories should also relate to the gingiva around an implant, because the mode of attachment of gingiva to a tooth or implant have been reported to be similar.[12,13]

An exudate indicates a peri-implantitis and consequent bone loss. The reduced amount of bone may in turn lead to secondary occlusal trauma. Therefore, stress criteria need to be evaluated and causative elements eliminated. In addition, short-term antibiotic treatment, use of chlorhexidine, and aggressive professional and patient care of the soft tissue is indicated. An exudate persisting for more than 1 to 2 weeks usually warrants force reduction and surgical management of the condition.

Percussion

Percussion is neither an indicator of clinical health nor of the state of rigid fixation. The "ringing" sound that occurs on percussion corresponds to the presence of "some" bone at the interface, inasmuch as 2 mm of bone and 16 mm of bone-implant interface sound almost identical.

Radiographic Evaluation

Radiographic interpretation is a most difficult way of assessing implant health, but often is used as an early indicator of clinical problems. The crestal bone region is usually the most useful diagnostic tool in determination of a healthy implant. Crestal bone loss is used primarily to determine the need for initial preventive therapy. Early loss of crestal bone is usually a result of stress at the permucosal site. A radiograph only illustrates the mesial and distal crestal levels of bone. Early bone loss most often occurs on the facial aspect of the implant. The radiographic height of bone represented usually is the higher, thicker lingual or palatal plate of bone, whereas the actual crestal bone usually slants toward the facial aspect in an inferior direction.

An absence of radiolucency around an implant does not mean bone is present at the interface, especially in the anterior mandible. As much as 40% decrease in trabecular bone is necessary to produce a radiologically evident difference in this region, because of the dense cortical bone.[13] However, the presence of a radiolucent region around an implant definitely represents the presence of fibrous tissue, although the amount cannot be determined precisely. It usually is greater than the radiolucent zone next to the implant.

Parallel periapical radiographs are more difficult to obtain for implants than teeth. The implant is often placed in bone inferior to the apex of the preexisting natural tooth. As a result, the inferior portion of the implant often is located below muscle attachments or in regions almost impossible to record with a parallel radiographic method. A foreshortened or elongated image compromises the radiographic interpretation of the crestal bone.

Implant Failure

An implant diagnosed as a clinical failure is easier to describe than one which is a "success." Horizontal mobility beyond 1 mm or any clinical observed vertical movement under less than 500-g force, rapid progressive bone loss regardless of the stress reduction and peri-implant therapy, or pain during percussion or function indicate failure and the need for implant removal. Whether the implant remains in the mouth or not, the implant has failed.

TABLE 3–2.

Implant Quality Scale*

Group	Clinical Conditions	Treatment
I (optimum conditions)	No pain or tenderness on palpation or function Rigid fixation; no horizontal or vertical mobility under 500-g load <1.5-mm original crestal bone loss <1.0-mm bone loss in preceding 3 years Stable probing (sulcus) depth No exudate No radiolucency	Normal maintenance
II (moderate health)	No pain or tenderness on palpation or function Rigid fixation; no horizontal or vertical mobility under 500-g load >1.5-mm original crestal bone loss <1.0-mm bone loss in preceding 3 years <3 mm increasing sulcus depth in preceding 3 years Past transient exudate history (+) or (−) No radiolucency	Reduce stresses Shorter intervals between hygiene Yearly radiographs
III (moderate implantitis)	No pain or tenderness on palpation or function Rigid vertical fixation; 0- to 1-mm horizontal mobility >3-mm crestal bone loss in preceding 3 years >3-mm probing depth in preceding 3 years History of exudate Slight radiolucency around portion of implant	Reduce stresses Drug therapy, antibiotics, chlorhexidine Surgical reentry Change in prosthesis and/or add implants
IV (clinical failure)	Pain on palpation or function >1-mm mobility horizontally; any vertical mobility or progressive bone loss Uncontrolled exudate Generalized radiolucency "Sleepers"	Removal of implant
V (absolute failure)	Implants surgically removed Implants exfoliated	Bone graft

*After James and Misch. See text.

When in doubt, the implant is treated similar to a natural tooth presenting the same conditions. Implementation of aggressive implant maintenance treatment is warranted with horizontal mobility of less than 1 mm, exudate, a pocket depth of 5 mm and increasing, a bleeding index 2 or above, or slight tenderness to percussion or function. The mobile implant is in greater need of treatment than natural teeth, whereas an implant with greater than 5 mm pocket depth may be stable, with further treatment not indicated.

The ultimate decision of implant "success" lies with the practicing dentist rendering continued dental therapy for the patient. A single tooth implant with 1 mm mobility is less at risk than a 12-unit fixed prosthesis implant abutment with 0.5-mm mobility. A "gray scale" of decision making exists, and absolute rules make for easy decisions, but not necessarily the correct ones for all patients.

IMPLANT QUALITY SCALE

A scale presented for implant quality based on clinical evaluation was first established by James (personal communication), and modified by Misch (Table

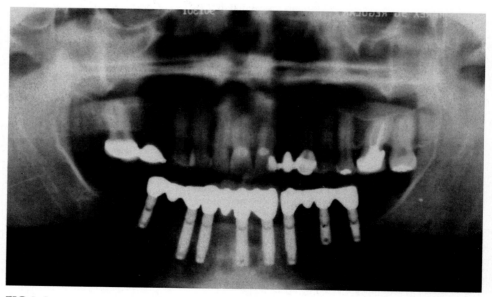

FIG 3–2.
Category 1 Quality Scale. Five-year postoperative radiograph demonstrates less than 1.5 mm crestal bone loss from the original implant surgery, and/or less than 1 mm bone loss in the preceding 3 years.

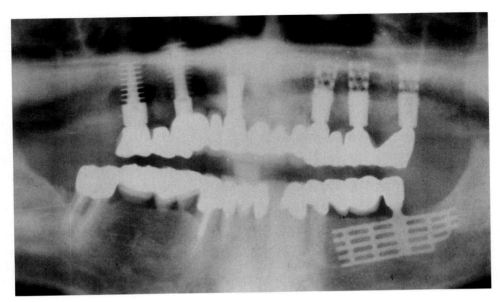

FIG 3–3.
Six-year postoperative radiograph demonstrates Quality Scale Category 2 for the plate form in the mandible, category 3 for the implant in maxillary right posterior, and category 2 for the root forms in the left posterior maxilla.

3–2). Group 1 represents optimum conditions. Ideally, the bleeding index is 0 to 1 and is an early indicator of soft tissue problems, but is not an essential component of category 1 implant health (Fig 3–2).

Group 2 implants are stable but show history of clinical problems. These implants may have a history of a transient exudate, but there is a lack of radiolucency, and the bleeding index may range from 0 to 2. Treatment consists of methods to reduce forces, preventive maintenance appointments, and annual radiographic study.

Group 3 implants correspond to questionable quality and warrants clinical therapy. Exudate may last more than 1 to 2 weeks in the preceding 3 years and may be accompanied with a slight radiolucency that may be evident around a portion of the implant. The bleeding index ranges from 1 to 3, but is more likely to be in the 2 range. If two or more of these signs exist, intervention is warranted (Fig 3–3).

Stress factors are first addressed. Modification of the occlusal scheme to decrease the forces in the afflicted regions includes occlusal adjustment or occlusal splint therapy. Antibiotics and local chemical agents such as chlorhexidine are indicated in presence of exudate. In rapid bone change the prosthesis may be changed from a fixed to a removable restoration. Additional implants to support the restoration may be indicated, especially if the patient is unwilling to wear a removable prosthesis.

Surgical management most often results in removal or exposure of a portion of the implant. Synthetic bone graft materials may be used in conjunction with these approaches around the implant. However, the method is usually not beneficial if the causative forces on implant failure are not reduced. Hence, a threefold approach is indicated for this category in the following order: (1) stress reduction, (2) antimicrobial therapy, and (3) surgical intervention.

The fourth degree of implant health is clinical failure. The implant should be removed under any of the five conditions listed in Table 3–2. Occasionally the patient will not permit removal of the implant. Whether the patient returns for implant removal, the implant is recorded as failure in all statistical data. The patient should be warned against irreversible damage to the surrounding bone with implants maintained in this condition. This category also includes implants surgically placed but unable to be restored ("sleepers"). Consideration should be given to their removal, because future treatment may be compromised (Fig. 3–4).

The fifth and last category for implant quality comprises implants surgically removed or exfoliated and no longer in the mouth. This condition is often treated

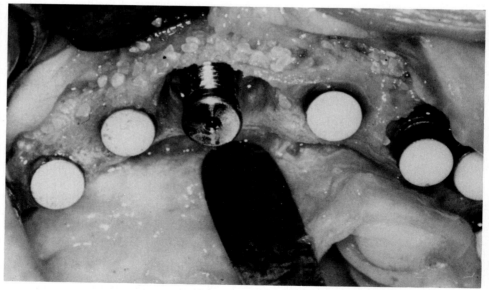

FIG 3–4.
Implant in the maxillary lateral region demonstrates Quality Scale Category 4. The implant should be removed because uncontrolled progressive bone loss has occurred. The implant in the left lateral region demonstrates category 2 because more than 1.5 mm of bone was lost since the initial surgery.

with autogenous and/or synthetic bone graft procedures, performed to replace the missing bone.

SUMMARY

The success or failure of an implant is as difficult to describe as the success criteria required for a tooth. The range from health to disease is similar in both conditions. The primary criteria for assessing implant quality are pain and mobility. The presence of either factor greatly compromises the implant, and removal is usually indicated.

Probing depth may be related to the presence of local disease or preexisting tissue thickness before the implant was inserted. Increasing probing depth is more diagnostic and signifies bone loss, gingival hyperplasia, or hypertrophy. Bone loss is usually evaluated best with probing rather than with radiographs. The most common cause of bone loss the first few years following an implant is exaggerated factors of stress.

The bleeding index is an easily observed phenomena and indicates inflammation of the gingiva. However, implant health status is not as related to sulcular inflammation as would be the case for a natural tooth.

Implant failure is easier to describe and may consist of a variety of factors. Any pain, vertical mobility, uncontrolled progressive bone loss, and/or generalized periradiolucency warrant implant removal.

REFERENCES

1. Council on Dental Care Programs: reporting periodontal treatment under dental benefit plans, *J Am Dent Assoc* 17:371–373, 1988.
2. *Dental implants: benefit and risks,* A National Institute of Health–Harvard Consensus Development Conference, Publication 81, 1531, Washington, DC, 1980, U.S. Dept. of Health and Human Services.
3. Ten Bruggenkate C, Van der Kwast WAM, Oosterbeek HS: Success criteria in oral implantology—a review of the literature, *Int J Oral Implant* 7:45–53, 1990.
4. Steflik DE, Koth DC, McKinney RV: Human clinical trials with the single crystal sapphire endosteal implant, *J Oral Implant* 13:39–53, 1986.
5. Lekholm U et al: Marginal tissue reactions at osseointegrated titanium fixtures, II: a cross-sectional retrospective study, *Int J Oral Maxillofac Surg* 15:53–61, 1981.
6. Lekholm U et al: Clinical evaluation of fixed bridge restorations supported by the combination of teeth and osseointegrated titanium implants, *J Clin Periodontol* 13:307–312, 1986.
7. Rams TE, et al: The subgingival microflora associated with human dental implants, *J Prosthet Dent* 5:529–539, 1984.

8. Helm FR et al: Percent mineralized interface of rigid endosseous implants, University of the Pacific and Veterans Administration Medical Center, San Francisco, Calif, Second International Congress on Prosthetic Surgery, Palm Springs, Calif, May 14–16, 1987.

9. McKinney RV Jr, Steflik DE, Koth DL: Peri or trans: a concept for improved dental implant terminology, *J Prosthet Dent* 52:267–269, 1984.

10. Stefani LA: The care and maintenance of the dental implant patient, *J Dent Hygiene* October 1988, pp 447–466.

11. James RA, Schultz RL: Hemidesmosomes and the adhesion of junctional epithelial cells to metal implants—a preliminary report, *J Oral Implant* 4:294, 1974.

12. Steflik DE, McKinney RV, Koth DL: Ultrastructural (TEM) observations of the gingival response to the single crystal endosteal implant, *J Dent Res* 61:231, 1982.

13. Goaz P, White SC: *Oral radiology: principles and interpretation,* St Louis, 1982, CV Mosby.

Chapter 4

Prosthetic Options in Implant Dentistry

Carl E. Misch

The ideal implant treatment plan is based on the patient's needs, desires, and financial commitment. Not all patients should be treated with the same restoration type or design. Traditional dentistry often provides limited treatment options for the edentulous patient. The dentist cannot add additional abutments, and the restoration design is directly related to present oral conditions. On the other hand, implant dentistry may provide a range of additional abutments. Bone augmentation further modifies the existing conditions and affects the final prosthetic design. As a result, a number of various treatment options are available to many partially and completely edentulous patients.

For determination of the initial prosthesis design, the existing problems are evaluated, to determine if a fixed or removable restoration is desired. An axiom of implant treatment is to provide the easiest, most cost effective, most predictable treatment that will satisfy the patient's needs and desires.

A removable implant–supported prosthesis offers several advantages over a fixed restoration in the completely edentulous patient:

1. Fewer implants are required.
2. Prosthodontic appointments are less complicated, and treatment is less expensive. There is improved hard and soft tissue evaluation and access for routine procedures.
3. Long-term maintenance or treatment of complications is facilitated, and daily homecare conditions are improved.
4. Esthetics are much easier to control for labial flange and denture teeth than customized metal or porcelain. The labial contours may replace lost bone width and height and support the labial soft tissues.

5. The prosthesis can be removed at night, to help treat parafunction or implant sensitivity.

The patient should not be forced to accept a fixed prosthesis if tested removable prostheses are available. However, some completely edentulous patients require fixed restoration because of desire or their oral condition.

A common axiom in traditional prosthodontics for partial edentulism is to provide a fixed partial denture whenever applicable. The fewer natural teeth missing the more a fixed partial denture is indicated. This scenario also is applied to implant prostheses in the partially edentulous patient. Ideally, the fixed partial denture is completely implant supported, because this necessitates the greatest use of implant surface area in the available bone.

The patient presents to the implant dentist for replacement teeth, not implants, but a definite relationship exists between the foundation and superstructure. The implants serve primarily as support to the intended restoration. As a consequence, the final restoration must be visualized at the onset. After this first important step, the individual areas of abutment support are determined. If natural teeth are present in those areas, they are evaluated with the same criteria of traditional prosthodontics. If no natural teeth are in the areas of primary support, the bone is evaluated to assess which types of implants may be placed to support the intended prosthesis. If inadequate natural or implant abutments exist or cannot be inserted, the existing oral conditions or the needs and desires of the patient must be changed. Therefore abutment location and number must satisfy the goals of the intended restoration; otherwise, the mind or mouth of the patient must be changed.

In 1988 Misch reported five prosthetic options available in implant dentistry (Table 4–1). [1,2] The first three choices are fixed restorations. They may replace partial or total dentition and may be cemented or screw-retained. Common to all fixed options is the inability of the patient to remove the prosthesis. These fixed restoration options depend on the amount of hard and soft tissue structures replaced. Two types of final restorations are removable, and depend on the amount of implant support. As most traditional removable prostheses, they are used primarily in full arch restorations.

FIXED PROSTHESES

FP-1

There are three kinds of fixed prosthesis (see Table 4–1). FP-1 is a fixed restoration, and appears to the patient to replace only the anatomic crown of the natural tooth. There usually has been minimal loss of hard and soft tissue. The volume and position of bone often permit ideal placement of the implant in a

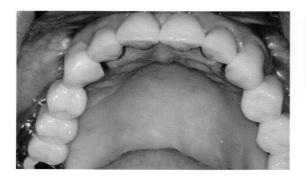

PLATE 1.
FP-1 prosthesis is fixed and appears to replace the anatomic crown of natural teeth. Volume and position of bone often permit ideal implant placement.

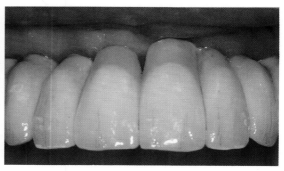

PLATE 2.
FP-2 prosthesis is fixed and replaces more than the anatomic crown. The teeth are hypercontoured, especially in the cervical region.

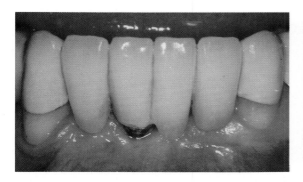

PLATE 3.
FP-2 or FP-3 prosthesis may have the implant abutment placed in an embrasure area, and the final restoration may still be constructed with normal crown width. This is much more difficult when only the anatomic crown is replaced.

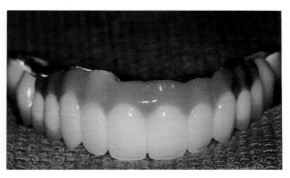

PLATE 4.
FP-3 prosthesis appears to replace tooth and gingival color. Materials used in this case are porcelain to metal.

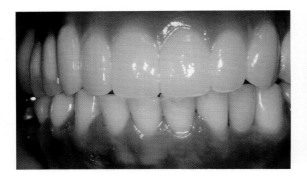

PLATE 5.
FP-3 prosthesis in Figure 4–4 in place. Color of the pink porcelain is shaded to appear similar to the interdental papillae in the apposing arch.

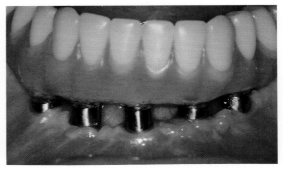

PLATE 6.
Materials used in this FP-3 restoration are metal, pink acrylic, and denture teeth. The more vertical bone replaced the more often this type of reconstruction is indicated.

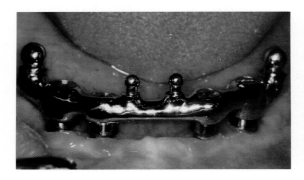

PLATE 7.
RP-4 restoration is completely implant supported. Superstructure in this patient is cantilevered distally from four anterior implants.

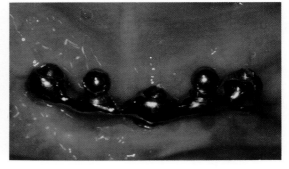

PLATE 8.
RP-5 removable prosthesis is supported by soft tissue in the posterior section, and implant supported or retained in the anterior section.

TABLE 4–1.

Prosthodontic Classification (Misch, 1988)

FP-1	Fixed prosthesis; replaces only the crown, looks like a natural tooth
FP-2	Fixed prosthesis; replaces the crown and a portion of the root; crown contour appears normal in the occlusal half, but is elongated or hypercontoured in the gingival half
FP-3	Fixed prosthesis; replaces missing crowns and gingival color and portion of the edentulous site; prosthesis most often uses denture teeth and acrylic gingiva, but may be porcelain to metal
RP-4	Removable prosthesis; overdenture supported completely by implant
RP-5	Removable prosthesis; overdenture supported by both soft tissue and implant

location similar to the root of a natural abutment. The final restoration appears very similar in size and contour to most traditional fixed prostheses used to restore or replace natural crowns of teeth (Plate 1).

The FP-1 prosthesis is most often desired in the maxillary anterior region. However, if width and/or height of bone at the crest of the edentulous site is lacking, augmentation is often required to achieve a natural looking crown in the cervical region. In addition, because there are no interdental papilla regions in edentulous ridges, gingiplasty is required after the abutment is positioned, so as to improve the gingival contour. Ignoring this step results in open triangular spaces (where papillae are usually present) that appear black in the patient with a high lip line when he or she smiles.

The final restoration appears to the patient to be a natural, healthy tooth. In reality, the implant abutment rarely can be treated exactly as a natural tooth prepared for a full crown. For example, posterior implant-supported prostheses often have narrower occlusal tables at the expense of the buccal contour, because facial bone loss requires that the implant be placed more lingual. The lingual contour is similar to that of natural teeth. The occlusal table is modified to conform to the implant size and position, and to direct vertical forces to the implant.

The diameter of a maxillary central incisor is approximately 8 to 10 mm, with an oval to triangular cross-section. The implant abutment is usually 3 to 4 mm in diameter and round in cross-section. In addition, the placement of the implant rarely corresponds exactly to the crown-root position of the original tooth. The thin labial bone lying over the facial aspect of a root remodels after tooth loss, and the crest width shifts lingually and decreases 40% to 60% within the first 2 years.[3] Thus the implant cannot be positioned exactly as the natural tooth had been, but instead is placed usually to the lingual.

To restore the implant abutment to ideal esthetic contour, the cervical portion of the tooth often needs to be repositioned facially. The restoring dentist is confronted with a similar esthetic decision for the pontics of a fixed prosthesis. The modified ridge lap pontic fulfills the esthetics and contour requirements of the missing teeth. In addition, the relief of the palatogingival region provides an acceptable means of oral hygiene.

Exactly the same pontic design may be used for an implant abutment in a palatal situation. An abutment hole on the lingual aspect of the "pontic" connects the implant abutment to the pontic-designed crown. Dental floss may be passed under the modified ridge lap (MRL) crown to remove plaque. A common mistake is to place the implant abutment coping or substructure margin subgingival on the labial portion of the pontic contour. This creates unaccessible areas for homecare maintenance at the level of the MRL crown contours. Therefore, supragingival margins on the labial metal substructure are usually indicated.

The restorative material of choice for an FP-1 prosthesis or crown is porcelain to noble metal. The noble metal allows the substructure to be separated and soldered if a passive fit does not exist at the metal try-in. The noble metals are also less likely to cause metal corrosion, especially when subgingival margins on a metal implant are present. Any history of exudate around a subgingival base metal margin will dramatically increase the corrosion effect.

FP-2

The fixed prosthesis FP-2 appears to restore the anatomic crown and portion of the root of the natural tooth. The quantity and location of available bone dictate a different vertical implant placement, which is slightly apical compared to the cemento-enamel junction of a natural root. As a result, to position the incisal edge in the correct position, the gingival third of the crown is overextended, usually apical and lingual to the position of the original tooth (Plate 2). These restorations are similar to teeth with gingival recession after periodontal bone loss. The patient and doctor should be aware from the onset of treatment that the final prosthetic teeth will appear longer than healthy natural teeth. If the lip lines during smiling or speech are favorable, the longer teeth are usually of no consequence, provided that the patient has been informed before treatment.

An implant placed in the embrasure region of two anterior teeth will often result in an FP-2 restoration. The most esthetic result usually requires the two crowns to be ideal in width (Plate 3), as if the implant was not there. The embrasure positioned implant placed too lingual is easier to restore than one inserted too facial. The material of choice for an FP-2 prosthesis is also noble metal to porcelain. A metal try-in is especially important for evaluation of the amount of unsupported porcelain in the final prosthesis.

FP-3

The FP-3 is a fixed restoration that appears to replace the crowns of the natural teeth and the color of the soft tissue. The original available bone height has been lost by natural resorption or osteoplasty at the time of implant surgery. In order to place the incisal edge of the teeth in proper position for esthetics, function, lip support, and speech, the excessive vertical dimension to be restored requires teeth that are unnatural in length. The addition of gingival-tone acrylic or porcelain for a more natural appearance is often indicated (Plates 4 and 5).

The more gingival tissue replaced in the final restoration, the more likely the materials used for fabrication are metal with acrylic and denture teeth. The cost, ease of construction, esthetics, weight, and ability to repair the restoration are all advantages. They may also provide a stress relief advantage over porcelain to metal, especially related to impact forces first generated when the teeth occlude (Plate 6).

Anterior edentulous areas with vertical bone loss also present loss of bone width. The implants are inserted to the lingual aspect of the natural crown, which dictates nonanatomic contours for the fixed prosthesis in height and cervical contour. The maxillary prosthesis is extended or juxtaposed to the tissue, so speech is not impaired. The mandibular restoration may be left above the tissue, similar to a sanitary pontic. This facilitates the patient to oral hygiene in the mandible, especially when the implant permucosal site is level with the floor of the mouth and the depth of the vestibule.

A skeletal Angle Class II or III malocclusion can be corrected with the FP-2 or FP-3 fixed prosthesis to recreate ideal occlusal and esthetic patterns. However, the anterior cantilevered prosthesis must be designed to allow hygiene procedures.

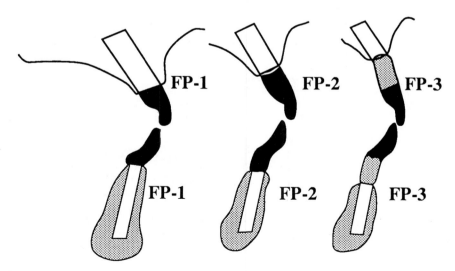

FIG 4–1.
FP-1 prosthesis has better biomechanics related to implant length than FP-3 restoration. More and/or greater diameter implants are required for FP-3 than for FP-1. The difference in FP-2 or FP-3 is related to lip position during smiling and/or speaking.

Selection of an FP-2 or FP-3 restoration often depends on the patient's maxillary high lip line position during smiling or mandibular low lip line position during speech. The restored gingival color and contours give the teeth a more natural appearance in size and shape. Implants placed too facial, lingual, or in embrasures are easier to restore when vertical bone has been lost and an FP-3 prosthesis is indicated, because even high lip lines do not expose the implant abutments. An FP-3 restoration usually has greater crown-implant ratios compared with other fixed types of prosthesis. A greater moment of force is placed on the implant cervical regions, especially during occlusal excursions. As a result, additional implant abutments should be considered to support an FP-3 restoration compared to FP-1 (Fig 4–1).

REMOVABLE PROSTHESES

There are two kinds of removable prosthesis (see Table 4–1). Patients are able to remove the restoration, but not necessarily the superstructure or attachments. The difference in these two categories of removable restorations is the amount of implant support. The most common removable implant prostheses are overdentures. Traditional removable partial dentures with clasps on implant abutment crowns have not been reported in the literature with any frequency. No long-term or short-term studies are currently available. On the other hand, complete removable overdentures have been reported to have acceptable longevity. As a result, the removable prosthetic options are primarily overdentures (Fig 4–2).

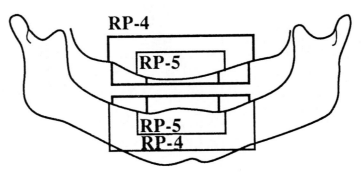

FIG 4–2.
Removable prostheses are related to the amount of implant support for the restoration. *RP-4* prosthesis has anterior and posterior superstructure support. *RP-5* restoration has primarily anterior implant support, and soft tissue support in the posterior region.

RP-4

RP-4 is a removable prosthesis and is completely supported by the implant and tooth. This prosthetic option is determined by the support, not the amount of hard or soft tissue replacement. The restoration is rigid when inserted, and attachments usually connect the removable prosthesis to a low-profile or tissue bar superstructure that splints the implant abutments (Plate 7). Usually five to six implants in the mandible and six to eight implants in the maxilla are required to fabricate completely implant-supported RP-4 prostheses in patients with adequate dental criteria.

The RP-4 prosthesis may have the same appearance as an FP-1, FP-2, or FP-3 restoration. A porcelain to metal prosthesis with attachments in selected abutment crowns may be fabricated for patients with the cosmetic desire of a fixed prosthesis, but with excess stresses requiring a removable restoration.

RP-5

RP-5 is a removable prosthesis combining implant and soft tissue support. The amount of implant support is variable. The completely edentulous mandibular overdenture may have two anterior implants splinted in the canine region to enhance retention (Plate 8), three implants in the premolar and central areas to also provide lateral stability, or four implants splinted with a cantilevered bar to reduce abrasions and limit the amount of the soft tissue coverage needed for support. The primary advantage of a RP-5 restoration is the reduced cost. The prosthesis is very similar to traditional overdentures.

The RP-4 or RP-5 removable restoration may allow modification of a preexisting acceptable prosthesis. The implant dentist may use the restoration as a guide for implant placement. The patient may wear the prosthesis during the healing stage. Once the implants are uncovered, the superstructure is fabricated within the guidelines of the existing restoration. A rebase then adapts the premade acceptable restoration to the connecting bar and soft tissue. This technique is especially indicated for patients difficult to satisfy with the esthetic result. A preimplant treatment traditional denture may be fabricated to ensure the patient's esthetic satisfaction. Once this is acquired, the existing prosthesis may be converted to the RP-5 restoration.

SUMMARY

In traditional dentistry the restoration reflects the existing oral conditions of the patient. Existing natural abutments are first evaluated, and a removable or fixed restoration is accordingly fabricated. Implant dentistry is unique because a foundation of support may be added for a desired prosthodontic result. The needs and desires of the patient are determined first. The prosthesis which satisfies these goals and eliminates the existing problems is then designed. The prosthesis may be fixed or removable.

If only one implant system is used for all patients, the same surgical and prosthetic scenario is invariably repeated. For example, if a traditional mandibular staple bone plate is used on all edentulous mandibles, not only are the implant and surgery similar regardless of intraoral or extraoral conditions, but a RP-5 prosthesis always results, regardless of the patient's needs and desires.

The real benefits of implant dentistry can be realized only when the prosthesis is first discussed and determined. An organized treatment approach based on the prosthesis permits predictable results of therapy. Five prosthetic options are available in implant dentistry. Three restorations are fixed and vary in the amount of hard and soft tissue replaced; two are removable and are based upon the amount of support for the restoration. The amount of support required for an implant prosthesis should initially be designed similar to traditional tooth-supported restorations. Once the intended prosthesis is designed, the implants and treatment surrounding this specific result can be established.

REFERENCES

1. Misch CE: Prosthodontic options for implant dentistry, *Dent Today* 8:39–44, 1989.
2. Misch CE: Prosthodontic options in implant dentistry, *Int J Oral Implant* 7:17–21, 1991.
3. Pietrokovski J: The bony residual ridge in man, *J Prosthet Dent* 34:456–462, 1975.

Chapter *5*

Medical Evaluation

Carl E. Misch

In this chapter the need for medical evaluation for patients considering implant therapy is emphasized. The chapter is developed in three major sections. The first focuses on the importance of the medical questionnaire and physical examination. The medical history includes those medical conditions most likely to influence implant treatment decisions. The physical examination consists of a hands-on evaluation and record of the patient's vital signs. In the second major section, titled Laboratory Evaluation, those laboratory tests of interest to implant dentistry are reviewed. These include a complete blood count, sequential multiple analysis, and bleeding disorder tests. The third major section relates the medical and dental implications of the most common systemic diseases found in an implant practice and having the greatest impact on implant dentistry.

The medical evaluation is more important in implant dentistry than in most other disciplines of dentistry, because systemic conditions that influence treatment are seen commonly. Implant treatment is primarily a surgical, prosthetic, and maintenance discipline for an older segment of the population. The need for implant-related treatment increases with the age of the patient,[1, 2] and as a result, the implant dentist treats more elderly patients than the other disciplines in dentistry.

An estimated 12% of the U.S. population is currently 65 years of age or older, but this number is expected to reach 21% (64.6 million) in the year 2030.[3] A 65-year-old person has a life expectancy of another 16.7 years, and an 80-year-old person can expect to live an additional 8 years.[4] These patients often request implant support in their removable prostheses. Therefore, the number of elderly patients in the dental practice will increase, and it is important to design the medical and physical evaluations to accommodate the special conditions of these patients.

PHYSIOLOGIC CHANGES IN THE ELDERLY

Physiologic changes associated with aging and their pharmacologic counterparts modify the physical, social, and economic life of the patient. Although important individual variations exist, the biological systems of the elderly patient must cope with a decrease in function and physiologic reserve. These physiologic changes may predispose or increase the aging patient's susceptibility to disorders such as the following:

- 50% lung function
- 80% blood flow
- 70% cardiac output
- 50% renal plasma flow
- 69% glomerular filtration
- Decreased elasticity of arterial system (increase in systolic blood pressure)
- 70% vital capacity
- Decreased gastric motility
- Decreased intestinal absorption
- Body weight often reduced
- Increase in body fat
- Drug distribution phase modified from increased water weight, decreased plasma albumin, and decreased cardiac output
- Decreased plasma albumin causes increase of free and active drug
- Decreased excretion of drug (from decreased renal function)
- Reduced immune response
- Increased sensitivity to central nervous system (CNS) depressant drugs
- Greater individual variations of drug effects
- Multiple disease states
- Drug reliance decreased

In general, a healthy senior citizen demonstrates only half the lung function of a healthy young adult. The blood flow of an older patient represents 80% of that of the healthy 30 year old, the cardiac output is only 70%, and the renal plasma flow and glomerular filtration are considerably less effective (respectively, 50% and 60%). A decrease in the elasticity of the arterial system is illustrated by an increase in systolic blood pressure. The vital capacity is reduced to 70% of that of a 17-year-old patient and corresponds to a decrease in arterial partial pressure of oxygen.[5] Gastric motility and intestinal absorption are also decreased.

The total body weight of the patient is often reduced, especially if masticatory deficiency from lack of teeth and bone is present. However, there is an increase in body fat. Consequently, any medications administered will follow modified pharmacokinetics and dynamics. Drug kinetics are modified, especially in the distribution phase, as a result of the increased water weight, decreased plasma albumin, and decreased cardiac output. The decreased plasma albumin concentration causes a greater percentage of the drug to remain free and active. The decreased ability to metabolize drugs, which is related to the decreased renal function, is responsible for the decreased excretion of the drugs. Therefore, the intervals between their administration should be longer, and dosage should be decreased, except for liposoluble drugs and antibiotics, to compensate, respectively, for the increase in body fat and the reduced immune response.

The decreased gastric motility of the elderly patient affects the use of oral analgesics, such as codeine. Pharmacodynamic alterations include an increased sensitivity to CNS-depressant drugs. The individual variations are greater than in other segments of the population, and the dosage should be assessed for each patient.

Chronic illness and multiple disease states are characteristic of aging. Patient surveys indicate that 80% of elderly people have at least one chronic disease. Also, half of people older than 65 years have arthritis, 39% have hypertension, 27% have other cardiovascular problems, and 28% have hearing impairment. Other conditions often associated with aging are the increased frequency of diabetes (9.8%), immune response problems, orthopedic (osteoporosis) problems (17%), and sensory deficiencies as well as degenerative diseases.[6] The influence of chronic disease states are double for people over 65 years of age and affect the way that pathologic processes and surgery may affect an individual's surgical risk and prognosis.

Elderly patients receive 25% of all prescription drugs, although they represent only 20% of the total population. They receive an average of 13 prescriptions a year, in addition to many over-the-counter drugs, mainly analgesics. The drugs most often prescribed are diuretics, anticoagulants (e.g., aspirin, warfarin), cardiac agents (digoxin), steroids (prednisone), thiazides, and anticholinergics. Those drugs are among those most often responsible for adverse drug reactions. Hence in the elderly, 30% of drug-induced illnesses are due to interactions between these medications. These interactions also account for 20% of hospital admissions in senior citizens.

The elderly patient's compliance is often decreased. Aging patients have a tendency to forget to take medications or to mistake dosage and frequency. Because of impaired hearing and vision, they may become confused more easily. Many follow an inadequate diet, which may further impair their condition and slow healing after surgery.

MANAGEMENT OF ELDERLY IMPLANT PATIENTS

Because of their age, even healthy older implant candidates should be considered as patients with mild systemic disease. As a result of a decrease in physiologic adaptability, the aged patient has less reserve to react to stress. If the limits of homeostatic reserve are reached, the patient may reach a critical condition.[7] The elderly patient can follow regular implant therapy provided a typical stress-reduction protocol is implemented. Monitoring of vital signs, modified dosage of medications, and special care during sedation because of an increased sensitivity to CNS depressants, are indicated. An increased dosage of antibiotics compensates for the decreased immune system. An increased dosage of liposoluble drugs is also suggested. Elderly patients are reportedly less sensitive to pain, so a reduced dosage of narcotic analgesics is recommended, especially because their gastric motility is reduced. The doctor should be aware of the eventual adverse drug reactions of the medications taken by these patients when combined with those prescribed for implant surgical procedures.

MEDICAL HISTORY AND PHYSICAL EXAMINATION

The medical history is often the first opportunity for the dentist to talk with the patient. The time and consideration taken at the onset will set the tone of the entire following treatment. This first impression should reflect a warm, caring practitioner, highly trained to help patients with complex treatments. A sincere interest and active note-taking process are beneficial. The practitioner should not underestimate the value of the medical evaluation interview. Asking questions which show an understanding of listed medical conditions and related common problems offers several benefits.

The three basic categories of information addressed during taking of the medical history include past medical history, social and family history, and a review of the patient's systemic health. The dental office uses a medical evaluation form to obtain most of this information (Fig 5–1). Of particular note is medication usage within the preceding 6 months, allergies, and a review of the systems of the body. The pathophysiology of the systems, the degree of involvement, and the medications being used to treat the condition are evaluated. It is important to review this form with the patient to ensure comprehension is adequate to answer all questions. The form should include all medical areas of interest to the implant dentist.

Extraoral and Intraoral Examinations

Once the medical history is reviewed, the medical physical examination begins. This is the first physical contact the office staff has with the patient. A gentle, caring approach should continue throughout. A complete evaluation of the head and neck is important initially and at all subsequent preventive maintenance (recall) appointments. Inform the patient of the need for periodic examination for cysts and for benign or malignant tumors, and that 26,000 cases of cancer are diagnosed in the head and neck region every year.

The extraoral and intraoral examinations are similar to those addressed in any oral evaluation text. A few specific areas are mentioned, since complications of implant treatment have been observed. The extraoral examination is performed first. Features and facial symmetry are observed, including the ears, nose, and eyes. If the midline, occlusal plane, or smile line of the natural teeth or existing prosthesis are not harmonious, the cause should be determined. Patients are most acceptable to critical evaluation and treatment limitations relating to facial esthetics before reconstruction begins. A similar discussion at the end of treatment is considered an excuse.

The submental, submandibular, parotid, and cervical areas are palpated for lymphadenopathy or unusual swelling. Sialoliths may be blamed on implant surgery, when in fact they were previously present. The area between the cricoid notch and the suprasternal notch is palpated for hypertrophy of the thyroid gland, as several hormones relating to its physiology influence bone metabolism and implant management.

Intraoral examination of the lips, labial and buccal mucosa, hard and soft palate, tongue, and oral pharynx is then performed. Any lesions or disease states must be further evaluated before implant procedures commence.

Vital Signs

The recording of vital signs (blood pressure, pulse, temperature, respiration, weight, and height) also is part of the physical examination. This information can

MEDICAL HISTORY		
For the following questions, circle yes or no, whichever applies. Your answers are for our records only, and will be considered confidential. These facts have a direct bearing on your dental health.	DATE __/__/__	DATE __/__/__
Sex.........Height.........Weight.............. Age .... Race.............................		
1. Are you in good general Health?..	Yes No	Yes No
2. Has there been any change in your general health within the year?...........................	Yes No	Yes No
3. My last physical examination was on (approx. date) _____		
4. Are you now under a physician's care?..	Yes No	Yes No
If yes, for what condition?_____		
5. The name and address of your physician is _____		
6. Have you had any serious illness or operation?..	Yes No	Yes No
If so, please list._____		
7. Have you been hospitalized or had a serious illness within the past five years?..........	Yes No	Yes No
If yes, reason		

© Misch Implant Institute, 1988

FIG 5–1.
Medical evaluation form.

Medical History (cont.)	DATE __/__/__	DATE __/__/__

Cardiovascular system

CV1. Do you have or have you ever had any of the following........Please circle one...............

A. Heart trouble, heart attack, stroke, coronary insufficiency, damaged heart valves, congenital heart disease ?.....................................	Yes No	Yes No
CV2. Rheumatic heart disease, Heart murmur?.....................................	Yes No	Yes No
CV3. Chest pain after exertion?.....................................	Yes No	Yes No
CV4. Shortness of breath after mild exercise?.....................................	Yes No	Yes No
CV5. Do your ankles swell?.....................................	Yes No	Yes No
CV6. Do you use extra pillows to sleep?.....................................	Yes No	Yes No
CV7. Do you have a cardiac pacemaker?.....................................	Yes No	Yes No
CV8. Do you have any blood pressure problems?.....................................	Yes No	Yes No
High.............Low.............		

Central Nervous system

CN1. Do you have or have you ever had

A. Epilepsy?.....................................	Yes No	Yes No
B. Fainting Spells?.....................................	Yes No	Yes No
C. Seizures?.....................................	Yes No	Yes No
D. Emotional disturbances?.....................................	Yes No	Yes No
CN2. Do you follow any treatment for a nervous disease?.....................................	Yes No	Yes No

Respiratory system

RE1. Do you have a persistent cough or cold?.....................................	Yes No	Yes No
RE2. Do you have or have you ever had Tuberculosis?.....................................	Yes No	Yes No
RE3. Is there any history of Tuberculosis in your family?.....................................	Yes No	Yes No
RE4. Do you have any sinusitis, sinus trouble?.....................................	Yes No	Yes No
RE5. Do you have Emphysema, Chronic Bronchitis, Asthma?.....................................	Yes No	Yes No

Digestive system

GI1. Do you have any stomach ulcers?.....................................	Yes No	Yes No
GI2. Do you have or have you ever had.....................................		
Hepatitis?.....................................	Yes No	Yes No
Jaundice?.....................................	Yes No	Yes No
Liver Disease?.....................................	Yes No	Yes No
GI3. Have you ever vomited blood?.....................................	Yes No	Yes No
GI4. Do you have any diarrhea?.....................................	Yes No	Yes No

Endocrine system

EN1. Do you have Diabetes?.....................................	Yes No	Yes No
EN2. Does anyone in your family have diabetes?.....................................	Yes No	Yes No
EN3. Do you urinate more than 6 times a day?.....................................	Yes No	Yes No
EN4. Are you thirsty very often or do you have a dry mouth?.....................................	Yes No	Yes No
EN5. Do you have Hypothyroidism or Hyperthyroidism?.....................................	Yes No	Yes No

FIG 5–1. (cont.)

| | DATE _/_/_ | DATE _/_/_ |

Medical History (cont.)

Hematopoietic system

HB1. Do you have Anemia, Sickle cell disease, Blood disorder?..................................	Yes	No	Yes	No
HB2. Is there any family history of blood disorders?..	Yes	No	Yes	No
HB3. Are you hemophilic?..	Yes	No	Yes	No
HB4. Have you had abnormal bleeding after any surgery, extraction, or trauma?...........	Yes	No	Yes	No
HB5. Have you ever had a blood transfusion?...	Yes	No	Yes	No

Allergies

AL1. Are you allergic to or have you acted adversely to.................................				
A. Local Anesthetics?..	Yes	No	Yes	No
B. Antibiotics, Penicillin, Sulfadrugs?................................	Yes	No	Yes	No
C. Barbiturates, sedatives, or sleeping pills?.........................	Yes	No	Yes	No
D. Aspirin?...	Yes	No	Yes	No
E. Iodine?..	Yes	No	Yes	No
F. Codeine or other narcotics?...	Yes	No	Yes	No
G. Other?_____.	Yes	No	Yes	No
AL2. Do you have Asthma or Hay Fever?..	Yes	No	Yes	No
AL3. Do you have or have you ever had Hives or Skin rash?................................	Yes	No	Yes	No

Genitourinary system

UR1. Do you have or have you ever had..				
A. Kidney Trouble?..	Yes	No	Yes	No
B. Syphilis, Gonorrhea?..	Yes	No	Yes	No
C. AIDS?	Yes	No	Yes	No

Bone-Joints

BJ1. Do you have..				
A. Arthritis?..	Yes	No	Yes	No
B. Inflammatory Rheumatism?..	Yes	No	Yes	No
C. Bone Infection?...	Yes	No	Yes	No
D. Osteoporosis?...	Yes	No	Yes	No

Neoplasms

TR1. Do you have or have you ever had..				
A. Tumor or malignancy?..	Yes	No	Yes	No
B. Chemotherapy, or Radiation Therapy?.................................	Yes	No	Yes	No
Do you have any disease, condition or problem not listed above that you think we should know about?_____	Yes	No	Yes	No
Are you regularly exposed to x-rays or any other ionizing radiation or toxic substances?....	Yes	No	Yes	No
Do you have Glaucoma? If yes, wide or close angle.......................................	Yes	No	Yes	No
Are you wearing, or do you wear, contact lenses?.......................................	Yes	No	Yes	No
Do you drink alcohol? If yes, how much and how often...................................	Yes	No	Yes	No
Do you smoke or use tobacco? If yes, how much and how often............................	Yes	No	Yes	No

Page 3

FIG 5–1. (cont.)

Medical History (cont.)	DATE __/__/__	DATE __/__/__

Medications

AL1.Are you taking any of the following medications? If yes, please list below..............................

A. Antibiotics or sulfa drugs?...	Yes No	Yes No
B. Anticoagulants?..	Yes No	Yes No
C. Medicine for high blood pressure?..	Yes No	Yes No
D. Tranquilizers?	Yes No	Yes No
E. Iodine?..	Yes No	Yes No
F. Codeine or other Narcotics?...	Yes No	Yes No
G. Other?_____	Yes No	Yes No

Women

1. Are you pregnant? or Nursing? If yes, please circle which...........................	Yes No	Yes No
2. Do you have any problems associated with your menstrual period?................	Yes No	Yes No
3. Are you taking oral contraceptives or hormonal therapy?.............................	Yes No	Yes No

Dental History

1. What is your chief dental complaint?_____

2. Are you experiencing any discomfort or pain at this time?...............................		
3. Are you satisfied with the appearance of your teeth?.....................................		
4. Are you able to eat and chew foods satisfactorlily?..	Yes No	Yes No
5. Do you have headaches, earaches, or neck pain?...	Yes No	Yes No
6. Do you frequently experience sinus problems?..	Yes No	Yes No
7. Have you had any serious trouble associated with any previous dental treatment?............	Yes No	Yes No
If yes, please explain._____	Yes No	Yes No
_____	Yes No	Yes No

Responsibility and Consent Statement

I hereby authorize and request the performance of dental services for myself or for

_____

I also give my consent to any advisable and necessary dental procedures, medications or anesthetics to be administered by the attending dentist or by his supervised staff for diagnostic purposes or dental treatment.
These records may include study models, photographs, x-rays, and blood studies.
I understand and acknowledge that I am financially responsible for the services provided for myself or the above named, regardless of insurance coverage.
Treatment plans involving extended credit circumstances are subject to a credit check. I also understand that the treatment estimate presented to me is only an estimate. Occasionally, the need may arise to modify treatment. In such a case, I will be informed of the need for additional treatment, and its fee.
To the best of my knowledge the information provided in this form is accurate.

Signature of Patient_____

Signature of Doctor_____

Date _____

Page 4

FIG 5–1. (cont.)

often be gathered by trained dental auxiliary personnel before the patient's history is reviewed by the dentist. If any findings are unusual, the doctor can repeat the evaluation as needed.

Blood Pressure

Approximately 10% of dental offices record the patient's blood pressure.[8] This proves worthwhile for the implant dentist, because surgery and long prosthodontic procedures are frequently required. The blood pressure is measured within the arterial system. The maximum pressure is the systolic and the minimum pressure is the diastolic. Blood pressure is influenced by the cardiac output, blood volume, viscosity of the blood, condition of blood vessels (especially the arterioles), and heart rate. There is a direct and indirect determination of blood pressure. The dentist will only use the indirect method. This technique was first developed by the Italian physician Riva-Rocca in the 19th century.[9] The sphygmomanometer consists of an inflatable bag covered by a cuff, and a manometer to register the force and rate of air within the bag. The two most common manometer systems use mercury gravity or aneroid gauges. The mercury system is more accurate in changing climates; once calibrated, it is consistent for many years. The aneroid manometer can be as accurate as the gravity type, but requires regular calibration.

The patient is seated comfortably and the inflatable bag is positioned over the bare upper arm at the level of the patient's heart, with his or her palm supine. The brachial or radial artery is palpated and the bag is inflated to obliterate the vessel, about 30 mm Hg above the estimated systolic pressure. The cuff is deflated 2 to 4 mm Hg at every heartbeat. Using a stethoscope over the brachial artery, the systolic pressure is recorded at the first tapping sound heard. When the sounds become muffled or inaudible the diastolic pressure is noted.

Hypertension is the abnormal elevation of the resting arterial systolic and/or diastolic blood pressure. Hypertension and arteriosclerosis account for about 40% of organic heart diseases. Yet, it is estimated that half of the cases of hypertension in the United States remain undiagnosed. A more thorough understanding of the impact of hypertension on implant therapy is reviewed in the section later in this chapter.

Pulse

Only about 3% of dentists record the pulse of their patients, yet much pertinent information is available from this simple procedure. The pulse represents the force of the blood against the aortic walls for each contraction of the left ventricle. The pulse wave travels through the arteries and reaches the wrist 0.1 to 0.2 seconds after each contraction. The actual blood flow takes longer to travel this distance.

The usual location at which to record pulse is the radial artery in the wrist. However other locations, such as the carotid artery in the neck and the temporal artery in the temporal region, are convenient during implant surgery or dental treatment. Pulse monitors are very easy to use and beneficial during surgery or long prosthetic appointments.

Pulse Rate.—The normal pulse rate varies from 60 to 90 beats per minute in a relaxed, nonanxious patient. The beats are both strong and regular. The normal cardiac rhythm originates in the sinoatrial (SA) node, and the pulse reflects the ventricular contractions. The upper limit of normal may be considered 100 beats/min, and people in excellent physical condition may have a pulse rate of 40 to 60 beats/min. A pulse rate less than 60 beats/min in the nonathlete, or above 110 beats/min should be suspect and warrants a medical consultation.

A decreased pulse rate of normal rhythm (less than 60 beats/min) signals sinus bradycardia. It is natural for some patients, and may reach as low as 40 beats/min, although most patients become unconscious below this rate. Inappropriate bradycardia may indicate impending sudden death.

During implant surgery, if the pulse rate of the patient decreases to less than 60 beats/min and is accompanied by sweating, weakness, chest pain, or dyspnea, the implant procedure should be stopped, oxygen administered, and immediate medical assistance obtained.

An increased pulse rate of regular rhythm (more than 100 beats/min) is called sinus tachycardia. This rate is normal if experienced during exercise or anxiety. However, in patients with anemia or severe hemorrhage, the heart rate increases to compensate for the depletion of oxygen in the tissues. Pulse rate and temperature are also related, the pulse rate increasing 5 beats/min for each degree as the temperature rises.

Hyperthyroidism and acute or chronic heart disease also may result in sinus tachycardia. A condition called paroxysmal atrial tachycardia (PAT) is characterized by episodes of very fast heart beats, which may last a few minutes or several weeks. All of these conditions affect the surgery or may increase postoperative swelling. The increased swelling favors the occurrence of infections and complications, not only during the first critical weeks after implant placement but also the subsequent years of implant service to the patient.

Pulse Rhythm.—Two types of abnormal pulse rhythm are noted: regular and irregular irregularities. A regular irregularity increasing during exercise can signal atrial fibrillation. This may be a consequence of hyperthyroidism, mitral stenosis, or hypertensive heart disease and should be considered before implant surgery. Stress-reduction protocols can be implemented, and implants may even be contraindicated if the causal conditions are severe.

Premature ventricular contractions (PVCs) are noticed as a distinct pause in an otherwise normal rhythm. This condition may be associated with fatigue, stress, or excessive use of tobacco or coffee, but is also observed during myocardial infarction and as a precursor to cardiac arrest. If during implant surgery, five or more PVCs are recorded within 1 minute, especially when accompanied by dyspnea or pain, the surgery should be stopped, oxygen administered, the patient placed in a supine position, and immediate medical assistance obtained. If the health history includes cardiovascular disease, including hypertension, the pulse rhythm especially should be recorded. Sudden death in persons older than 30 years with PVC are six times more frequent than in younger persons.[8]

Pulse Volume.—The patient's pulse rate and rhythm may be normal, yet the volume may vary in strength. The pulse may alternate between strong and weak beats, which indicates pulsus alternans and severe myocardial damage. Implant surgery is contraindicated and medical consultation with electrocardiographic examination is needed to confirm the diagnosis. After a diagnosis of pulsus alternans is diagnosed, a patient's lifespan rarely extends 1 or 2 years.

Temperature

The thermometer, invented by Galileo, was first used clinically by Santorio of Padua in the 17th century.[9] Normal body temperature ranges from 96.8°F to 99.4°F in a healthy individual. It is usually lowest in the morning and highest during late afternoon or evening. An oral temperature of 99.5°F or higher is considered in the febrile range. For every degree of fever, the pulse rate rises about five beats per minute and the respiratory rate increases about four per minute.

The usual cause of elevated body temperature is bacterial infection and its toxic byproducts. Other causes can be exercise, hyperthyroidism, myocardial infarction, congestive heart failure, and tissue injury from trauma or surgery. Dental conditions causing an elevated temperature include severe dental abscess, cellulitis, and acute herpetic stomatitis. Low body temperature may be found in hypothyroidism.

In general, no elective surgery (including implants) should be performed on febrile patients. The cause of the fever may complicate the postsurgical phase of healing. In addition, because elevated temperature increases the patient's pulse rate, the risks of hemorrhage, edema, infection, and postoperative discomfort are greater.

Respiration

Respiration is noted while the patient is at rest. The normal rate in the adult varies between 16 to 20 breaths per minute and is regular in rate and rhythm. If the patient uses accessory muscles in the neck or shoulders for inspiration, whether before or during surgery, dyspnea should be suspected. Many intravenous drugs, including narcotics, cause dyspnea. Congestive heart failure, bronchial asthma, and advanced pulmonary emphysema also impair breathing. If dyspnea occurs during surgery, the pulse should immediately be evaluated to rule out the presence of PVC or myocardial infarction.

Hyperventilation is the result of both an increased rate and depth of respiration and may be preceded by frequent sighs, such as seen in the anxious patient. A respiratory rate greater than 20 breaths per minute requires investigation. Anxiety may increase this rate, in which case sedatives or stress-reduction protocols are indicated prior to implant surgery. Other causes for an increased respiration rate are severe anemia, advanced bronchopulmonary disease, and congestive heart failure. All three may affect the surgical procedure and/or healing response of the implant candidate.

LABORATORY EVALUATION

Routine laboratory screening of patients in a general dental setting who previously reported a normal health history have shown that 12% to 18% have undiagnosed systemic diseases.[10, 11] Many of these disorders may influence implant surgery protocol or long-term success rates. The percentage of implant patients with unreported systemic illness is most likely higher, because the average implant patient is older than in these general studies. Implant therapy comprises an elective surgery involving a considerable financial investment by the patient. Therefore, clinical laboratory tests are often used to supplement diagnosis and treatment planning. Laboratory screening is also of benefit in helping one to recognize oral manifestations of systemic diseases. However, preoperative testing should not be considered mandatory for all patients. Justification of the laboratory procedures should relate to the specific type of surgery and patient conditions.

The most common laboratory evaluation for implant dentistry may include a complete blood cell count (CBC), sequential multiple analysis (SMA), and bleeding disorder tests.[12] The dentist should select the tests needed to assist in the diagnosis of systemic diseases affecting implant treatment.

Urinalysis

In the healthy adult, approximately 180 L of fluid are filtered through the glomeruli of the kidneys each day. The glomeruli filter the plasma, and the tubules selectively reabsorb water and substances useful to the body. They leave undesirable substances behind, or secrete them into the urine. The urinary constituents can be altered in the presence of systemic disease or infection, or focal urinary track infection.

Urinalysis is not indicated as a routine procedure for all dental patients, and is rarely used in implant dentistry. It is primarily a screening test for diabetes, deficiencies or irregularities in metabolism, renal disease, or suspected infection. The most frequent use of urinalysis by the dentist concerns suspicion of or screening for diabetes mellitus, which is the most common cause of glucosuria.

However, other conditions such as pregnancy, Cushing disease, Graves disease, intracranial tumor, and coronary thrombosis can modify this level. In addition, a diabetic patient with high glucose blood levels may not spill glucose into the urine. Examination of the blood, on the other hand, indicates more precisely the patient's glucose metabolism and is a more reliable test. Therefore, urinalysis is rarely indicated specifically for oral implant surgery.

Complete Blood Cell Count

The CBC consists of several individual measurements on a single sample of blood. These tests include the number of erythrocytes and leukocytes, leukocytic differential, cellular morphology and maturity, hemoglobin determination, hematocrit, and platelet count. Indications for a CBC are suspected dyscrasia, glucocorticoid therapy within 1 year, chemotherapy, renal diseases, or major blood loss expected. Asymptomatic patients do not require a CBC unless major blood loss is possible with surgery. The CBC has a more definite indication if any dyscrasia is suspected, when glucocorticoid therapy has been used within the preceding year, and when chemotherapy and/or renal diseases are listed in the present medical history.

Evaluation of the CBC can be limited to three clinical situations for implant dentistry: erythrocytic disorders, leukocytic disorders, and bleeding disorders.[13]

White Blood Cell Count

The normal white blood cell (WBC) count ranges from 5,000 to 10,000/mL and often varies with diseases. An increase in WBCs, or leukocytosis, is not specific to one white blood cell type. A decrease in number of WBC is referred to as leukopenia. One or all the WBC elements may be decreased.

The determination of an inflammatory process is often important for the implant dentist and often occurs without leukocytosis. An increased count of band neutrophils indicates inflammation. Segmented neutrophils phagocytize bacteria and increase in times of infection. Therefore, if a WBC count is ordered to determine if infection around an implant is affecting the patient's overall health, a differential of WBC types is evaluated, not just the number of leucocytes present.

Red Blood Cell Count

Red blood cells (RBC) are responsible for the transport of oxygen and carbon dioxide throughout the body and for control of the blood pH. They compose the largest segment of the formed elements of the blood. The normal RBC count is higher in men than women. Increases may result from polycythemia, congenital heart disease, or Cushing's syndrome. The most common finding is a decreased count and usually indicates anemia.

Hemoglobin

Almost 95% of the dry weight of an RBC is hemoglobin. It is responsible for the oxygen-carrying capacity of the blood. The normal level of hemoglobin is 13.5 to 18 g/dL in men and 12 to 16 g/dL in women. The preoperative threshold of 10 g/dL is often used as a minimum baseline for surgery. However, many patients can undergo surgical procedures safely at 8 g/dL. The threshold is related to the underlying conditions of the patient and the anticipated blood loss.[14]

Hematocrit

The hematocrit represents the packed cell volume and indicates the percentage of red blood cells in a given volume of whole blood. It is the prime indicator of anemia or blood loss. Therefore, if one of these conditions is suspected, the hematocrit is evaluated.

Bleeding Tests

One of the most critical conditions encountered in surgery is bleeding disorders. The platelet count may reflect this complication; however, it does not provide enough information to determine potential bleeding disorders. The patient's medical history provides a better detector (see Bleeding Time).

An understanding of the normal clotting process is necessary to determine which bleeding test to evaluate. Whenever the integrity of a vessel wall is altered surgically, hemostasis is achieved by vascular spasm, blood coagulation, and, finally, growth of fibrous tissue to close the defect in the vessel. For hemostasis to be maintained or achieved, the blood vessels must be normal, functional platelets must be present in sufficient numbers, and the coagulation mechanism of the blood must be intact. In summary, three phases are necessary for hemostasis, involving the vessels; the platelets; and coagulation, both extrinsic (outside blood vessels) and intrinsic (inside blood vessels).

The vascular phase corresponds to the vasoconstriction and retraction of the arteries that have been severed and an extravascular pressure from the blood loss around the injured site. This occurs immediately following injury.

The platelet phase begins a few seconds after vessels are severed. The circulating functional platelets become "sticky," allowing them to adhere to the endothelium of the damaged vessels, to the collagen in the surrounding tissues, and to each other. Formation of a "platelet plug," which seals off the opening of the vessels, requires several seconds to minutes to occur.

The blood coagulation phase takes place more slowly than the previous two steps. It has been described in many ways, but the easiest way to correlate the necessary information to the clinical setting is to describe it as being initiated by two separate mechanisms. The extrinsic system and the intrinsic system both lead to completion of hemostasis along a common pathway. Both systems are necessary for normal coagulation. The extrinsic system is activated outside the blood vessels; the intrinsic system is activated within the blood vessels.

Three ways to detect potential bleeding problems are the medical history, physical examination, and screening clinical laboratory tests. Over 90% of bleeding disorders can be diagnosed on the basis of the medical history alone. The history should include questions covering five topics placed on the past medical history form:

1. Bleeding problems in relatives
2. Spontaneous bleeding from the nose, mouth, or other apertures
3. Bleeding problems after operations, tooth extractions, or trauma
4. Use of medications that may cause bleeding disorders
5. Past or present illness associated with bleeding disorders.

Bleeding problems in relatives are significant because they indicate inherited coagulation disorders. Hemophilia and Christmas factor disease are the most common. Spontaneous bleeding from the nose, gingiva, and/or joint, may indicate either inherited disease or illness with bleeding disorders (for example, acute leukemia). If no problems resulted from any previous surgery, then no significant inherited disorder is present and no acquired disorders were present at that time.

Medications causing increased bleeding are the most common causes of bleeding resulting from platelet disorders. These iatrogenic factors are seen primarily with three types of drugs: anticoagulants, aspirin, and long-term antibiotics. Past or present illnesses that may present associated bleeding disorders include leukemia, anemia, thrombocytopenia, hemophilia, and hepatic diseases. In approximately half of patients with liver disease there is a decrease in platelets secondary to hypersplenism, and therefore potential bleeding disorders.[15]

The second method by which the implant dentist may detect a patient with a bleeding disorder is the physical examination. The exposed skin and oral mucosa must be examined for objective signs. Petechiae, ecchymoses, spider angioma, or jaundice may be observed in liver disease patients with bleeding complications. Intraoral petechiae, bleeding gingiva, ecchymoses, hemarthroses, and hematomas may be present in patients with genetic bleeding disorders. Patients with acute or chronic leukemia show signs of ulceration of the oral mucosa, hyperplasia of the gingiva, petechiae or ecchymoses of the skin or oral mucosa, and/or lymphadenopathy.

The third option by which to detect a bleeding disorder is clinical laboratory testing. If a patient's health history does not include potential bleeding disorders, routine screening with a coagulation profile is not indicated. However, if extensive surgical procedures are expected, a coagulation profile is indicated. Four tests are typically used to screen patients for bleeding disorders. These include the platelet count, bleeding time, partial thromboplastin time (PTT), and prothrombin time (PT).

The platelet count is obtained in the CBC, and normal values range between 200,000 and 300,000/mL. A clinical manifestation usually does not occur until the platelet count is below 80,000/mL. The Ivy bleeding time is an excellent test by which to determine adequate platelet function and may also test the vascular phase.

Coagulation Tests

The PTT is used to determine the ability of the blood to coagulate within the vessels. Therefore, it tests the intrinsic and common pathways of coagulation. The PT determines the ability of the blood to coagulate outside the vessels and therefore tests the extrinsic and common pathways of coagulation. Both systems are necessary for normal coagulation.[16]

The patient's history and physical examination can now be related to the appropriate clinical laboratory tests.[17] For example, for patients who have been taking aspirin, a bleeding time and PTT should be obtained. One 5-grain tablet of aspirin can affect platelet agglutination for 3 days. If four or more tablets a day are taken for a period longer than 1 week, both the bleeding time and PTT can be affected and should be suspect.

If the patient is taking an anticoagulant medication because of recent myocardial infarction, cerebrovascular accident, or thrombophlebitis, the PT should be checked. Oral anticoagulants are mainly coumarin derivatives. The coumarins are vitamin K antagonists that interfere with the synthesis of prothrombin complex factors. Their action usually begins within 8 to 12 hours, with a peak effect in about 36 hours. Two or 3 days of a reduced level of coumarin are required before a decrease in PT is observed. If the PT is still greater than twice normal, the dosage of anticoagulant should be reduced again by the physician, and another test reordered 2 or 3 days later. The amount of reduction and time sequencing for these changes should be determined by the physician administering the medications.

When heparin is the anticoagulant, usually prescribed for renal dialysis, a PTT should be scheduled for the day of surgery. Heparin is a short-acting anticoagulant. Therefore, this test and the surgery should be scheduled 24 hours after heparin administration. Kidney dialysis patients often experience healing and maintenance complications with their natural teeth; thus implants are usually contraindicated in these patients. However, the dentist may have to treat a dialysis patient who has previously had implant therapy.

Long-term antibiotic therapy can affect the intestinal bacteria that produce the vitamin K necessary for prothrombin production in the liver. Therefore, if long-term administration of antibiotics has been used by the implant patient, a PT should be obtained to evaluate possible bleeding complications.

Bleeding disorders should be suspected in a patient who is alcoholic or shows signs of liver dysfunction. Most coagulation factors are produced in the liver, and 50% of patients with liver disease have hypersplenism resulting from the destruction of platelets. The PT is the single most useful test in the evaluation of impaired hepatocyte synthesis of prothrombin complex factors and to assess hemostasis in patients with liver disease. The bleeding time and PT should therefore be evaluated.

The PT and PTT may be used together to determine coagulation factor defects. A normal PT and abnormal PTT suggests hemophilia. An abnormal PT and a normal PTT suggest Factor VII deficiency. If both PT and PTT are longer, a deficiency of Factors II, V, X, or fibrinogen are considered.

No surgical procedures should be performed in a patient suspected of having a bleeding problem based on history, examination, and clinical laboratory tests, without proper preparation, understanding, and management by the dentist. If the bleeding problem has been previously undiagnosed, the underlying cause should be addressed before the implant surgical procedures.

Biochemical Profiles

The tenets of laboratory diagnosis must be understood, particularly as they relate to implant dentistry. The interpretation of biochemical profiles and the ability to communicate effectively with medical consultants will enhance the treatment of many patients.

Oral implant treatment may be affected by the results of biochemical profiles, by either contraindicating the procedure completely, altering the type of implant surgery and reconstruction, postponing the treatment until therapy controls the disease entity, or simply changing the sequence of medications normally used during the treatment. Biochemical sanguine profiles are a more necessary part of the medical evaluation for an implant candidate in the presence of systemic diseases and/or advanced surgical procedures.[18] They are not indicated for every potential implant patient.

Dentists have been trained to take a careful medical history, perform a thorough dental examination, and on occasion, order laboratory tests that will either confirm or exclude a provisional diagnosis. However, with biochemical profiles, such as the SMA-12/60, the opportunity exists to evaluate many different biochemical parameters reflecting the patient's health.

To become comfortable in interpreting the biochemical profile, some time must be spent in learning the pattern of systemic diseases. This pattern recognition is similar to the tissue patterns a pathologist looks at during a biopsy. In fact, the SMA profile has been described as a "biochemical biopsy" of the blood. It includes normal and abnormal values that have interrelationships in the diagnosis of systemic diseases. It would not be wise to single out one value from which to establish a diagnosis. The data should be related with other values obtained in the profile before further determinations are rendered.

More than 20 different tests are available for the selection of this profile, from which each laboratory and its referring physicians choose. Therefore, the use of different laboratories makes it difficult to develop interpretative skills. It is suggested the dentist use the same laboratory consistently, which highlights the abnormal values for an individual test. The dentist is not responsible to treat the many systemic diseases that the biochemical profile will reveal. However, it is necessary to know the consequences of a disease on the implant treatment.

Normal Range

The normal values found on the SMA represent a statistical norm. Any population characteristically shows a bell-shaped curve for a particular measurement. It has been shown that 56% of a sample falls within one standard deviation of the mean and 95% fall within two standard deviations. The normal value in the biochemical profile represents two standard deviations. Thus, "normal" in the statistical sense does not necessarily mean healthy; the word merely describes the typical range of values expected in any given population. Approximately one in 20 results will be outside the two standard deviation range. The further from the average value a particular value falls, the more certain its clinical significance. Different laboratories may have different "normal" results.

As biochemical profiles are accumulated for an individual patient over several years, the deviation in a given test may indicate a radical change for that individual, although the result never deviates from the "normal" population range. The implant dentist should remember that the healthy patient of today may have a systemic disease in the future. Therefore, when evaluating long-term complications, it is of interest to relate a recent biochemical profile to the one first reviewed before the initial surgery.

The patient should fast before the blood is collected to avoid artificial elevations of blood glucose and depressed inorganic phosphorus. Most of the other elements of the profile will not be affected. This chapter will limit the discussion to those factors of most benefit to the implant dentist (Table 5–1): glucose, calcium, inorganic phosphorus, alkaline phosphatase, lactic dehydrogenase (LDH), creatinine, and bilirubin.

TABLE 5–1.

Laboratory Evaluation of Disease Indicators

Chemistry	Disease
Glucose	Diabetes, steroid dysfunction
Calcium	Renal disease, diet, bone diseases, (carcinoma, parathyroid disease, Paget disease)
Inorganic phosphorus	Renal disease, endocrine (parathyroid, thyroid, steroids), antacids
Alkaline phosphatase	Liver disease, bone diseases (Paget disease, metastases, fractures, hyperparathyroidism)
Lactic dehydrogenase	Hemolytic disorders, liver disorders, myocardial infarction
Creatinine	Renal function
Bilirubin	Liver disease

Glucose

The normal range of glucose found in the blood, 70 to 100 mg/mL, is maintained within fairly narrow limits. Hyperglycemia is a relatively common finding, and the most common cause of this condition is diabetes mellitus. If high glucose values are found, referral to a physician for glucose tolerance tests after a glucose loading dose is recommended, except when inorganic phosphorus values are depressed. Depressed inorganic phosphorus usually indicates the patient has eaten before the blood was drawn and the elevated glucose is then related to digestion. Cushing's disease and other conditions related to excess production of adrenal corticoids are also considered in the differential diagnosis with hyperglycemia. Hypoglycemia is unusual and related to varied causes, for example Addison's disease, bacterial sepsis, and excessive insulin administration.

Calcium

The implant dentist may be the first to detect diseases affecting the bone. Chemical confirmation is primarily dependent on the patient's serum levels of calcium, phosphorus, and alkaline phosphatase. Over 98% of the calcium in the body is stored in the skeleton and teeth. Calcium ions are responsible for neuromuscular excitability, normal blood coagulation, and the activation of several enzymes. Serum calcium levels are influenced by the parathyroid hormone and calcitonin. Serum calcium levels are increased by bone resorption, intestinal absorption, and renal reabsorption of calcium.

Decreased levels of calcium are primarily seen in hypoproteinemic conditions and in renal disease. Renal disease is much more common, but the diet of the potential implant patient may be severely affected by the lack of denture comfort and stability. The cause and treatment of hypocalcemic serum levels should be addressed before implant reconstruction.

Elevated levels of serum calcium are associated with carcinoma in bones, dietary or absorptive disturbances, and hyperparathyroidism. The osteoporosis that may accompany this disorder has been observed in the mandible. Hyperparathyroidism also causes hypophosphatemia. Hypercalcemia associated with a significant elevation of alkaline phosphatase suggests Paget's disease of bone. All other biochemical values being normal, an elevated calcium value may be the result of laboratory error.[19] If phosphorus and/or alkaline phosphatase levels are also affected, medical evaluation and treatment is indicated before implant surgery.

Inorganic Phosphorus

Inorganic phosphorus levels maintain a ratio of 4 to 10 compared with calcium, and there usually is a reciprocal relationship, so when the level of one increases, the other decreases. The most common cause of elevated phosphorus is chronic glomerular disease, indicated by elevated blood urea nitrogen (BUN) and creatinine values.

In the absence of significant glomerular disease (normal BUN and creatinine values), phosphorus level abnormalities are usually associated with the endocrine system or bone metabolism. If an increase in phosphorus is associated with a decrease in calcium and normal renal function, hypoparathyroidism is suspected. Other endocrine disorders associated with an increased phosphorus level include hyperthyroidism, increased growth hormone secretion, and Cushing syndrome.

Decreased levels of phosphorus may appear in hyperparathyroidism patients, especially when associated with hypercalcemia. The chronic use of antacids containing aluminum hydroxide also may induce hypophosphatemia and warrants investigation for a peptic ulcer.

Alkaline Phosphatase

Serum alkaline phosphatase determination helps evaluate hepatobiliary diseases and bone diseases. The normal levels for this enzyme in adults are derived primarily from the liver, so extremely high levels of alkaline phosphatase are often associated with hepatic disease.

In the absence of liver disease, elevations of alkaline phosphatase are often a sign of osteoblastic activity in the skeletal system. Therefore bone metastases, fractures, Paget disease, and hyperparathyroidism often increase the level of this serum enzyme. Serum alkaline phosphatase is generally normal in patients with adult osteoporosis. Low levels of alkaline phosphatase are usually not of clinical significance for the dentist.

Lactic Dehydrogenase

Lactic dehydrogenase (LDH) is an intracellular enzyme present in all tissues. False elevated LDH levels occur as a result of hemolyzed blood specimens. Therefore, if all other blood values are normal, LDH testing should be repeated before further investigation.

The highest elevations of this enzyme are seen in patients with myocardial infarction, hemolytic disorders such as pernicious anemia, and liver disorders. Lactic dehydrogenase, aspartate aminotransferase (AST [SGOT]), bilirubin, uric acid, and total protein are indicators of hematologic and reticuloendothelial disorders. Blood disorders are particularly important to the implant surgeon. When LDH values are elevated, the complete blood count is evaluated for blood abnormalities.

Creatinine

Creatinine is an anhydride of creatine used in muscle metabolism. It is freely filtered by the glomeruli and not reabsorbed. The constancy of formation and excretion permits creatinine levels to be an index of renal function. This important system should not be impaired during implant surgery. Kidney dysfunction may lead to osteoporosis and decreased bone healing, because the kidney is required for complete formation of vitamin D. Medications may alter pharmacokinetics, and normal healing may also be affected with kidney disease.

Bilirubin

While seven of 12 tests in the SMA are indicative of liver function (total protein, albumin, cholesterol, bilirubin, LDH, alkaline phosphatase, AST), primary hepatic disease is typically reflected in elevations of bilirubin and enzymes as SGOT. Therefore, for the evaluation of liver disease, the measurement of bilirubin is of primary importance. Approximately 80% of the bilirubin comes from the degradation of red blood cells. The liver is responsible for hundreds of chemicals and proper body functions. This organ should be adequate for proper healing, drug pharmacokinetics, and long-term health.

SYSTEMIC DISEASE AND ORAL IMPLANTS

Most implant patients have some remaining teeth, and systemic diseases may affect this natural dentition. Most physicians are unaware of the wide range of treatments performed in oral implantology. Some conservative surgery and prosthetic implant procedures are rarely contraindicated based on systemic conditions, whereas other complex treatments must be excluded for the same condition. Therefore it is the responsibility of the implant dentist to understand the interrelationship of systemic diseases and implant dentistry.

Common conditions that may affect the implant treatment are discussed in three sections. The first section describes the entity in general. The second section discusses dental implant implications and the last section reviews dental implant management.

Systemic diseases have a range of effects on a patient, depending on their severity. The diseases discussed are classified as mild, moderate, or severe (Fig 5–2). A disease entity affects the host related to the intensity of the process. Hence a range of diabetes may permit implants in the mild form, yet the same disease may contraindicate most implant therapy in the severe expression of the disease. A general format may be established with most expressions of systemic disease. The systemic conditions addressed are those most commonly observed in the implant practice and do not include all conditions encountered:

1. Cardiovascular
   a. Hypertension
   b. Angina pectoris
   c. Myocardial infarction
   d. Congestive heart failure
   e. Bacterial endocarditis

Procedure

RISK		Type 1	Type 2	Type 3	Type 4
Mild	ASA II	+	Sedation Stress Reduction Protocol	IV Sedation Stress Reduction Protocol	
Moderate	ASA III	+	IV Sedation Stress Reduction Protocol Physician		Hospitalization
Severe	ASA IV	+	Postpone All Elective Procedures		

FIG 5–2.
Systemic diseases should be evaluated as to severity. Typical patterns of treatment in patients with mild, moderate, and severe disease are shown. See Table 5–2 for explanation of procedures included in types 1 through 4.

2. Endocrine
   a. Diabetes mellitus
   b. Thyroid
   c. Adrenal glands
   d. Pregnancy
3. Hematologic
   a. Erythrocyte
      (1) Polycythemia
      (2) Anemia
   b. Leukocyte
4. Pulmonary
   a. Chronic obstructive pulmonary disease
5. Hepatic
   a. Cirrhosis
6. Bone
   a. Osteoporosis
   b. Vitamin D disorders
   c. Hyperparathyroidism
   d. Fibrous dysplasia
   e. Osteitis deformans
   f. Multiple myeloma

7. Central nervous system
   a. Seizures
8. Prosthetic joints

In addition to the range of disease expression, a variety of implant treatments may be delivered to a patient. In Table 5–2, four levels of surgical and prosthetic treatment are established. A systemic condition may contraindicate one class of treatment, yet a more simple implant procedure may still be performed. The four levels of treatment vary from noninvasive procedures with little or no risk of gingival bleeding, to those which are most complicated and invasive.

Type 1 procedures can usually be performed on almost every patient regardless of systemic condition. Type 2 procedures are more likely to cause gingival bleeding or bacterial invasion of the bony structures. Type 3 procedures are surgical procedures that require more time and technique. Type 4 procedures are advanced surgical procedures.

Cardiovascular Conditions

Hypertension

Hypertension (and arteriosclerosis) accounts for about 40% of all organic heart diseases. Hypertension is the abnormal elevation of resting arterial systolic blood pressure above 140 mm Hg and/or above 90 mm Hg diastolic blood pressure. Approximately 20% of the U.S. adult population and 40% of the black adult population are affected. A 35-year-old person with untreated hypertension may have a life span 17 years shorter than average.[20] And yet, it is estimated that half of the cases of hypertension in the United States are undiagnosed.

Hypertension is usually asymptomatic, accelerates atherosclerosis, and is the major risk factor for cardiovascular morbidity and mortality for people over 50 years. Ninety percent of hypertensive patients have essential or idiopathic hypertension of unknown cause. Patients with essential hypertension are

TABLE 5–2.

Classification of Dental Treatments

Type I	Examinations, radiographs, study model impressions, oral hygiene instruction, supra-gingival prophylaxis, simple restorative dentistry
Type II	Scaling, root planning, endodontics, simple extractions, curettage, simple gingivectomy, advanced restorative procedures, simple implants (endodontic root forms)
Type III	Multiple extractions, gingivectomy, quadrant periosteal reflections, impacted extractions, apicoectomy, plate form implants, multiple root forms, ridge augmentation, subantral augmentation, unilateral subperiosteal implants
Type IV	Full arch implant (complete subperiosteal implants, ramus frame implants, full-arch endosteal implants); orthognathic surgery; autogenous bone augmentation; bilateral subantral augmentation

candidates to develop three times as much coronary disease, four times as much cardiac failure, and seven times as many strokes as patients with a normal blood pressure.

Essential hypertension is often treated with medications, many of which alter implant therapy because of their numerous side effects: orthostatic hypotension, dehydration, sedation, xerostomia, and depression. These side effects may alter treatment or require special precautions. For example, hypotension affects a patient brought from a supine to upright position. The patient may feel lightheaded or even faint, so the dental chair should be uprighted gradually. Xerostomia decreases the valve seal of soft tissue–borne removable prostheses and increases the risk of abrasions and sore spots.

In addition, severe hypertension can lead to angina pectoris, congestive heart failure, or even a cerebrovascular event from a rapid increase in the blood pressure during an injection or surgery. Cerebral hemorrhage, myocardial infarction, retinal hemorrhage, and kidney failure are other serious complications.

When a patient indicates hypertension on the medical history form, the date of the diagnosis, complications, and medications should be reviewed. The medications are a strong indicator as to the severity of the disease. Single diuretic drugs that treat mild hypertension cause the fewest complications that may modify implant treatment. Combination drugs indicate more severe hypertension, and a stress-reduction protocol is indicated. Patients taking clonidine have more severe hypertension,[21] and medical consultation is necessary before complicated implant surgery procedures. Additional medication or close follow-up following surgery may be indicated.

Dental Implant Management (Fig 5–3).—Anxiety often affects the blood pressure; therefore, a stress-reducing protocol is indicated for the hypertensive patient. A medication such as flurazepam (Dalmane) 30 mg or diazepam 5 to 10 mg may be prescribed to help the patient sleep quietly the night before a procedure. An early appointment also is beneficial, because the medication may still have an effect in the elderly patient. Additional premedication often is indicated at the time of the procedure. If the patient is taking a diuretic to help control mild hypertension, it should not be taken in the morning if conscious sedation or aseptic surgical techniques are used. Otherwise, the increased frequency of urination complicates the procedure.

The patient with controlled or mild hypertension (up to 160/105 mm Hg) and no other systemic disease can tolerate all nonsurgical and single implant surgical type 1 and type 2 procedures. Oral or conscious sedative techniques are beneficial for the more involved implant surgery (types 3 and 4).

Patients with moderate hypertension (up to 190/125 mm Hg) should be referred to their physician for a review of the medical management and more aggressive therapy. When this is done early in the course of treatment, the patient's blood pressure may be reduced prior to surgery. Nonsurgical procedures

RISK		Type 1	Type 2	Type 3	Type 4
Mild	140/90 mm Hg ASA II	+	+	Sedation	
Moderate	160/105 mm Hg ASA III	+	Sedation		Outpatient Hospitalization
Severe	190/125 mm Hg ASA IV	+	Postpone All Elective Procedures		

FIG 5–3.
Dental implant management in patients with hypertension.

(type 1) can be performed during early evaluation and treatment by the physician. Sedation techniques should be used with long restorative appointments or simple implant procedures (type 2). Intermediate or advanced surgical procedures are preferably performed in an outpatient hospital setting (types 3 and 4). A urinary catheter may be indicated for longer surgical appointments under general anesthetic. Complications include more bleeding, decreased vision, more swelling, and discomfort. More frequent monitoring of vital signs should occur during surgery or long restorative appointments. Orthostatic hypotension is common with many of the drugs used to control the moderate hypertensive state. These patients should take their medications the morning of surgery to help decrease the blood pressure during surgery, in spite of the complications of frequent urination.

The severe hypertensive (blood pressure 190/125 or greater) may only follow examination or maintenance therapy (type 1). Referral to the physician is indicated. If the patient becomes severely hypertensive years after implant surgery and prosthodontics, 3-month preventive/maintenance (recall) appointments are indicated to decrease the risk of severe complications and minimize the effect of dental prophylaxis appointments.

Angina Pectoris

Angina pectoris, or "chest pain" or cramp of the cardiac muscle, is a form of coronary heart disease. Occasionally the myocardium needs more oxygen-laden blood than it can receive. Transient myocardial available oxygen demand is in excess of supply. Atherosclerosis of the coronary vessels is the usual cause, although anemia or hypotension also may be involved. The symptom of retrosternal pain often develops during stress or physical exertion, radiates to the shoulders, left arm, or mandible, and is relieved by rest. Episodes last 3 to 5 minutes after the stress or exercise is halted. Sublingual nitroglycerin is beneficial. When retrosternal pain occurs, myocardial infarction is part of the differential diagnosis. This pain is similar in region, but is more intense, does not cease within 3 to 5 minutes, and is not relieved by nitroglycerin. Risk factors for angina pectoris are smoking, hypertension, high cholesterol, obesity, and diabetes.

If a patient reports a history of angina, the severity of the disease is evaluated by the frequency and severity of attacks and the medications prescribed. Like hypertension, the disease may be classified as mild, moderate, or severe. The patient with mild angina has one or fewer attacks each month; the patient with moderate angina may suffer infrequent but predictable attacks, even in the absence of excessive stress or exertion; patients with severe angina have almost daily attacks. The major concern for the implant dentist is the precipitation and/or management of the actual angina attack.

Dental Implant Management (Fig 5–4).—The dental emergency kit should include nitroglycerin tablets (0.3 to 0.4 mg), which are replaced every 6 months because of their short shelf life. During an angina attack all dental treatment should be stopped immediately. Nitroglycerin is then administered sublingually, and 100% oxygen given at 6 L/min, with the patient in a semi-supine or 45-degree position. Blood pressure should be monitored after nitroglycerin is administered, because transient hypotension may occur. If the systolic blood pressure falls below 100 mm Hg, the patient's feet should be elevated. If the pain is not relieved in 8

RISK		Type 1	Type 2	Type 3	Type 4
Mild	≤1/Month ASA II	+	+	Sedation Supplemental Oxygen	
Moderate	≤1/Week ASA III	+	Sedation Premedicate Nitrates Supplemental Oxygen		Premedicate Sedation Outpatient Hospitalization
Severe	Daily/More ASA IV Unstable	+	Physician	Elective Procedures Contraindicated	

FIG 5–4.
Dental implant management in patients with angina pectoris.

to 10 minutes with the use of nitroglycerin at 5-minute intervals, the patient should be transported by ambulance to a hospital.

Patients with mild angina (up to one attack per month) may undergo most nonsurgical dental procedures performed with normal protocol (type 1). Advanced restorative procedures and minor implant surgery often are performed with nitrous oxide or oral sedation (type 2). For more advanced implant procedures, appropriate sedation techniques should be used (types 3 and 4). Appointments should be as short as possible. This may require more than one surgical or restorative appointment.

Patients with moderate angina (up to one attack per week) tolerate examination and most simple operative procedures (type 1). Prophylactic nitroglycerin (0.3 to 0.4 mg) or long-acting nitrates are given sublingually just before advanced operative or simple to moderate implant surgery (types 2 and 3). Advanced surgical procedures may require a hospital setting (type 4).

Patients with severe angina (daily episodes) are limited to examination procedures performed under normal protocol (type 1). Medical consultation is recommended for any additional treatment. Usually, simple operative procedures can be performed with prophylactic nitrates. Elective implant surgical procedures are usually not performed on these patients.

The side effects of nitroglycerin are important to recognize, because prophylactic administration is in order for the patient with moderate to severe angina. There is a decrease in blood pressure, which causes a decrease of the blood flow to the brain. Fainting is possible; therefore the patient should be lying down during administration. The heart attempts to compensate for the decreased blood pressure; the pulse rate may increase to as much as 160 beats/min. Blushing of the face and shoulders is common after administration of nitroglycerin. If the patient has been taking long-acting nitrates, tolerance to the drug may occur, and two tablets may be needed at a time. Headache may occur after administration, and analgesics often are indicated.

Myocardial Infarction

Myocardial infarction (MI) is prolonged ischemia or lack of oxygen that causes injury to the heart. Approximately 10% of patients 40 years or older undergoing noncardiac surgery in a hospital setting give a history of previous MI.[22] The implant dentist primarily treats patients in this age group, and therefore sees many such patients.

The patient usually has severe chest pain in the substernal or left precordial area during an MI episode. It may radiate to the left arm or mandible. The pain is similar to angina pectoris but more severe. Cyanosis, cold sweat, weakness, nausea or vomiting, and irregular and increased pulse rate are all signs and symptoms of MI.

The complications of MI include arrhythmias and congestive heart failure. The larger the ischemic area the greater the risk of heart failure or life-threatening arrhythmias. Any history of MI indicates significant problems in the coronary vessels. Recent infarctions correspond to higher morbidity and death rates with even simple elective surgery. Approximately 18% to 20% of patients with a recent history of MI will have complications of recurrent MI, with a high mortality rate of 40% to 70%. After 12 months the incidence of recurrent MI stabilizes at about 5%.[23]

Dental Implant Management (Fig 5–5).—The dental evaluation should include the dates of all episodes of MI, especially the latest, and any complications. Medical consultation should preclude any extensive restorative or surgical procedure. Patients with a MI in the preceding 6 months may have dental examinations (type 1) without any special protocol. Any treatment should be postponed if possible for 6 months. Patients who experienced a MI 6 to 12 months preceding consultation may have examination, nonsurgical procedures, and simple emergency surgical procedures performed after medical consultation. Longer procedures should be sectioned into several shorter appointments whenever possible. Stress reduction protocol is indicated. Elective implant procedures should be postponed for at least 12 months following MI. Elective hospitalization is an accepted modality for all advanced surgical procedures, regardless of the time elapsed after a MI, and is almost mandatory if general anesthesia is required.

Congestive Heart Failure

Congestive heart failure (CHF) is a chronic heart condition in which the heart is failing as a pump. Approximately 2.5 million people have CHF; 40,000 deaths

RISK		**Type 1**	**Type 2**	**Type 3**	**Type 4**
Mild	>12 Months	+	+	Physician	Physician Hospitalization if General Anesthesia Required
Moderate	6–12 Months ASA III	+	Postpone All Elective Procedures		
Severe	< 6 Months ASA IV	+	Postpone All Elective Procedures		

FIG 5–5.
Dental implant management in patients with myocardial infarction.

per year are directly due to CHF, and it contributes indirectly to another 230,000 deaths.

The heart pumps about 2,000 gallons of blood per day to the other organs and body tissues. It coordinates the function of two pumps simultaneously: the left side, the larger of the two sides, pushes the blood out into the body, and the right side sends the blood to the lungs for oxygenation.

When the heart has been damaged the blood begins to back up in the lungs or body. The heart will attempt to compensate by increasing the rate of contraction and stretching the muscle to accommodate a larger volume of blood so that it can contract with a greater force and eject more blood (Starling's Law).

Both of these techniques maintain circulatory needs in the short term, but they exact a long-term price. Beating faster leaves the heart with less time to refill, so that less blood is circulated, while the extra effort increases the heart muscle's demand for oxygen. When this need is unmet the heart rhythms can become dangerously abnormal (arrhythmic) and lead to death.

Compensatory measures are taken by other parts of the body to counteract the insufficient circulation. The kidneys retain water and salt. In the case of heart failure, this only further strains the heart by increasing the amount of blood it must pump. At the same time, the retained fluid may seep into the body tissue.

The symptoms of CHF include

1. Abnormal tiredness or shortness of breath (dyspnea) brought on by slight activity or even occurring at rest. These symptoms are due to excess fluid in the lungs and partly to the excess work required of the heart.
2. Wheezing, caused by fluid in the lungs (pulmonary edema).
3. Edema, or swelling of the ankles and lower legs.
4. Frequent urination at night.
5. Paroxysmal nocturnal dyspnea (PND), the sensation of being unable to breathe, which may interrupt sleep. This symptom is primarily due to the effect of gravity on fluid that has spent the day down at the feet. As the fluid flows back up, it may pool in the lungs, causing a feeling of suffocation.
6. Excessive weight gain, as much as 20 to 30 pounds, with no change in diet. This increase, purely from fluid retention, gives some indication of how poorly the heart is pumping.

While heart failure affects both sides of the heart, one side tends to be more weakened, so the condition is often referred to as left-sided or right-sided failure. Left-sided failure is most common. The fluid backs up into the lungs and brings on the symptom of breathlessness. Right-sided heart failure causes fluid backup in the veins that return blood to the heart, leading to swelling of the extremities and the liver.

Medications prescribed for CHF are loosely classified as the 3-Ds: digitalis, diuretics, and dilators. Digitalis (e.g., Lanoxin) increases the heart's pumping action; diuretics (e.g., Lasix) eliminate excess salt and water; vasodilators (e.g., ACE) expand the blood vessels so that pressure is decreased and blood can flow more readily. Because digitalis is such a common drug for treating CHF, the side effects should be realized, as they are very common.

The lethal dose of digitalis is only twice the treatment dose. The dentist who recognizes the more common side effects (i.e., nausea, vomiting, anorexia) should report them to the treating physician. The heart rate is decreased because the drug decreases the effect of the atrioventricular node and stimulates the vagus nerve. Premature ventricular contractions (PVC) are more common because the heart rate is decreased. Less common side effects (e.g., abnormal color vision, a halo around objects) may be reported. Trigeminal neuralgia symptoms may occur with use of digitalis. Although very uncommon, this condition has been reported to the author, and decrease of the medication dose partially relieved the symptoms.

Bacterial Endocarditis

Bacterial endocarditis is an infection of the heart valves or the endothelial surfaces of the heart. It is the result of the growth of bacteria on altered cardiac surfaces. The microorganisms most often associated with endocarditis following dental treatment are α-hemolytic *(viridans)* streptococci, and less frequently staphylococci and anaerobes. The disorder is serious, with a mortality rate of about 10%.[21] Dental procedures causing transient bacteremia are a major cause of bacterial endocarditis. As a result, the implant dentist should identify the patient at risk and implement prophylactic procedures (Table 5–3).

Altered surfaces of the heart have many causes. The best known to the dental profession is the mitral valve defect from rheumatic fever. Acquired valvular lesions, roughened areas of the heart from septal defects, and prosthetic heart valves also increase the risk of endocarditis. Patients with prosthetic heart valves develop endocarditis with an incidence of 4% per year. The chance of reoccurrence is significantly increased in patients with a history of endocarditis. Any patient with one previous episode of endocarditis has a 10% per year risk of a second infection. Once the second infection occurs, the risk factor increases to 25%.

The risk of bacterial endocarditis increases with the amount of soft tissue trauma. For example, there is a correlation between the incidence of endocarditis and the number of teeth extracted, or the degree of a preexisting inflammatory disease of the mouth.[24] A six times higher incidence of bacteremia is found for a patient with severe periodontal disease.[25] If scaling and root planing are performed before subsequent soft tissue surgery, the risk of endocarditis is greatly reduced. Bacteremia after traumatic tooth brushing, endodontic treatment, and chewing paraffin has also been reported.[26] Endocarditis may even occur in an edentulous patient with denture sores.[27] Chlorhexidine painted on isolated

TABLE 5–3.

Incidence of Bacterial Endocarditis

High
   Previous endocarditis
   Prosthetic heart valve
   Surgical systemic pulmonary shunt
Significant
   Rheumatic valvular defect
   Acquired valvular disease
   Congenital heart disease
   Intravascular prostheses
   Coarctation of the aorta
Minimum risk
   Transvenous pacemaker
   Rheumatic fever history and no documented rheumatic heart disease
Least risk
   Innocent or functional heart murmur
   Uncomplicated atrial septal defect
   Coronary artery bypass graft operations

gingiva or irrigation of the sulcus 3 to 5 minutes prior to tooth extraction reduces postextraction bacteremia.

Several additional conditions predispose patients to endocarditis. Most congenital cardiac malformations, rheumatic and other acquired valvular defects, hypertrophic cardiomyopathy, and mitral valve prolapse with audible valvular regurgitation are specific examples.

Dental Implant Management (Fig 5–6).—The implant dentist must be familiar with the antibiotic regimens for heart conditions requiring prophylaxis. A similar regimen is suggested for any person requiring antibiotic coverage. The standard regimen may be administered orally or parenterally. The oral regimen in adults is 3.0 g amoxicillin 60 minutes prior to the dental appointment, followed by 1.5 g amoxicillin 6 hours later. If the patient is allergic to penicillin-like antibiotics, erythromycin ethylsuccinate 800 mg or erythromycin stearate 1.0 g is administered orally 2 hours prior to the procedure, followed by one-half the dose 6 hours later. Clindamycin 300 mg 1 hour before the appointment followed by 150 mg 6 hours later also is an acceptable protocol for the patient allergic to penicillin.

The antibiotic may be administered by the parenteral route prior to the dental procedure for patients unable to take oral medications. Ampicillin 2.0 g intravenously or intramuscularly is administered 30 minutes prior to the procedure. The implant dentist may choose to let the patient's physician administer these drugs, because anaphylactic reactions are more severe by the intramuscular or intravenous route. Intravenous or intramuscular ampicillin 1.0 g or oral amoxicillin 1.5 g is then administered 6 hours later. For patients allergic

ANTIBIOTIC REGIMEN
FOR DENTAL/ORAL PROCEDURES
1. Standard regimen in patients at risk (includes those with prosthetic heart valves and other high-risk patients):*

Amoxicillin 3.0 g PO 1 hour before procedure, then 1.5 g 6 hours after initial dose

a. For amoxicillin/penicillin-allergic patients:

Erythromycin ethylsuccinate 800 mg or erythromycin stearate 1.0 g PO 2 hours before procedure, then half dose 6 hours after initial administration

or

Clindamycin 300 mg PO 1 hour before procedure, then 150 mg 6 hours after initial dose

2. Alternate Regimens in Patients At Risk:

a. For patients unable to take oral medications:

Ampicillin 2.0 g IV (or IM) 30 minutes before procedure, then ampicillin 1.0 g IV (or IM) or amoxicillin 1.5 g PO 6 hours after initial dose

or

b. For amoxicillin/ampicillin/penicillin-allergic patients unable to take oral medications:

Clindamycin 300 mg IV 30 minutes before a procedure, then 150 mg IV (or PO) 6 hours after initial dose

c. For patients considered at high risk who are not candidates for the standard regimen:

Ampicillin 2.0 g IV (or IM) plus gentamicin 1.5 mg/kg IV (or IM) (not to exceed 80 mg) 30 minutes before procedure, then amoxicillin 1.5 g PO 6 hours after initial dose. Alternatively, parenteral regimen may be repeated 8 hours after initial dose

d. For amoxicillin/ampicillin/penicillin-allergic patients considered at high risk:

Vancomycin 1.0 g IV administered over 1 hour, starting 1 hour before procedure. No repeat dose necessary

---

*Initial pediatric doses are as follows: Follow-up oral dose should be half initial dose. Total pediatric dose should not exceed total adult dose.

Amoxicillin (see Note)	50 mg/kg	Vancomycin:	20 mg/kg
Clindamycin	10 mg/kg	Ampicillin:	50 mg/kg
Erythromycin ethylsuccinate		Gentamicin:	20 mg/kg
or stearate:	20 mg/kg		

NOTE: The following weight ranges also may be used for initial pediatric dose of amoxicillin:
<15 kg (33lb): 750 mg
15–30 kg (33–66 lb): 1,500 mg
> 30 kg (66 lb): 3,000 mg (full adult dose)

FIG 5–6.
Antibiotic regimens for patients with heart conditions requiring prophylaxis. (Data from American Heart Association, Dallas.)

to penicillin-related antibiotics, clindamycin 300 mg may be given intravenously 30 minutes before the procedure, and 150 mg intravenously or orally 6 hours after the initial dose.

For patients considered at high risk who are not candidates for the standard regimen, 2.0 g ampicillin intravenously (or intramuscularly) plus gentamicin 1.5 mg/kg intravenously IV (or IM) not to exceed 80 mg is administered 30 minutes before the procedure, followed by amoxicillin 1.5 mg orally 6 hours after the initial dose. Alternatively, the parenteral regimen may be repeated 8 hours after initial dose.

In some patients implant therapy may be contraindicated because of high risk for endocarditis. Edentulous patients with implants now must contend with transient bacteremia from chewing, brushing, or peri-implant disease. As a result, patients with limited oral hygiene potential with a history of requiring prophylaxis, as well as those with a history of some strokes, may be contraindicated for implants. In addition, intramucosal inserts may be contraindicated for many of these patients, since a slight bleeding may occur on a routine basis for several weeks during the initial healing process. Endosteal implants, with an adequate width of attached gingiva, are the implants of choice for patients with this condition who need implant-supported prostheses.

Endocrine Disorders

Diabetes Mellitus

Diabetes mellitus is related to an absolute or relative insulin insufficiency. It is the third leading cause of death in the United States, the most common metabolic disorder, and the major cause of blindness in adults. There is a 12- to 17-year decrease in lifespan when diabetes onset is between the ages of 10 and 30 years.[21] Almost 2% of individuals 25 to 44 years old in the United States are diabetic, and 8% of these are older than age 65. Because the implant dentist primarily treats patients older than 40 years, more than 5% of patients will have diabetes. In addition, an estimated half of diabetic patients are undiagnosed.

The major symptoms of diabetes are polyuria, polydypsia, polyphagia, and weight loss. The patient's medical history should report increased thirst, urination, and appetite or recent weight loss. Almost every cell membrane needs insulin to enable glucose penetration, with the exception of those cells in the brain and spinal cord. With insulin deficiency, the glucose remains in the bloodstream, hence the increased blood glucose level. Diabetic patients are prone to develop infections and vascular complications. Protein metabolism is decreased, healing of soft and hard tissue is delayed, nerve regeneration is altered, and angiogenesis is impaired.

The implant dentist will confirm or discover diabetes by the presence of glucose levels above 120 mg/dL. Ninety percent of these patients have adult-onset diabetes mellitus, which develops after age 40. Juvenile diabetes usually appears before age 25 and induces more insulin-related complications. Implant dentistry is not contraindicated in most diabetic patients; however, patient care should be as controlled as possible. A fasting glucose or even postprandial test may not determine if the patient's glucose level is usually controlled. A glycohemoglobin determination test often is indicated. A percentage of hemoglobin is glycohemoglobin, and the level is determined over a 3-month period. Although not always completely accurate, the glycohemoglobin test is a good indicator of a diabetic's long-term blood glucose level.

Dental Implant Management (Fig 5–7).—The most serious complication for diabetic patients during dental procedures is hypoglycemia, which usually occurs as a result of excessive insulin level, hypoglycemic drugs, or inadequate food intake. Weakness, nervousness, tremor, palpitations, and/or sweating are all signs of hypoglycemia. Mild symptoms can be treated with sugar in the form of orange juice or candy. If the symptoms are not addressed, they may evolve from confusion and agitation to seizure, coma, and death.

Patients at low risk of complications related to diabetes are those who are asymptomatic and have good metabolic control. Their blood glucose levels are less than 200 mg/dL (average, 100 mg/dL). These patients may be treated with a normal protocol for all nonsurgical appointments (type 1). For surgical procedures, these patients need a little more care and attention. Need for a stress reduction protocol, diet evaluation before and after surgery, and control of the risk of infection are all addressed. Sedative procedures and antibiotics are often used for implant or advanced surgical procedures (types 3 or 4). Corticosteroids, often used to

RISK		Type 1	Type 2	Type 3	Type 4
Mild	≤ 200 mg/dL ASA II Glyc. 0–1+ Ketonuria 0	+	+	Sedation Premedication Diet/Insulin Adjustment	
Moderate	≤ 200 mg/dL ASA III Glyc. 0–3+ Ketonuria 0	+	+	Sedation Premedication Diet/Insulin Adjustment Physician	Diet/Insulin Adjustment Physician Hospitalization
Severe	Uncontrolled > 250 mg/dL ASA IV Glyc. 3+ Ketonuria 0	+	Postpone All Elective Procedures		

FIG 5–7.
Dental implant management in patients with diabetes.

decrease edema, swelling, and pain, are not used in the diabetic patient because of their effect on blood sugar levels. Insulin therapy is adjusted to half the dose in the morning of surgery if oral intake is expected to be compromised. Intravenous conscious sedation and infusion of glucose and saline solution (D_5W) may be used for lengthy procedures.

Patients at moderate risk show periodic manifestations of the disease but are in metabolic balance because few complications of diabetes are present. Their blood glucose levels are below 200 mg/dL. Diet control, stress reduction protocol, aseptic technique, and antibiotics are more important for these individuals than for those in the low-risk group. Most nonsurgical procedures can follow a normal protocol (type 1). Oral sedation may be considered for some restorative procedures. Medical consultation should precede moderate or advanced surgical procedures (types 3 and 4), and the insulin dosage is often altered. Sedative techniques and hospitalization should be considered for advanced surgical procedures (type 4).

Patients at high risk report a history of frequent hypoglycemia and show multiple complications of diabetes. Their fasting blood sugar fluctuates widely, often exceeding 250 mg/dL. These patients can follow type 1 procedures when a conscious effort is made to decrease stress. All other procedures, whether nonsurgical or surgical, require medical consultation. If possible, any treatment should be deferred until the medical condition is stabilized. The patient's diet needs careful attention in relationship to insulin dosages postoperatively.

In general, all diabetic patients are subject to a greater incidence and severity of periodontal disease. Approximately 75% of these patients suffer from periodontal disease and exhibit increased alveolar bone loss and inflammatory gingival changes. An increase in caries is also evident as a result of xerostomia. Tissue abrasions are more likely in denture wearers, because the depletion in oxygen tension decreases the rate of epithelial growth and decreases tissue thickness.

Thyroid Disorders

Thyroid disorders are the second most common endocrine problem, affecting approximately 1% of the general population, principally women. Because the vast majority of patients in implant dentistry are women, a slightly higher prevalence of this disorder is seen in dental implant practice.

The major function of the thyroid gland is the production of the hormone thyroxine (T_4). Thyroxine is responsible for the regulation of carbohydrate, protein, and lipid metabolism. In addition, the hormone potentiates the action of other hormones, such as catecholamines and growth hormones.

Abnormalities in the anterior pituitary gland or the thyroid can result in disorders of thyroxine production. Excessive production of thyroxine results in hyperthyroidism. Symptoms of this disorder include increased pulse rate, nervousness, intolerance to heat, excessive sweating, weakness of muscles, diarrhea, increased appetite, increased metabolism, and weight loss. Excessive thyroxine may also cause atrial fibrillation, angina, and congestive heart failure. Palpitation of the patient's neck often reveals an enlarged thyroid gland between the cricoid cartilage and the suprasternal notch.

An insufficient production of thyroxin results in hypothyroidism. The related symptoms are a result of a decrease in metabolic rate. The patient complains of cold intolerance, fatigue, and weight gain. Eventually hoarseness and decreased mental activity occur, which may lead to coma. Thyroid function tests also are used to confirm the diagnosis of hypothyroidism.

Dental Implant Management (Fig 5–8).—Patients with hyperthyroidism are especially sensitive to catecholamines, as epinephrine in local anesthetics and gingival retraction cords. When exposure to catecholamines is coupled with stress (often related to dental procedures) and tissue damage (dental implant surgery), an exacerbation of the symptoms of hyperthyroidism may occur. The result is termed thyrotoxicosis or "thyroid storm." The result is very high temperature, CNS alterations such as agitation and psychosis, and a high risk of life-threatening arrhythmias and/or congestive heart failure.

The hypothyroid patient is particularly sensitive to CNS depressant drugs, especially narcotics and sedative drugs such as diazepam or barbiturates. The risk of respiratory depression and/or cardiovascular depression or collapse must be considered.

The most common thyroid disorder patient seen by the implant dentist is the one with known and treated thyroid disease. Any patient with a medical examination in the preceding 6 months who reports normal thyroid function and

RISK		Type 1	Type 2	Type 3	Type 4
Mild	Med Exam <6 Months Normal Fct Last 6 Months	+	+	+	+
Moderate	No Symptoms No Med Exam No Fct Test	+	Decrease Epinephrine, Steroids CNS Depressants	Physician	
Severe	Symptoms	+	Postpone All Elective Procedures		

FIG 5–8.
Dental implant management in patients with thyroid disorders.

has no symptoms of the disease is at low risk. A normal protocol may be followed for all dental implant surgery and restorative appointments (types 1 to 4).

The thyroid disorder patient who has no symptoms related to thyroid disorders but has not had a physical or thyroid function test recently is placed in the moderate-risk category. This patient may follow a normal protocol for type 1 procedures. Stress-reduction protocol with or without sedation is suggested for simple to advanced operative appointments and simple surgical procedures (type 2). The use of epinephrine and of CNS depressants such as narcotic analgesics, barbiturates, and diazepam should be limited. For moderate to advanced implant procedures or surgery (types 3 and 4), medical laboratory reexaminations are often indicated. Once thyroid control is established, these patients are placed in the low-risk category and normal protocol is adopted.

Undiagnosed thyroid disease is rare, and the thyroid problems usually are related to previously treated thyroid disease. Therefore, a patient with a past history of thyroid disorders should be asked about temperature sensitivity, recent weight gain or loss, tremors, or changes in appetite. The pulse and respiration are carefully noted. A symptomatic patient is at high risk, regardless of when the last medical evaluation was performed.[28] Such patients should have only examination procedures performed (type 1); all other treatment is deferred until a medical and laboratory evaluation confirms control of the disorder.

Adrenal Gland Disorders

The adrenal glands are endocrine organs located just above the kidneys. Epinephrine and norepinephrine are produced by chromaffin cells in the adrenal medulla, which forms the central portion of the gland. These hormones are largely responsible for the control of blood pressure, myocardial contractility and excitability and general metabolism.[29] The outer portion of the gland or adrenal cortex produces three different types of hormones. Glucocorticoids regulate carbohydrate, fat, and protein metabolism and also help decrease inflammation. They may be used by the implant dentist to decrease swelling and pain.[30] The mineralocorticoids maintain sodium and potassium balance. The third category are the sex hormones. The hypothalamus, the anterior pituitary gland and the adrenal glands all interact to regulate glucocorticoid production. The mineralo-corticoids are regulated by reninangiotensin hormone, the anterior pituitary gland, and serum potassium levels.

Addison disease corresponds to a decrease in adrenal function. These patients show symptoms of weakness, weight loss, orthostatic hypotension, nausea, and vomiting. The implant dentist should require a medical consultation. These patients cannot increase their steroid production in response to stress, and in the midst of surgery or long restorative procedures may have cardiovascular collapse. During the physical examination, the dentist can notice hyperpigmented areas on the face, lips, and gingiva.[31] An increase in serum potassium level (hyperkalemia) and decrease in serum glucose level are characteristic of Addison disease.

Patients with hyperfunction of the adrenal cortex may have Cushing syndrome. The characteristic changes associated with this disease are moon facies, truncal obesity or "buffalo hump," muscle wasting, and hirsutism. Patients usually are hypertensive, and long-term excess function of the cortex decreases collagen production. These patients bruise easily, have poor wound healing, experience osteoporosis, and are also at increased risk for infection. These elements are especially noteworthy to the implant dentist. Laboratory studies show an increase in blood glucose as related to an interference with carbohydrate metabolism. The complete blood count often shows a slight decrease in eosinophil and lymphocyte counts.

Corticosteroids are potent anti-inflammatory drugs used to treat a number of systemic diseases and are one of the most prescribed drugs in medicine. Steroids are used for arthritis, collagen and vascular disorders, kidney diseases, asthma, and dermatologic disorders. However, the continued administration of exogenous steroids suppress the natural function of the adrenal glands and cause a condition equivalent to Cushing's disease. As a result, patients under long-term steroid therapy are placed on the same protocol as patients with hyperfunction of the adrenal glands.

Dental Implant Management (Fig 5–9).—Patients with a history of adrenal gland disease, whether hyperfunctioning or hypofunctioning, face similar problems related to dentistry and stress. The body is unable to produce increased levels of steroids during stressful situations, and cardiovascular collapse may occur. As a result, additional steroids are prescribed for the patient just prior to the stressful situation. These doses are stopped within 3 days. The healthy patient

RISK		Type 1	Type 2	Type 3	Type 4
Mild	Equiv. Prednisone Alternate Day > 1 year	+	Surgery on Day of Steroids	Sedation and Antibiotics Steroids <60 mg Prednisone Day 1 Dose ×/2 Day 2 Maintenance Dose Day 3	
Moderate	Equiv. Prednisone >20 mg or >7 Days in Past Year	+	Sedation and Antibiotics 20–40 mg Day 1 Dose ×/2 Day 2 Dose ×/4 Day 3	60 mg Day 1 Dose ×/2 Day 2 Dose ×/4 Day 3	
Severe	Equiv. Prednisone 5 mg/day	+	Elective Procedures Contraindicated		

FIG 5–9.
Dental implant management in patients with adrenal disorders.

will accelerate steroid production 3 to 5 times higher than regular levels to respond to the stress of surgery or dental procedures. Therefore for patients with known adrenal disorders, the physician should be contacted for consultation. The nature of the disorder and recommended treatment should be evaluated.

The patient on regular maintenance doses of steroid in excess of prednisone 5 mg/day is at high risk of adrenal suppression. Consultation with the patient's physician is indicated. For simple to advanced operative procedures and simple extractions, periodontal or implant surgery (types 1 and 2), the steroid dose should be doubled up to 60 mg prednisone or equivalent (10 mg dexamethasone). The day after the procedure, the maintenance dose is returned to normal. Oral or intravenous conscious sedation is utilized to reduce stress. For moderate to advanced implant surgery or the very anxious patient, general anesthesia may be indicated. The day of the procedure 60 mg prednisone is administered. This dose is reduced by 50% each day over a 2- to 3-day period to the maintenance dose. Antibiotics are also prescribed for 3 to 5 days.

Patients at significant or moderate risk for adrenal suppression are those formerly on steroid therapy of 20 mg prednisone or more, longer than 7 days within the preceding year. Simple to complex restorative procedures or simple surgery (types 1 and 2) suggest administration of 20 to 40 mg prednisone the day of the procedure. Sedation techniques and antibiotics for 3 to 5 days are suggested. The following day, the steroid dose is reduced 50% and the third day the dosage is reduced by an additional 50% or returned to normal. For type 3 and 4 moderate to advanced surgical procedures, the protocol is further modified. Prednisone 60 mg or equivalent is administered the day of the surgery. This dose is reduced 50% the following day, and another 50% on the third day. General anesthesia may be used to reduce anxiety, especially in the apprehensive patient.

Patients at low risk for adrenal suppression are those on alternate-day steroid therapy or those whose steroid therapy ended 1 year or more prior to the implant procedure. For these, dental procedures are scheduled the day steroids are taken or up to 60 mg prednisone is administered. On the second day the dose is reduced 50%, and on the third day the patient resumes the alternate day schedule. Sedation and antibiotics are also used.

Steroids act in three different ways that affect implant surgery. They decrease inflammation and are useful in decreasing swelling and related pain. However, steroids also decrease protein synthesis and therefore delay healing. In addition, they decrease leukocytosis and thereby reduce the patient's ability to fight infection. Therefore, whenever steroids are given to patients for surgery, it is reasonable to prescribe antibiotics. After a loading dose, penicillin V or erythromycin 500 mg are given four times a day for 3 to 5 days.

Pregnancy

Implant surgery procedures are contraindicated for the pregnant patient. Not only is the mother the responsibility of the dentist, but so is the fetus. The radiographs or medications that may be needed for implant therapy and the increased stress are all reasons the elective implant surgical procedure should be postponed until after childbirth. However, after implant surgery has occurred, the patient may become pregnant while waiting for the restorative procedures, especially as modalities may require 3 months to a year of a healing phase.

Periodontal disease is often exacerbated during pregnancy. All elective dental care, with the exception of dental prophylaxis, should be deferred until after the birth. The only exceptions to this are caries control or emergency dental procedures. In these instances, medical clearance should be given for all drugs, including anesthetics, analgesics, and antibiotics. Usually lidocaine, penicillin, erythromycin, and acetaminophen (Tylenol) are approved. Aspirin, vasoconstrictors (epinephrine), and drugs that cause respiratory depression (e.g., narcotic analgesics) are usually contraindicated. Diazepam (Valium), nitrous oxide, and tetracycline are almost always contraindicated.

Almost 15% of pregnancies are terminated by spontaneous abortion or miscarriage during the first trimester. Dental prophylactic appointments are suggested in the second or third trimester. The hygienist and dentist should realize that in the middle to late third trimester hypotension can occur in a supine mother as a result of pressure of the fetus on the inferior vena cava.

Hematologic Diseases

Erythrocytic Disorders

In a healthy patient 4 to 6 million RBCs per milliliter of blood are in circulation. Red blood cells make up the largest portion of the formed elements in the blood. There are two main categories of erythrocyte disorders: polycythemia (increased erythrocyte count) and anemia (decrease in hemoglobin).

Polycythemia.—Polycythemia is a rather rare chronic disorder characterized by splenic enlargement, hemorrhages, and thrombosis of peripheral veins. Death usually occurs within 6 to 10 years, and complicated implant or reconstruction procedures are usually contraindicated.[13]

Anemia.—Anemia is the most common hematologic disorder. Almost all blood dyscrasias may at one time or another be associated with anemia. Anemia is not a disease entity; rather, it is a symptom complex that results from a decreased production of erythrocytes, an increased rate of their destruction, or from a deficiency in iron. It is defined as a reduction in the oxygen-carrying capacity of the blood and usually results from a decrease in the number of erythrocytes or abnormality of hemoglobin. There are a number of different types of anemia, the most common being iron deficiency anemia and relative bone marrow failure. Iron deficiency anemia may be due to a decreased intake of iron, a decreased absorption of iron, or an increase in bleeding. Vitamin C increases the absorption of iron. The female patient may normally be anemic in menses or pregnancy. Mild anemia in a man, however, indicates a serious underlying medical problem. The most common causes of anemia in men are peptic ulcers or carcinoma of the colon. These serious complications warrant medical evaluation of any male patient found anemic.

The general symptoms and signs are all a consequence of either a reduction of oxygen reaching the tissues or alterations of the red blood cell count. The symptoms of mild anemia include fatigue, anxiety, and sleeplessness. Chronic anemia is characterized by shortness of breath, abdominal pain, bone pain, tingling of extremities, muscular weakness, headaches, fainting, change in heart rhythm, and nausea. The general signs of anemia may include jaundice, pallor, spooning or cracking of the nails, increased size of liver and spleen, and lymphadenopathy. The oral signs of anemia primarily affect the tongue, and symptoms include a sore, painful, smooth tongue; loss of papillae; redness; loss of taste sensation; and paresthesia of the oral tissues.

Anemia Complications.—Complications in the implant patient may affect both short-term and long-term prognoses. Bone maturation and development are often impaired in the long-term anemic patient. A faint, large trabecular pattern of bone may even appear radiographically, which indicates at least a 40% loss in trabecular pattern. Therefore, the character of the bone needed to support the implant can be affected significantly. The decreased bone density affects the initial placement and may influence the initial amount of mature lamellar bone forming at the interface of an osteointegrated implant. The time needed for a proper interface formation is longer in poor density bone.[32]

Abnormal bleeding is also a common complication of anemia and during extensive surgery, a decreased vision from the hemorrhage, or difficulty in bone impressions for subperiosteal implants, may be encountered. Increased edema and subsequent increased discomfort postsurgically are common consequences. In addition, the excess edema increases the risk of postoperative infection and its consequences. Not only are anemic patients prone to more immediate infection from surgery, they are also more sensitive to chronic infection throughout their lives. This may affect the long-term maintenance of the proposed implant or abutment teeth.

Approximately 0.15% of the black population has sickle cell anemia.[33] Patients with such a disorder usually show marked clinical manifestations, and often die before the age of 40 years. Secondary infections are a common consequence, and complicated implant surgical procedures are contraindicated. This is not to be confused with sickle cell trait, which occurs in 9% of the black population. Black patients can be screened for sickle cell trait by using the "Sickledex test," which is simple enough to be performed in the dental office. These individuals show symptoms with low concentrations of oxygen. It is wise to use at least 50% oxygen during nitrous oxide/oxygen administration and to avoid diffusion hypoxia at the termination of the procedure by administering 100% oxygen at the conclusion of nitrous oxide administration.

The laboratory tests needed to diagnose anemia or polycythemia are in the CBC. The most accurate test for anemia is the hematocrit, followed by the hemoglobin, the least accurate being the red blood cell count. The hematocrit indicates the percentage of a given volume of whole blood made up of erythrocytes. The normal values for men range from 40 to 54%; those for women, from 37 to 47%. Hemoglobin makes up almost 95% of the dry weight of red blood cells. Abnormal hemoglobin may result from its combination with substances other than oxygen (for example, carbon monoxide) or genetic diseases (for example, sickle cell diseases). Normal values for men are 13.5 to 18 g/dL; those for women, 12 to 16 g/dL. The usual minimum baseline recommended for surgery is 10 mg/dL, especially for elective implant surgery.

For the vast majority of anemic patients, implant procedures are not contraindicated. However, preoperative and postoperative antibiotics should be administered, and the risk of bleeding not potentiated by aspirin. Hygiene appointments may be scheduled more frequently for these patients.

Leukocytic Disorders

Leukocyte disorders are an important consideration of hematologic diseases. The WBC count normally ranges from 5,000 to 10,000/mm^3 in the adult. Leukocytosis is defined as an increase in circulating WBCs in excess of 10,000/mm^3. The most common cause of leukocytosis is infection. Leukemia, neoplasms, acute hemorrhage, and diseases associated with acute inflammation or necrosis (for example, infarction and collagen diseases) are more serious causes of leukocytosis. Physiologic conditions such as exercise, pregnancy, and emotional stress may also lead to leukocytosis.

Leukopenia is defined as a reduction in the number of circulating WBCs to less than 5,000/mm^3. A decreased leukocyte count may accompany certain infections (as infectious hepatitis), bone marrow damage (from radiation therapy), nutritional deficiency (vitamin B$_{12}$ and folic acid), and blood diseases (anemia).

In the potential implant candidate with leukocytosis or leukopenia, many complications may compromise the success of the implant prosthesis. The most common complication is infection, not only during the initial healing phase, but also several years later. Delayed healing is also a consequence of WBC disorders. For most implant procedures, the first few months are very critical for long-term success. Extended healing periods increase the risk of secondary infection.

Severe bleeding may also illustrate leukocyte disorders. It may be related to a thrombocytopenia (decreased platelet count) or to the associated anemia. In either condition, the surgical procedure is complicated, with increased edema, postoperative discomfort, and increased chance for secondary infection.

Most oral implant procedures are contraindicated for the patient with acute or chronic leukemia. Acute leukemia is an almost inevitably fatal disease. Nearly all of these patients experience serious oral problems either secondary to the disease process or as complications following chemotherapy. The patient with chronic leukemia will experience anemia and thrombocytopenia. Although the infection is less severe than in acute leukemia, radiolucent lesions of the jaws, oral ulcerations, hyperplastic gingiva, and bleeding complications develop in these patients.

Treatment planning modifications should shift toward a conservative approach when dealing with leukocyte disorders. Complications are more common than in erythrocyte disorders. If the condition is temporary, as an acute infection, surgical procedures should be delayed until the infection has been controlled and the patient has returned to a normal condition.

Pulmonary Disease

Chronic Obstructive Pulmonary Diseases

The two most common forms of chronic obstructive pulmonary disease (COPD) are emphysema and chronic bronchitis. Chronic obstructive pulmonary disease is the second most common cause of death, after cardiovascular disease. It accounts for 50,000 deaths in the United States each year, and 3% of the population has COPD. This disease primarily affects men over the age of 40 and is closely related to smoking.

The usual course of COPD is progressive and results in a decline in pulmonary function over a span of many years. Respiratory failure is usually precipitated by pulmonary infection and leads to death.[34]

Patients with COPD may present a combination of many symptoms. They include chronic cough, sputum production, or shortness of breath. The examination evaluates tachycardia, tachypnea, wheezing, use of accessory respiratory muscles, cyanosis, an increase in the anterior-posterior diameter of the chest (barrel chest), prolonged expiration, and failure of the right side of the heart.

Dental Implant Management (Fig 5–10).—Patients treated with COPD should be evaluated for the severity of their disease. If a patient has been hospitalized for respiratory difficulties, a medical consultation is warranted. The dentist should especially inquire as to the carbon dioxide retention of these patients. Patients who retain carbon dioxide have a severe condition and are prone to respiratory failure when given sedatives, oxygen or nitrous oxide, and oxygen analgesia.

Patients with difficulty breathing only on significant exertion and normal laboratory blood gases are at minimal risk and may follow all restorative or surgical procedures with normal protocols (types 1 to 4). Patients with difficulty breathing upon exertion in general are at moderate risk, as are patients on chronic bronchodilator therapy or recent use of corticosteroids. These patients may follow examination procedures with normal protocol (type 1). A recent medical

RISK		Type 1	Type 2	Type 3	Type 4
Mild	ASA II	+	+	+	+
Moderate	ASA III	+	Physician	Physician/ Moderate Treatment	
Severe	ASA IV	+	Postpone (Hospitalization)	Elective Procedures Contraindicated	

FIG 5–10.
Dental implant management in patients with chronic obstructive pulmonary disease.

examination is recommended for all other procedures. If the patient is on bronchodilators, no epinephrine or vasoconstrictors should be added to the anesthetics or gingival retraction cord. Adrenal suppression should be evaluated for any patient on steroid therapy within the past year.

Patients at high risk are those with previously unrecognized COPD, acute exacerbation (as respiratory infection), patients with dyspnea at rest, or those with a history of carbon dioxide retention. Examination procedures may be performed under normal protocol (type 1). Elective moderate procedures or advanced surgical or prosthetic procedures are usually contraindicated. However, if needed they should be performed in the hospital. The use of epinephrine should be limited. Drugs that depress the respiratory function, such as sedatives (including nitrous oxide), tranquilizers, and narcotics should be discussed with their physician.

Hepatic Disorders

Cirrhosis

Cirrhosis is the third leading cause of death in young men between the ages of 35 and 54 years. It occurs as a result of injury to the liver with resultant loss of liver cells and progressive scarring. The major cause is alcoholic liver disease.[35] If the patient's response is yes to the question, "Do you drink?", there is a one in six chance of active alcoholism.

The liver is a major organ. Two more important functions to the implant dentist are the synthesis of clotting factors and the ability to detoxify drugs. Fifty percent of patients with liver disease have a prolonged PT time and clinical bleeding. The inability to detoxify drugs may result in oversedation or respiratory depression. The laboratory evaluation of the implant candidate gives much insight to hepatic function. Many SMA tests are associated with the liver; however, the tests that relate most specifically to liver disorders are bilirubin and albumin. In addition, the CBC, PT, and even PTT tests will be affected. Therefore a history of abnormal bleeding may indicate liver dysfunction.

Dental Implant Management.—Patients with no abnormal laboratory values for SMA, CBC, PTT, and PT are at low risk. A normal protocol is indicated for all procedures (types 1 to 4).

Patients with an elevated PT less than one and one-half times control value or bilirubin slightly affected are at moderate risk. These patients should have a physician consultation. The use of sedatives and tranquilizers needs physician clearance. Nonsurgical and simple surgical procedures may follow normal protocols (types 1 and 2); however, strict attention to hemostasis is indicated. For example, bovine collagen (such as Collatape), topical thrombin, or sutures may be indicated. Moderate to advanced surgical procedures may require hospitalization (types 3 and 4). Postsurgical close surveillance is indicated. Elective implant therapy is relatively contraindicated in the active alcoholic patient with symptoms.

Patients with a PT greater than 1.5 times control value, mild to severe thrombocytopenia (platelets under 100,000/ml), or several liver-related enzymes or chemicals affected (bilirubin, albumin, alkaline phosphatase, SGOT, and serum glutomic pyruvic transaminase) are at high risk. Elective dental procedures are usually contraindicated. If surgical procedures must be performed, hospitalization is recommended. Fresh frozen plasma may be used to correct PT to under 0.5 control value. Platelet transfusion may also be required for even scaling procedures and administration of mandibular nerve blocks.

Bone Diseases

Diseases of the skeletal system and specifically the jaws, often influence decisions regarding treatment in the field of oral implants. Bone and calcium metabolism are directly related. Approximately 99% of the calcium in the body is held in the bones and teeth. Calcium equilibrium is decided by the calcium metabolism of the body, and this affects the bones. Alveolar bone responds to systemic bone active agents.[36]

Parathyroid hormone is the most important regulator of extracellular calcium concentrations. Vitamin D, prostaglandins, lymphocytes (through osteoclast activating factors), insulin, glucocorticoids, and estrogen also are involved in this complex balance. Prostaglandins act as a local factor and may cause osteolysis and hypercalcemia and therefore bone resorption.

Osteoporosis

The most common disease of bone metabolism the implant dentist will encounter is osteoporosis. Past the age of 60, almost one third of the population has this disorder; it occurs in twice as many women as men.[21] This condition is especially common in postmenopausal women or those with a history of ovariectomy. The lack of estrogen increases the likelihood of osteoporosis and the addition of estrogen is the single most effective treatment to increase the absorption of calcium in these women.

The osteoporotic changes in the jaws are similar to other bones in the body. The structure of the bone is normal; however, the cortical plates become thinner, the trabecular bone pattern more discrete, and advanced demineralization occurs.[37] Oral bone loss related to osteoporosis may be expressed in both the dentate and edentulous patient. In one study of osteoporotic women who had their teeth at age 50, 44% had a complete denture by the age of 60, whereas only 15% of nonosteoporotic women had dentures.[38] A strong correlation was shown between periodontal disease and skeletal osteoporotic changes.

The loss of trabecular bone is accelerated in the edentulous patient, since the factors involved in resorption are already established. Osteoporosis affects the trabecular bone mass loss to a greater extent than cortical bone.[39]

By the age of 65 years, half of all women present bone mineral density below the normal fracture threshold of a 20-year-old woman. It is estimated that 133,000 hip fractures occur every year as a result of osteoporosis. Most patients fail to recover normal activity, and 20% die within the first year from complications related to the fracture.

Bone remodeling is a continuous process; however, bone mass increases during youth and diminishes with aging. The peak bone mass is usually reached by the age of 35 to 40 years and is usually 30% higher in men than in women. In the first 3 to 10 years after menopause, bone loss is most rapid. Trabecular bone loss in women 80 years old reaches 40% while only reaching 27% in men. Persons most at risk are thin, postmenopausal white women with a history of poor dietary calcium intake, cigarette smoking, and British or Northern European ancestry.

The actual diagnosis and treatment of osteoporosis should be accomplished by the physician. The implant dentist can benefit the patient by noting the loss of trabecular bone and early referral. Treatment of osteoporosis remains controversial. Its management concentrates on prevention. Regular exercise has shown to help maintain bone mass and increase bone strength. Adequate dietary calcium intake is essential. The advanced demineralization and consequent increase in bone loss of the complete edentulous may lead to a vicious circle. The denture becomes less secure, and the patient may not be able to follow a diet to maintain proper calcium absorption levels.

The recommended calcium intake is 800 mg/day. The average person in the United States ingests 450 to 550 mg. In postmenopausal women 1,500 mg may be required to maintain a positive calcium balance.[40] Calcium supplements of 1 to 2 g of elemental calcium per day have been shown in several studies to reduce the rate of bone loss. However, there is no evidence that these supplements lead to recovery of bone mass. Plain calcium carbonate tablets contain the greatest fraction of elemental calcium and are relatively inexpensive. It is insoluble and is absorbed after conversion into calcium chloride by the gastric hydrochloric acid. Patients with achlorhydria (lack of hydrochloric acid) should be given other salts than calcium carbonate. If the patient has a lactate deficiency, lactate salts are contraindicated. Several food-drug interactions have been reported. Tetracycline or iron do not work effectively with calcium doses. Patients should also avoid phosphate (found in some dairy products) or oxalic acid (in spinach and rhubarb) and the phytic acid in bran and whole grains, as these decrease calcium absorption. Patients with a history of renal calculi should avoid calcium supplements. Patients with renal dysfunction especially need periodic serum and urine calcium levels and serum pH monitored to avoid hypercalcemia and metabolic alkalosis.

Estrogen therapy can halt or retard severe bone demineralization caused by osteoporosis and can reduce fractures by about 50% compared with the fracture rate of untreated women. However, long-term estrogen therapy has been linked to a slight increase of endometrial cancer.

Vitamin D Disorders

Vitamin D is a hormone synthesized by the body in several steps that involve the skin, liver, kidney, and intestine. It is activated by the kidney in conjunction with parathyroid hormone. The deficiency of vitamin D in the adult leads to osteomalacia. Vitamin D increases calcium and phosphate absorption from the intestine and kidney reabsorption. The major cause of osteomalacia is dietary vitamin D deficiency or lack of exposure to sunlight.[21] The homebound elderly patient who is unable to wear dentures or who is a strict vegetarian is more at risk. Anticonvulsant drugs, especially diphenylhydantoin and phenobarbital, may give drug-induced osteomalacia. Many gastrointestinal disorders also may result in osteomalacia.

The oral findings of osteomalacia are usually not dramatic. A decrease in trabecular bone, indistinct lamina dura, and an increase in chronic periodontal disease have been reported.[45]

Hyperparathyroidism

The clinical manifestations of this disease vary widely, depending on the severity. Mild forms may be asymptomatic. Renalcolic disorders often occur with moderate disease. Severe hyperparathyroidism may result in bone, renal, and gastric disturbance. It has been noted, that when skeletal depletion occurs as a result of stimulation by the parathyroid gland, alveolar bone may be affected prior to rib, vertebrae, or long bones.

For the most part oral changes related to this disorder occur only with advanced disease. The loss of lamina dura is the most significant finding.

Clinically, patients with this disorder develop loose teeth. Altered trabecular bone pattern with the appearance of ground glass may also occur. In animals, secondary hyperparathyroidism affects alveolar bone loss greater than any other bone of the skeleton.[41] Intrabone or extrabone giant cell tumors may also develop.

Fibrous Dysplasia

Fibrous dysplasia is a disorder in which fibrous connective tissue replaces areas of normal bone. It is found twice as often in women than men. It may affect a single bone or multiple bones. The single bone disorder is more common in the adult and it is present in the jaws about 20% of the time. The condition in the maxilla is twice as common as in the mandible. The monostotic (single bone) fibrous dysplasia begins as a painless, progressive lesion. The facial plate usually expands. The teeth may move as a consequence of the progression. Radiographically, the appearance of fibrous dysplasia is a noted increase in trabeculation which gives a "mottled appearance." A ground-glass appearance may also be noted.[42] Roots of the teeth may be displaced, but external resorption is rare. The polyostotic (multiple lesions) fibrous dysplasia may affect one or virtually all bones. A predisposition to fracture may occur with this entity.

Excision of fibrous dysplasia areas is often the treatment choice. Radiation therapy has been used but may be responsible for the transformation of fibrous dysplasia into osteosarcoma or chondrosarcoma. Implant dentistry is contraindicated in the regions of this disorder. The lack of bone and increased fibrous tissue decrease rigid fixation of the implant, is more susceptible to local infection processes. These local infections may spread through the bone and result with more advanced complications.

Osteitis Deformans (Paget Disease)

Osteitis deformans, or Paget disease, is a slowly progressing, chronic bone disease. Both osteoblasts and osteoclasts are involved in this disorder, but osteoblastic activity is predominant. Men are affected slightly more than women, and patients are usually over 40 years of age.

Paget disease is marked by high elevations of serum alkaline phosphatase and normal calcium and phosphate levels. The jaws are affected in approximately 20% of the cases.[21] The maxilla is more often involved than the mandible. Increased tooth mobility is often reported. Edentulous patients are often unable to wear their prostheses without discomfort.[43] Radiographs reveal a cotton or wool appearance to the bone. Bony enlargements may often be palpated. Spontaneous fractures are relatively common as the increase in osseous vascularity is significant.

There is no specific treatment for Paget disease and these patients are predisposed to develop osteosarcoma. Oral implants are contraindicated in the regions of this disorder.

Multiple Myeloma

Multiple myeloma is a plasma cell neoplasm that originates in the bone marrow. It causes hypercalcemia, immune suppression, anemia, and thrombocytopenia as it causes widespread bone destruction. The disease is usually found in patients between 40 and 70 years of age. Usually it affects several bones in the body with symptoms of skeletal pain. Pathologic fractures may occur. Punched-out lesions appear radiographically. Oral manifestations of the disease are common (80%) and may affect either/or both the maxilla and mandible. Paresthesia, swelling, tooth mobility, and movement may occur. Gingival enlargements are also possible. Plasma cell malignancy, Bence-Jones proteins in the urine, and anemia are possible laboratory findings associated with this disorder. There is no treatment for multiple myeloma, and the condition is usually fatal, 2 to 3 years after onset. Implants are contraindicated.

Central Nervous System

Seizure Disorders

Epilepsy is estimated to occur in 0.5 to 2% of the population. Symptoms range from altered consciousness and/or motor activity to aberrant sensory phenomena and behavior. The most common form of seizure is the grand mal or generalized seizure. Of patients with seizure disorders, 90% have grand mal at some phase of the disorder and 60% have this form of seizure exclusively. Petit mal seizures are the second most common seizure disorder. Only 4% of patients have petit mal seizures exclusively. The third most common type of seizure is psychomotor seizures.[19] These seizures are partial in nature, and usually there is no loss of consciousness. As with most types of seizures, these patients may also experience grand mal seizures.

The medical evaluation of the patient with seizure disorders includes a past history of medications prescribed and the frequency of seizures while on medication. The majority of patients with seizure disorders are on phenobarbital and/or phenytoin (Dilantin) and should have very infrequent seizures.[44]

Phenytoin therapy may induce gingival hyperplasia in approximately 50% of patients on long-term therapy. It is more common among younger patients. The level of plaque formation is critical, since gingivitis is favored in its presence. Hyperplasia around dental implants has not been reported.

Dental Implant Management.—A patient with a history of seizure but no recent occurrence in the recent several years is at low risk. Dental restorative and surgical procedures (type 1 to 4) may follow normal protocol.

Patients at moderate risk are those who are on medication, but with no symptoms for over 1 year. Non-narcotic analgesics are preferred for patients receiving the CNS depressant drugs phenobarbital and primidone. Tetracyclines are relatively contraindicated for patients on phenytoin, phenobarbital, or primidone, since they accelerate hepatic degradation.[19] Frequent prophylaxis is indicated against gingival hyperplasia. Dental implants and related prosthetics are not contraindicated. However, gold or metal occlusal surfaces may be indicated to decrease the risk of fracture of porcelain and additional implants are indicated to improve excess stress distribution and decrease abutments fracture.

Patients with grand mal seizures more frequently than once per month are at high risk. They are contraindicated for implant supported prostheses.

Prosthetic Joints

Approximately 100,000 artificial hip joints and 40,000 total knee replacements are performed every year in the United States, and more than 60% are performed on patients over the age of 65.[45] Approximately 1% to 2% of these prostheses will become infected each year. The literature reports an association between prosthetic joint infection and dental treatment. It is hypothesized that bacteria from the dental treatment may seed the prosthesis and produce infection. The evidence for this often seems circumstantial or coincidental.[21] Reported cases related to the mouth have involved regions of established suppuration, such as a dental abscess or tonsillitis, rather than procedure-induced transient bacteremia. It is prudent to use prophylactic antibiotics in these patients prior to dental treatment. However, there is no agreement about the need for prophylaxis, the drugs, dosage, and duration of coverage.

The antibiotic regimen for patients with prosthetic joints is usually similar for those patients with risk of endocarditis. However, the most offending bacteria in a prosthetic joint space may be resistant to penicillin. Therefore it is suggested a better regimen is the use of dicloxacillin, cephaloxin (Keflex), or clindamycin. These agents are taken 1 hour to one-half hour prior to dental treatment and maintained for as long as 48 hours after surgery.

CONCLUSION

Systemic diseases have a broad effect. They usually may be separated into mild, moderate, and severe expressions of the disorder. Implant therapy also has a broad range of treatment. Four categories have been established. The overlay of implant therapy and general expressions of disease are often similar. Patients with mild diseases may have all types of treatment, and a stress reduction protocol is suggested for more advanced treatment. Patients with moderate disease usually require more monitoring and hospital assistance is usually required for the more advanced procedures. Severe diseases generally contraindicate elective implant therapy.

REFERENCES

1. Misch CE: Medical evaluation of the implant candidate, *J Oral Implant* 9:556–570, 1981.
2. Misch CE: Analysis of medical history pinpoints conditions that contraindicate implants, *Dentist*, March 23–24, 1989.
3. Dycht K: *Age wave: the challenges and opportunities of an aging America*, New York, 1988, St Martin's Press.
4. U.S. Bureau of the Census: *Population reports, population estimates*, Washington, DC, 1988, 1024:25.
5. Zamost B, Benumof JL: Anaesthesia in geriatric patients. In Katz J, Benumof JL, Kadis LB, editors: *Anaesthesia and uncommon diseases: pathophysiologic and clinical correlation*, ed 2, Philadelphia, 1976, WB Saunders, p 315.
6. Alder M, Kitchen S, Jrion A: *Data book on the elderly: a statistical portrait*, Washington, DC, U.S. Department of Health and Human Services, 1987.
7. Gilbert GH, Minaker KL: Principles of surgical risk assessment of the elderly patient, *J Oral Maxillofac Surg* 48:972–979, 1990.
8. McCarthy FM: Vital signs—the six-minute warning, *J Am Dent Assoc* 100:682–691, 1980.
9. Halstead C, editor: *Physical evaluation of the dental patient*, St Louis, 1982, CV Mosby, pp 74–81.
10. Sabes WR, Green S, Craine C: Value of medical diagnostic screening tests for dental patients, *J Am Dent Assoc* 80:133–136, 1970.
11. Sones ST et al: Comparison of the nature and frequency of medical problems among patients in general specialty, and hospital dental practices, *J Oral Med* 38:58, 1985.
12. American Academy of Implant Dentistry, Implant criteria workshop, Dearborn, Michigan, June 1978.
13. Misch CE: Medical evaluation of the implant candidate, Part II, *Int J Oral Implant* 2:11–18, 1982.
14. Corman L, Bolt RJ, editors: Medical evaluation of the pre-operative patient, *Med Clin North Am* 63:6, 1979.
15. Sherlock S: *Diseases of the liver and biliary system*, Oxford, 1975, Blackwell Scientific.
16. Little JW, Falace DA, editors: *Dental management of the medically compromised patient*, St Louis, 1980, CV Mosby, pp 176 16–188.
17. Bennett B: Coagulation pathways: inter-relationships and control mechanisms, *Semin Hematol* 14:301, 1977.
18. Misch CE: Medical evaluation of the implant candidate, Part III, SMA 12/60, *J Oral Implant* 9:556–570, 1981.
19. Raslavicus PA, Mei Shen E: Laboratory diagnosis by chemical methods, *Dent Clin North Am* 18:155–170, 1974.
20. Hypertension Detection and Follow-up Program Co-operative Group: Five year findings of the hypertension detection and follow-up program, I: reduction in mortality of persons with high blood pressure, including mild hypertension, *JAMA* 242:2562, 1979.
21. Sones S, Fazio R, Fang L, editors: *Principles and practice of oral medicine*, Philadelphia, 1984, WB Saunders.

22. Humphries JO: Survival after myocardial infarction: prognosis and management. *Mod Concepts Cardiovasc Dis* 46:51, 1977.

23. Pell S, D'Alonzo CA: Immediate mortality and five year survival of employed men with a first myocardial infarction, *N Engl J Med* 270:915, 1964.

24. Burkett LW, Burn CG: Bacteremias following dental extraction: demonstration of source of bacteria by means of a non-pathogen *(Serratia marcescons)*, *J Dent Res* 16:521, 1937.

25. Korn VA, Schaffer EM: A comparison of the postoperative bacteremias induced following different periodontal procedures, *J Periodontol* 33:226, 1962.

26. Bender IB, Seltzer S, Yermish M: The incidence of bacteremias in endodontic manipulation, *Oral Surg* 13:353, 1960.

27. Cameron IW: SBE in an edentulous patient: a case report, *Br Med J* 1:821, 1971.

28. Irvine WJ, Toft AD: The diagnosis and treatment of thyrotoxicosis, *Clin Endocrinol* 5:687, 1976.

29. Liddle GW, Melmon KC: The adrenals. In Williams RH, editor: *Textbook on endocrinology,* ed 5, Philadelphia, 1974, WB Saunders.

30. Misch CE, Moore P: Steroids and the reduction of pain, edema, and dysfunction in implant dentistry, *Int J Oral Implant* 6:27–31, 1989.

31. Dummett CO, Barens C: Oromucosal pigmentation: an updated literary review, *J Periodontol* 42:726, 1971.

32. Misch CE: Density of bone: effect on treatment plans, surgical approach, healing and progressive bone loading, *Int J Oral Implant* 6:23–31, 1990.

33. Konotey-Ahuke FI: The sickle cell diseases, *Arch Intern Med* 133:611, 1974.

34. Burrows B: Physiologic variants of chronic obstructive lung disease, *Chest* 58(suppl 2):415, 1970.

35. Conn HO: Cirrhosis. In Schiff L, editor: *Diseases of the liver,* ed 45, Philadelphia, 1975, JB Lippincott.

36. Baglink DJ et al: Systemic factors in alveolar bone loss, *J Prosthet Dent* 31:486, 1977.

37. Lindsey R et al: Bone response to termination of estrogen treatment.

38. Cann CE et al: Quantitative computed tomography for prediction of vertebral fracture risk, *Bone* 6:1, 1985.

39. Wakley GK, Baylink DJ: Systemic influences on the bone response to dental and orthopedic implants, *J Oral Implant* 14:285–311, 1988.

40. Farley JR, Wergedal JE, Baylink DJ: Fluoride directly stimulates proliferation and alkaline phosphatase activity of bone forming cells, *Science* 222:330, 1983.

41. Henrikson P: Periodontal disease and calcium deficiency: an experimental study in the dog, *Acta Odontol Scand* 26(suppl 50):1–132, 1968.

42. Obisesan AA, et al: The radiologic features of fibrous dysplasia of the craniofacial bones, *Oral Surg* 44:949, 1977.

43. McGousar DA: Clinical problems in Paget's disease affecting the jaws, *Br J Oral Surg* 11:230, 1974.

44. Tharp BR: Recent progress in epilepsy: diagnostic procedures and treatment, *Calif Med* 119:19, 1973.

45. Salvati EA et al: Infections associated with orthopedic devices. In Sugarman B, Young EJ, editors: *Infections associated with prosthetic devices,* Boca Raton, Fla, 1984, CRC Press, pp 181–218.

Chapter **6**

Diagnostic Evaluation

Carl E. Misch

RADIOGRAPHIC EXAMINATION

A variety of radiographic views enable one to evaluate and treat patients with dental implants adequately. The most common diagnostic roentgenograms include periapical, panoramic, and lateral cephalometric views, along with conventional radiographs and computed tomographic images. This section briefly describes the inherent qualities of each of these radiographic modalities for evaluation during dental implant diagnosis.

Intraoral Techniques

Periapical Radiographs

Periapical radiographs provide detailed information regarding the dimensions in length and height of available bone in small sections. They are indicated during treatment planning for single tooth implant, but are of limited value for more extensive edentulous sites.

The "paralleling technique" described by McCormack for teeth in 1920 should be used when obtaining periapical radiographs.[1] The procedure is modified so the x-ray film is positioned parallel to the final implant body position. This technique minimizes geometric distortions, provides better resolution, and produces anatomically truer images.

When the implant position has not been determined, the film should be placed parallel to the lingual cortical plate of bone, because the angulation of the implant osteotomy often depends on this structure. Usually in the maxillary anterior and mandibular posterior edentulous sites, the bone angulation in relation to the crowns of the replacement teeth is greater than that of the roots of the natural teeth. In these regions, because of the anatomy, the central ray needs to be oriented 10 degrees more positive (superior) than for its dentate counterpart.

Correct positioning of the radiographic film is more difficult in edentulous regions of the mouth. If the crest of the ridge is more than 10 mm apical to the occlusal plane, interfering landmarks may impair proper positioning. The floor of the mouth is sometimes above the edentulous mandibular ridge, which may further complicate correct positioning.

These compromising anatomic conditions may cause significant foreshortening of the image and prevent visualization of the opposing landmarks of the edentulous site. As a result, implant height is often incorrectly assessed with periapical radiographs. The location of the mandibular canal is difficult to assess in the first molar region of the mandible, and the mental foramen is visible in only 50% of these films.[2]

The use of radiopaque millimeter lines on periapical radiographs does not permit a true assessment of bone quantity. There are many disadvantages to this technique. The anatomic detail becomes more difficult to interpret. The millimeter grid is applied to the x-ray film, not to the edentulous ridge; as a result, the millimeter lines appear 1 mm apart, regardless of foreshortening or elongation of the image.

Occlusal Radiographs

An occlusal projection is an intraoral radiographic technique used to visualize the maxilla and mandible. The film is intraorally placed and the patient's head is rotated so the film is at a right angle to the floor. The primary beam is then directed at a right angle to the film to provide a cross-sectional image.

The buccolingual width of the mandible depicted on an occlusal film is the distance between the points located on extreme boundaries of the buccal and lingual cortical plates, but not necessarily in the horizontal plane.[3, 4] For this reason, occlusal radiographs are of very limited use in implant dentistry.

Extraoral Techniques

Lateral Cephalograph

Periapical and panoramic radiographs provide a two-dimensional image of height and length of the edentulous regions for implant dentistry. When adequate height for endosteal implants is present, the width of available bone is the most important criteria for implant selection and success. The angulation of bone is also very important. Neither the width nor angulation can be visualized on most traditional radiographs.

A lateral cephalograph or skull projection may be used as a tomogram, or section, of the midsagittal region of the maxilla and mandible. The magnification ranges from 6% to 15% and provides a more accurate representation than panoramic radiographs of vertical height, width, and angulation of bone at the midline. In addition, a lateral projection of the skull can help evaluate a loss of vertical dimension, skeletal arch interrelationship, anterior crown-implant ratio, anterior tooth position in the prosthesis, and resultant moment forces.

Panoramic Radiograph

The panoramic radiograph produces a single image of the maxilla and mandible and their supporting structures in a frontal plane. This type of radiograph is the most utilized diagnostic element in implant dentistry today. Panoramic images offer several advantages:

1. Opposing landmarks are easily identified.
2. The vertical height of bone initially can be assessed.
3. The patient is exposed to a relatively low radiation dose.
4. The procedure is performed with convenience, ease, and speed.
5. Gross anatomy of the jaws and any related pathologic findings can be evaluated.[5]

The main disadvantage of the panoramic radiograph is that the image does not resolve the fine anatomic detail that is seen with other types of radiographs. Other drawbacks include nonuniform magnification, geometric distortion, and overlapping of images.

Panoramic Distortion.—Control of radiographic distortions is particularly important in implant dentistry treatment planning because the amount of vertical and horizontal edentulous bone available determines the design of the implant. Distortion may be divided into vertical and horizontal components. The dimensions of the vertical image are dependent on the x-ray source as the focus. The horizontal dimensions are affected by the rotation center of the beam as the focus.

The degree of distortion of the vertical dimension depends on the distance of the patient's arches from the film. Because the panoramic beam is angled from below the edentulous arches and the width of bone increases toward the base, overlapping planes of the radiograph are displaced in relation to each other. As a result, the vertical height of bone is increased, especially in the maxilla. The wider the crest of the mandibular ridge, the more acute this effect in the lower arch.

The horizontal dimension changes dramatically in relation to the object-film distance. The horizontal magnification decreases as the object is brought closer to the film. This relationship is more critical in the anterior region. However, if one side of the patient is closer to the film than the other, the farther object will have greater magnification than the corresponding decrease in object size. A varied focus-to-object distance around an edentulous arch results in varied magnifications in different regions of the film. Horizontal dimensions are very unreliable for obtaining accurate measurements, especially in the anterior arch. Vertical dimensions are more accurate as long as the object is near vertical in position. The posterior maxilla is the most vertical region, and available bone under the antrum can be assessed with as little as 10% error. The maxillary anterior edentulous region is often oblique to the film. Combined with an anterior position, the maxillary anterior height and length are the most difficult areas to assess correctly. Dimensions of inclined objects cannot be relied upon in panoramic radiographs.

Lund and Manson-Hing,[6] in conducting studies on numerous panoramic X-ray units, have concluded that objects in front of and behind the focal trough were either blurred, magnified, reduced in size, or distorted to the extent of being unrecognizable. Fifty percent to 70% magnifications occurred in the horizontal dimension, and 10% to 32% in the vertical axis.[6]

Magnification can be determined by placing two or more ball bearings or wires along the edentulous sites during the panoramic radiograph exposure (Fig 6–1). The amount of magnification can be determined by a ratio established in the region between the actual dimension of the ball bearing and that observed on the image. Therefore, a 5-mm diameter ball, which measures 6 mm in vertical and 8 mm in horizontal, can help determine the amount of available bone in the region. In Figure 6–1 there is a 20% vertical magnification and 60% horizontal magnification in the edentulous region. Ideally, the ball bearings or wires should

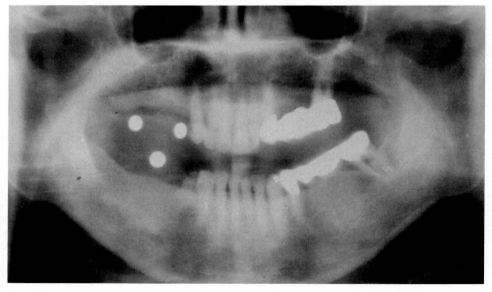

FIG 6–1.
Magnification may be evaluated on a panoramic film by placing 5-mm ball bearings on the crest of the ridge in the region of the future implants.

be placed into position before the first diagnostic panoramic radiograph. Otherwise, a second x-ray exposure is required for this procedure. Diagnostic casts and a stent may be made before the first radiograph, but this requires additional time and expense for all new patients.

An alternative is to position the ball bearings in rope wax in the edentulous regions during radiography. The ball bearings should rest directly on the edentulous ridge; otherwise, the acrylic or wax under the bar may be misinterpreted, and available bone height misdiagnosed.

Guidelines for Obtaining Panoramic Radiograph.—Completely edentulous patients should not wear their dentures during presurgical diagnostic panoramic radiography. The anterior denture teeth are usually anterior to the ridge, and when used as a guide for arch placement show increased distortion and magnification of the underlying bone. The patient's tongue should be placed against the roof of his or her mouth during the entire exposure, otherwise, a dark radiolucent shadow will appear above the apices of the maxillary teeth. This will obscure the images of the maxillary sinus and will make vertical available bone height measurements difficult to obtain.

The lead apron should not be positioned above the clavicles of the patient. The resulting radiopaque artifacts will create difficulty in reading the radiograph. The voltage (kVp) and/or intensity (mA) factors should be reduced one setting for the edentulous patient, unless the patient has darker skin pigmentation or heavy soft tissue and/or bone structure. Edentulous patients with small, narrow facial bones may require further reduction in the exposure factors.[7]

Anterior arch position is the most sensitive region for proper head positioning when obtaining panoramic radiographs. The anterior edentulous arch is a primary site for endosteal implants. Since the maxilla often presents an anterior angulation of 15 to 25 degrees, the anterior occlusal plane should be tilted downward to improve vertical orientation. Although the anterior plane is positioned more inferior, the patient's neck must remain straight, or the spinal column may obstruct the lower anterior segment of the film, making the image undiagnostic. In addition, if the occlusal plane is parallel to the floor (1) the palate line appears lower on the image,[7] and the maxillary available bone height may appear decreased in the anterior, and (2) the posterior floor of the antrum is often difficult to interpret.

Panoramic Landmarks

Crest of Ridge.—For the determination of available bone for possible implant sites, the crest of the ridge should first be evaluated. If a radiopaque line is present, this is representative of cortical bone and a very stable condition. However, this is rarely seen, and if present is usually a sign of advanced residual ridge resorption.

Opposing Landmarks.—After determination of the crest of the ridge, the opposing landmark is evaluated to determine the amount of available bone present. In the maxilla, the opposing landmarks to determine available bone height are

- *Anterior:* Inferior piriform aperture of the nares
- *Canine/premolar region:* Lateral piriform aperture of the nares and anterior border of the maxillary sinus
- *Posterior:* Floor of the maxillary sinus

Often the anterior nasal spine, palate, and inferior piriform aperture coalesce in the anterior region, and as a result, anterior bone height may be difficult to ascertain in the midline.

In the mandible, the opposing landmarks to determine available bone height are

- *Anterior:* Inferior border of the symphysis
- *Canine/premolar region:* Mental foramina and anterior loops of the mandibular canals
- *Posterior:* Mandibular canal

Radiographic Examination of Specific Structures

Maxilla

Incisive Foramen.—The incisive foramen lies in the midline on the palatal aspect of the maxillary central incisors. The extent of the foramen should be noted because if it is encroached upon by implant placement, soft tissue may proliferate around the implant instead of bone. Rarely is this structure a concern for paresthesia or surgical complications.

Maxillary Sinus.—The sinus shows considerable variability, as the anterior border has been observed as far as the midline. More common is the posterior migration of the sinus which expands toward the posterior wall of the maxillary process.

The innominate line is often mistaken for the posterior border of the maxillary sinus. This is seen as a thin, vertical, radiopaque line in the posterior aspect of the sinus. This is a radiographic artifact resulting from superimposition of two separate bones, the posterior surface of the zygomatic process of the maxilla and the posterior surface of the frontal process of the zygoma.[7]

Often the maxillary sinus is transversed by radiopaque lines called septa. Septa represent folds of cortical bone oriented vertically; these vary in number, thickness, and length.[3] These folds of bone complicate sinus elevation with subantral augmentation procedures.

Tuberosity.—The maxillary tuberosity represents a very poor prosthetic location for implant insertion. Rarely are third and fourth molar abutments indicated in a prosthesis. However, the bone in this region is easily accessible to harvest for intraoral autogenous bone grafts. The amount of bone available is highly variable, and the panoramic radiograph is an excellent way of assessment.

Canine Region.—The available bone height in the canine region is usually greater than in any other maxillary location. A column of bone between the lateral piriform aperture and the anterior border of the maxillary sinus is usually present. However, the antrum often extends over this canine region, thus limiting available bone height.

Mandible

In the anterior mandible, landmarks of primary importance in implant dentistry include the location of the mandibular canal and foramen and the inferior border of the mandible.

Anterior Mandible.—The maximum available mandibular bone is found between the mental foramina or the anterior loops, if present. The mandibular canine region is strongly influenced by the anterior loop. An anterior loop of the mandibular canal occurs when the neurovascular complex proceeds anterior and below the mental foramen, then rotates up and posterior to meet and exit the mental foramen. The presence of an anterior loop occurs in approximately 12% of patients, and when present usually extends five mm anterior to the foramen.[8]

The anterior bone height measured is greater than the actual available bone height, even after correction of the magnification. The angulation of the anterior bony region usually requires that the implants be placed against the lingual cortical plate, above the radiographic inferior border. A lateral cephalogram helps determine the angulation of implant insertion and the amount of actual anterior available bone height.

Posterior Mandible.—The posterior mandible demonstrates a radiographic line which represents the external oblique of the mandible. If the bone has resorbed at or below this structure, the buccinator muscle will usually have migrated toward the crest of the ridge, which results in a lack of attached tissue in the region. These conditions cause more incision line opening as immediate postoperative complications. Rarely is there adequate bone height in the posterior mandible for endosteal implants when the external oblique line represents the highest point of the residual ridge. When adequate width is present, the height of bone available in the posterior mandible is measured from the crest of the edentulous ridge to the upper limit of the mandibular foramen and/or canal.

Several clinical approaches to the posterior mandible have been proposed using radiographic techniques. In the first molar region, the mandibular canal often is difficult to identify because of the submandibular fossa, in which the facial and lingual cortical plates approximate, leading to an increase in density that obscures the superior cortical lining of the mandibular canal.

Yosue and Brooks[2] determined that the mental foramen could always be identified on a panoramic radiograph; however, only 28% of studies showed its accurate position. The majority of panoramic radiographs illustrate the mental foramen significantly closer to the inferior border of the mandible than its actual position. In addition, the appearance of the foramen varied with the positioning of the mandible in relationship to the focal length used while obtaining the radiograph.[2]

A panoramic radiograph is often used to determine the height of bone available over the canal. A 25% manufacturer-supplied magnified image of the implant is placed over the radiograph, enabling one to select the desired size of implant to be inserted in the abutment position. However, panoramic radiographs do not have a predictable magnification rate. Additional variables such as the patient's head position may significantly alter magnification.

The usual vertical height from the inferior border of the mandible to the mental foramen is approximately 10 to 12 mm, and the mandibular canal approximately 8 to 10 mm from the inferior border (anterior to the first molar). Occasionally, the position of the mental foramen may be difficult to observe. Therefore, if 20 to 24 mm of total vertical height of bone is observed in the mandibular body, adequate height is often available for endosteal implants. The distance from the foramen or canal to the inferior border represents one third of the original height of bone in this region. As a result, the percentage of vertical bone height loss can be estimated.

Zone of Safety.—A zone of safety for the placement of posterior mandibular endosteal implants was established by Misch in 1980 by the evaluation of 530 consecutive panoramic radiographs of partially edentulous patients.[8] In 1989 this evaluation was confirmed by Crawford with an additional 324 consecutive panoramic radiographs. The zone of safety is defined as an area within the bone in which implants may be placed safely, without fear of impingement on the neurovascular bundle. The result of these studies indicated the radiographic prevalence of the mandibular canal below a line drawn parallel to the plane of occlusion and at the height of the mental foramen (Fig 6–2).

A zone of safety was observed in 100% of radiographs mesial to the middle of the mandibular first molar. In the region of the distal half of the first molar, the mandibular canal was below this line in 97.5% of radiographs. In the region of the mesial half of the second molar, it was below the second parallel line in 43% of studies, and in the distal half of the second molar in 5.5% of studies (see Fig 6–2). The most common position of the canal anterior to the mid first molar region was 2 mm or more inferior to the parallel line drawn from the top of the foramen, representing a gray zone of additional surgical safety.

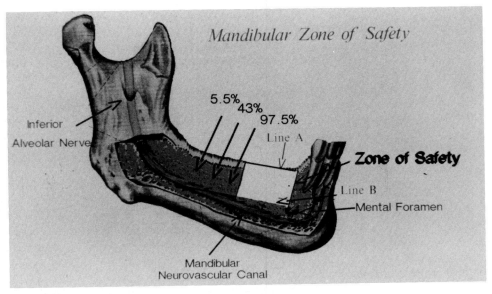

FIG 6–2.
Mandibular zone of safety. Draw an imaginary line parallel to the plane of occlusion at the crest of the posterior ridge *(line A)*, and another parallel line at the top of the foramen *(line B)*. The height of bone between these lines is in the zone of safety to the mid–first molar region.

As a result of these groups of measurements, a zone of safety for endosteal implant placement has been established for implants placed anterior to the mid first molar area. Radiographic estimates of vertical bone height are made prior to surgery, using calibrated ball bearings or wire ratios of magnification, or an arbitrary 25% magnification.[8]

Tomography

Conventional Tomography

Conventional tomography is a radiographic technique in which a "slice," or section of a given internal body structure, is made in a predetermined plane. Tomography will reveal the quality and quantity of bone in a predetermined implant location. In conventional tomography, the x-ray source moves in one direction while the film or recording medium moves in the opposite direction. The tube and film move simultaneously in a constant relationship that is maintained by a connecting system which rotates about an axis lying in the plane of the section to be projected. Planes other than the sections to be projected are blurred. The degree of blurring depends on the distance of the other planes from the projected plane.[9] With the use of conventional tomography, the clinician can accurately evaluate the cortical and trabecular bone along with vital structures in the region desired for implant placement.

If the conventional tomographic unit has a constant fulcrum system, all images will exhibit a constant degree of magnification because of the constant distance from the radiation source and the film to the object being imaged. Thus direct measurements can be made with a known correction factor. Several investigators have shown that conventional tomography exhibits an accurate assessment of bone quantity after magnification correction.[10,11]

Intraoral alignment stents can be made with mouthguard acrylic, using ball bearings, amalgam plugs, or gutta-percha to help align the unit to achieve true cross-sections at specific sites along the curvature of the mandible.

The average radiation exposure during a tomographic series is less than that for a full mouth radiographic survey.[12] The average dose per tomographic exposure is 1 to 6 mrad, or 50 mrad for the entire tomographic examination or series of films.[13]

Computed Tomography

Computed tomography, or computer-assisted tomography (CT), was first introduced to the medical field by Hounsfield in 1942. CT produces digital data from the amount of x-ray transmission through an object. By rotating the x-ray tube and detectors around the object being imaged, data on the density characteristics in the object are obtained. Through the use of a computer, the image of the object is reconstructed.

For optimum placement of implants, a knowledge of the cross-sectional anatomy of the alveolar ridges is needed. For many years, techniques utilizing CT failed to provide true cross-sections through the desired location in the bone. Only cross-sectional scans perpendicular to the long axis of the body can be obtained with ease. These scans are not true cross-sections and are only approximations due to the curvature of the bone. Through the use of special reformatting programs, a series of true cross-sectional images can now be created by the CT data. The computer may also create multiple panoramic and three-dimensional images.[14] Thus recently there has been extensive interest in the use of CT scanning in the field of oral implantology.

The advantages of CT scans in implantology are numerous. Superimposition of objects does not occur, and all tissues irradiated can be displayed. Cross-referencing with tick marks is used to reveal specific locations instead of the use of stents. Direct measurements can be made from the cross-sectional images with a millimeter ruler or calipers (Fig 6–3). However, artifacts from metallic dental restorations, lack of availability to CT scanning units, and the cost of a scan series are some of the drawbacks of this technique.[14] The most common indication for CT scanning is in the region of the premaxilla, as treatment plans and anatomic assessment are most difficult to obtain in this area.

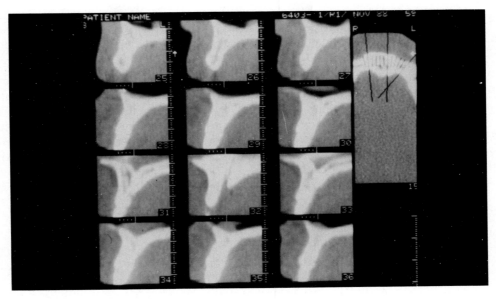

FIG 6–3.
CT study of an anterior maxillary arch.

Magnetic Resonance Imaging

Magnetic resonance imagers recently have become popular in the medical field. As of this time, MRI has limited use in oral implantology diagnosis. Although there is a total absence of radiation with this technique and no special reformatting programs are needed, there are several disadvantages. The interpretation of the quality of cortical and trabecular bone is very difficult, metal restorations cause artifacts, there is limited availability of imaging units, and the cost is approximately double that of CT units.[15]

DIAGNOSTIC CASTS, TREATMENT PROSTHESES, AND SURGICAL STENTS

Diagnostic Casts

The value of diagnostic casts or study models is often very critical in oral implantology as in any other restorative treatment. Many patients have been partially edentulous for long periods of time. The combination of edentulous bone loss and dentition changes related to missing teeth increase the number of factors that must be considered for oral rehabilitation compared with traditional prosthodontic treatment. The final prosthesis, and the number and location of ideal and optional abutment sites are selected before surgery. Diagnostic casts enable the dentist to evaluate several prosthodontic criteria in the absence of the patient. These casts permit an open discussion of treatment with other practitioners and/or laboratory technicians for consultation. Surgical stents are often designed from the diagnostic casts, or after wax-up of the designed prosthesis. They assist with implant site selection and angulation requirements during the surgical phase. The casts may be used as a permanent record of pretreatment conditions for dental-legal issues, since nonreversible procedures may be performed. The diagnostic casts and pretreatment set-ups may be used for presentations to motivate patient's acceptance of the proposed treatment.[16]

Diagnostic casts mounted with an accurate record of centric jaw relationship and maxillomandibular occlusion on an adjustable articulator provide 16 items of information related to treatment,[17] all of which influence the final prosthesis treatment plan:

1. Occlusal relationships, both interarch and interdental
2. Edentulous ridge relationships to adjacent teeth and opposing arches
3. Tooth position of potential abutments, including inclination, rotation, extrusion, spacing, and esthetic considerations
4. Tooth morphology, structure of potential abutments, and overall conditions
5. Direction of forces in future implant sites
6. Present occlusal scheme
7. Edentulous soft tissue angulation, length, width, locations, and permucosal esthetic position
8. Interarch space
9. Overall occlusal curve of Wilson and curve of Spee
10. Arch relationships
11. Opposing dentition
12. Existing occlusion
13. Number of missing teeth
14. Arch location of future abutments
15. Arch form
16. Parallelism of abutments

A duplicate diagnostic cast may be mounted on an articulator for selective alterations and prewaxing to determine the desired occlusal scheme and esthetic aspects of the final restoration. A face-bow transfer, centric and eccentric occlusal records should help mount these casts on a semiadjustable articulator. Occasionally a panographic recording of mandibular movements and a fully adjustable articulator may be indicated when oral reconstruction is extensive and/or temporomandibular relationships are of specific concern.

The diagnostic wax-up usually is prescribed in detail, and performed by the laboratory technician. The specific laboratory communicative processes are thereby begun before actual treatment, and may be modified during treatment as required. These considerations include occlusal plane correction, edentulous ridge position and its effect on implant placement and occlusion, esthetic considerations, and interarch distance. The altered diagnostic wax-up casts may also be used to provide a guide for provisional restorations, and may be evaluated during the provisional stages of reconstruction.

Treatment Prostheses

A treatment prosthesis may be indicated for the following reasons:

1. To improve hard and/or soft tissues
2. To evaluate esthetics and hygiene considerations
3. To determine final vertical dimensions
4. To determine placement of the superstructure bar
5. To evaluate the patient's psychologic health and attitude
6. To determine conditions for patient management

Treatment Sequence

The sequence of treatment for implant-supported reconstructions is as follows:

1. Initial appointment
   a. Past medical and dental history
   b. Dental evaluation and x-ray examinations
   c. Treatment plan; case presentation and alternatives
   d. Diagnostic casts
   e. Extra-office diagnostic orders (e.g., set-up, CT scans, tests for medical evaluation, consultation with team members)
2. Confirmation appointment
   a. Diagnostic wax-up of final results on duplicate diagnostic casts
   b. Final treatment plan and alternatives
   c. Laboratory tests
   d. Prescriptions and postoperative instructions
   e. Consent forms and request for treatment forms
   f. Pictures of existing conditions
3. Presurgical restorative appointment
   a. Initial caries removal, extractions, temporary teeth
   b. Periodontal treatment
   c. Occlusal plane correction
   d. Transitional prosthesis and/or diagnostic try-in; tissue conditioning
   e. Impression for surgical guide stent (if oral condition altered from initial diagnostic cast)

4. Implant surgery
   a. Stage I: implant placement
   b. Healing phase
   c. Stage II: secondary permucosal extension, initial loading
5. Prosthodontics: Progressive bone loading
   a. Initial abutment preparation and impression
   b. Final abutment preparation and impression
   c. Metal try-in or waxed teeth try-in
   d. Initial delivery
   e. Final delivery
6. Maintenance
   a. First year: every 3 to 4 months
   b. Radiographs at 6 months, then annually for 3 years, then as required
   c. Home care education
      (1) Fluoride on teeth
      (2) Chlorhexidine on implants
      (3) Home care instrumentation

The final treatment plan and patient's physical and mental evaluation should be assessed before implant surgery. If the restoring dentist is not sure the planned final prosthesis is compatible with the desires of the patient, or the patient's attitude and demand do not seem usual, further evaluation is required. A treatment prosthesis provides additional appointments and time for these evaluations.

The vertical dimension of occlusion may gradually decrease, especially in the completely edentulous patient, as a result of bone loss and prosthesis occlusal attrition. Temporomandibular joint and myofacial dysfunction may be related to this condition. A treatment prosthesis helps determine the patient's specific needs regarding the dysfunction. As the vertical dimension decreases, the anterior mandibular jaw positions become more prognathic. Subperiosteal implants require the design of the prosthetic superstructure at the same time as the implant substructure. Hence, a treatment prosthesis can establish the correct vertical and tooth position prior to placement of the implant and fabrication of the superstructure bar.

Esthetic evaluation may be related to a host of factors. These include tooth size and position, tooth color, and lip support. A fixed restoration design must allow access for proper hygiene procedures around the teeth and implants. A high or low lip line position may affect the patient's speech and also influence the gingival contour of the restoration. A treatment prosthesis may help determine if an implant supported removable prosthesis will be required to satisfy the patient's goals and desires.

The soft tissue supporting a removable prostheses often become abused. Hyperplasia, hypertrophy, increased mobility, and/or abrasions of soft tissue may occur. A soft tissue conditioner may be used to restore proper occlusion and vertical dimension, while acting as a resilient base to improve soft tissue health. A treatment prosthesis may be required in addition to tissue conditioning when occlusal and vertical dimensions are significantly affected.

The maxillary vermillion border is usually altered by the loss of the maxillary anterior teeth. Once bone is also lost, the support of the entire lip is deficient. Under these conditions, the anterior acrylic flange of a removable prosthesis is required to restore proper contour. A fixed partial denture may require an anterior cantilever away from the soft tissue in a horizontal and vertical relation to provide this support. A treatment prosthesis can provide the information required to determine if a fixed prosthesis will compromise esthetics, support, or hygiene in this region.

Surgical Guide Template

The surgical guide template is fabricated by the restoring dentist after the presurgical restorative appointment(s), the final prosthesis design, optional abutment number and location, occlusal scheme, and implant angulation have been determined.

Several methods of fabricating the surgical guide template are available. The requirements are more relevant than the options of fabrication. The template should be stable and rigid when in correct position. Two suggestions help achieve those criteria. If the arch treated has remaining teeth, the template should fit over and/or around enough teeth to stabilize and position the guide stent (Fig 6–4). When no remaining teeth are present, the template should extend onto unreflected soft tissue regions, that is, the palate and tuberosities in the maxilla, or the retromolar pads in the mandible (Fig 6–5). In this way, the guide template may be used after the soft tissue has been reflected from the implant site, and during preparation for the implant osteotomy.

Prosthodontic goals of FP-1 or FP-2 restorations require more ideal implant placement. In a FP-3 restoration, the abutments may be placed independently from the actual replacement crowns, because the gingival replacement contours separate the crowns from the implant abutment. The restoring dentist should decide if the final restoration will be cement or screw-retained. The edentulous ridge crest usually is more medial than its dentulous counterpart when teeth were present. If a cemented final restoration is planned, the implant abutment should ideally be placed under the stamp cusp of the opposing posterior tooth, or within the body of an anterior tooth. For a screw-in prosthesis, the implant should ideally be aligned with the centric fossa of the posterior teeth. In this way, the access opening is in a different position than the primary contact of the abutment tooth. The retention screw should not emerge through the stamp cusp for obvious occlusal considerations.

An implant placed adjacent to a natural tooth should remain greater than 2

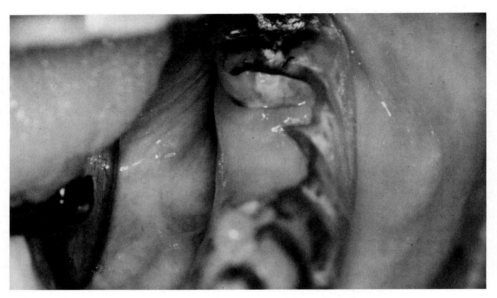

FIG 6–4.
Surgical guide template in a partially edentulous mouth should engage the teeth for stability. The facial contours of the replacement teeth are represented. The lingual aspect should provide maximum surgical freedom.

mm away from the crown or roots. Therefore the pilot hole should be at least 4 to 5 mm away from the natural tooth. This location is not in the mid-tooth position of a missing maxillary lateral incisor or any mandibular incisor adjacent to a natural tooth.

The ideal angulation for implant insertion should be visualized during surgery and requires at least two reference points for each implant. For that purpose, the surgical guide must be elevated above the edentulous site. The distance between the occlusal surface of the abutment crown and the crest of the ridge represents 8 mm or more. As a result, these two points of reference correspond to the path of ideal implant insertion. The ideal angulation is perpendicular to the occlusal plane and parallel to the most anterior abutment joined to the implant.

A maxillary anterior implant for a FP-1 result requires the most precise pretreatment planning and implant placement. The incisal edge of the crown, facial profile, and labial cervical position are all related to implant position. The ideal implant position results with a straight abutment slightly lingual to the incisal edge of the final crown for a cemented prosthesis. Screw-retained prostheses should have the implant emerging more toward the cingulum of the anterior tooth.

An implant in the maxillary first premolar position must consider mesial angulation when a natural canine is present. The 11-degree average distal inclination of the canine root places the apex of the root and first premolar implant in the same area. Therefore the implant should be angled to follow the root of the canine and prevent contact and/or perforation of the natural root.

The surgical template should relate the ideal gingival contour position. Many edentulous ridges have lost bone and gingival width at the expense of the facial contour. This may be replaced during implant insertion by an onlay graft of dense hydroxylopatite and demineralized freeze-dried bone. The amount of augmentation required to support the tissue can be determined by the surgical template.

The easiest method to construct the implant surgical template is to use a modification of Preston's clear splint for the diagnosis of tooth contours, tooth position, and occlusal form.[18] The diagnostic wax-cast is completed to determine tooth size, position, contour, and occlusion in the edentulous regions where implants will be inserted. No selective grinding or modification is performed on any teeth that have not been altered prior to surgery; otherwise, the template will not fit correctly in the mouth. A full arch irreversible hydrocolloid impression is made and poured in dental stone. On the duplicate cast of the wax-up teeth, a vacuum acrylic shell is pressed and trimmed to fit over the teeth and gingiva contours of the buccal aspect of the ridge. If no natural teeth remain, the posterior

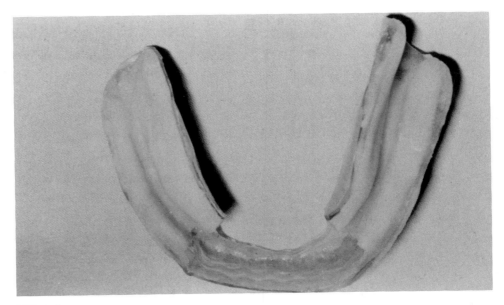

FIG 6–5.
Template for a completely edentulous patient extends to unreflected regions of the jaws.

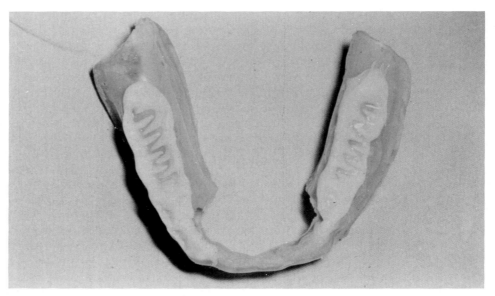

FIG 6–6.
Surgical template for the completely edentulous patient has an opposing occlusal index. This ensures that the template is seated in the correct mesiodistal and faciolingual position.

portion of the template should be maintained and cover the retromolar pads or tuberosities to aid in positioning.

The occlusal acrylic is removed over the ideal and optional implant sites, maintaining the facial and facio-occlusal line angle of the surgical template. This provides maximum freedom for implant placement, yet communicates the ideal tooth position and angulation during surgery. In the edentulous arch the vacuum form may be of the existing removable prosthesis, if within accepted guidelines. A soft tissue liner may then be added in the tuberosity or retromolar pad regions and other soft tissue areas not involved in surgery. Acrylic is then added over the occlusal portion of the stent where no implants are planned. The patient then occludes into this index. In this manner the template may be correctly positioned over the edentulous ridge once the tissue is reflected. Otherwise, template position too far facial or off to one side is likely (Fig 6–6).

REFERENCES

1. McCormack FW: A plea for a standardized technique for oral radiology with an illustrated classification of findings and their verified interpretations, *J Dent Res* 2:467–510, 1920.

2. Yosue T, Brooks SL: The appearance of mental foramina on panoramic and periapical radiographs, *Oral Surg Oral Med Oral Pathol* 68:488–492, 1989.

3. Wheeler RC: *Dental anatomy and physiology and occlusion,* St Louis, 1974, CV Mosby.

4. DuBrul EL:*Sicher's oral anatomy,* ed 7, St Louis, 1980, CV Mosby.

5. Goaz PW, White SC: *Oral radiology: principles and interpretation,* St Louis, 1982, CV Mosby.

6. Manson-Hing L: Radiation exposure and distribution measurements for three panoramic x-ray machines, *Oral Surg* 313–318, 1977.

7. Langland OE: *Panoramic radiology,* ed 2, Philadelphia, 1989, Lea & Febiger.

8. Misch CE, Crawford EA: Predictable mandibular nerve location—a clinical zone of safety, *Int J Oral Implant* 7:37–40, 1990.

9. Rosenberg HM: Laminography: methods and application in oral diagnosis, *J Am Dent Assoc* 74:88–96, 1967.

10. Petrokowski CG, Pharoah MJ: Presurgical radiographic assessment of implants, *J Prosthet Dent* 61:59–64, 1989.

11. Fernandes RJ, Azarbal M, Ismail YH: A cephalometric tomographic technique to visualize the buccolingual and vertical dimensions of the mandible, *J Prosthet Dent* 58:466–470, 1987.

12. Richards A, Colquitt W: Reduction in dental x-ray exposure during the past 60 years, *J Am Dent Assoc* 103:713–718, 1981.

13. Borglin K et al: Radiation dosimetry in tomography of the teeth and jaws using a multi-film cassette, *Acta Radiol* 26:739–743, 1985.

14. Engelman MJ, Sorenson JA: Optimum placement of osseointegrated implants, *J Prosthet Dent* 59:467–473, 1988.

15. Zabalegui J, Gil JA, Zabalegui B: Magnetic resonance imaging as an adjunctive diagnostic aid in patient selection for endosseous implants: preliminary study, *Int J Oral Maxillofac Implant* 5:283–288, 1991.

16. Thompson EO: Constructing and using diagnostic models. *Dent Clin North Am* 67–84, 1963.

17. Laney WR: Critical aspects of removable partial denture service. In Goldman HM, et al, editors: *Current therapy in dentistry,* St Louis, 1968, CV Mosby, pp 3:287–304, 1968.

18. Preston JD: A systemic approach to the control of esthetic form, *J Prosthet Dent* 35:393–402, 1976.

Chapter 7

Divisions of Available Bone

Carl E. Misch

Long-term success in implant dentistry requires the evaluation of unique dental criteria. Once adequate education is achieved in implant surgery and related prosthodontics on the part of the dentist, the two major variables of treatment are the condition of the individual patient's mouth and teeth and the related treatment options based upon thorough evaluation. More than 50 dental criteria influence implant treatment planning.[1] The doctor and patient must be aware that success rates with implants vary widely. The training and experience of the doctor and the amount and quality of available bone in the patient are primary determining factors in predicting individual success. Once the prosthodontic needs and desires of the patient have been determined, if implants are needed to support the intended prosthesis, the most important element in the implant region is the available bone. Greenfield already appreciated its importance in 1913.[2]

LITERATURE REVIEW

This chapter describes the three-dimensional concept of available bone and the implant treatment options for each type of bone anatomy. Weiss and Judy[3] developed a classification of mandibular atrophy and its influence on subperiosteal implant therapy in 1974. Louisiana State University and Kent presented a classification of alveolar ridge deficiency designed for alloplastic bone augmentation in 1982.[4] Another classification was proposed by Zarb and Lekholm[5] in 1985 for residual jaw morphology with the insertion of Branemark fixtures. They described five stages of jaw resorption, ranging from minimal to extreme. All classifications used the same implant modality and surgical approach. In 1985 Misch and Judy established four basic divisions of available bone for implant dentistry, which follow the natural resorption phenomena.[6–8] These four classes have been expanded to offer an organized approach to implant treatment options

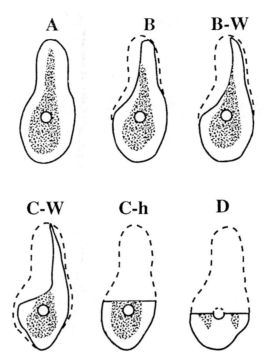

FIG 7–1.
Classification of available bone (Divisions A, B, C, and D) follows the natural patterns of bone resorption in the jaws. Each division presents unique surgical and prosthetic approaches. h = Inadequate height; w = inadequate width.

for surgery and prosthodontics (Fig 7–1).[9] The ability to organize the available bone of the potential implant site into specific related categories of common treatment options and conditions is of major importance. Improved communication among health professionals and the collection of relevant specific data for each category are some of the benefits. The following terminology has facilitated these processes during the past several years within the profession, university and private implant programs, and international implant societies.

AVAILABLE BONE

The category and design of the final prosthesis is first determined. The abutments necessary to support the restoration are then established. If no natural teeth are in the indicated regions, an implant (or implants) is considered. Available bone describes the amount of bone in the edentulous area considered for implantation. It is measured in width, height, length, angulation, and crown-implant body ratio (Fig 7–2).

As a general guideline, 2 mm is maintained between the implant and any adjacent landmark. This is especially applicable when the opposing landmark is the mandibular nerve. Experience has demonstrated that the implant may proceed without complication through the cortical plate of the maxillary sinus or inferior border of the mandible, or next to the cribriform plate of a natural tooth. However, if the implant should become mobile or affected by peri-implant disease, the adjacent landmark may be adversely involved.

Manufacturers describe the root form implant in dimensions of width and length. The length corresponds to the height of available bone. Therefore, this text will refer to implant height rather than length. The width of a root form implant is related to the width and mesiodistal length of available bone. The width of a plate form implant is related to the width of bone, the length of the implant corresponds to the mesiodistal length of available bone, and the height is related to the height of bone.

Many factors justify the use of maximum available bone at the implant-bone interface. All teeth are not equal when considered as abutments for a prosthesis. The restoring dentist knows how to evaluate the surface area of the natural abutment roots. A maxillary first molar with over 450 mm^2 root surface area constitutes a better abutment for a fixed prosthesis than a mandibular lateral incisor with 150 mm^2 of root support. Likewise, all implants are not equal abutments.

The greater the surface area of the implant-bone system, the less concentrated the force transmitted to the bone, and the better prognosis of the implant abutment. For a root form implant, with each 0.25-mm increase in diameter, the surface area increases approximately 10%. Therefore, for a root form implant 1 mm greater in diameter, the total surface area increases approximately 40% (Fig 7–3). In addition, the greater diameter decreases the amount of stress at the crestal bone–implant interface.

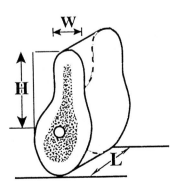

FIG 7–2.
Available bone in the region of a potential implant abutment is evaluated by height *(H)*, width *(W)*, and length *(L)*. Also considered are crown-implant body ratio and the direction of force to the implant body.

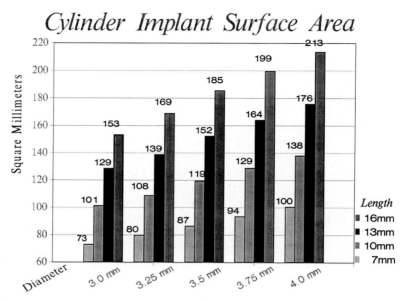

FIG 7–3.
Generic surface areas of root form implants in heights of 7, 10, 13, and 16 mm. Diameters range from 3.0 to 4.0 mm (x-axis). Surface area (y-axis) is increased approximately 10% for each 0.25-mm increase in diameter when the height remains similar.

The height of an implant also affects the total surface area. An implant that is 3 mm higher provides more than 10% increase in surface area. The significance in increased length is not found at the crestal bone interface but rather in initial stability, in amount of bone-implant interface, and in long-term resistance to the moment force (Fig 7–4). The maximum height of implant in the available bone also provides healing, with decreased risk of movement at the interface. The opposing anatomic landmark is often composed of cortical bone. Cortical bone may remodel quickly at the periosteal and endosteal surface of callous formation and at a 50 to 100 times slower rate within the cortical bone than the trabecular bone, which initially heals with woven rather than lamellar bone. As a result, the cortical bone holds the implant while the trabecular woven bone forms. The remodeled trabecular bone may then keep the implant rigid while the cortical bone remodels. In this way, the implant is more inclined to maintain a direct bone-implant interface.

Available Bone Height

The height of available bone is measured from the crest of the edentulous ridge to the opposing landmarks, such as the maxillary sinus or mandibular canal in the posterior regions. The anterior regions are limited by the maxillary nares or the inferior border of the mandible. The maxillary canine eminence region offers greater height of available bone than the maxillary anterior or posterior regions. The mandibular canine or first premolar region may present reduced height of available bone compared with the anterior region, because of the anterior loop of the mandibular canal as it passes below and proceeds superior, then distal, before it exits through the mental foramen (Fig 7–5).

The dilemma of available bone in implant dentistry involves the existing anatomy of the edentulous mandible and maxilla. The opposing landmarks limit the available bone height more in the posterior regions. As a result, in the areas where most of the forces are generated and the natural dentition has two or three roots for each tooth, the shortest implants, if any, must be used. It is not unusual in the mandible to place anterior implants and distally cantilever the prosthesis. The anatomy in the posterior region may be modified, as in the maxilla, which is often altered with subantral augmentation to permit the placement of posterior endosteal implants into newly created bone height.

The available bone height is first estimated by radiographic evaluation in the edentulous ideal and optional regions where implant abutments are required for the intended prosthesis. A panoramic radiograph is the most common method used for this purpose.

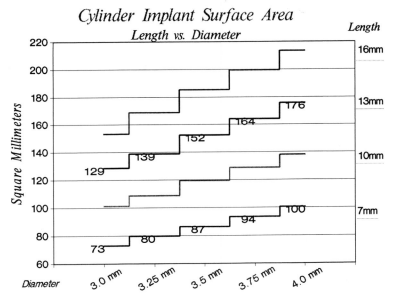

FIG 7–4.
Surface area (y-axis) of an implant is related to the height of the implant body. Increase in height to the next size improves surface area more than 10%.

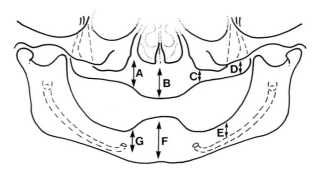

FIG 7–5.
Height of available bone is measured from the crest of the edentulous ridge to the opposing landmark. The opposing landmark may be in the maxillary canine region *(A)*, floor of the nares *(B)*, maxillary sinus *(C)*, tuberosity *(D)*, mandibular canine region *(G)*, anterior mandible *(F)*, or bone above the inferior mandibular canal *(E)*.

The minimum bone height for predictable long-term endosteal implant survival approaches 10 mm. In 1983 Branemark stated that 10 mm was the major implant height necessary to obtain predictable success.[10] This philosophy has been redeveloped, and as much as 20 mm bone height is now used when possible. However, the 10-mm height minimum has remained a valuable criterion. The inexperienced dentist may wish to have 12 mm of bone height to place a 10-mm-high implant body before proceeding with the surgery. This precaution allows 2 mm surgical error, or permits an osteoplasty to gain additional width of bone. The 10-mm height minimum applies to most endosteal implant designs. This height requirement may be reduced in the very dense bone of the symphysis of an atrophic mandible, or increased in the very porous bone of the posterior maxilla.[11, 12] The final prosthodontic design, the experience and training of the dentist, the density of the bone, and the other elements of the dental evaluation all contribute to the treatment plan options when available bone is limited.

Available Bone Width

The width of available bone is measured between the facial and lingual plates at the crest of the potential implant site. The crest of an edentulous ridge is supported by a wider base. The triangular-shaped cross-section permits an osteoplasty in order to obtain greater width of bone, although of reduced height. Crest reduction affects the location of the opposing landmark, with possible consequences for surgery, implant height selection, appearance, and the design of the final prosthesis.

Once adequate height is available for implants, the primary criteria affecting long-term survival of endosteal implants is the width of available bone. Root form implants of 3.75-mm diameter usually require 5 mm or more of bone in width to ensure sufficient bone thickness and blood supply around the implant for predictable survival. Plate form implants 1.25 mm wide require at least 2.5 mm of available bone width for predictable results. These dimensions ensure more than 0.5 mm bone on each side of the implant at the crest. Because the bone usually widens toward the base, this minimum dimension rapidly increases. For root form implants, bone width is critical only in the midfacial and midlingual areas of the crestal area exclusively (Fig 7–6).

Available Bone Length

The mesiodistal length of available bone in an edentulous area is often limited by adjacent teeth or implants. The length of available bone necessary for endosteal implant survival depends on the width of bone. For bone 5 mm wide or more, a minimum mesiodistal length of 5 mm is usually sufficient for each implant. A width of bone 2.5 mm to 5 mm requires a greater length for implant support. In this narrower ridge, the necessary length reaches 15 mm to achieve sufficient implant-bone surface area to compensate in length for the deficiency in width of the implant.

Available Bone Angulation

Bone angulation is the fourth determinant for available bone. Ideally, it is aligned with the forces of occlusion and is parallel to the long axis of the clinical crowns used in the prosthodontic restoration. The incisal and occlusal surfaces of the teeth follow the curve of Wilson and curve of Spee. This results in the roots

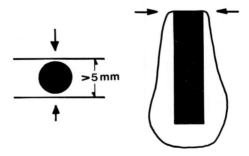

FIG 7–6.
The minimum bone width for a 3.75-mm root form is 5 mm in the midfacial and lingual region, because the round implant design results in more bone in all other dimensions (width and height).

of the maxillary teeth being angled toward a common point approximately 4 inches away. The mandibular roots flare, so the anatomic crowns are more medial in the posterior and facial in the anterior, compared to the corresponding roots. The first premolar cusp tip is usually vertical to its root apex.

The alveolar bone angulation follows the root trajectory to the occlusal plane. Rarely does this bone angulation remain the same after the loss of teeth, especially in the anterior edentulous maxillary arch. In addition, the maxillary anterior natural teeth are less perpendicular to occlusal forces than any other teeth. In this region, labial undercuts and resorption after tooth loss mandate greater angulation of the implants. In the posterior mandible, the submandibular fossa mandates implant placement with increasing angulation as they progress to the distal. Hence, in the premolar region the angulation may be 10 degrees to the occlusal plane; in the first molar area, 15 degrees; and in the second molar region, 20 to 25 degrees.

The limiting factor of angulation of force between the body and the abutment of an implant is correlated to the width of bone. In edentulous areas with a wide ridge, root form implants may be selected. Such implants allow modifications up to 30 degrees divergence with the adjacent implant(s), natural teeth, or axial forces of occlusion. The greater diameter implant decreases the amount of stress transmitted to the crestal bone. In addition, the greater width of bone permits some latitude in angulation at implant placement. The implant body may be inserted so as to reduce the divergence of the abutments. Therefore, the bone angulation in the wider ridge may be as much as 30 degrees.

The narrow yet adequate width ridge often indicates a narrower design root form or plate form implant. Compared with a larger diameter root form implant, a smaller diameter design has greater crestal stress and may not offer the same range of custom abutments. In addition, the narrower width of bone does not allow as much latitude in placement regarding its angulation within the bone. Bending the neck of the plate form implant aligns the abutment with the adjacent natural teeth. The implant neck should not be bent beyond 20 degrees, as this may compromise the fatigue strength of the metal. This limits the acceptable angulation of bone in the narrow ridge to 20 degrees from the axis of the adjacent clinical crowns or a line perpendicular to the occlusal plane.

Crown-Implant Body Ratio

The crown-implant body ratio impacts the appearance of the final prosthesis and the amount of moment of the force on the implant and the crestal surrounding bone. The crown height is measured from the occlusal or incisal plane to the crest of the ridge and the endosteal implant height from the crest of the ridge to its apex. The greater the crown-implant ratio, the greater the moment of the force with any lateral force. In addition, the prosthesis is less likely to replace only the anatomic crowns of natural teeth.

DIVISIONS OF AVAILABLE BONE

Division A

Division A corresponds to abundant available bone in all dimensions (Table 7–1; Fig 7–7). The bone is 5 mm wide or greater, the height is greater than 10 mm, and the mesiodistal length of bone is greater than 5 mm. The angulation does not exceed 30 degrees between the occlusal plane and the implant body. The crown-implant body ratio requirement of bone Division A usually requires the implant height to be greater than 12 mm, especially in the anterior regions of the mouth.

TABLE 7–1.

Divisions of Available Bone

Division	Dimension	Treatment Options
A	> 5 mm width > 10–12 mm height > 5 mm length < 30° angulation C/I ratio < 1	Division A root form
B	2.5–5 mm width >10–12 mm height > 15 mm length < 20 angulation C/I ratio < 1	Osteoplasty *Division A root form* Augmentation *Demanding esthetics* *Great force factors* Narrow implant *Division B root form* *Plate form*
C	Unfavorable in: Width C-w Height C-h Length Angulation C-a C/I ratio > 1	Osteoplasty (C-w) Augmentation *Fixed prosthesis* *Demanding esthetics* *Great force factors* Endosteal *Root form* *Ramus frame* Subperiosteal *Arch form* *Angulation* *Cost* *Time*
D	Severe atrophy Basal bone loss Flat maxilla Pencil mandible	Augmentation *Treatment of choice* Endosteal *Root form* *Ramus frame* Subperiosteal

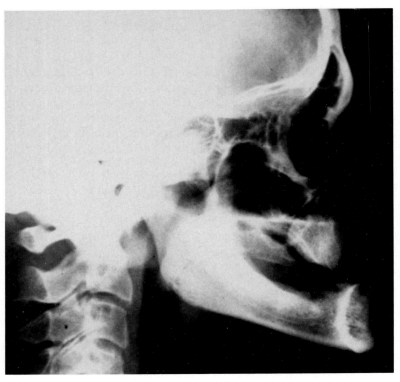

FIG 7–7.
Lateral cephalogram of a bone Division A mandible and maxilla.

Division A is most often restored with root form implants. A plate form implant has 1.5 times more surface area in contact with bone than a root form implant of similar height. However, for several reasons a root form implant is indicated over a plate form design (Table 7–2).

Stress distribution advantages of root forms include greater total surface area and implant diameter, and the design and density of surrounding bone. A plate form implant requires at least 15 to 20 mm of available bone in length for bone support, even in wide available bone. Two to four root form implants may be inserted in the same length. As a result, the overall surface area is greater with more than one root form implant (Fig 7–8). The greater the permucosal implant abutment and body diameter, the less stress transferred to the crestal surrounding bone, where implant bone loss is first observed. The diameter of a root form implant is approximately twice that of plate form implants and permits a dramatic decrease in crestal bone stress. Root form implants are in closer approximation and often engage the lateral cortical bone. This results in a greater amount of lamellar bone at the implant interface, bone bridging from trabecular bone to cortical bone, and an implant interface more stable to occlusal loads (Fig 7–9).

Prosthodontic-related advantages of root form implants compared with plate forms are listed in Table 7–2. Root form implants may provide independent support of a prosthesis or may be splinted to natural teeth and/or implants. Plate form implants must be joined to additional implants and/or teeth because they use the length of bone of two or more teeth for support. Neither a single plate nor root form implant should replace two or more teeth.

The greater diameter of the root form implant abutment permits better esthetics of the abutment crown. Root form implants have greater diameter abutments and compare more favorably to the 7- to 10-mm cervical diameter of a natural crown.

The root form systems provide a number of prosthodontic abutment options. Straight and angled abutments for cement or screw, attachment abutments, and custom cast abutments are a few examples. Plate form implants primarily have abutments for cement which are bent at the time of surgery, to be parallel to the natural teeth.

Uncemented or unretained screw prostheses are one of the three most common causes of prosthesis-related failure. The root form abutments provide greater retention and resistance than the smaller diameter plate form cement

TABLE 7–2.

Advantages of Root Form Implants Over Plate Forms in Division A Restorations

Stress distribution
   Greater surface area
   Greater post diameter
   Greater bone density
Prosthodontics
   Treatment options
   Esthetics
   Abutment designs
   Fewer pontics
   Greater retention
   Less fracture
Skill required
   Calibrated round drills
   No bending required
   Constant inserting angle
   Less modification of technique
Healing
   Insertion and crest of bone
   Preparation of bone

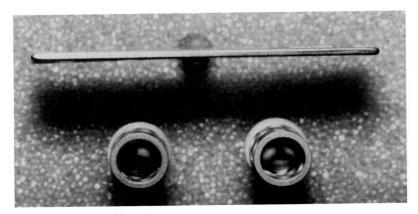

FIG 7–8.
Plate form implant requires 15 mm or more length for adequate surface area, even in Division A bone. Two or more root forms may be placed in an area of this size, which results in greater implant surface area.

abutments. The greater the abutment surface area, the greater the retention of the crown. Several root form abutments increase the number of retentive elements, compared with the one or two posts of the plate form design. The flexibility of a prosthesis increases relative to the cube of the distance between abutments. A fixed prosthesis with two pontics flexes 8 times more than a one pontic restoration. The additional root forms placed in an edentulous site decrease the number of pontics. A larger post diameter is also less likely to fracture under heavy loads or suffer from fatigue fracture under repeated lighter horizontal stresses.

The skill necessary to place root form implants is much less than to place a plate form implant. Root forms require a round osteotomy of specific depth, width, and angulation prepared with a series of calibrated rotating drills. Plate form implants need a free-hand osteotomy that often cannot be straight in length or angulation. The implant is then custom bent to follow the osteotomy and tapped into position. Placement of a root form implant requires less than half the time required for placement of a plate form implant. The plate form surgery not only requires more skill but may also present more complications that require modification of technique. As a result, more training and experience are necessary for placement of the plate form implant.

The root form implant may be inserted level or below the crest of the edentulous ridge. The neck of the plate form implant extends above the bone and is often exposed within the mouth during the healing phase. As a result, the plate form implant is more at risk from trauma during healing, which may cause movement at the bone-implant interface. If movement occurs, fibrous tissue and increased risk of mobility result. The root form implant may be prepared with a slow speed handpiece and a more controlled bone temperature. Plate form implant osteotomies require a higher speed drill, and the bone temperature increase is more variable.

In some cases the wide posterior ridge presents bone too soft to achieve initial stability of the root form implant upon initial insertion. In these rare circumstances, a Division A root form/plate form combination implant may be inserted. The combination implant provides extended length and surface area for improved primary stability.

The prosthetic options for Division A span the full gamut. An FP-1 restoration is more achievable with this ridge anatomy than any other division. However, an FP-2 prosthesis is often the result obtained in the anterior mandible, because osteoplasty is often required before the Division A width criterion is obtained. An FP-3 prosthesis is most often the option selected in the anterior Division A when the maxillary smiling lip position is high or a mandibular low lip line during speech exposes regions beyond the natural anatomic crown position. For RP-4 or RP-5 restorations in Division A, the final position of the tooth must be evaluated before designing the superstructure bar attachment. A limited intraoral space is more common in Division A and may contraindicate O-ring attachments or superstructures placed several millimeters above the tissue for hygiene considerations.

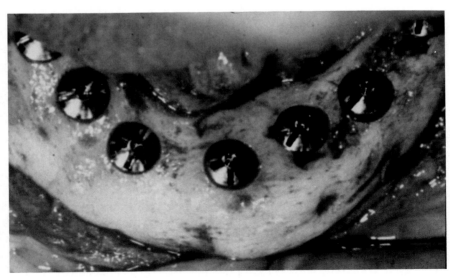

FIG 7–9.
Root forms placed in a Division A mandible.

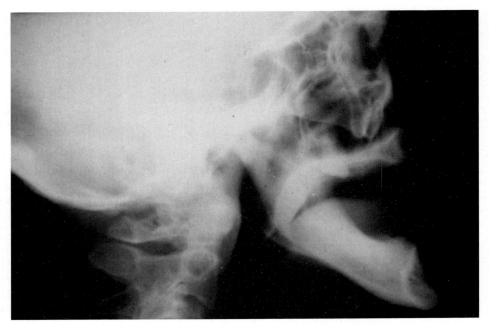

FIG 7–10.
Lateral cephalogram of a Division B maxilla and mandible.

Division B

As the bone resorbs, the width of available bone first decreases at the expense of the facial cortical plate. The cortical bone is thicker on the lingual aspect of the alveolar bone, especially in the maxilla. There is a 40% decrease in bone width within the first 1 to 3 years after tooth extraction.[13] As a result, the narrower ridge is often inadequate for most root form implants. Slight to moderate atrophy is often used to describe this clinical condition.

Division B offers sufficient available bone (see Table 7–1). The height of bone is at least 10 mm, as in Division A, but the bone width ranges from 2.5 to 5 mm (Fig 7–10). The length of available bone in the edentulous site should be greater than in Division A and at least 15 mm to ensure adequate surface area at the implant-bone interface, because the width is decreased. The body of the implant must bisect the bone angulation in the narrower ridge. A smaller diameter faciolingual implant abutment is used in the narrower bone, which increases the amount of stress at the permucosal implant bone interface. If a plate form design is selected, the implant neck may be bent at the time of surgery to compensate for lack of abutment parallelism. Plate form implants must be joined to additional implants and/or teeth, because they use the length of bone of two or more teeth for support. As a consequence, the bone angulation in this division is limited to

20 degrees, to prevent consequences of long-term fatigue fracture of bent metal or increased force from horizontal loads on narrower abutments. The crown-implant ratio is less than 1, to decrease the moment of the force within lateral or offset loads in Division B, especially because the abutment is smaller in diameter.

Three treatment options are available for the Division B edentulous ridge:

1. Modify the existing Division B ridge to another division by osteoplasty to permit the placement of root form implants
2. Insert a narrow plate or root form implant
3. Modify the existing Division B by augmentation

The most common approach is to modify the narrower Division B ridge to another bone division by osteoplasty. The edentulous ridge crest may be reduced, thereby increasing the width of the ridge. If the remaining height of available bone is not reduced below 10 mm and the crown-implant ratio is still less than 1, the ridge division is changed into a Division A with a width greater than 5 mm. If the ridge height is reduced below 10 mm or the crown-implant ratio is greater than 1, the division is not changed to a Division A. Instead, it has been altered to a Division C and is not as predictable for endosteal implant placement as Division A.

When a Division B ridge is changed to a Division A by osteoplasty procedures, the final prosthesis design has to compensate for the increased clinical crown height. For example, the restoring dentist may wish to fabricate a fixed prosthesis similar to a natural tooth–supported prosthesis (FP-1). Prior to surgery, the height of the remaining available bone may be at the proper vertical dimension for this prosthetic design. However, if at the time of surgery the ridge is found deficient in width for implant placement, an osteoplasty may be performed. In the anterior edentulous region it is not unusual to remove 3 to 6 mm before reaching a Division A width. This means the final restoration will require an additional 3 to 6 mm in height. Hence, it may result in an extended tooth or teeth and gingiva (FP-2, FP-3) restoration rather than the fixed porcelain to metal bridge originally planned (Fig 7–11).

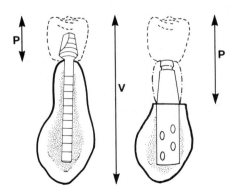

FIG 7–11.
Division B ridge may have a narrow implant and prosthesis that is closer to the anatomic crown (FP-1) *(left)*, or osteoplasty with Division A root forms and extended crown heights (FP-2 or FP-3) *(right)*.

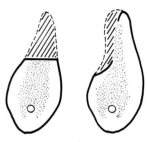

FIG 7–12.
Division B ridge may be converted to Division A by augmentation *(right)* or osteoplasty *(left)*. The augmentation requires 4 to 6 months, but can result in improved crown-implant ratio and more natural looking abutments. Implants may be placed at the same time as osteoplasty, but the crown-implant ratio is increased.

The second main treatment option for the Division B narrow available bone is the plate or small-diameter root form implant. The original plate form implants were designed for a soft tissue interface and slight clinical mobility.[14] The author coordinated a surgical and healing approach for direct bone interface and rigid fixation of plate form implants in 1983 (See Chapter 23).[15] This technique slightly modifies the surgical and healing approach established by Branemark for root form implants. A plate form multiple abutment design with greater abutment

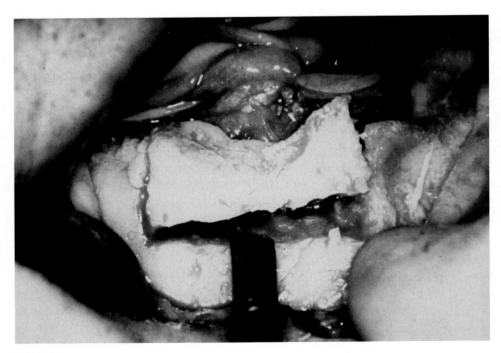

FIG 7–13.
Block osteoplasty is performed to convert the bone Division B to a bone Division A condition in the mandible. (Same patient as in Fig 7–10.)

length and width (Ultimatics) was designed for long-term rigid fixation in 1985 and further modified in 1988.

Smaller diameter root form implants are also designed for Division B. The overall surface area of a 3-mm-diameter implant is 30% to 40% less than the 3.75- to 4-mm root forms placed in Division A bone. In addition, greater stresses are transferred to the crestal bone. As a result, the angulation of bone for small diameter root forms should be less than 20 degrees, and more than one implant or natural teeth should be included in almost all prostheses that replace more than one tooth. These conditions are similar to plate form implants.

The third alternative to change the Division B ridge into a Division A consists of grafting the edentulous ridge with autogenous and/or demineralized freeze-dried bone (DFDB) and/or synthetic bone substitutes (Fig 7–12). If this graft is intended for implant placement, a healing period of at least 4 to 6 months is needed for maturation of the graft and before endosteal implants can be placed. A predictable Division B alloplastic augmentation technique in the anterior maxilla or mandible requires the periosteum not to be in contact with the graft. One technique is an intrapositioned graft. A narrow osteotomy is made between the bony plates, and bone spreaders are tapped into the edentulous site. The ridge may be increased to 6 mm using this technique. The expanded osteotomy is then filled with autogenous material and/or DFDB and the tissue approximated. Four to 6 months later the site may be treated as Division A bone. The success of

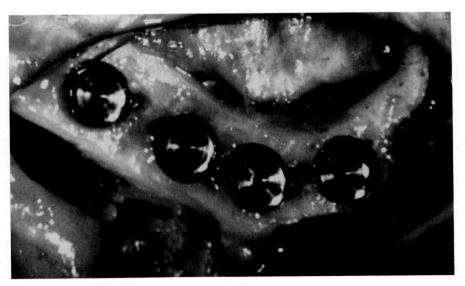

FIG 7–14.
Series of anterior root forms are placed in the converted Division A mandible.

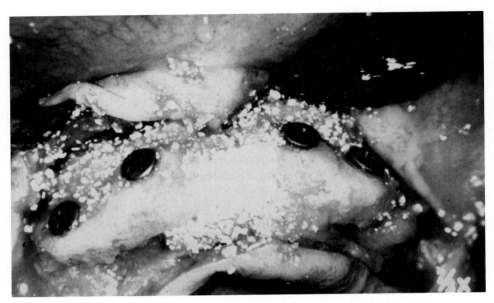

FIG 7–15.
Blocks of bone harvested from the anterior mandible are fixed on the labial aspect of the Division B maxilla with DFDB and calcium phosphate to augment the width to Division A.

alloplastic materials for augmentation correlates with the number of osseous walls in contact with the material. Hence a socket with five walls heals with bone at a much faster and predictable rate than an onlay graft.

If the ridge contour should be altered for improved prosthodontic relationships, an onlay graft of autogenous bone is indicated. The graft may be harvested from the mental protuberance and placed along the lateral aspect of the ridge that corresponds to ideal arch form. Division A root form implants may be placed 4 months after the block membranous bone graft (Figs 7–13 to 7–15).

An alternative approach of augmentation uses guided tissue regeneration concepts. The tissue barrier is placed over the grafted bone and prevents the soft tissue from invading the implant or onlay graft. These materials improve DFDB onlay attempts at augmentation. The implant should be placed after the augmentation process to permit ideal implant placement and to ensure complete bone formation before placing the implant, because the crest of bone usually determines implant health in the long term.

The prosthetic options for Division B require more planning than those for the previous bone category. An FP-1 prosthesis usually requires the combination of augmentation and root form implant, or a smaller diameter implant and modified ridge lap crown, or a smaller diameter implant and dense hydroxylapatite (HA) to augment the facial aspect of the ridge to decrease the overcontouring of the cervical region of the crown. An FP-3 restoration may be required if the patient has a high maxillary smile lip line or low mandibular speech lip position. Removable prostheses (RP-4, RP-5) usually require osteoplasty and Division A root form implants. When a complete removable prosthesis is selected with plate form implants, an RP-4 treatment plan (totally implant support overdenture) is indicated. An RP-5 overdenture with anterior plate form(s) is usually contraindicated, because the moment of force overstresses the permucosal posts, implant interface, or both.

The surgical options of osteoplasty, augmentation, or smaller diameter implants as plate form implants are most frequently influenced by the final prosthesis design. An FP-3 or RP-5 prosthesis usually requires osteoplasty, whereas an FP-1 often mandates ridge augmentation.

Division C

The resorption of the available bone occurs first in bone width, and then in height. As a result, the Division B ridge continues to resorb in width and becomes

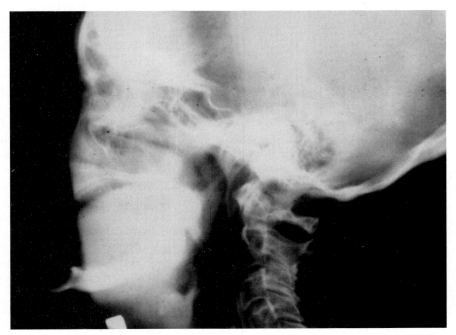

FIG 7–16.
Lateral cephalogram of a bone Division C-a anterior mandible.

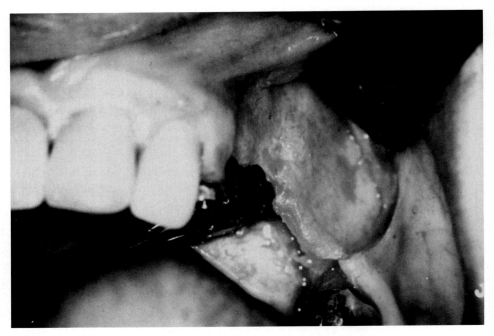

FIG 7–17.
Maxillary canine and premolar region demonstrates bone Division C-w. A fixed prosthesis is desired.

inadequate for endosteal implants. This process continues, and the available bone is then reduced in height. Once the alveolar bone is reduced in height, the basal bone usually begins to decrease in width, followed by a decrease in height. Moderate to advanced atrophy may be used to describe the clinical conditions of Division C. The floor of the mouth is often level with the residual crest of the ridge. During swallowing, the floor of the mouth may prolapse over the residual crest and implant sites, causing constant irritation of the permucosal posts and impairing proper design of the superstructures.

The Division C available bone is deficient in one or more dimensions (width, length, height, angulation, or crown-implant ratio) (see Table 7–1). Therefore, the width may be less than 2.5 mm even after osteoplasty, the height less than 8 mm in the atrophic anterior mandible or 10 mm in most other areas, or the angulation greater than 30 degrees regardless of the position of the implant body into the edentulous site.

The Division C edentulous ridge does not offer as many elements for predictable endosteal implant survival or prosthodontic management compared with Divisions A or B. Anatomic landmarks to determine implant position are usually not present; thus, greater surgical skill is required. The doctor and patient should realize that Division C ridge implant–supported prostheses are more complex and are slightly less predictable in healing, prosthetic design, or long-term maintenance. However, the patient usually is in greater need for

increased prosthodontic support. Therefore treatment plans are often warranted, because the benefits outweigh the risks.

The edentulous site may be deficient in one or more anatomic dimensions. There are two common subcategories of Division C: a ridge with inadequate width, or Division C-w; and a potential implant site with inadequate height or Division C-h, which usually denotes more overall resorption than in C-w. In addition, the crown-implant ratio is greater than 1. The posterior maxilla or mandible are the most common examples of this condition, because the maxillary sinus or mandibular canal limit vertical height sooner than in the anterior regions.

There is one uncommon subcategory of Division C, namely C-a. In this category, available bone is adequate in height and width, but angulation is greater than 30 degrees regardless of implant placement. This condition is most often observed in the anterior mandible or maxilla (Fig 7–16).

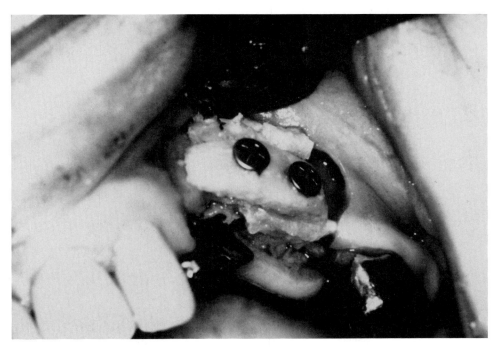

FIG 7–18.
Block of membranous bone harvested from the symphysis is fixated to the lateral aspect of the C-w maxilla.

There are four treatment options for Bone Divisions C. These include osteoplasty, root form implants, subperiosteal implants, and augmentation procedures. These methods of treatment require greater skill than similar treatment methods in Division A or B.

A C-w ridge may be treated by osteoplasty or augmentation. An osteoplasty converts the ridge to a width suitable for root forms. The most common available bone division after osteoplasty of C-w is C-h available bone, not Division A, because the crown-implant ratio becomes greater than 1. Augmentation of C-w is most often used when prosthetic guidelines require a FP-1 restoration or excess force factors require greater surface area of implants or improved biomechanics of the prosthesis (Figs 7–17 to 7–19).

The Division C-h available bone may be restored in several ways. Endosteal implants, subperiosteal implants, or ridge augmentation combined with endosteal implants are the three most common options. When endosteal root form implants shorter than 10 mm are used in Division C-h bone, additional implants should be placed to increase the overall implant-bone surface area and the prosthesis should load the implants in a vertical direction (Figs 7–20 and 21). Another option is to design prostheses with stress relief, because the crown-implant ratio is greater than 1. Reduced long-term predictability is expected if additional implants or less stressful prosthesis are not used, because a greater moment force is transmitted to the implants with the increased crown height and decreased surface area of support (Fig 7–22).

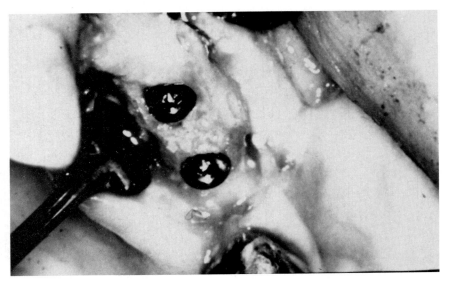

FIG 7–19.
Two root form implants placed in the augmented ridge site 4 months after augmentation.

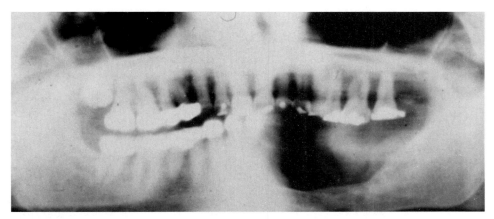

FIG 7–20.
Panoramic radiograph of a bone Division C-h posterior mandible.

An alternative to endosteal implants in the partially or completely edentulous Division C-h arch is the subperiosteal implant (Figs 7–23 and 24). The permucosal posts may be designed and cast at almost any angulation necessary for proper prosthodontic reconstruction. This implant may be fabricated from a direct bone impression or from a model obtained from computer generated (computed tomographic) scanning systems. This implant modality is more predictable in the mandibular arch.

Subperiosteal implants may be indicated as a result of anatomy, cost, time, or decreased surgical risk. The superstructure and abutment posts for the subperiosteal implant are designed and cast before implant placement. The permucosal

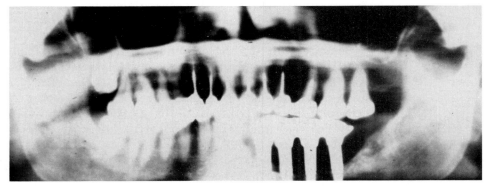

FIG 7–21.
Three-year postoperative panoramic radiograph of the final prosthesis, which is loaded only in a vertical direction to the implants.

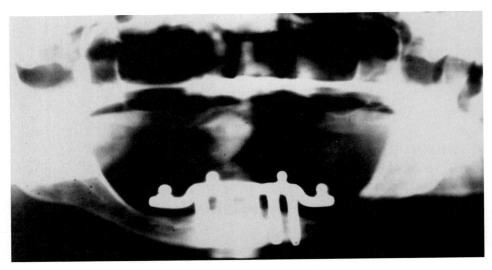

FIG 7–22.
Removable implant-supported prosthesis (RP-4) is designed for bone Division C-h rather than a fixed restoration. The restoration may be removed at night to reduce parafunction and decrease stress to the implant system.

posts may be positioned with greater latitude than endosteal implants. As such, when anterior angulation is unfavorable, the abutments of root form implants may be positioned too far lingual for prosthodontic support, speech, and/or hygiene (Fig 7–25).

A square arch form may not permit a superstructure to be cantilevered to the distal when anterior root forms are placed. An RP-4 prosthesis is contraindicated with root forms in a square arch form with only anterior support. A subperiosteal implant provides anterior and posterior bone support, and the square arch form does not affect an RP-4 prosthesis.

The doctor's cost for the subperiosteal implant is less than for root forms to support the same RP-4 prosthesis. Five root forms are usually required in Division C for an RP-4 implant-supported removable prosthesis. The implants, abutments, impression transfers, screws, and construction of the mesobar are more than twice the cost of a subperiosteal implant that already includes the superstructure.

The overall treatment time required for subperiosteal implants and root forms also differs. Endosteal implants require 3 to 4 months to osteointegrate, and six appointments are required to fabricate a mesobar and final prosthesis over an additional 2 to 4 months based on bone density. A subperiosteal implant and prosthesis may be completed within 2 months, although a regular diet is delayed until several months later.

Endosteal implants placed in the posterior Division C mandible require

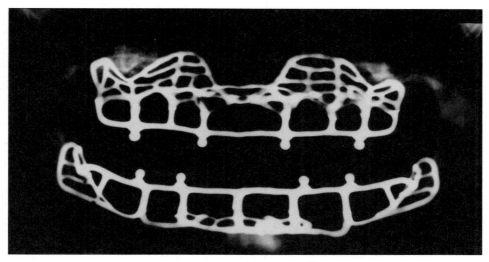

FIG 7–23.
Maxillary and mandibular complete subperiosteal implants include the superstructure for the RP-4 prosthesis.

autogenous grafts and/or nerve repositioning. The increase in treatment time, surgical risks and postoperative complications (such as paresthesia) are to be thoroughly discussed with the patient. Circumferential or unilateral subperiosteal implants permit the placement of posterior prosthodontic units without risks of paresthesia from nerve repositioning or lengthened treatment time associated with autogenous bone grafts and endosteal implants.

Additional training is required for subperiosteal implants. Direct bone impressions or computed tomography, implant designs, and laboratory fabrica-

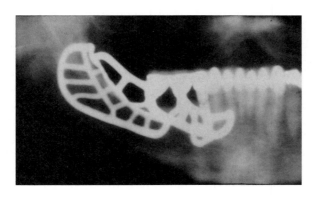

FIG 7–24.
Unilateral superiosteal implant in the posterior bone Division C-h mandible, joined to a root form implant in the first premolar, with an independent fixed prosthesis.

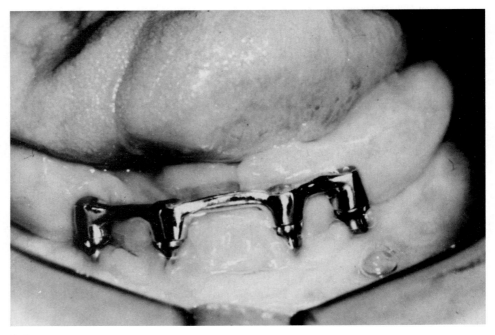

FIG 7–25.
Root form implants placed in a bone Division C-a may result in too lingual placement. Prosthodontic support, speech, and hygiene are compromised.

tion require specific techniques not used in any other implant modality. The overall implant survival may be greater for Division C bone with subperiosteal implants. However, soft tissue complications are more common.

In general, implants placed in Division C edentulous arches should receive additional prosthodontic consideration gained from splinting additional implants or teeth, cross-arch stabilization, stress equalizers, opposing a removable prosthesis, or a combination. Treating the Division C ridge requires more experience, caution, and training than the previous two divisions; however, excellent results may be achieved.

Another treatment option is to alter the Division C with autogenous, demineralized, or resorbable synthetic bone, or a combination of these, in order to upgrade the division and place endosteal implants. Use of autogenous bone for this procedure is more predictable in the Division C arch. After the ridge is augmented, it is treated with the options available in the acquired division. The patient who desires a fixed prosthesis, with a conventional fixed appearance (FP-1) often requires an autogenous graft for lip support, ideal crown height, and restored vertical dimension in the anterior edentulous arch (Figs 7–26 to 7–28). An alternative method of treatment in Division C arches is to change the division with nonresorbable HA. This treatment option is often indicated for a traditional maxillary denture with a limited premaxilla support. Rarely is nonresorbable augmentation material used for additional support for a mandibular denture or used for endosteal implant support.

In conclusion, the final prosthesis often determines the treatment option. For mandibular RP-4 restorations, a subperiosteal implant or five root forms may be used. An RP-5 prosthesis may be fabricated with anterior root form implants. Augmentation is often required for a fixed prosthesis if stress cannot be reduced.

Division D

The long-term bone-resorption process may result in complete alveolar process loss accompanied by basal bone atrophy. Severe atrophy describes the clinical condition of the Division D ridge. Basal bone loss results in a completely flat maxilla or pencil-thin mandible. Resorption of the nasal spine and the palate to the level of the zygomatic arch may have occurred in the maxilla. The mandibular arch presents with mental foramina and portions of the mandibular

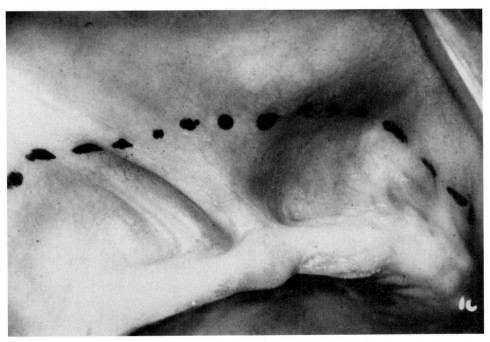

FIG 7–26.
C-w edentulous premaxilla. The patient desires a fixed prosthesis.

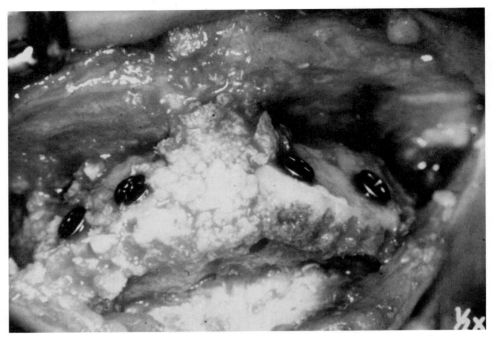

FIG 7–27.
An autogenous iliac crest bone graft is placed on the anterior maxilla. Bilateral subantral augmentations were also performed in the posterior maxilla.

canal dehiscent. Therefore it is not infrequent that these patients complain of paresthesia of the lower lip, especially during mastication. In the mandible, the superior genial tubercles are the most superior aspect of the ridge. The mentalis muscle has lost much of its attachment and the inferior portion attaches near the crest of the resorbed ridge. The buccinator muscle may approach the mylohyoid muscle above the body of the mandible. The crown-implant ratio is greater than 5 (Fig 7–29).

The completely edentulous Division D patient is the most difficult to treat in implant dentistry. Benefits must carefully be weighed against the risks. Although the practitioner and patient often regard this condition as the most drastic possible, these patients do not usually have oral antral fistulae or deviated facial features. If implant failure occurs, the patient may become a dental cripple, unable to wear any prosthesis. Therefore, autogenous bone grafts to upgrade the division are strongly recommended prior to any implant treatment initiated. Once autogenous grafts are in place and allowed to heal for 6 months, endosteal or subperiosteal implants may be inserted, depending on the division of bone obtained (Figs 7–30 and 7–31).

The autogenous grafts are not intended for improved denture support. If soft tissue–borne prostheses are fabricated on autogenous grafts, 90% of the grafted bone resorbs within 5 years as a consequence of accelerated resorption.[16] Additional augmentation to compensate for this resorption is not indicated. Repeated relines, highly mobile tissue, sore spots, and patient frustration are a consequence. Autogenous bone grafts in conjunction with implant placement are maintained long term.

A patient classified as maxillary posterior Division D who has healthy anterior teeth and/or implants may undergo graft procedures with a combination of local autogenous bone, DFDB, and calcium phosphate bone substitutes. Sinus elevation and subantral augmentation are usually indicated, because the interarch space is rarely sufficient for onlay grafts and endosteal implants of adequate height. After 8 to 10 months, the Division D posterior maxilla has usually been improved to Division A, and root form implants may be inserted for posterior prosthodontic support.

The completely flat maxilla may also be augmented with DFDB and HA to improve the division. A conventional denture may then be fabricated with improved support. However, because no ridge form exists to guide the placement

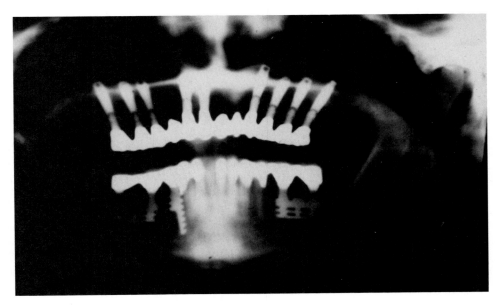

FIG 7–28.
Anterior and posterior root forms are placed after healing and after rigid fixation was fabricated in the maxilla. The mandible had posterior Division B and plate form implants inserted. These were joined to the teeth after healing and rigid fixation for a fixed prosthesis.

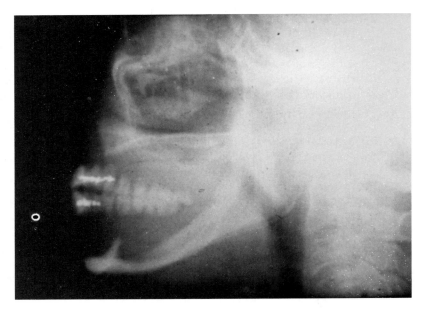

FIG 7–29.
Lateral cephalogram of a patient with Division D mandible. The genial tubercle is the most superior aspect of the anterior mandible. The crown-implant ratio is greater than 5.

of the material, migration of the graft at the time of surgery, or in the future after healing, is a more frequent sequel.

Past beliefs regarding subperiosteal implants indicated their use on atrophied bone over any other type of implant support and that the less bone available, the more ideal the indication for a subperiosteal implant. On the contrary, adequate bone should also be present for this implant modality. The maxilla rarely provides enough support in the Division D ridge for a subperiosteal or root form implants of any design. If adequate mandibular anterior bone is present, root form implants, tripodal subperiosteal implants, or ramus frame implants may be used cautiously in the edentulous mandible. However, idiopathic fracture during surgery, or from implant failure and/or removal, is a more likely complication than in other divisions. Hence, practitioners who treat Division D mandibles should be able to manage complications, which may be extensive.

Endosteal root form implants without autogenous grafts may be used on occasion in the anterior Division D mandible when the remaining bone is dense and the opposing arch is preferably edentulous. Care must be taken during placement, because mandibular fracture at insertion or during postoperative healing is a significant complication. The crown-implant ratio may be greater than

5 to 1, and the number of implants four or less. An RP-5 removable restoration is usually indicated for these conditions, in spite of atrophic masticatory muscles and reduced occlusal force.

The Division D arch requires more training to treat, and results in more frequent long-term complications. Thus treatment options include a guarded prognosis and are offered in situations that can tolerate failure without devastating results. The choice to render treatment is the doctor's, not the patient's. Do not compromise the implant-support approach when implant failure results in significant risks.

SUMMARY

In implant dentistry the type of prosthesis that will obtain optimal results and satisfy the patient's needs and desires is first determined. This may range from a completely fixed prosthesis to one with primarily soft tissue support. Once the final prosthesis has been decided, the number and location of abutments necessary to satisfy prosthodontic requirements can be established. The primary determinant in the selection of the type, number, and location of the implant

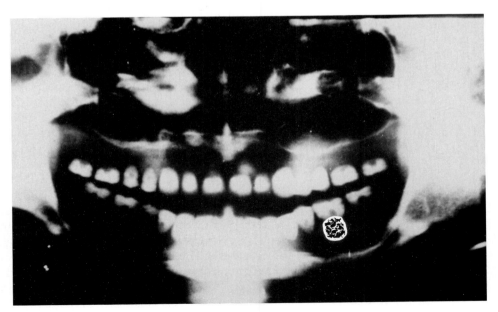

FIG 7–30.
Panoramic radiograph of a Division D mandible in a patient desiring a fixed prosthesis.

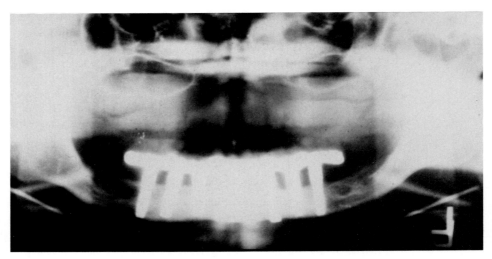

FIG 7–31.
Two-year postoperative radiograph shows formation of new mental foramina, seven root form implants, and a fixed prosthesis.

abutment is the amount of available bone. The author and Judy[6-8] have developed four divisions of available bone, based on the width, height, length, angulation, and crown-implant ratio of the bone in the edentulous site. Once the bone division has been determined, consistent implant treatment plan procedures elaborated for each category may be followed.

The Division A edentulous ridge offers abundant bone in all dimensions. Root form implants are optimally utilized as independent support for the prosthesis, although rigid connection to healthy natural teeth is often indicated. Division B provides adequate width for narrower plate form or small-diameter root form endosteal implants. The decreased width and surface area usually requires splinting teeth or other implants in the related final prosthesis. The second option for Division B is to change the condition to a Division A by augmentation or osteoplasty. Root form implants may then be used. The edentulous ridge with moderate resorption and limited elements for predictable endosteal implants is Division C. The decision to restore with additional endosteal implants, to use subperiosteal implants, or to upgrade by augmentation before implant placement is influenced by the prosthesis. The Division D edentulous ridge corresponds to basal bone loss and severe atrophy, resulting in dehiscent mandibular canals or a completely flat maxilla. The patient often requires augmentation with autogenous bone before implant prosthodontic reconstruction.

After the available bone is determined in the regions where prosthetic abutments are needed, the type and conditions of implant design are related to the original concept of prosthesis design. If conditions do not exist for a predictable end result, the patient's mind or mouth must be modified. For example, the expectations of the patient must be reduced so the prosthesis may be changed from FP-1 to FP-3 or RP-4, or the bone must be augmented to improve the height and width and change the division so that implant support and prosthetic design will be harmonious.

REFERENCES

1. Misch CE, Judy KWM: Patient dental-medical implant evaluation form. International Congress of Oral Implant, 1987.
2. Greenfield EJ: Implantation of artificial crown and bridge abutments, *Dent Cosmos* 55:364–369, 1913.
3. Weiss CM, Judy KWM: Severe mandibular atrophy: biological considerations of routine treatment with complete subperiosteal implants, *J Oral Implant* 4:431–469, 1974.
4. Kent JN: Correction of alveolar ridge deficiencies with non-resorbable hydroxyapatite, *J Am Dent Assoc* 105:99–100, 1982.
5. Zarb G, Leckholm U: Tissue integrated prostheses. In Branemark PI, editor: Chicago, 1985, Quintessence, pp 199–209.
6. Misch CE: Treatment planning and implant dentistry (abst). Misch Implant Institute, 1985.
7. Misch CE, Judy KWM: Classification of partially edentulous arches for implant dentistry, *Int J Oral Implant* 4:7–12, 1987.
8. Misch CE: Available bone influences prosthodontic treatment, *Dent Today* February 1988, pp 44, 75.
9. Misch CE: Divisions of available bone in implant dentistry, *Int J Oral Implant* 7:9–17, 1990.
10. Branemark PI: Osseointegration and its experimental background, *J Prosthet Dent* 50:399–410, 1983.
11. Misch CE: Bone character: second vital implant criterion, *Dent Today* June/July 1988, pp 39–40.
12. Misch CE: Density of bone: effect on treatment plans, surgical approach, healing and progressive bone loading, *Int J Oral Implant* 6:23–31, 1990.
13. Pietrokowski J: The bony residual ridge in man, *J Prosthet Dent* 34:456–462, 1975.
14. Linkow L: The multipurpose Blade-Vent implant, *Dent Dig* 1967.
15. Misch CE: Osteointegration and the submerged Blade implant, *J Houston District Dent Assoc* January 1988, pp 12–16.
16. Wang JH, Eaite DE, Steinhauser E: Ridge augmentation: an evaluation and follow-up report, *J Oral Surg* 34:600–602, 1976.

Chapter 8

Dental Evaluation: Factors of Force

Carl E. Misch

Several elements observed during the dental evaluation may be the source of additional forces on implant abutments. The implant-bone interface and the stability of the prosthetic connection are affected by these additional loads. These increased forces must be accounted for in the treatment planning and in the design of the final prosthesis.

Stress is a particular entity that is expressed as *force*. As a result, any dental influence that increases force magnifies the stress. The amount of force variation from one individual to another is easier to appreciate than the area over which the force is transmitted. Dental factors that affect stress primarily include

1. Parafunction
2. The position of the abutment in the arch
3. Masticatory dynamics
4. The nature of the opposing arch
5. The direction of load forces
6. Crown-implant ratio
7. The density of bone

These conditions are first discussed; their management is then addressed.

FACTORS CREATING STRESS

Normal Bite Force

The origin of the forces naturally occurring on the teeth were described by Picton et al.[1, 2] The greatest natural forces exerted against teeth, and thus against implants, occur during mastication. These forces are primarily directed perpendicular to the occlusal plane in the posterior region, are of short duration, occur only during brief periods of the day, and range from 5 to 44 lb for natural teeth. The actual force on each tooth during function has been recorded on strain gauges in inlays.[3] A force of 28 psi was needed to chew a raw carrot, and 21 psi to chew meat.[1] The actual time during which chewing forces are applied on the teeth is about 9 minutes each day. The perioral musculature and tongue exert a more constant, yet lighter, horizontal force on the teeth or on implants. These forces reach as high as 3 to 5 lb during swallowing. A person swallows 25 times per hour while awake, and 10 times per hour while sleeping, or a total of 480 times each day.[4] Therefore the bite forces against the teeth are less than 30 psi and for less than 30 minutes for all normal forces of deglutition and mastication (Table 8–1).

The maximum bite force differs from mastication force, varies widely among individuals, and depends on the state of the dentition and masticatory musculature. There have been many attempts to quantify the normal maximum bite force. In 1681 Borelli suspended weights on a thread over the molars while the mandible was open. The maximum load recorded for which the person was still able to close ranged from 132 to 440 lb. A force of 165 lb was recorded on a gnathodynamometer, the first instrument to record occlusal force, which was developed by Patrick and Dennis in 1892. G.V. Black further improved this early design and recorded average forces of approximately 170 lb.[5] More recent studies indicate vertical biting forces can range from 45 to 550 lb.[6] The forces on the chewing side and the opposite side appear very similar in amplitude.[7]

TABLE 8–1.

Normal Forces Exerted on Teeth

Bite forces
  Perpendicular to occlusal plane
  Short duration
  Brief total period (9 min/d)
  Force on each tooth: 20 to 30 psi
  Maximum bite force: 50 to 500 psi
Perioral forces
  More constant
  Lighter
  Horizontal
  Maximum when swallowing (3 to 5 psi)
  Brief total swallow time (20 min/d)

Parafunction

Parafunctional forces on teeth or implants are represented by repeated or sustained occlusion and have long been recognized as harmful to the stomatognathic system.[8, 9] The most common cause of implant bone loss or lack of rigid fixation during the first year after implant treatment, is the result of parafunction. These implant-related conditions occur with greater frequency in the maxilla because of decrease in bone density and increase in the moment force. The lack of rigid fixation during healing is primarily a result of parafunction of soft tissue–borne prostheses overlying the submerged implant. Hence, the presence of these conditions must be carefully noted in implant dentistry.

Nadler has classified the causes of parafunction or nonfunctional tooth contact into six categories[10]:

1. Local
2. Systemic
3. Psychological
4. Occupational
5. Involuntary
6. Voluntary

Local factors include tooth form or occlusion, as well as soft tissue changes such as ulcerations or pericoronitis. Systemic factors include cerebral palsy, epilepsy, and drug-related dyskinesia. Psychological causes occur with the greatest frequency and include the release of emotional tension or anxiety. Occupational factors concern professionals such as dentists, athletes, and precision workers, as well as the seamstress or musician who develops altered oral habits. The fifth cause of parafunctional force is involuntary movement that provokes bracing of the jaws, such as during lifting of heavy objects or sudden stops while driving. Voluntary causes include chewing gum or pencils, bracing the telephone between the head and shoulder, and pipe smoking.

Bruxism

Bruxism is the vertical and horizontal, nonfunctional grinding of teeth. The forces involved are in excess of normal physiologic masticatory loads (up to 1,000 psi). Bruxism may affect teeth, muscles, joints, or all three. These forces may occur while the patient is awake or asleep, and may generate several hours per day of increased force upon the teeth. Bruxism is the most common oral habit.[11] The maximum biting force of bruxers is usually greater than average. A 37-year-old patient with a long history of bruxism recorded a force of more than 990 psi.[12]

Bruxism does not represent a contraindication for implants, but does influence treatment planning. The first step is to recognize the condition before the treatment is rendered. Many clinical signs warn of excessive grinding. The occurrence of nonfunctional wear facets on the occlusal surfaces may occur on both natural or replacement posterior teeth. Attrition of anterior teeth appear on the incisal edge and there may be notching of the cingulum. It is most significant when found in the posterior region when posterior implants will be placed. Posterior wear patterns are more difficult to manage, because greater forces are generated in this area. Consequently, the occlusal plane, the anterior incisal guidance, or both may need modification to eliminate all posterior contacts during mandibular excursions. Isolated anterior wear is not as much of a concern if all posterior teeth contacts can be eliminated in excursions, because lesser forces are generated in absence of posterior contacts.[13, 14]

The muscles of mastication may be tender to palpation and have undergone hypertrophy in the bruxing patient. The masseter and temporalis muscles are easily examined at the initial appointment. Hyperactive muscles are not always tender to palpation, but tender muscles in the absence of trauma or disease are a sign of excess use or incoordination between muscle groups. The lateral pterygoid muscle is always overused by the bruxing patient but is difficult to palpate. The ipsilateral medial pterygoid muscle provides more reliable information in this region. It acts as the antagonist to the lateral pterygoid in hyperfunction and, when tender, provides a good indicator of overuse of the lateral pterygoid.[15]

Muscle evaluation for bruxism also includes deviation on opening the jaw, limited opening, and tenderness of the temporomandibular joint. Limited opening is easily evaluated. The normal opening should be at least 38 to 40 mm from the maxillary incisal edge to the mandibular incisal edge in an Angle Class I patient. If any horizontal overjet or overlap exists, its value in millimeters is subtracted from the 40-mm minimum opening measurement.[16] The range of opening without regard for overlap or overjet has been measured to be 38.74 to 65 mm for men and 36.67 to 60.45 mm for women, from incisal edge to edge.[17]

Increased mobility of teeth may be an indication of a force beyond physiological limits, bone loss, or their combination. This not only requires further investigation in regard to bruxism, but is also very important if the implant may be joined to the teeth within the prosthesis. Fremitus, a vibration type of mobility of a tooth, is often present in the bruxing patient. To evaluate this condition, the dentist's finger barely contacts the facial surface of one posterior tooth at a time, while the patient taps the teeth together. Fremitus is symptomatic of the local excess occlusal loads. Tooth sensitivity to cold is also a consequence of bruxism.

Cervical erosion is a sign of parafunctional bruxism. In the past, G.V. Black analyzed the eight most popular theories for gingival ditching of the teeth, finding all inconclusive. This observation has frequently been called "tooth brush abrasion." McCoy has reported this condition on every other tooth, only one tooth, and even the teeth of some animals. Bruxism was the common link between patients presenting with this condition.[18] The notched appearance of the cervical

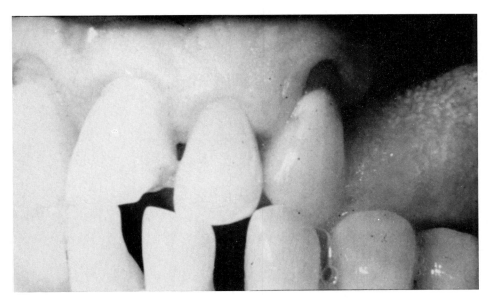

FIG 8–1.
Cervical erosion of the maxillary right central incisor and left canine. Patient also demonstrates unilateral posterior tongue thrust when swallowing.

portion of the tooth directly correlates with the concentration of forces shown in three-dimensional finite analysis[19] and photoelasticity studies (Fig. 8–1).[20] Other signs of fatigue encountered in bruxing patients include occlusal invaginations, stress lines in enamel, stress lines in alloy restorations (lines of Luder), and material fatigue (Figs 8–2 through 8–4). A study of a noninstitutionalized elderly population revealed that cervical abrasion was present in 56% of the participants.[21] Fremitus can be noticed clinically on many cervically eroded, nonmobile teeth. Not all gingival erosions are caused by bruxism. However, when present, the occlusion should be carefully evaluated, as well as other signs of excess force. If excessive forces appear to be the cause, the condition is referred to as McCoy notches or cervical abfraction.

Clenching

Clenching is the force exerted from one occlusal surface to the other without any movement. The forces on the teeth and implant abutments that result are similar to bruxism in amount and duration; however, several conditions differ in clenching from other parafunctions. The forces are directed more vertically to the plane of occlusion, at least in the posterior regions of the mouth. Wearing of the teeth is not likely; therefore, clenching often escapes notice during the intraoral

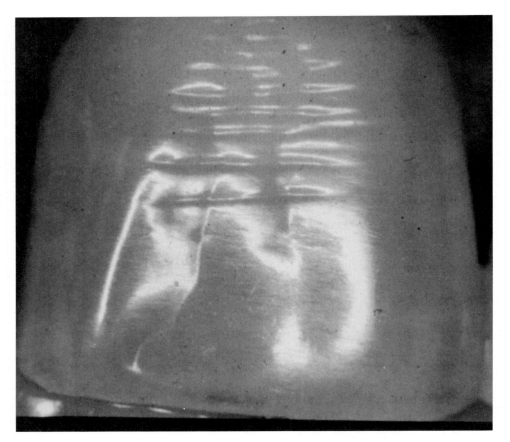

FIG 8–2.
Stress lines in the enamel of a patient who demonstrates parafunction.

examination. However, tooth mobility and/or greater temperature sensitivity, muscle tenderness and/or hypertrophy, deviation upon opening, limited opening, stress lines in enamel, McCoy notches, and material fatigue are all associated clinical signs. In addition, a common clinical finding is a scalloped border of the tongue (Fig 8–5). The tongue is often braced against the lingual surfaces of the teeth during clenching, exerting lateral pressures and resulting in the scalloped border.

Tongue Thrust and Size

Parafunctional tongue thrust is the unnatural force of the tongue against the teeth during swallowing.[22] A force of approximately 41 to 709 g/cm^2 on the anterior and lateral areas of the palate has been recorded during swallowing.[23] In orthodontic movement, a few grams of constant force are sufficient to displace teeth. Eight different types of tongue thrust have been identified; anterior, posterior unilateral, and posterior bilateral are the most common.

Although the force of tongue thrust is of lesser intensity than in other parafunctional forces, it is horizontal in nature, and can increase stress at the pergingival site of the implant. In addition, it can lead to tooth movement or mobility, which is of consequence when joined to implants in the same prosthesis. If the natural teeth were lost as a result of an aberrant tongue position or movement, the implant is at risk during initial healing and early prosthetic loading.

To evaluate this condition, the doctor holds the lower lip down and asks the patient to swallow. A patient with an anterior tongue thrust is not able to create the vacuum needed to swallow, if a seal is not achieved with the lower lip. A posterior tongue thrust is evaluated by retracting one cheek at a time away from the posterior teeth with a mirror or tongue blade, and asking the patient to swallow. Visual evidence of the tongue during deglutition may also be accompanied by pressure against the instrument, and confirms a lateral force.

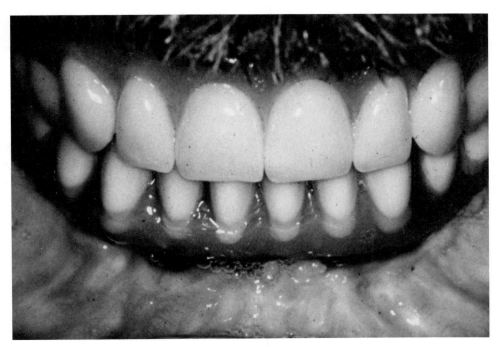

FIG 8–3.
Material fatigue evident on cervical of mandibular FP-3 implant prosthesis. The maxillary arch also has an FP-3 implant–supported restoration.

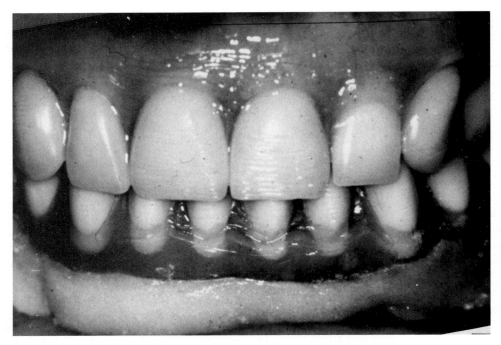

FIG 8–4.
Patient in Figure 8–3 2 years later shows signs of material fatigue from parafunction in the maxilla and mandible. Five implant abutments in the mandible were fractured at the cervical margin, and the restoration has a temporary soft liner.

The size of the tongue may increase with the loss of teeth. The tongue often accommodates the available space. As a result, a patient not wearing a mandibular denture often presents with a larger than normal tongue. The placement of implants and prosthetic teeth in such a patient results with an increase in lateral force, which may be continuous. In addition, the patient complains of inadequate room for the tongue, and may bite it during function. The lingual cusp of the restored mandibular posterior teeth should follow the curve of Wilson and include proper horizontal overjet to protect the tongue during occlusion.

Position Within the Arch

The maximum biting force is greater in the molar region and decreases as measurements progress anteriorly. Forces in the anterior incisor region correspond to approximately 35 to 50 psi; those in the canine region range from 47 to 100 psi; whereas those in the molar area vary from 127 to 250 psi.[6] Mansour et al. evaluated occlusal forces and moments mathematically using a Class III lever arm, the condyles being the fulcrum and the masseter and temporalis muscles supplying the force.[24] The force at the second molar was 10% higher than at the first molar, indicative of a range from 140 to 275 psi. The anterior biting force is decreased in the absence of posterior tooth contact and greater in the presence of posterior occlusion or eccentric contacts.[13, 14]

Masticatory Dynamics

Masticatory muscle dynamics are responsible for the amount of force exerted on the implant system. The force is related to the amount of function. For example, chewing paraffin wax for 1 hour each day for 1 month can increase the biting force in men from 118 lb to 140 lb. Eskimos, whose diets include extremely tough substances, reached values of about 300 lb maximum force.[25] Parafunctional bruxism or clenching often lead to hypertrophy of the muscles of mastication and increased force. Large athletic men can generate greater forces; patients of weak physical condition often develop less force than athletic patients. In general, the

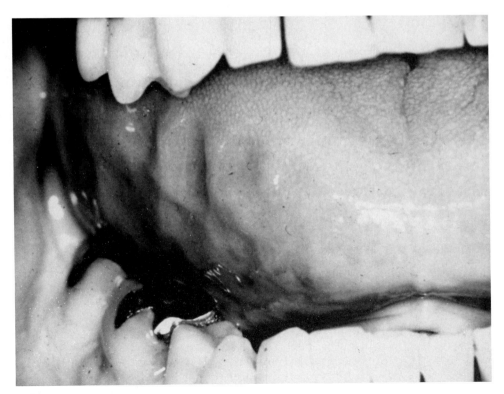

FIG 8–5.
Scalloped tongue border is a common observation in patients who have clenched the teeth for extended periods.

forces recorded in women are 20 lb less than those in men. Older patients record lower bite force than young adults. In addition, the younger patient needs the additional implant support for the prosthesis for a longer period of time. An 80-year-old patient will need implant support for far fewer years than one 20 years old, all other factors equal.

The maximum bite force decreases as muscle atrophy progresses throughout years of edentulousness. A maximum force of 5 lb may be the result of 30 years without natural teeth.[26] This force may increase 300% in the 3 years following implant placement.[27] Therefore sex, muscle mass, exercise, diet, state of the dentition, physical status, and age may all influence muscle strength, masticatory dynamics, and therefore maximum bite force.

Opposing Arch

Natural teeth transmit greater forces through occlusal contacts than do complete dentures. The maximum occlusal force of patients with complete dentures ranges from 5 to 26 lb.[26] The force is usually greater in recent denture wearers, and decreases with time. Muscle atrophy, thinning of the oral tissues with age or disease, and bone atrophy often occur in the edentulous patient as a function of time. Partial denture patients record forces of approximately 26 lb, which is intermediate between that of natural teeth and complete dentures and depends on the location and condition of the remaining teeth, muscles, and joints.[28] Overdentures improve the masticatory performance and permit a more consistent return to centric relation during function. The maximum force is related to the amount of tooth or implant support. In the partially edentulous patient with implant-supported fixed prostheses, force ranges are more similar to those of natural dentition. Completely edentulous patients may recover 300% of the forces after a few years with implant-supported prostheses.[26, 27] However, because long-term edentulism may result in muscle atrophy and a maximum force as low as 5 lb with a denture, an improvement of 300% may represent a final maximum force of only 15 lb (Fig 8–6).

Direction of Load

Failures of natural teeth as a result of excessive abnormal stress are attributed primarily to leverage and torque rather than to overload.[30] The direction of the occlusal load also results in significant differences in the amount of force exerted on an implant. Forces are tensile, compressive, or shear to the implant system (see Chapter 15). There is much less tensile and compressive stress with vertical loads. Three-dimensional stress analysis has shown that almost all the stresses occur in the coronal half of the implant and bone.[30, 31] Lateral forces represent approximately a 50% increase in stress compression compared with vertical loading, and tensile stresses and horizontal stresses increased more than tenfold in compres-

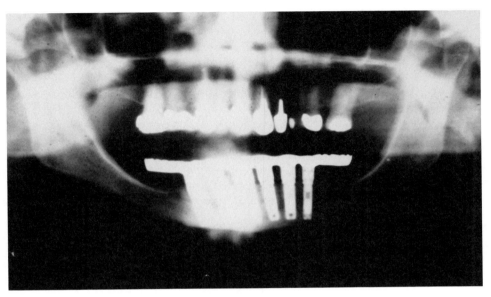

FIG 8–6.
This patient desired a fixed prosthesis in the mandible. The opposing arch is of natural teeth. The mandibular bone division required six implants. The posterior cantilevers do not occlude in any excursion. The last molar on each side was added after the prosthesis was functioning for 1 year, to improve the bone density before additional force was added to the system.

sion and in tension.[32] The direction of forces may be one of the most critical factors to be evaluated during implant treatment planning (see Chapter 15).

Maxillary anterior teeth or implants are rarely placed perpendicular to occlusal forces. After tooth loss, the bone is resorbed from the labial aspect first, and labial concavities are often present in this region. Therefore the implant apex must be placed with a palatal angulation. Mandibular posterior implants are often placed with a facial inclination of the implant apex, to avoid perforation of the submandibular fossa. These anatomic configurations affect implant angulation and the final treatment plan. If the forces of occlusion are not axial to the implant body, additional implants, stress relievers in the prosthesis, or overdentures should be considered.

Crown-Implant Ratio

The crown-implant ratio also affects the amount of forces distributed to the implant-prosthetic system, especially in the presence of lateral forces. Lateral forces result in a moment of the force on the implant and an increase in horizontal stresses. Implants placed in the anterior maxilla experience more frequent complications because of lateral stresses and the moment forces. The greater the crown-implant ratio, the greater the moment of the force under lateral loads. The vertical distance from the occlusal plane to the opposing landmark for implant insertion is typically a constant in an individual. Therefore, as the bone resorbs, the crown height becomes larger but the available bone height decreases. An indirect relationship is found between the crown and implant height. The Misch-Judy Bone Division C-h has a crown-implant ratio greater than 1, and results in greater forces being applied to the crestal bone with lateral force than in Division A bone, in which the crown-implant ratio is less than 1. A linear relationship exists between the applied load and internal stresses.[33, 34] Therefore, the greater the load applied, the greater the tensile and compressive stresses transmitted at the bone interface and to the prosthetic components.

Bone Density

Stress is defined as force over area. The density of bone is in direct relationship with the amount of implant-bone contact. The very dense bone of a resorbed anterior mandible (D-1) or of lateral cortical bone in the anterior mandible has the highest percentage of lamellar bone in contact with an endosteal implant. The percentage of bone contact is significantly greater in cortical bone than in trabecular bone. The initial bone density not only provides mechanical immobilization during healing, but also permits better distribution and transmission of stresses from the implant-bone interface. The mechanical distribution of stress occurs primarily where bone is in contact with the implant. Open marrow spaces or zones of unorganized fibrous tissue do not permit force dissipation or controlled physiologic increases in the density of the supporting bone (Fig 8–7). The sparse trabeculae of the bone often found in the posterior maxilla (D-4) offer less areas of contact with the body of the implant. Consequently, greater implant surface area is required to obtain the same amount of implant-bone contact there than for an anterior mandibular implant (see Chapter 21). The less area of bone contacting the implant body the greater the overall stress, if all other factors are equal. Progressive bone loading changes the amount and density of the implant-bone contact. The body is given time to respond to a gradual increase in occlusal load. This increases the quantity of bone at the implant interface, improves the bone density, and improves the overall support system mechanism[35] (see Chapter 28).

EFFECTS ON TREATMENT PLANNING

Once the implant dentist has identified the sources of additional force on the implant system, the treatment plan is altered to contend with, and lower, their

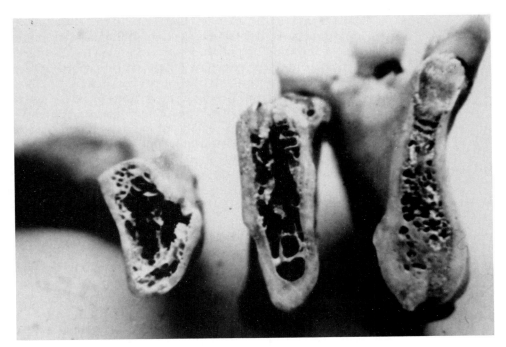

FIG 8–7.
Density of bone in the posterior mandible ranges from D-2 *(far right)* to D-4 *(far left* if an osteoplasty was required). The amount of stress to the implant increases in D-4 bone, because fewer regions of bone contact are present.

negative impact on the implant, bone, and final restoration. Under these conditions, a consistent solution is an increase in implant-bone surface area. Additional implants are the solution of choice to decrease stress, rather than only an increase in implant height or width. Use of more implants decreases the number of pontics and the associated mechanics and strains on the prosthesis (see Chapter 15), and also dissipates stresses more effectively to the bone structure, especially at the crest. The retention of the final prosthesis or superstructure is also further improved with additional implant abutments. The amount of bone in contact with the implant is increased as a multiple of the number of implants. An increase in implant width is preferable to implant length if the bone density is similar. The supplemental implant support gained from additional implants, preferably of greater diameter, decreases stress and the likelihood of implant fracture. An increase of 0.5 mm of the abutment post diameter may increase the fatigue strength by over 30%. In addition, the greater the diameter of the permucosal implant, the less stress transmitted to the surrounding crestal bone.

Forces from bruxism are often the most difficult extra forces to contend with on a long-term basis. Crestal bone loss, unretained abutments, and fatigue stress fractures of implants or prostheses are more likely a result of this condition. Informed consent of the patient is helpful to gain cooperation in eliminating or reducing the parafunction. If the opposing arch is a soft tissue–supported removable prosthesis, the effects of the noxious habit are greatly diminished.

The implant treatment plan is modified primarily in two ways when implants are inserted in the posterior region. Additional implants and occlusal considerations are both important. The elimination of posterior lateral occlusal contacts during excursive movements is recommended if the opposing dentition is an implant-supported or tooth-supported fixed prosthesis. This is beneficial in two aspects. Because lateral forces dramatically increase stress at the implant-bone interface, the elimination of posterior contacts diminishes the negative effect of bruxism. In addition, during excursions in the absence of posterior contacts, fewer fibers of the temporalis and masseter muscles are stimulated and the forces applied on the anterior implant-teeth system are reduced as much as two-thirds. In the presence of posterior contacts during excursions, almost all fibers of these two muscles may contract, as well as the external pterygoid muscle.[14, 15] The anterior teeth may need modification to create the proper incisal guidance to avoid posterior contacts during excursions.

Use of a night guard is helpful for the bruxism patient with a fixed prosthesis, to transfer the weakest link of the system to the removable acrylic appliance. Anterior guided disclusion in excursions is strongly suggested in the night guard, which may be designed to fit the maxilla or mandible. Clenching affects the treatment plan in a similar fashion to bruxism. However, the vertical forces are less detrimental than horizontal forces, and the anterior occlusal scheme is not as important to modify as with the bruxing patient. Night guards are also less effective. However, a soft night guard, which is slightly relieved over the implants is often beneficial to a patient with clenching.

A common cause of implant failure during healing is parafunction found with a patient wearing a soft tissue–supported prosthesis over a submerged implant. The tissue overlying the implant is compressed during the parafunction and loads the implant. The premature loading may cause micromovement of the implant body in the bone, after which a fibrous tissue interface will develop. The tissue over the implant often becomes dehiscent when an overlying soft tissue–borne restoration exerts pressure as a result of parafunction. A pressure necrosis of the tissue develops, and the implant becomes exposed within the oral cavity. The higher rate of failure reported when submerged implants become exposed is not corrected by surgically covering the implant with soft tissue. The soft tissue over the implant does not affect the bone interface. The problem is early loading through the soft tissue because of parafunction. Therefore the soft tissue support region over the implant is generously removed from the prosthesis during the healing period whenever parafunction is noted.

A removable partial denture over a healing implant is especially of concern. These patients often have many teeth remaining and higher forces transmitted to the soft tissue regions that support the restorations. The abutment teeth also maintain the prosthesis in place against the tissue with greater frequency. The acrylic between the soft tissue–borne region and metal substructure is less than 2 mm thick. Removing the thin acrylic over the implant is often not sufficient. Instead, a hole through the metal substructure is indicated. In this manner, a bruxing patient will not load the submerged implant during healing.

The time intervals between prosthodontic restoration may be increased to provide additional opportunity for the progressive bone loading techniques to produce load-bearing bone around the implants. Anterior implants submitted to lateral parafunction forces require further treatment considerations. Additional implants are indicated, preferably of greater diameter. The excursions are canine guided if natural, healthy canines are present. Mutually protected occlusion, with additional anterior implants and/or teeth distributing the force, is developed if the implants are in the canine position, or if this tooth is restored as a pontic. A healthy first premolar may also disclude the remaining posterior teeth when the patient is a skeletal Class II, or when anterior implants are small in size or number.

The skeletal Class III patient is primarily a vertical chewer, and generates vertical forces with little excursive movement. However, some patients appear as pseudo Class III as a result of anterior bone resorption or loss of posterior support reduced vertical dimension and anterior rotation of the mandible. These patients demonstrate lateral excursive movements when the incisal edge position is restored to its initial position.

A lateral tongue thrust is most detrimental if horizontal forces are applied to the implant during the early stages of interface formation. Submerged, two-phase, rigid, fixated implants are indicated. The posterior mandible with unavailable bone height that has been restored with a unilateral subperiosteal implant is most at risk from a posterior lateral tongue thrust. Inadequate bone height prevents extension of the implant substructure, and the greater extended permucosal abutment posts are subjected to increased lateral oral forces. Myofunctional therapy or autogenous bone grafts to modify the bone division prior to implant placement, cantilevered bridges, or conventional removable partial dentures are often indicated.

The prosthesis may be designed to improve the distribution of stress throughout the implant system. Centric vertical contacts should be aligned with the long axis of the implant whenever possible. The restoring dentist should mark the desired contacts on the opposing cast and communicate precise requirements to the laboratory technician. The posterior occlusal tables may be narrowed in order to prevent inadvertent lateral forces, to decrease the forces necessary for mastication and food penetration, and to leave greater space for the tongue. Enamoplasty of the cusp tips of the opposing natural teeth is indicated to help improve the direction of vertical forces and to achieve posterior horizontal overjet for tongue and cheek biting protection, within the guidelines of the intended occlusion.

If the patient applies significant extra forces to the implant system, and anatomic conditions do not permit the placement of additional implants, a removable overdenture (RP-4 or RP-5) should be considered. The RP-4 or RP-5 prostheses may be removed during periods conducive to noxious habits. Stress distributors may be used in the attachment system. Additional soft tissue support with attachments that allow movement, decrease the amount of force and may be indicated.

REFERENCES

1. Picton DC: Johns RB, Wills DJ: *Oral Sci Rev* 5:3–21, 1971.
2. Picton DC: In Melcher AH, Bowen WH, editors: *Biology of the periodontium,* New York, 1969, Academic Press, pp 363–419.
3. Scott I, Ash MM Jr: A six-channel intra-oral transmitter for measuring occlusal forces, *J Prosthet Dent* 16:56, 1966.
4. Profitt WR et al: Intra-oral pressures in a young and adult group, *J Dent Res* 43:555, 1966.
5. Black GV: An investigation of the physical characters of the human teeth in relation to their diseases, and to practical dental operations, together with the physical characters of filling materials, *Dent Cosmos* 37:469, 1895.
6. Craig RG: In *Restorative dental materials,* ed 6, St Louis, 1980, CV Mosby, p 60.
7. Anderson DJ: Measurements of stress in mastication, *J Dent Res* 35:664, 671, 1958.
8. Ramfjord SP, Ash MM: *Occlusion,* ed 2, Philadelphia, 1971, WB Saunders, pp 99–140.
9. Graf H: Bruxism, *Dent Clin North Am* 13:659–665, 1969.
10. Nadler SC: Bruxism, a clinical and electromyographic study, *J Am Dent Assoc* 62:21, 1961.
11. Alderman MM: Disorders of the temporomandibular joint and related structures. In Burket LW, editor: *Oral Medicine,* ed 6, Philadelphia, 1971, JB Lippincott.
12. Gibbs CH et al: Limits of human bite force, *J Prosthet Dent* 56:226–229, 1986.
13. Williamson EH, Lundquist DO: Anterior guidance: its effect on electromyographic activity of the temporal and masseter muscles, *J Prosthet Dent* 49:816–823, 1983.
14. Belser H: The influence of altered working side occlusal guidance on masticatory muscles and related jaw movement, *J Prosthet Dent* 53:3, 1985.
15. Dawson PE: *Differential diagnosis, and treatment of occlusal problems,* ed 2, St Louis, 1989, CV Mosby, pp 457–460.
16. Tanaka TT: Recognition of the pain formula for head, neck, and TMJ disorders: the general physical examination, *Calif Dent Assoc J* 44–49, 1984.
17. Mezitis M, Rallis G, Zachariatdes N: The normal range of mouth opening, *J Oral Maxillfac Surg* 47:1028–1029, 1989.
18. McCoy G: On longevity of teeth, *J Oral Implant* 11:1983.
19. Selna LG, Shillingburg HT Jr, Kerr PA: Finite element analysis of dental structures—asymmetric and plane stress idealizations, *J Biomed Mater Res* 9:235–237, 1975.

20. Hood JAA: Experimental studies on tooth deformation: stress distribution in Class V restorations, *NZ Dent J* 68:116–131, 1968.
21. Hand ASJ, Hunt A, Reinhardt JW: The prevalence and treatment implications of cervical abrasion in the elderly, *Geriodontics* 2:167–170, 1986.
22. Kydd WL, Toda JM: Tongue pressures exerted on the hard palate during swallowing, *J Am Dent Assoc* 65:319, 1962.
23. Winders RV: Forces exerted on the dentition by the peri-oral and lingual musculature during swallowing, *Angle Orthod* 28:226, 1958.
24. Mansour RM, Reynik RJ, Larson PC: Piezoelectric transducers for biting force measurements (Ph.D. Thesis). In abstracts of the 27th A.C.E.M.B., 1974.
25. Howell AH, Bruderold F: Vertical forces used during chewing of food, *J Dent Res* 29:133, 1950.
26. Carr AB, Laney WR: Maximum occlusal forces in patients with osseointegrated oral implant prostheses and patients with complete dentures, *Int J Oral Maxillofac Implant* 2:101–108, 1987.
27. Carlsson GE, Haraldson T: Functional response in tissue-integrated prostheses osseointegration. In Branemark PI, Zarb GA, Albrektsson T, editors: *Clinical Dentistry,* Chicago, 1985, Quintessence, pp 155–163.
28. Klaffenback AO: Gnathodynamics, *J Am Dent Assoc* 23:371–383, 1936.
29. Howell AH, Bruderold F: Vertical forces used during chewing food, *J Dent Res* 29:133, 1950.
30. Ismail YH, Fleming J, Pahoutis L: Comparison of two-dimensional and three-dimensional finite stress analysis of the blade implant, *Int J Oral Implant* 4:25–31, 1987.
31. Ismail YH: A comparison of current root form implants—biomechanical design and prosthodontic application, *NY State Dent J* 55:34–36, 1989.
32. Misch CE: A three-dimensional finite stress analysis of two blade implant neck designs (thesis), University of Pittsburgh School of Dental Medicine, 1989.
33. Kakudo Y, Amano N: Dynamic changes in jaw bones of rabbit and dogs during occlusion, mastication, and swallowing, *J Osaka Univ Dent Soc* 6:126–136, 1972.
34. Kakudo Y, Ishida A: Mechanism of dynamic responses of the canine and human skull due to occlusal, masticatory, and orthodontic forces, *J Osaka Univ Dent Soc* 6:137–144, 1972.
35. Misch CE: Density of bone: effect on treatment plans, surgical approach, healing, and progressive bone loading, *Int J Oral Implant* 6:23–31, 1990.

Chapter 9

Natural Abutment Evaluation

Carl E. Misch

EVALUATION AND TREATMENT PLANNING

Implant dentistry is often indicated to create the additional abutments necessary to rehabilitate the partially edentulous patient with fixed prostheses. The implants may be used as independent support for the restoration or in conjunction with natural teeth in the same prosthesis. The treatment plan is strongly influenced by the dental evaluation of the potential natural abutments. The natural teeth may require additional therapy before the final prosthesis may be completed. It is best to communicate with the patient regarding all required treatment involved in the restoration of the patient's mouth before the implants are surgically inserted. Otherwise, treatment outcome and cost may conflict with the originally projected result and lead to dissatisfaction, the need to modify the original treatment plan, and/or poorer prognosis.

The dental criteria addressed in this section include abutment mobility, crown size, crown-root ratio, endodontic status, root configuration, tooth position, parallelism, arch position, caries and periodontal factors. In addition, criteria usually not considered in traditional prosthetic therapy are discussed. These include the anatomy of the edentulous ridge adjacent to the natural abutment, the decision to extract the adjacent questionable teeth and place additional implant abutments, and options for prosthesis abutments.

Adjacent Bone Anatomy

The bone in an edentulous area adjacent to a natural tooth is variable in height, width, length, and angulation and is dependent on the dental history of the former tooth. If the bone is not ideal for endosteal implant placement in the immediate abutment site, the consideration of an adjacent pontic is indicated. An osteoplasty needed to obtain adequate bone width in the area may compromise the adjacent natural root support of the tooth, increase the crown height of the final restoration, and affect the esthetic final result. If a prosthodontic abutment must be positioned adjacent to the natural tooth and inadequate bone width is available, augmentation of the edentulous site prior to implant insertion may improve the bone anatomy without compromising the natural abutment.

Inadequate bone height as a result of crestal bone loss offers a poorer prognosis for augmentation adjacent to a tooth. The selection of implant support farther than one tooth from the natural tooth is usually a better option. If the bone is inadequate for predictable implant insertion within the edentulous span of two teeth, the natural tooth should be considered as one of the abutments for the fixed partial denture. If one endosteal implant is placed for two or more missing teeth, the natural tooth should also be considered for abutment support.

Extraction of Natural Teeth

Implant dentistry has modified the treatment plan selection in periodontal therapy. Advanced periodontal disease may be addressed with extraction more frequently, provided that the resulting edentulous area offers sufficient bone for predictable endosteal implant placement and a more predictable prognosis. "Herodontics" are discouraged when the prognosis is poor, and failure of treatment may result in inadequate bone for implant placement. The cost of the questionable periodontal treatment may result in the inability of the patient to later afford the more predictable implant therapy. Endodontics, root amputation, post and core placement, and a nevertheless remaining angled root with poor root surface area are cost prohibitive for the service provided. On the other hand, the recent trend to extract teeth with good prognosis for periodontal treatment is discouraged. The success of implants is not 100% predictable, and implants should not be substituted for natural teeth presenting a good or even fair prognosis. The decision-making protocol can be summarized as follows:

Prognosis:

>10 Years:
   a. Keep tooth and restore as indicated.

5–10 Years:
   a. Make independent implant restoration.
   b. If abutment must be included, make coping and retrievable prosthesis.
   c. Make tooth a "living pontic" by adding more implants or splinting to additional teeth.

<5 Years:
   a. Extract and graft.
   b. Consider implant in site after healing.

Natural abutments may be independent of or connected to implant abutments. If the natural tooth has a favorable prognosis for more than 10 years, treatment plans including the natural tooth may be indicated. If the natural tooth prognosis is in the 5- to 10-year range, an independent implant-supported prosthesis is more justified. If the edentulous region does not permit an independent restoration, then maintenance of the tooth and placement of additional implants with treatment alternatives that permit removal of the tooth without sacrificing the restoration are indicated. Copings are usually placed on these teeth, and the final restoration is fabricated with the ability to remove the prosthesis. Copings on natural teeth often require additional removal of tooth structure in the preparation to prevent an overcontoured crown. This may require endodontic therapy for the ideal result. Less than 5-year prognosis warrants extraction of the tooth and the planning of additional implant abutment support.

Implant or Tooth Abutment Options

An edentulous segment offers several options for adequate restoration. Under ideal conditions, there are several advantages to placing implant abutments in sufficient numbers to fabricate a completely implant-supported prosthesis. The most common cause of failure of tooth-supported fixed prostheses is caries of the abutment teeth.[1] Unrestored natural teeth do not decay as often as restored teeth, and implant abutments do not decay. As a result, this may be one of the reasons why 10-year survival rates indicate a 15% higher rate for implant prostheses over natural abutments. In addition, natural teeth are easier to clean, less sensitive, and less subject to periodontal inflammation than restored teeth.

Natural teeth respond to occlusal forces differently from implants. A light force produces most of the recorded movement of a tooth, whereas the amplitude of implant movement is directly related to the force applied.[2] In arches with both implant and natural abutments, occlusal forces are easier to adjust when the prostheses are independent.

Treatment plans that provide enough implants for an independent prosthesis are encouraged. An increase in implant abutment number increases the implant-bone interface and improves the ability of the fixed restoration to withstand forces. In addition, because the additional retentive units support the prosthesis, uncemented or unretained restorations occur with less frequency. However, completely implant-supported fixed prostheses in partially edentulous patients are not always feasible. Therefore, the natural tooth may be considered a potential abutment.

The decision to splint implant(s) and natural teeth within the same prosthesis should be considered when the surface area of the implant support does not permit replacement of the total number of missing teeth. For example, a Division B ridge may only permit the placement of a plate form implant in the posterior mandible. Because the implant is narrow, the span of two or more teeth is needed to obtain the surface area necessary for predictable replacement. As a result of its geometry, the implant should be joined by a rigid connector to natural teeth or other implants within the prosthesis. A root form implant may be placed in an edentulous span of two or more teeth and require pontic(s) in the prosthesis. The pontic(s) should not be cantilevered off one implant. As a result, the root form implant and natural tooth may be considered abutments for a fixed prosthesis.

NATURAL TOOTH ABUTMENTS AND IMPLANTS

Mobility

The actual mobility of potential natural abutments may influence the treatment more than any other factor. In the implant-tooth rigid fixed prosthesis, four important components may contribute movement to the system: the implant, bone, tooth, and prosthesis. The tooth has normal physiologic movements in vertical, horizontal, and rotational directions.[3] The amount of movement found in a natural tooth is related to the surface area and design of its supporting system. Therefore, the number and length of the roots; their diameter, shape, and position; and the type and amount of surrounding bone influence the physiologic mobility of the tooth.

A natural posterior tooth has zero clinical mobility in a vertical direction. Actually, initially the tooth can be depressed approximately 28 μ.[4] The rebound of the tooth is approximately 8 μ, so additional forces within 4 hours move the tooth far less than the original force. The vertical movement of a rigid implant has been measured as 2 to 3 μ under a 10-lb force.[2] The fixed prosthesis that connects to the tooth and implant also illustrates movement.[5] Under a 25-lb vertical force, a single pontic prosthesis fabricated in base metal flexes 5.5 μm; two pontics, 44 μm; and three pontics, 150 μm movement. The same force applied to a noble metal prosthesis results in a 12 μm movement for one pontic, 97 μm for a two-pontic span, and 330 μm with three pontics (R. Phillips, personal communication, 1990). Therefore the fixed prosthesis compensates for any difference in vertical mobility of a healthy tooth and implant.

Horizontal tooth mobility is greater than vertical movement. The initial mobility of a healthy "nonmobile" posterior tooth is less than for an anterior tooth and ranges from 56 to 75 μ, which is 2 to 9 times vertical movement. Initial horizontal mobility is greater in anterior incisor teeth and ranges from 90 to 110 μ.[4]

The implant-to-bone interface also exhibits lateral movement. Sekine et al. evaluated the movement of endosteal implants with rigid fixation and found a range of 12 to 66-μ movement in the labiolingual direction,[2] and Komiyama found 40 to 140-μ movement in the mesiodistal direction under a force of 2,000 g, or about 4.5-lb.[6]

The clinical assessment of tooth mobility is recorded as 0 to 3 +. Posterior and canine teeth often have zero horizontal clinical mobility, yet as previously stated, actually move 56 to 75 μm. The implant and noble metal fixed prosthesis can permit mesiodistal movement from 52 to 470 μm if one pontic or more is present. Therefore, zero clinical mobility of the natural abutment allows rigid connection between fixated implant and tooth, since the implant, bone, and prosthesis compensates for the slight tooth movement.

Anterior incisor teeth are often recorded as (+) mobility. The range of movement is 90 to 110 μ in these anterior teeth. Therefore, clinical evaluation can detect movement above 90 μm. When the natural abutment presents clinical horizontal movement, or conditions promote horizontal forces against the abutment tooth, options can be selected for the final prosthesis. The first, and option of choice, is to place additional implants and to avoid the use of natural abutments. The other options are to improve stress distribution by splinting additional natural abutments until zero clinical mobility is observed, use mobile metal in the prosthesis, and/or add pontics between the implant and natural teeth.

Splinting natural teeth does not significantly decrease the mobility of a tooth once the prosthesis is removed. However, the overall prosthesis movement is decreased, especially when forming an arc. If posterior contacts cannot be eliminated in lateral excursions as a result of skeletal relationships or when opposing a removable prosthesis, splinting often is safer to reduce the risk of long-term complications. In addition, splinting natural abutments also decrease the amount of load to each abutment. Therefore a 150-lb load is distributed to both splinted abutments, and the resultant force on each abutment is less. The number of teeth splinted is related to prosthesis movement. The initial dental evaluation may include acid etching and bonding potential mobile implant abutments to each other, to determine how many teeth must be joined to reduce the prosthesis mobility to clinical zero.

If additional implants cannot be placed and the implant must be joined to clinically mobile natural teeth of (+) to 1+, a plate form implant is considered. The plate form implant may function in either a slightly mobile fibrous tissue-implant interface or a direct bone-implant relationship. The fibrous tissue plate form implant is more likely to accommodate the moment of forces from the slightly mobile teeth. However, in these conditions use of independent rigid fixed implant prostheses or additional splinted teeth is usually indicated in the treatment plan. A nonrigid connector in a unilateral prosthesis is rarely indicated because it adds cost, creates overcontoured abutments, leads to more difficult hygiene, and does not decrease the clinical tooth movement.

If the natural teeth are too mobile in relation to the implant in the same prosthesis, several complications may present. If the prosthesis is cemented, movement may break the cement-implant attachment. Cement does not adhere as well to titanium as to dentine. In addition, the mobile tooth will move, rather than break the cement seal. In a screw-in prosthesis the coping screw will often loosen or break in the implant. Once the prosthesis is loose from the implant, more stress is applied to the natural tooth abutments.

Until the implant retainer attachment is lost, the greatest stress will be transmitted through the prosthesis to the implant and bone section. Crestal bone loss or implant breakage from fatigue are then possible complications.

Pier Abutments

When an implant serves as a pier abutment between two natural teeth, the differences in movement between implant and tooth may be more meaningful. Because of its decreased movement, the implant acts as the fulcrum of a lever. This is more important if one abutment tooth shows clinical mobility. An uncemented abutment, usually the least retentive crown or least mobile tooth, is then a more common occurrence. In conventional fixed prostheses, the "male" portion of a nonrigid attachment is usually located on the mesial aspect of the posterior pontic, while the "female" is in the distal of the natural pier abutment tooth. This prevents mesial drift from unseating the attachment.[7] However, an implant is unlikely to undergo mesial movement during function, so the nonrigid connector location can be more variable. Of greater concern is the difference in mobility when the implant abutment is rigidly joined to a clinically mobile natural tooth. A stress-breaking element placed in the least retentive crown, or between the mobile terminal abutment and implant, often is indicated to prevent prosthesis uncementation. This often results with the stress breaker positioned between the anterior abutment and the implant because it usually is more mobile and less retentive. On the other hand, when a natural tooth is the pier abutment between two implants, a stress breaker is rarely indicated. The tooth may then act as a living pontic, contributing less to the support, provided the number of pontics is limited and the implants are of sufficient dimension (see Chapter 29).

Terminal Natural Splinted Abutment

The adjacent natural abutment connected to a rigid fixated implant or the last natural tooth secondary abutment in a fixed prosthesis should not exhibit clinical mobility or poor retentive form. Implant prostheses often use additional secondary natural abutments to decrease the movement of the prosthesis, so rigid fixation of the implant will not be compromised. However, if the last abutment is mobile, it does not serve the intended purpose, but further burdens the adjacent abutment. A general guideline is to not end a fixed prosthesis on the weakest abutment. The weak tooth does not offer additional support, and further burdens the healthier abutment(s). In addition, if cement failure occurs, or the restoration needs retrieval, the mobile abutment is more difficult to uncement from the partial retained prosthesis. Crown fracture and other complications are more frequent in attempting to remove the restoration.

The retentive form of the terminal natural splinted abutment is also important. Tensive forces are applied to the ends of a fixed prosthesis when more than two abutments are present. Dental cements are weak in tension compared with their compression characteristics. For example, zinc phosphate cement has a compressive strength of 12,000 psi, but only 600 psi in tension. As a result, a poor retentive terminal abutment will become uncemented and the tooth segment of the bridge will be more mobile, leading to additional force on the implant. This condition also results with increased risk of decay on the abutment.

Crown Size

Uncemented restorations are the second most common complication of fixed prostheses.[1] Once a natural tooth becomes uncemented, a significant concern is caries. This may proceed rapidly and result in loss of the abutment, endodontics, post and core, a new prosthesis, or an abutment with even poorer retention. These same conditions exist if the natural retainer becomes uncemented from an implant-tooth restoration. In addition, the implant is at greater risk. The fixed prosthesis then acts as a lever, with a dramatic increase in moment of the force. Crestal bone loss, coping screw fracture, implant fracture, or mobility of the implant are all possible consequences.

The retention of a crown is influenced by the diameter and height of the abutment. Molars are more retentive than premolars because of their increased surface area, all other factors being equal. Crown height may be affected when interarch space is limited. Splinting teeth with limited crown height to improve retention often compromises access for hygiene in the interproximal areas. Instead, crown lengthening is often indicated with decreased interarch space to improve the retention of the prosthesis as well as the esthetic result and homecare. Crowns of reduced size require minimal tapering and additional retentive elements such as grooves or boxes to limit the path of insertion and direction of dislodgement.[8] These fundamental criteria apply to both natural and implant abutments. For example, the implant abutment selected should use a screw-retentive system if interarch space does not provide sufficient surface for cementation. Additional implant abutments to increase retention may also be considered. A crown height reduction of 2 mm may decrease the retention as much as 40% when the implant abutment is only 4 mm in diameter.

Crown-Root Ratio

The crown-root ratio represents the height of the crown of the tooth—from the most incisal or occlusal height, to the crest of the alveolar ridge around the tooth—compared with the height of the root within the bone. The crown-root ratio is correlated with crown size and abutment mobility. A patient with a history of periodontal disease may show no abutment mobility, yet an increased crown-root ratio. These teeth show more long-term risk of mobility. Lateral forces are more detrimental in this situation because of an increased moment of the force.

Splinting may be indicated and occlusal schemes modified to protect these abutment teeth from horizontal stresses. In addition, teeth with an increased crown-root ratio are often restored with FP-2 or FP-3 prostheses. A high lip line during smiling and low lip line during speech should be carefully evaluated. The most ideal crown-root ratio for a fixed prosthetic abutment is 1:2, but this is rarely observed.[9] A more common condition is 2:3, and a 1:1 ratio is the minimum requirement opposing natural teeth and serving as an abutment for an implant-tooth prosthesis.

Tooth Position

When adjacent teeth have been missing for a long time the remaining tooth abutment has often drifted from its ideal position. Tipping, tilting, rotation, exfoliation, and/or extrusion are often observed. Their correction should be considered in the original treatment plan for the partially edentulous patient. Treatment may consist in modification of the crown preparation, endodontic therapy before restoration, or orthodontic movement. Orthodontic therapy is more indicated when interarch corrections or gross occlusal correction is indicated, skeletal patterns require improvement, or esthetic improvement of anterior teeth position is required for patient's satisfaction. This treatment should be planned in conjunction with the healing phase for rigid fixated implant(s). The teeth adjacent to the selected natural abutment often need coronoplasty for improved occlusal force direction, interproximal contact position, esthetics, and/or path of insertion of the prosthesis.

Parallelism

Implant dentistry often treats patients with dentition lost to periodontal disease. As such, abutment teeth often display some mobility, associated with an increased crown-root ratio, which requires splinting of natural abutments. As a result, the splinting of mandibular incisors is more common in implant dentistry. These teeth are often crowded or rotated. Some mandibular anterior teeth show very wide incisal edges and narrow cervical portions, especially if recession of the gingiva has occurred. In addition, the path of insertion of a prosthesis that includes anterior and posterior dental units often requires more extensive tooth preparation. Past periodontally involved teeth are more at risk of disease conditions of the pulp after tooth preparation. All these factors result in endodontic therapy in greater incidence. If this is not explained to the patient before treatment begins and endodontic therapy is required, the patient often feels inadequate treatment has been rendered. Endodontic therapy or posts and crowns of overlapping anteriors may still provide inadequate embrasures for hygiene, and not only compromise esthetics but also result in the loss of more than one tooth. Selective extraction of incisor(s) may be indicated if rotations or overlapping of teeth represent impossible conditions for oral hygiene after restoration.

Caries

All carious lesions should be eliminated before implant placement, even when the teeth will be restored with crowns for the final prosthesis. The rigid fixation implants require several months of healing after initial placement before the final restoration. The progression of the decay may alter the final treatment plan, with a decrease in retention and the need for additional endodontic therapy, posts, cores, or even loss of a desired abutment. If the caries are eliminated at the same time as implant therapy, this should be performed before any tissue is reflected. An increased risk of implant infection exists when caries are excavated under conditions favoring bacteria invasion under the soft tissue or in the implant osteotomies.

Root Configuration

The root configuration of a natural abutment may affect the amount of additional stress the tooth may withstand without potential complications.[10] Tapered or fused roots and blunted apecies are examples of decreased ability to withstand occlusal loads. The maxillary second molar very often presents these varied root configurations. On the other hand, dilacerations or curvatures of roots improve the prosthodontic support of an abutment tooth. However, this anatomy may be very difficult to negotiate if endodontic therapy is indicated. The maxillary canine often has a distal curvature to the root. An implant placed in the first premolar region may be placed into the canine root apex when this condition is not appreciated.

Teeth with roots circular in cross-section do not represent as good a prosthodontic abutment, as those with an ovoid cross-section. Therefore, the maxillary premolar is a better abutment than the maxillary central incisor, although their surface areas are similar. The maxillary lateral incisor may exhibit less lateral mobility than the central incisor, as a result of its cross-sectional anatomy.[8]

Root Surface Area

In general, the larger the root surface area of a proposed abutment tooth, the greater the support. Posterior teeth offer greater periodontal surface area and provide greater support than anterior teeth. Teeth affected by periodontal disease lose surface area and represent poorer support elements for a prosthesis. For a maxillary first molar, bone loss to the beginning of the furcation, corresponds to a root surface area reduced by 30%. Ante's law requires the root surface area of the abutment teeth to be equal to or greater than that of the teeth replaced by the pontics of the fixed restoration.[11] Although this statement was originally presented without research documentation, it has stood the test of time and serves as a clinical guideline. This evaluation process is one of the original requirements to determine if implants and natural teeth are required in the fixed restoration to replace missing teeth.

Endodontic Evaluation

The natural abutment included in a mixed tooth and implant prosthesis should present a stable pulpal condition or a successful root canal obturation. Lesions of endodontic origin are evaluated before implant surgery, because an exacerbation of the lesion during healing may result in the adjacent implant failure. If the pulpal or endodontic status of an abutment is questionable, the prudent treatment is endodontic therapy. In this way, the abutment crown may be evaluated for retention, need for post and/or core, and any other related criteria before final prosthodontic treatment. Apicoectomy procedures, when indicated, are best performed without use of amalgam retrograde filling, to avoid corrosion byproducts in the area, which may contaminate metal implants.

Periodontic Evaluation

The periodontal evaluation of natural abutments to be connected to implants is identical to evaluation of other tradition fixed partial dentures. However, unique situations do exist. The adjacent implant site may be contaminated by bacteria around the tooth during surgery, and the incision line for implant placement often includes the abutment teeth. The implant surgeon should decide if periodontal therapy is indicated on the abutment teeth at the same time as implant placement. A reduction in the number of surgical procedures is a benefit to the patient; however, active infection should be kept to a minimum. The pathologic condition of the abutment teeth is addressed before the soft tissue is reflected in the region of the implant osteotomy. Therefore, initial preparation of the natural teeth prior to implant placement is indicated if any exudate is present. In addition, tetracycline is administered before implant surgery to decrease the sulcular flora, which may contaminate the implant site.

CONCLUSION

An axiom in traditional prosthodontics is to provide a fixed prosthesis whenever possible. A removable restoration is indicated when posterior abutments are not present, the edentulous span too long, or the natural abutments inadequate. Implant dentistry permits the scope of fixed prosthetics in the partial edentulous to be expanded.

The ideal restoration is completely implant supported and has several advantages. However, when insufficient implant support is present, the natural teeth must be evaluated for potential abutment(s). The most important natural tooth criteria for implant-tooth supported restorations is tooth mobility. A clinical assessment of zero mobility allows a rigid connection between the tooth and implant. However, if mobility is present, the tooth-supported aspect of the prosthesis should find a means to return to zero mobility, or an independent implant restoration is considered. Splinting natural teeth is the usual method of reducing mobility. If this is not possible, grafting the edentulous site and use of additional implants often is indicated.

Several additional factors are important to evaluate for a potential implant–natural abutment. These include crown size, crown-root ratio, tooth position, parallelism, caries, root configuration, root surface area, endodontics, and periodontic evaluation. Although these same criteria are important for any fixed restoration, each has a unique aspect in implant prostheses.

REFERENCES

1. Walton JN, Gardner FM, Agar JR.: A survey of crown and fixed partial denture failures: length of service and reason for replacement, *J Prosthet Dent* 56:416–421, 1986.
2. Sekine H et al: Mobility characteristics and tactile sensitivity of osseointegrated fixture-supporting systems, in van Steenberghe D, editor: *Tissue integration in oral maxillofacial reconstruction,* Excerpta Medica, Amsterdam, Elsevier, 1986; pp 306–332.
3. Muhlemann HR: Tooth mobility: a review of clinical aspects and research findings, *J Periodontol* 38:686, 1967.
4. Parfitt GS: Measurement of the physiologic mobility of individual teeth in an axial direction, *J Dent Res* 39:68, 1960.
5. Bruski JB: Biomechanics of oral implants: future research directions, *J Dent Res* 52:775, 1988.
6. Komiyama Y: Clinical and research experience with osseointigrated implants in Japan, in Albrektsson T, Zarb G, editors: *The Branemant, Osseointigrated Implant,* Chicago, 1989, Quintessence.
7. Shillingburg HT, Fisher DW: Nonrigid connectors for fixed partial dentures, *J Am Dent Assoc* 87:1195–1199, 1973.
8. Shillingburg HT, Hobho S, Whitsett LD: *Fundamentals of fixed prosthodontics,* ed 2, Chicago, 1981, Quintessence.
9. Penny RE, Kraal JH: Crown to root ratio: its significance in restorative dentistry, *J Prosthet Dent* 42:34–38, 1979.
10. Laney WR, Gibelisco JA: *Diagnosis and treatment in prosthodontics,* Philadelphia, 1983, Lea & Febiger, p 169.
11. Ante IH: The fundamental principles of abutments, *Mich Dent Soc Bull* 8:14, 1926.

Chapter 10

Prosthodontic Considerations

Carl E. Misch

PROSTHETIC EVALUATION IN IMPLANT DENTISTRY

The prosthodontic evaluation of the patient's condition closely resembles traditional dentistry. However, several specific conditions modify the course of implant treatment and should be evaluated before the final treatment plan is presented to the patient. These conditions are

1. Interarch space
2. Implant permucosal position
3. Existing occlusal plane
4. Arch relationship
5. Arch form
6. Existing occlusion
7. Existing prosthesis
8. Number and location of missing teeth
9. Lip line
10. Mandibular flexure

Interarch Space

The amount of interarch space is variable in an edentulous region. An increase in space results from the vertical loss of alveolar bone. Consequently the replacement teeth are elongated and often need the addition of gingival tone materials in esthetic regions. The increased crown height results in an increased moment of the force on implants, and an increased risk of material fracture, especially on cantilevered sections of fixed restorations, or provokes the fracture of unsupported occlusal material due to inadequate metal substructure design. In addition, this also may result in enlarged interproximal areas that entrap food debris in the posterior areas during function, or affect speech patterns in the anterior segments.

The amount of interarch space may be decreased by the addition of autogenous or alloplastic grafts prior to or in conjunction with implant placement. Autogenous grafts offer the advantage of a resultant increase in implant-bone surface area and concomitant decrease in crown-implant ratio because wider or longer implants may be inserted. However, they require an additional surgical donor site. On the other hand, alloplastic materials have not predictably generated the formation of bone when layed upon an edentulous ridge; instead, a mixture of fibrous tissue and alloplast is usually present. The esthetics of the final prosthesis are improved, but the moment of the forces related to lateral stresses remain similar to the initial conditions, dependent on the amount of actual bone contact with the implant. In addition, pocket depth around the implant may increase if bone does not form and may influence anaerobe bacteria formation and future bone loss.

A decrease in interarch space may be present opposing the edentulous implant site as a result of unopposing natural dentition. The exfoliation or extrusion of posterior teeth is a common condition under these circumstances. The alveolar process may follow the exfoliating teeth, and after their loss the alveolar crest is closer to the occlusal plane. Earlier tooth abrasion, attrition, and skeletal insufficiencies may also lead to a decreased interarch space. The consequences include a decrease in abutment height, which may lead to an inadequate retention of the restoration, inadequate bulk of restorative material for strength or esthetics, and poor hygiene conditions compromising long-term maintenance. The retention and resistance difference between a 3 mm and a 5 mm preparation in height may be 40%. In addition, the final restoration deflects or bends inversely to the cube of the thickness of material.[1] A fixed prosthesis half as thick, will bend eight times as much, and further result in broken cement seals, loosening of fixation screws and/or porcelain fracture.

If the opposing arch should not be altered, the limited interarch space may be improved with osteoplasty and soft tissue reduction, provided adequate bone height remains after the procedure for predictable implant support. These surgical procedures may be performed at the time of implant placement, to reduce the time and number of surgical interventions for the patient.

Countersinking of the implant is usually indicated in these cases, because the osteoplasty eliminates the cortical plate and crestal bone loss can be expected after an osteoplasty (Fig 10–1).

Implant Permucosal Position

The permucosal position of the implant abutment is of particular importance for FP-1 prostheses. An implant placed in the improper position can compromise the final results in esthetics, biomechanics, and hygiene maintenance. The most

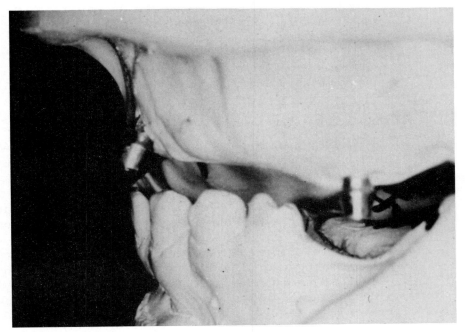

FIG 10–1.
Lack of interarch space was not evaluated prior to implant placement. The abutment for screw are now in the implant body and the final restoration cannot be fabricated. In addition, too few implants and too long a span is present to properly restore this patient.

compromising position for an implant is too facial. The resulting final restoration often is compromised in esthetics, phonetics, lip position, and function. An angled abutment may help improve the condition if the improper placement is not severe, but the facial gingival contour remains compromised. Also, the angled abutment does not affect the increase in forces exerted at the crest of the bone. The labial cortical plate is much thinner than the lingual, and the thin cortical bone must resist greater force. Cervical bone loss is common under these conditions.

A lingually positioned implant is easier to correct in the final restoration. The forces are usually directed more longitudinal to the implant body, and the thicker lingual cortical bone provides initial stability and denser bone for improved force transfer at the implant-bone interface. Because the implant body is often half the diameter of the adjacent teeth, the final crown is not necessarily overcontoured on the lingual aspect.

An implant placed too far mesial or too distal is of less consequence if the lip position does not expose the cervical third of the restoration. The final restoration is constructed with the interproximal area ideal for esthetics, independent of implant placement. This may place the interproximal region directly over the implant abutment post. Hygiene is compromised, but can be maintained with modified conventional approaches of brushing and flossing.

The use of presurgical stents for implant placement is strongly suggested in anterior edentulous regions requiring an FP-1 prosthesis. This stent should provide both ideal implant permucosal placement and angulation information.

Existing Occlusal Plane

The natural dentition opposing a partially edentulous ridge must be carefully examined and often needs modification. The opposing teeth have often drifted as a result of improper or missing opposing contacts. In addition, the partially edentulous ridge may require implant insertion more medial in relation to the original central fossa of the natural dentition. Enameloplasty of the opposing teeth is often indicated to redirect occlusal forces over the long axis of the implant body.

A curve of Spee and curve of Wilson are indicated for proper esthetics and to prevent posterior lateral interferences during excursions. The occlusal plane is evaluated in relationship to the final implant position. Odontoplasty, endodontic therapy, and/or crowns are indicated to remedy tipping, extrusions, and/or

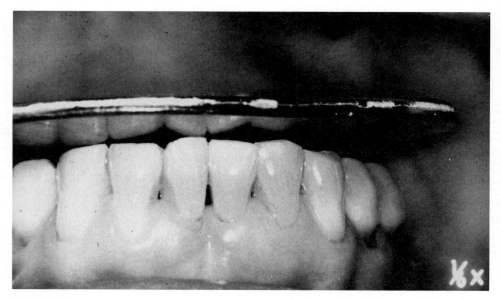

FIG 10–2.
The existing occlusal plane opposing a implant reconstruction is irregular. A Misch Occlusal Analyzer based on a 3⅞-, 4-, or 4⅛-inch sphere is used to demonstrate the condition.

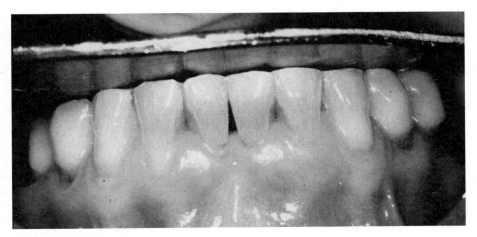

FIG 10–3.
After enameloplasty the occlusal plane is restored to follow a curve of Wilson and a curve of Spee demonstrated with the Misch Occlusal Analyzer.

exfoliations. A pretreatment diagnostic wax-up is strongly suggested to evaluate these needed changes before implant placement.

An occlusal plane analyzer may be used on diagnostic casts to evaluate pretreatment conditions and intraoral occlusal plane correction. A Misch Occlusal Analyzer (MOA) is fabricated in three sizes. The medium size corresponds to a 4-inch sphere and provides a starting point for ideal curves of Wilson and Spee. The larger plane for bigger skeletal patterns corresponds to a 4⅛-inch sphere and the smaller occlusal plane analyzer is a 3⅞-inch sphere for smaller arches. Any discrepancy observed on the cast may be corrected in the mouth. The thickness of the MOA is 2 mm and corresponds to the ideal thickness of porcelain in a porcelain-metal restoration. The MOA may be used over the opposing arch and the metal framework constructed to touch the MOA. Once removed, 2 mm clearance for porcelain is present (Figs 10–2 and 10–3).

Arch Relationship

Several conditions relate to arch position. An improper skeletal position may be modified by orthodontics, surgery, or both. It is far better to discuss these options with the patient before treatment, because implant surgery may be performed at the same time as orthodontic treatment. Compromises of the final result should be discussed with the patient when orthognathic surgery or orthodontic therapy is not used for patients with skeletal complications.

Arch relationship often concerns the anterior regions of the maxilla and mandible. The anterior edentulous maxilla resorbs toward the palate. The width of the alveolar ridge decreases 40% within a few years, primarily at the expense of the labial plate.[2] Consequently, implants are often placed lingual to the original incisal or central fossa tooth position. The final restoration is overcontoured in the gingival third to place the incisal two-thirds in the ideal tooth position for esthetics. The incisal edge tooth position is facial to the remaining bone. This results in a cantilevered force on the anterior implant body. The maxilla is affected more than the mandible, because the incisal edge position cannot be modified and is dictated by esthetics, speech, lip position, and occlusion. Anterior cantilevered teeth require additional implants to control the increase in lateral loads and moment of the force.

The anterior cantilever in the mandibular arch may correct an Angle Skeletal Class II jaw relationship. The maxillary teeth support the lower lip at rest. A complete denture cannot extend beyond the bone support or neutral zone of the lips without less stability of the prosthesis. Implants can permit the teeth to be placed in more ideal esthetic and function position. However, the arch form and posterior edentulous region should provide more dental implant support and greater numbers to compensate for the anterior cantilever (Fig 10–4).

Arch Form

The description of an edentulous arch form includes ovoid, tapering, and square. The ovoid arch form is the most common, followed by the square arch

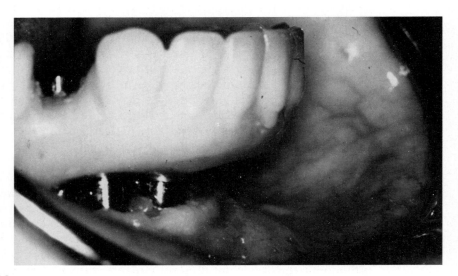

FIG 10–4.
A wax try-in of a mandibular FP-3 restoration which is cantilevered to the anterior to correct a skeletal class II relationship. This requires greater implant support to compensate for the offset loads.

form, then by the tapered form. The tapering arch form is more often found in skeletal Class II patients or as a result of oral parafunctional habits during growth and development. The square arch form may result from the initial formation of the basal skeletal bone. However, the formation of a square arch form is very often the result of labial bone resorption of the premaxilla region when anterior teeth are lost earlier than the canine and posterior teeth.

In the maxilla, anterior endosteal implants may not be inserted in their ideal location as a result of labial plate resorption and inadequate bone width at the implant site. This requires implant placement lingual to the original natural teeth, or in the canine locations in more advanced atrophied arches. The anterior restoration results in a fixed prosthesis placed with a greater cantilever in an original tapered arch form compared with the square arch form, all other factors being identical. The tapered arch form requires the support of additional implants of greater length and number to counteract the increase in lateral load and moment of the force, caused by the increased anterior lever arm replacing the anterior teeth. The distance between a line drawn through the middle of the posterior implant and a line drawn at the anterior part of the anterior implant serves as a guideline to the extent of the cantilever. The anterior cantilever should not extend more than 1 times the distance between the lines in the maxilla, or 1.5 times in the mandible.

The arch form is also a determinant when anterior implants are used to cantilever the restoration to the distal posterior regions. For these conditions, a square arch form provides a poorer prognosis than the tapered arch form. The anterior implants in the tapered arch form are able to offset the distal cantilevered force. The distance from the center of the most anterior implant to a line joining the bilateral distal aspect of the most distal implants provides an indication of the amount of posterior cantilever. The cantilevered posterior restoration should not exceed two and one-half times the anteroposterior distance and, depends on implant length and number. Therefore the most ideal biomechanical arch form depends on the restorative conditions. The tapering arch form is a favorable factor for anterior implants with posterior cantilevers. The square arch form is better when canine and posterior implants are used to support anterior cantilevers. The ovoid arch form has qualities from both tapered and square arches (Fig 10–5).

Existing Occlusion

The existing occlusion must be evaluated before implant placement. Partially edentulous patients often present occlusal interferences as a result of tooth migration. Deflective contacts are identified and eliminated before the implant prosthodontic phase. The occlusion may require complete rehabilitation to eliminate potential unfavorable forces against the implant(s). Both arches may require prosthodontic treatment to establish the desired occlusal schemes and forces. Parafunctional forces or an opposing single denture are the most common conditions which mandate more involved opposing dentition modification. The

Maxilla

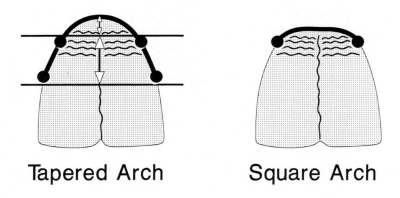

Tapered Arch   Square Arch

Mandible

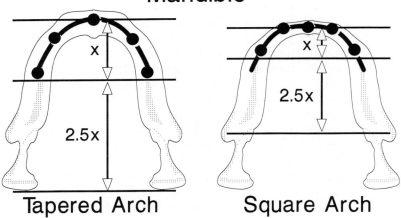

Tapered Arch   Square Arch

FIG 10–5.
Top, replacement of maxillary anterior teeth in a tapered arch form requires more posterior implants than in a square arch form with less offset loading of the mandibular teeth. **Bottom,** in the anterior mandible a tapered arch form permits greater cantilever length than does a square arch form, which has less anteroposterior distance. The maximum cantilever under ideal conditions is two and one-half times the anteroposterior distance *(X)*.

first condition often indicates a need to increase the anterior guidance, while the second warrants bilateral balance.

Existing Prostheses

When present, existing prostheses are evaluated for proper design and clinical requirements, function and compatibility with the proposed restoration, and similarity to natural teeth. A removable partial soft tissue–supported restoration opposing the proposed implant supported prosthesis is of particular interest. The occlusal forces vary widely as the underlying bone remodels. The patient may not even wear the removable partial denture in the future, which will dramatically modify the occlusal conditions. Constant maintenance and follow-up are indicated, including relines and occlusal evaluation.

The patient is asked if the esthetics of the existing prosthesis which will be replaced by the implant-supported restoration are acceptable. If unacceptable, the reasons for patient's dissatisfaction are noted. The contour, arrangement, and

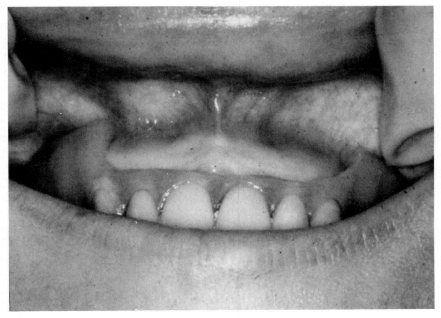

FIG 10–6.
The labial flange of the denture is removed and the patient lip support evaluated prior to the completed treatment plan of a fixed restoration. If additional lip support is required, an onlay graft of hydroxylapatite can increase labial tissue thickness for proper lip support.

position of the teeth in the existing restoration may all influence the future implant prosthesis design. A preexisting maxillary removable prosthesis which will be replaced with a fixed implant prosthesis is used as a template and guide for implant reconstruction. The thickness of the labial flange is observed, and it often removed to observe the difference in lip position and support. If additional lip support is needed once the labial flange is eliminated, a hydroxylapatite (HA) and demineralized freeze-dried bone onlay graft on the labial maxillary bone is usually indicated. This graft is not intended for implant support or replacement, but to advance the labial alveolar mucosa and improve maxillary lip support (Fig 10–6).

MISSING TEETH: NUMBER AND LOCATION

The number and location of missing teeth influences the prosthodontic treatment plan of the patient. For the most part, the second molar is not replaced in a posterior implant-supported prosthesis. The maxillary first molar is designed to occlude with the mesial cusp of the opposing natural mandibular second molar to prevent exfoliation, which might result in occlusal interference during mandibular excursions.

This philosophy is based on several observations. Ninety percent of the masticatory efficiency is generated anterior to the mesial half of the mandibular first molar, so function is rarely a reason to replace the second molar.[3] The tooth most likely to cause lateral balancing interferences in an anterior guidance occlusal scheme is the second molar. An incorrect articulator mounting results with the most significant premature centric contact on the second molar.[4] A 10% greater occlusal force is found on the second molar than on the first molar[5] and is especially important during parafunction, when occlusal forces are greater and implant abutment fatigue fracture or bone loss is more likely. The mandibular canal begins its ascent, and the maxillary sinus is larger in the second molar region, so endosteal implants are of reduced height and surface area.

In addition, the location of the mandibular canal anterior to the mid first molar corresponds predictably to the position of the mental foramen.[6] Implant placement in this region is safe and free of paresthesia risk when placed above the height of the foramen. However, in the region of the second molar the mandibular canal position becomes highly variable, and the risk of paresthesia is much greater. The bone in the second mandibular molar region is often less dense than in other regions of the mandible. The submandibular fossa is more accentuated in this region and mandates greater angulation of the implant body compared to the direction of occlusal forces. The interarch space is more limited in the second molar location. As a result, the posts are shorter and the cement surface area decreased, thus reducing the retention to the prosthesis. If the restoration is screw-retained, access for screw placement or removal is most difficult, especially with an opposing natural dentition. Hygiene and maintenance procedures are more difficult in this limited access region. Biting the cheek is more common in this region because the edentulous region may have buccinator muscles and soft tissue extension from the long-term edentulous condition. The opposing occlusion is more likely to be in cross-bite opposing an implant prosthesis constructed on a resorbed posterior maxilla. Finally, the cost of an additional implant and/or additional prosthesis unit to replace the second molar is greater for the patient.

A greater span between abutments in the prosthesis increases the flexibility.[2] The deflection or bending of a fixed prosthesis varies directly with the cube of the length. Therefore, a fixed prosthesis with one pontic deflects eight times less than one with two pontics, and 27 times less than a restoration with three pontics, all other factors being equal. This greater movement increases the occurrence of cement breakage or screw loosening in the restoration. Three posterior pontics can be replaced with a fixed prosthesis only under ideal conditions; however, such conditions rarely exist. Therefore, for all practical reasons, the number of pontics in a fixed restoration should not extend beyond two in the posterior areas of the mouth.

To limit the effect of the "law of beams," several factors may be considered. An additional implant may reduce the number of pontics while increasing simultaneously the number of abutments and distributing the forces more effectively and improving prosthesis retention. The thickness of the metal may also be increased. The flexibility is also related to the cube of the occlusal-gingival dimension. Therefore, a fixed prosthesis twice as thick deforms 8 times less. Because nonprecious metals deform approximately half less than high noble alloys, they may be selected for long-span restorations. However, corrosion factors may be a concern with nonprecious alloys, especially for subgingival margins. Additional grooves on the facial and lingual aspects of the implant abutment or the natural teeth also limit the effects of metal distortion under occlusal loads.[7]

A fixed prosthesis replacing a canine tooth is more at risk than most other replacement teeth. The maxillary lateral incisor is the weakest anterior tooth, and the first premolar is the weakest posterior tooth. A fixed prosthesis is not indicated if a canine and more than one adjacent tooth are missing.[7–9] Therefore, implants are warranted whenever a canine, lateral incisor, and first premolar; or canine, lateral and central incisors; or canine, first premolar, and second premolars is missing, if a fixed prosthesis is to be fabricated. An implant is usually placed in the canine region, and an additional implant is placed in the more posterior edentulous site. This results with an anterior cantilever when the missing teeth include incisors. The anterior bone is usually more narrow and the incisive canal may intrude into the central region. Dense HA augmentation may be placed on the labial of the anterior edentulous region to improve esthetics and pontic contour.

LIP LINE

Lip positions are evaluated as resting lip line, maxillary high lip line, and mandibular low lip line. The resting lip line is especially noted if maxillary anterior teeth are to be replaced. Removable prosthetic guidelines for incisal edge position established relative to esthetics, phonetics, and occlusion are applied.

The maxillary high lip line is determined while the patient displays a natural, broad smile. The determination between an FP-2 and FP-3 fixed prosthesis is often based solely on this evaluation. If a patient has a high lip position during smiling, the prosthodontic requirements are more demanding and may require modification of the patient's soft tissue prior to reconstruction. The cervical third of the maxillary premolars is also observed. The position of these teeth may be too palatal in a resorbed maxilla and therefore affect the esthetic result. It is not unusual with a high lip line to reveal the cervical third and gingival region of the premolars, and these teeth should not appear too short or unnatural in height.

The mandibular low lip position is often neglected, with disastrous esthetic results. Although the high lip line is evaluated during smiling, the low lip position is observed during speech. In pronunciation of the "s" sounds or sibilants, some patients may expose the entire anterior mandibular teeth and gingival contour. Patients are often unaware of this preexisting lip position and blame the final restoration for the display of the mandibular gingiva or complain the teeth look too long.

MANDIBULAR FLEXURE

The mandibular arch may require total reconstruction for the partially or completely edentulous patient. If the treatment plan consists of bilateral posterior implants to serve as abutment support, considerations concerning splinting these elements is mandatory. The mandible has considerable movement toward the midline upon opening.[10–13] This is primarily from the medial attachment of muscles and ligaments on the ramus and angle of the mandible. As a result, the medial movement occurs primarily distal from the position of the mental foramen. The farther posterior from the foramen, the more medial movement is observed. The amount of movement is variable and is dependent upon the density of bone, the division of bone, and the amount of opening of the jaws. The amount of this opening has been measured as 0.8 mm in the first molar region, to as much as 1.5 mm in the ramus area. Posterior rigid fixated implants splinted to each other in a full arch restoration would receive considerable bucco-lingual force upon opening. The difference in movement between the implant and bone range from 10 to 30 times. As a consequence, this factor is much more important to evaluate than whether an implant should be joined to a natural tooth (which usually differs in movement by less than a factor of 5).

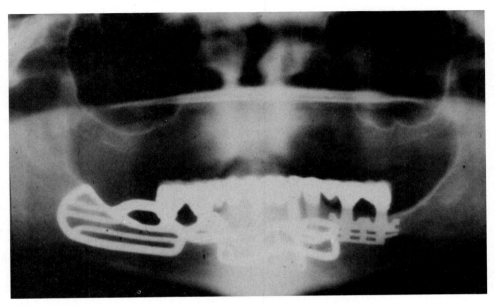

FIG 10–7
Bilateral posterior implants should not be splinted to each other because of mandibular flexure. Additional anterior implants were placed so three independent prosthesis may be fabricated. The canine joins the posterior plate form or unilateral subperiosteal implant. A separate anterior implant supported fixed prosthesis replaces the anterior incisors.

Splinting cross-arch posterior rigid fixated implants to each other is usually contraindicated in the mandible. The flexure of the mandible is still present even with the prosthesis.[14] The results include bone loss around the implants, loss of implant fixation, material fracture which may include implant or prosthesis components, unretained restorations, and/or discomfort upon opening.

If treatment plan options include bilateral posterior implants, several options exist. The span between posterior implants and anterior abutments may be increased. More flexible metals may be used in the superstructure, or the design may decrease faciolingual dimension and increase flexibility. A nonrigid facial-lingual connector(s) may be used anterior to the mental foramen. In this way the posterior implant receives vertical anterior support, but the medial movement on one side is independent from the contralateral posterior implant. Of course, additional implants may be placed to permit two or more independent prostheses. This is usually the best option, since it also increases implant surface area and retention components for the prosthesis (Fig 10–7).

CONCLUSION

The prosthodontic evaluation of the implant candidate borrows several conventional criteria from the evaluation of natural abutments. In addition, many of these situations require a unique approach for implant prosthodontics and may influence the implant treatment plan. The goal of the implant surgeon is to achieve predictable rigid fixation of endosteal implants. The restoring dentist's responsibility is to maintain the implant-bone interface, in an environment that satisfies all the traditional prosthodontic criteria.

REFERENCES

1. Smyd ES: Mechanics of dental structures: guide to teaching dental engineering at undergraduate level, *J Prosthet Dent* 2:668–692, 1952.
2. Pietrokovski J, Masseler M: Alveolar ridge resorption following tooth extraction, *J Prosthet Dent* 17:21–27, 1967.
3. Yurkstas AA: The effect of missing teeth on masticatory performance and efficiency, *J Prosthet Dent* 4:120–123, 1954.
4. Weinberg LA: Arcon principle in the condylar mechanism of adjustable articulators, *J Prosthet Dent* 13:263–268, 1963.
5. Mansour RM, Reynik RJ, Larson DC: Piezoelectric transducers for biting force measurements. Abstract presented at the 27th ACEMB, 1974.
6. Misch CE, Crawford EA: Predictable mandibular nerve location—a clinical zone of safety, *Int J Oral Implant* 7:37–44, 1990.
7. Shillingburg HT, Jacobi R, Brackett SE: *Fundamentals of tooth preparation,* Chicago, 1987, Quintessence, p 360.
8. Tylman SD: *Theory and practice of crown and bridge prosthesis,* ed 3, St Louis, 1954, CV Mosby.
9. Laney WR, Gibilisco JA: *Diagnosis and treatment in prosthodontics,* Philadelphia, 1983, Lea & Febiger, pp 164–165.
10. Picton DCA: Distortion of the jaws, *Arch Oral Biol* 7:573, 1962.
11. Goodkind RJ, Heringlake CB: Mandibular flexure in opening and closure movements, *J Prosthet Dent* 30:134–138, 1973.
12. DeMarco TL, Paine S: Mandibular dimensional change, *J Prosthet Dent* 31:482–485, 1974.
13. Fishman B: The rotational aspect of mandibular flexure, *J Prosthet Dent* 64:483–485.
14. Fishman BM: The influence of fixed splints on mandibular flexure, *J Prosthet Dent* 35:643–667, 1976.

Chapter 11

Classification of Partially and Completely Edentulous Arches in Implant Dentistry

Carl E. Misch

PARTIALLY EDENTULOUS ARCHES

Numerous classifications exist for partially edentulous arches. Their use allows the profession to visualize and communicate the relationship of hard and soft structures. Because there are over 65,000 possible combinations of teeth and edentulous spaces in a single arch, no universal agreement exists regarding the use of any one classification system. The purpose of this chapter is to introduce a classification for diagnosis and treatment planning for partially edentulous patients requiring implant prostheses. Because many possible combinations of hard and soft tissues are possible, a basic classification is warranted.

HISTORY

The classifications of partially edentulous arches that are most familiar to the profession include those originally proposed by Cummer,[1] Kennedy,[2] and Bailyn.[3] In addition, other classifications have also been proposed by Neurohr,[4] Mauk,[5] Godfrey,[6] Beckett,[7] Friedman,[8] Austin and Lidge,[9] Skinner,[10] Applegate,[11] and Avant.[12] None of these systems has been universally accepted or used. The Kennedy classification, however, is taught in most American dental schools.

The Kennedy classification divides partially edentulous arches into four classes.[2] Class I has bilateral posterior edentulous spaces. Class II has a unilateral posterior edentulous space. Class III has an intradental edentulous area, and Class IV has an anterior edentulous area which crosses the midline.

The Kennedy classification is difficult to use in many situations without certain qualifying rules. The eight Applegate (1954) rules are used to help clarify the system.[11] They may be summarized in three general principles. The first principle is that the classification should include only natural teeth involved in the final prosthesis and follow rather than precede any extractions of teeth that might alter the original classification. This concept, for example, considers whether second or third molars are to be replaced in the final restoration. The second rule is that the most posterior edentulous area always determines the classification. The third principle is that edentulous area(s) other than those determining the classification are referred to as modifications and are designated only by their number. The extent of modification is not considered.

CLASSIFICATION

The Implant Dentistry Classification developed by Misch and Judy builds on the four classes of partial edentulism described in the Kennedy-Applegate system.[12] This facilitates communication among the large segment of practitioners already familiar with this classification, and enables use of the common treatment methods and principles established for each Class.

The Implant Dentistry Classification for partially edentulous patients also includes the same four available bone divisions discussed in Chapter 7 for the edentulous site(s), which determine the class. Other intradental edentulous regions not responsible for the Kennedy-Applegate class determination present are not specified within the available bone section of the Misch-Judy system if implants are not considered in the modification region. However, if the more anterior intratooth edentulous span has an implant-support system option, the modification is listed, followed by the available bone division (Table 11–1).

TREATMENT PLANNING

The Implant Classification for partially edentulous patients allows several prosthodontic and implant principles to be applied in each Class and/or Division. A common axiom of prosthodontics in the partially edentulous patient is to provide fixed restorations when possible, which are preferred to removable partial dentures. This position is only modified and extended in implant dentistry. The

TABLE 11–1.

Implant Dentistry Classification of Partially Edentulous Arches

Class I: Partially edentulous arch with bilateral edentulous areas posterior to remaining natural teeth.
  Division A:
  1. Edentulous areas have abundant bone height (10 mm) and length (5 mm) for endosteal implant(s).

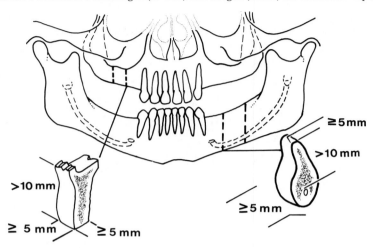

  2. Direction of load is within 30 degrees of implant body axis.
  3. Crown-implant ratio is <1.
  4. Root form implants and independent prostheses often are indicated.

  Division B:
  1. Edentulous areas have moderate available bone width (2.5 mm) and at least adequate bone height (10 mm) and length (15 mm).

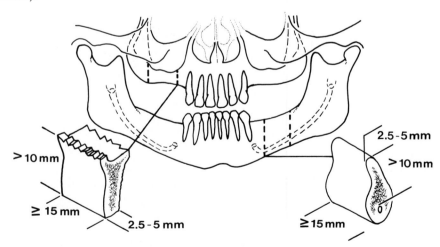

  2. Direction of load is within 20 degrees of implant body axis.
  3. Crown-implant ratio is <1.
  4. Surgical options include osteoplasty, small-diameter implants, and/or augmentation.

TABLE 11–1. (cont.)

Division C:
1. Edentulous areas have inadequate available bone for endosteal implant(s) with a predictable result, because of too little bone width (C-w), length, height (C-h), or angulation of load.

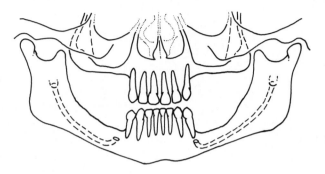

2. Crown-implant ratio often is >1.
4. Surgical options for C-w include osteoplasty or augmentation; for C-h, subperiosteal implants or augmentation. Root forms may be considered with augmentation and/or nerve repositioning.

Division D:
1. Edentulous areas have severely resorbed ridges, involving a portion of the basal or cortical supporting bone.

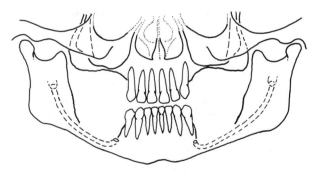

2. Crown-implant ratio is >5.
3. Surgical options usually require augmentation before implants can be inserted.
NOTE: If the bilateral edentulous areas are not within the same division, the right side is described first (e.g., Class I, Division A, B).

more healthy teeth present, the greater incidence of fixed partial denture treatment. If the prosthodontic treatment of a patient's dental condition requires additional support, implant dentistry often should be considered. The greater the number of missing teeth, the larger and/or more implants required to improve long-term success of the implant prosthodontic system.

TABLE 11–1. (cont.)

Class II: Partially edentulous arch with unilateral edentulous area posterior to remaining teeth.
  Divisions A to D same as for Class I.

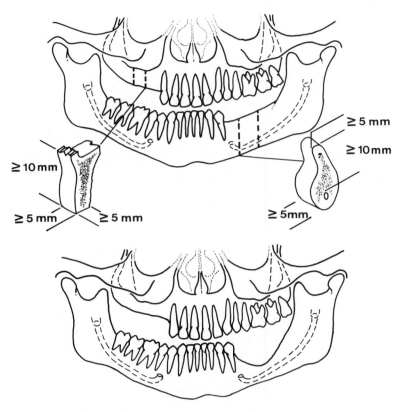

Class I

Class I patients still have natural anterior teeth to provide a vertical occlusal registration on natural teeth to distribute forces throughout the mouth in centric relation when posterior implants support the restoration. These anterior teeth also permit excursions during mandibular movement to disclude the posterior implant-supported prostheses and protect them from lateral forces.

Class I patients more often have mobile anterior teeth, because long-term lack of bilateral posterior support has resulted in an overload to the remaining dentition. Therefore these patients often require the posterior implant prostheses to be independent from the mobile natural teeth. This requires more implant support in each posterior section compared with most Class II or III patients.

TABLE 11–1. (cont.)

Class III: Partially edentulous arch with unilateral edentulous area with natural teeth remaining anterior and posterior.
Divisions A to D same as for Class I.

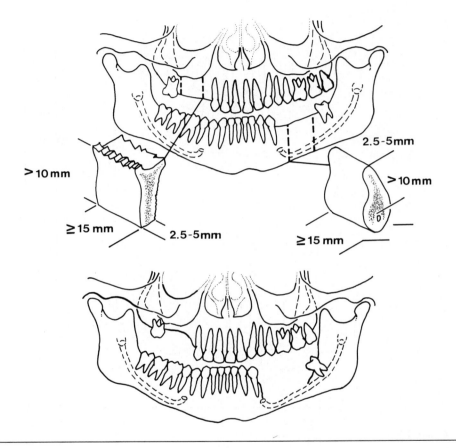

Financial concerns may require one posterior section to be restored several years in advance of the contralateral side. The posterior region with the greatest amount of bone usually is restored first. In this manner, the implants of greater size and surface area can resist the unilateral posterior forces while the patient waits for future treatment. However, if many years pass before implants are to be inserted in the less available bone, continued resorption may result in augmentation procedures prior to reconstruction.

The Class I patient is more likely to wear a removable partial denture than Class II and III patients because mastication and support of the upper

TABLE 11–1. (cont.)

Class IV: Partially edentulous arch with edentulous area anterior to remaining natural teeth, and crosses the midline.
Divisions A to D same as for Class I.

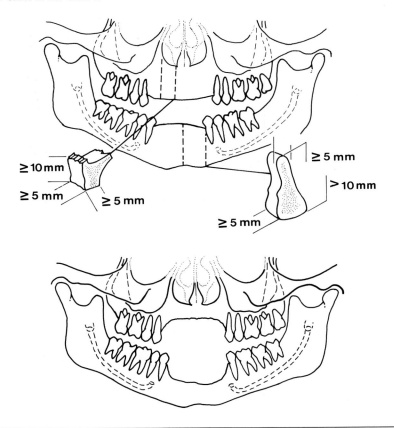

dentition/prostheses is more difficult with bilateral edentulism. The removable prosthesis often accelerates the posterior bone loss. A partial denture that is not well designed or maintained distributes additional loads to abutment teeth and may even contribute to poor periodontal health. These combinations of conditions lead to less bone in the edentulous regions and poorer adjacent natural abutments.

The treatment plan must consider the factors of force previously identified and relate them to the existing condition. Augmentation procedure may be required to improve posterior bone volume so there is greater surface area for implants and an independent implant restoration can result.

Osteoplasty cannot be as aggressive in the Class I patient to increase bone width because the opposing anatomic landmarks (maxillary sinus or mandibular canal) are closer to the crest of the ridge compared with the anterior sections of the mouth.

Class II

The Class II partially edentulous patient is missing teeth in one posterior segment. These patients are often able to function without a removable restoration and are less likely to tolerate or overcome the minor complications of wearing the prosthesis. As a result, they are not as likely to wear a removable restoration. The available bone is therefore often adequate for endosteal implants, even when long-term edentulism has been present. However, the local bone density is decreased. Endosteal implants with minimum osteoplasty is a common surgical indication for prosthetic support.

Natural teeth have often exfoliated or extruded into the posterior edentulous region. The occlusal plane should be evaluated and the final occlusion should disclude in excursions and not load the implants in a lateral direction.

Class III

A Class III patient who is a candidate for an implant typically has a long posterior span or anterior missing single tooth. A posterior edentulous region most often is splinted to a posterior tooth if an independent implant restoration is not feasible. The posterior tooth has less mobility, and posterior disclusion is possible on the restoration. An anterior tooth abutment has more mobility and more lateral forces in excursions.

An anterior single tooth implant replacement is indicated primarily when patient desires do not permit crowns on the adjacent teeth. However, this type of restoration is one of the more difficult restorations in an implant practice.

Class IV

The Class IV patient has an anterior space which crosses the midline. Traditional fixed partial dentures are often the treatment of choice when the canines are present. A lack of anterior bone is common, and bone grafts prior to implant placement are typical. The implants are often placed more lingual than the natural tooth roots. This causes a cantilever with the anterior incisor edge. The moment of a force is anterior to the arch in the maxilla and also is greater than the mandibular counterpart. The premaxilla is one of the more difficult regions of the mouth to predictably treat.

Division A Treatment Plans

Class I or II Division A patients have posterior edentulous space(s) and anterior teeth. When an implant is used in these categories, an independent implant-supported fixed prosthesis is usually indicated. Two or more endosteal root form implants are required to replace independent molar prostheses. The greater the number of teeth missing, the larger the size and/or number of implants required. Posterior available bone is limited in height by the mandibular canal in the mandible or the maxillary sinus in the maxilla. The first premolar positioned implants must angle to the distal to avoid encroachment upon the apex of the canine root and yet avoid the anterior loop of the mandibular canal or maxillary sinus. Partial dentures should be generously relieved or not worn at all during the healing process, especially if parafunction is present.

Class III Division A patients often have endosteal root form implant(s) placed when two or more missing teeth are in the edentulous space. This situation is also indicated when occlusal forces are too great for the natural abutment teeth to act as support for a fixed prosthesis. Single tooth replacement is more indicated in the maxillary anterior region. Implant placement is often anterior to the mandibular foramen or maxillary sinus in order to obtain maximum available height of bone. As a general rule, the final prosthesis may be implant supported only if two implants support each section of three missing teeth. Mobile natural teeth adjacent to the edentulous span cause greater incidence of unretained implant abutment, implant bone loss, or fracture when joined to the more rigid implant. Therefore, independent implant prostheses are often indicated.

Division B Treatment Plans

The Class I or II Division B patients have narrow bone in posterior edentulous spaces and anterior teeth. A fixed prosthesis is also indicated in these categories. Endosteal plate form implants or small-diameter root form implants are placed in the posterior Division B edentulous ridge. The greater the number of teeth missing, the larger the length and depth of the required implant(s). A double-headed plate form implant is indicated for improved load distribution and cement retention of the final prosthesis. Available bone height is restricted by the mandibular canal or maxillary sinus. As a result, osteoplasty to increase width of bone has limited application. If narrow-diameter root forms are used, more numbers are indicated than the Division A condition.

Division B implants usually require the use of natural teeth for a fixed prosthesis. The patient who is missing molars may have one double-headed plate form or two narrow-diameter root forms placed in the edentulous molar area. The final prosthesis should be splinted to a nonmobile second premolar. If tooth mobility is present, the implants should be splinted to additional natural abutments until the natural tooth segment has zero clinical mobility.

A similar treatment plan is applicable when molars and the second premolar are missing and the first premolar is not mobile. However, when the first premolar has clinical mobility, splinting the canine in the final prosthesis introduces lateral forces to the implant-tooth prosthesis when the patient goes into excursions. As a result, an additional Division B root form and an independent restoration is indicated. If an additional implant cannot be placed, lack of parafunction and good clinical health of the canine permit its splinting to the slightly mobile first premolar.

The patient missing molars and both premolars requires additional implant support. Three or four Division B root forms may result in an independent fixed partial denture, depending on the other stress factors. If a plate form implant is required, the location in front of the mandibular foramen or sinus is evaluated for osteoplasty with Division A root form insertion. The posterior plate form may then be splinted to the root form and support an independent fixed restoration. This scenario is also indicated with posterior Division B root forms. If the osteoplasty distal to the canine does not result in an edentulous region suitable for endosteal implants, the canine is joined to the posterior implants within the prosthesis. A mobile canine requires additional anterior splinting. However, incisors often have clinical mobility, especially when the canine is mobile. As a result, the splinting may require all anterior teeth, including the contralateral canine.

Molar endosteal implants should not be rigidly cross-splinted to each other in the Class I patient, even when anterior teeth are mobile. Flexure of the mandible during opening may cause a rigid splint to exert lateral forces on the posterior implants. Stress breakers, additional pontics with precious metal, or independent restorations are indicated.

Class III Division B patients may have narrow-diameter endosteal implants placed in the middle of a long-span edentulous space, or near the weakest abutment tooth. This treatment plan is primarily used for fixed prosthodontic treatment when the span is too long or occlusal forces are too great for the natural abutments to act as sole support for the final prosthesis. Plate form implants are used more often in the posterior region, whereas Division B root forms are inserted in the anterior narrow edentulous ridge. The final prosthesis may use the abutment tooth on the distal side of the edentulous region if it is not mobile. If one tooth is mobile the implant is placed next to it, and only the nonmobile tooth is joined to the implant. If the rigid implant is splinted to a mobile abutment, a pier abutment with additional complications result.

The Class IV Division B patient is treated very similar to the previous Class III Division B treatment. If the ridge is Division B and inadequate in width for root form implants, narrow-diameter root forms or single-tooth plate form implants may be selected. Bone augmentation is more often used in anterior edentulous regions with narrow bone, so Division A implants may be used. Single tooth replacement may remain independent. Two or more pontics are rarely indicated, and natural abutment support is usually necessitated. The canine is a prime abutment. When the canine is missing, the final prosthesis includes both anterior and posterior natural abutments. This compromises the occlusal scheme. A hydroxylapatite (HA) graft is often placed on the labial of the Division B edentulous ridge for increased soft tissue contouring, proper cervical tooth position, and improved lip support for esthetics.

Division C Treatment Plans

If inadequate bone exists in height, width, length, or angulation or if crown-implant ratios are greater than 1, the practitioner must consider several options. The first is to not use implant support, but instead to insist on conventional removable partial prostheses. The second is to utilize bone augmentation procedures. If the intent of the bone graft is to change a Division C to a Division A or B for endosteal implants, autogenous bone and demineralized freeze dried bone with a resorbable membrane may be utilized. After augmentation, endosteal implants provide abutment support. Augmentation is used most often in the Class I or II maxilla, where subantral grafts may use allografts and do not require as much autogenous bone as other regions. Implants may be placed at the same time as the subantral graft, and the treatment plan follows the options previously addressed.

If bone augmentation is performed for improved ridge contour and soft tissue support only, nonresorbable HA is recommended. A conventional soft tissue–borne prosthesis is then indicated unless adequate natural teeth exist for a fixed prosthesis and the HA is used for esthetic soft tissue support in the pontic areas.

The third option for the Division C patient is to place a subperiosteal implant. This implant has been used with greater clinical success in the mandible than in the maxilla. Mandibular circumferential (around the teeth) subperiosteal implants may be considered in the differential treatment plans for Class I patients. The circumferential subperiosteal implant may be treated as the root form implant for prosthetic design. Independent fixed prostheses, with no attachment to natural teeth, are possible.

The unilateral subperiosteal implant and the associated permucosal abutment heads are treated very similar to a plate form implant in Class II patients. This is usually joined to at least one healthy tooth or implant and may require cross-arch stabilization if serving as support for both premolars and molars. Subperiosteal implants are rarely used in the treatment plans for Class III or IV partially edentulous patients. Augmentation is the method of choice prior to endosteal implant placement.

Division D Treatment Plans

The bone in Division D is severely atrophied. No alveolar bone is present, and part of the basal bone is also resorbed. Class I or II Division D patients usually exhibit the long-term edentulous maxilla. Subantral augmentation is usually performed many months prior to implant placement. This condition is rarely found in the mandibular partially edentulous patient. The most common occurrence is from trauma or tumor surgery. These patients often need autogenous bone grafts to improve implant success and prevent pathologic fracture before prosthodontic reconstruction. After the graft is mature and the available bone improved, the patient is evaluated and treated similar to other patients who have improved available bone. Grafts made of HA for soft tissue contour do not work as well in Division D patients as in the other three divisions.

COMPLETELY EDENTULOUS ARCHES

The completely edentulous patient has few treatment options in conventional dentistry other than a complete removable denture. However, when implants are considered, treatment plans range from a two-implant overdenture to a completely implant-supported prosthesis. Whenever implants are considered for prosthetic support, the available bone in the regions of the potential abutments becomes paramount.

A history of edentulous classifications primarily includes the augmentation classification of Kent and the Louisiana Dental School.[14] This classification treats all regions of an edentulous arch in similar fashion and does not address regional variation. In addition, the classification was for ridge augmentation with hydroxylapatite and a conventional denture. Misch developed a more precise organization system for the completely edentulous arch in 1986.[15] The divisions of bone described in Chapter 7 are the basis of this classification.[16] This chapter presents a classification of the completely edentulous arch to organize the most common implant options of prosthodontic support.

CLASSIFICATION

The edentulous jaw is divided into three regions. In the mandible, the right and left posterior sections extend from the mental foramen to the retromolar pad, and the anterior area is located between the mental foramina. The right and left posterior regions of the edentulous maxilla begin in the second premolar region where the maxillary sinus most often determines the height of available bone. The anterior section of the maxilla extends in the region between the first premolars and is usually anterior to the maxillary sinus (Fig 11–1).

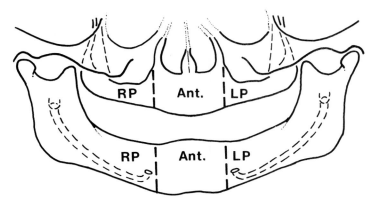

FIG 11–1.
The completely edentulous jaw is divided into three segments. The anterior component *(Ant)* is between the mental foramina or in front of the maxillary sinus. The right *(RP)* and left *(LP)* posterior segments correspond to the patient's right and left sides.

The classification of the edentulous jaw is then determined by the division of bone in each section of the edentulous arch. The three areas of bone are evaluated independently from each other. Hence the edentulous arch may have one, two, or three different divisions of bone. The term *type* is used in the completely edentulous classification, rather than class, as in the partially edentulous classification.

Type 1

In the Type 1 edentulous arch the division of bone is similar in all three anatomic segments. Therefore, four different categories of Type 1 edentulous arches are present. The Type 1 Division A ridge has abundant bone in all three sections. The patient may use as many root forms as needed, and wherever desired to support the final prosthesis (Fig 11–2).

The Type 1 Division B edentulous ridge has adequate bone in all three sections in which to place narrow-diameter root form or plate form implants. It is a common scenario to change the anterior section of bone by osteoplasty to a Division A and to place full size root form implants in this region. It is more unusual to have enough posterior height in either the maxilla or mandible to permit osteoplasty to improve the division. Therefore if posterior implants are needed, narrow implants are often indicated. Augmentation by bone spreading may be indicated if the patient desires an FP-1 prosthesis, especially when opposing natural teeth.

Type 1 Division C-w edentulous arches have inadequate bone width for implantation. If the patient desires a removable prosthesis, an osteoplasty

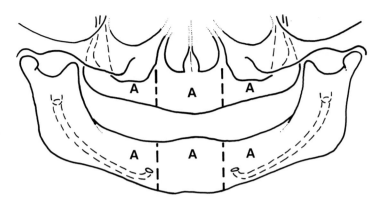

FIG 11–2.
The Type I Division A arch has Division A bone *(A)* in all three regions. Once the prosthesis is determined, the potential abutment sites may have root forms inserted.

converts the ridge to C-h. The treatment plan then follows a Type 1, C-h formula. An FP-1 restoration requires an onlay graft of autogenous bone to improve the bone category to Division A.

Type 1 Division C-h edentulous arches do not have all essential requirements for as predictable long-term endosteal implant treatment plans (Fig 11–3). An implant-supported RP-4 or RP-5 removable prosthesis is often indicated to reduce occlusal loads. The mandibular arch may be treated with a complete subperiosteal

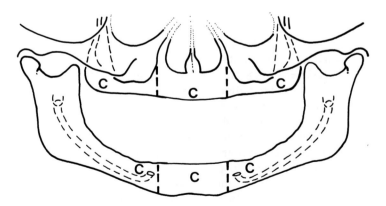

FIG 11–3.
Type I Division C-h has a crown-implant ratio greater than 1. The biomechanics of this prosthesis may indicate a removable restoration to improve long-term success. Augmentation can improve the division, and is most common in the posterior maxilla with subantral augmentation. Subperiosteal implants or root forms anterior are most often performed in the mandible.

implant or root form implants in the anterior section. The prosthesis is completely implant supported (RP-4) for the subperiosteal implant, and may have an RP-4 or combination support of implant and soft tissue for anterior root forms (RP-5) (see Chapter 12).

The maxillary prosthesis is often treated with a conventional removable prosthesis. If this denture needs additional retention or stability, HA and demineralized freeze-dried bone is used to augment the premaxilla on the lingual slope of the edentulous ridge. This squares the ridge shape and provides resistance to occlusal excursions during function. Intramucosal inserts may also be used to increase the retention of the removable complete denture. If the prosthesis of the maxillary Type I Division C patients needs more rigid implant support, a complete subperiosteal implant may be considered if other dental evaluation criteria permit. Subnasal augmentation and root form implants in the canine eminence region and subantral augmentation with posterior implants for an implant-supported overdenture may be considered. Implants can usually be placed in the posterior maxilla at the same time as the subantral augmentation. However, additional surgical training is required for these last two alternatives, and they have a greater incidence of complication. The prosthesis that needs complete fixed support may need autogenous grafts to change the division and improve success and esthetics.

The edentulous arches classified Type 1 Division D present the greatest challenge to traditional and implant dentistry (Fig 11–4). If an implant fails in a Type 1 Division D patient, pathologic fractures or almost unrestorable conditions may result. Yet, these are the patients who need the most help for support of their prosthesis. The benefits versus risks must carefully be weighed for each patient.

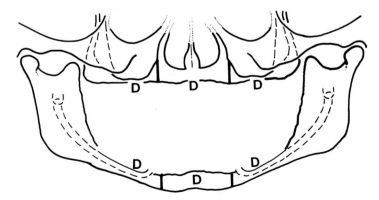

FIG 11–4.
Type I Division D arches *(D)* offer the greatest challenge to implant dentistry. An implant failure at the time of placement or many years later may result in mandibular fracture or oral-nasal fistula. Bone augmentation before implant placement or conventional dentures should be strongly considered.

Occasionally, in the mandibular arch with dehiscent canals and adequate width still present, a modified subperiosteal implant design may be selected. Endosteal implants may also be placed in the anterior mandible. However, the unfavorable crown-implant ratio is often greater than 5 to 1, and mandibular fracture during implant placement or after implant failure may result in significant complications.

Often the best solution is to change the division with autogenous grafts, then reevaluate the improved conditions and treat appropriately. The Type 1 Division D ridges use the autogenous iliac crest and particulate graft in conjunction with two or more root form implants. After 6 months a total of six to ten implants may be placed in the anterior and posterior regions (see Chapter 13).

Type 2

In the Type 2 completely edentulous arch the posterior sections of bone differ from those of the anterior segment. The most common arches in this category present less bone in the posterior regions, under the maxillary sinus, or over the mandibular canal, than in the anterior segment in front of these structures.

These types of edentulous ridges are described in the completely edentulous classification with two Division letters following Type 2, with the anterior segment listed first. Therefore, a mandible with a Division C ridge posterior to the mandibular foramen and Division A bone between the foramina is called a Type 2 Division A, C arch. The anterior region often has the greatest volume of bone in the arch. The anterior region is often the only segment used for implant support. In addition, the anterior portion is more critical for the overall treatment plan and success rate.

The edentulous arch described as Type 2 Division A, B has posterior sections that may be treated with narrow-diameter implants, while the anterior section is adequate for root form implants to support the prosthesis (Fig 11–5). The posterior Division B section may be changed into Division A by osteoplasty, but this is not always possible, because the height reduction during osteoplasty often encroaches closer to the opposing landmark, resulting with short endosteal implant support. Synthetic onlay augmentation is not as predictable or timely as Division B endosteal implants, and autogenous grafts are often too debilitating and healing periods too extended, for the benefit of increased width of posterior bone.

The Type 2 Division A, C edentulous ridge presents two primary modes of implant treatment. The most common mandibular situation is to utilize only the anterior section for implant support, with splinted root form implants. The maxillary arch may incorporate sinus elevation and subantral augmentation to upgrade the division, followed by endosteal implant placement if additional posterior support is required for the prosthesis. Because the bone density of the mandible is superior to that of the maxilla, and the moment of the force is within the arch form, rarely does the mandible require additional posterior support with grafts or circumferential subperiosteal implants.

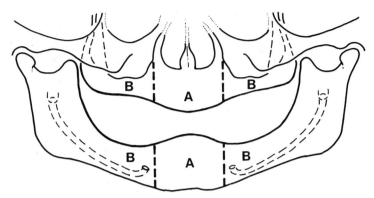

FIG 11–5.
The Type 2 Division A, B arch has an anterior section classified as Division A *(A)* and posterior sections as Division B *(B)*. The anterior region dominates the overall treatment plan in all edentulous arches and usually has greater volume of bone than the posterior.

The condition of the edentulous ridge with severe bone loss in the posterior and abundant bone in the anterior is rare, but may occur in the maxilla. The Type 2 Division A, D patient is treated very similar to the previous case of the Type 2 Division A, C arch.

The Type 2 Division B, C edentulous arch corresponds with two main treatment options (Fig 11–6). The anterior section may be changed to Division A

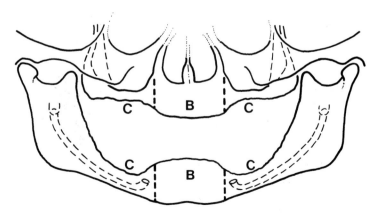

FIG 11–6.
The Type 2 Division B, C *(B* and *C)* arch has two main treatment options, as anterior Division B is not adequate for most treatment plans. An osteoplasty may convert the anterior ridge to Division A or C, and posterior treatment varies according to the maxilla or mandible.

if anatomic conditions permit. These patients are then treated exactly as the previously described Type 2 Division A, C. It is possible, especially in the anterior maxilla, that the ridge does not present sufficient height after osteoplasty to upgrade the division. In these cases the posterior divisions may be changed by sinus elevation and subantral augmentation with synthetic bone substitutes and the whole arch treated in the same manner as Type 1 Division B to Type 2, Division B, A. If this same anatomic limitation exists in the mandible, synthetic grafts are much less predictable. Instead, the anterior division may be changed to a Division C by osteoplasty, and a mandibular complete subperiosteal implant or anterior root forms and RP-4 or 5 prosthesis may be selected, as in Type 1 Division C mandibular patients.

Patients who present with advanced atrophy in the posterior segments and adequate ridge width and height in the anterior, may be described as Type 2 Division B, D. This condition almost never occurs in the mandible, but can be found on occasion in the maxilla. These patients are treated very similar to the Type 2 Division B, C previously described. The major difference is that the posterior graft is more extensive and requires additional months for healing before prosthodontic reconstruction.

Type 3

In Type 3 edentulous arches, the posterior sections of the maxilla or mandible differ from each other. This condition is less common than the other two types and is found more frequently in the maxilla than mandible. When this condition exists, the anterior is listed first, then the right posterior, followed by the left posterior segment. Therefore, the edentulous maxilla with no bone available for implants in the left posterior section, abundant bone in the anterior section, and adequate bone in the right posterior segment is a Type 3 Division A, B, D edentulous arch (Fig 11–7).

The patient whose mandible has adequate bone in the right posterior segment, inadequate bone on the other side, but abundant bone in the anterior is a Type 3 Division A, B, C edentulous ridge. A plate form implant may be placed in the right posterior, and root forms in the anterior section as indicated by the prosthesis. If additional prosthetic support is needed in the left mandibular region, usually additional anterior root forms are placed and splinted, and the teeth or bar cantilevered without implant support on the left posterior region. The Type 3 Division A, C, B patient is treated as a mirror image of Type 3 Division A, B, C.

The Type 3 Division A, D, C or Division A, C, D patient receives a treatment plan similar to the plans discussed under Type 2 Division A, C. Endosteal root form implants are used in the anterior section, and if the prosthesis needs additional posterior support, grafts are considered, especially in the posterior maxilla. The Type 3 arches with Division B or C in the anterior are treated similar

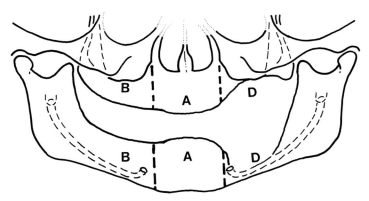

FIG 11–7.
The Type 3 Division A, B, D arch has abundant anterior bone *(A)*, moderate bone in the posterior right *(B)*, and severe atrophy in the left posterior segment *(D)*. Sinus augmentation is a common treatment if posterior implants are required in the maxilla. However, bone augmentation in the posterior mandible is more unusual, and additional anterior implants with a cantilever are more typical.

to the corresponding Type 2 patients with an anterior Division B or C. The Type 3 edentulous ridge may be Division B, C, D or Division C, D, B, for example.

When the posterior sections are different, the arch is Type 3, even when the anterior region is similar to one of the posterior sections. For example, the Type 3 Division C, D, C ridge has Division C in the anterior, severe atrophy on the right

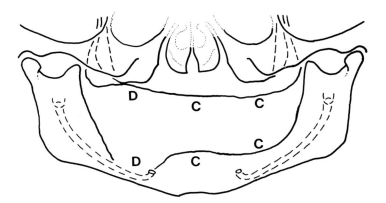

FIG 11–8.
The Type 3 Division C, D, C patient has mandibular treatment of anterior root forms or a subperiosteal implant and RP-4 prosthesis. The maxilla often uses posterior sinus augmentation and subnasal elevation for endosteal implants. A RP-4 restoration permits improved hygiene and esthetics, as well as improved force transfer because the patient can remove the restoration at night and decrease the risk of parafunction overload.

section, and moderate atrophy in the left section (Fig 11–8). The mandibular arch often uses the anterior section only, although a subperiosteal implant may be indicated. The maxilla usually has posterior and anterior treatment as subantral augmentation and subnasal elevation, because the moment of the force and bone density is poorer than the mandibular counterpart.

The anterior section is the primary region that determines the treatment plan. Rarely are posterior implants inserted without any anterior implant support. Kennedy-Applegate Class I, Modification I partially edentulous patients with anterior missing teeth are often restored with an anterior fixed partial denture and posterior removable partial denture in traditional dental treatment. Rocking of the prosthesis is reduced during anterior function, and less moment of the force is distributed to the abutments. Conventional prosthetics dictates that a fixed partial denture is not indicated when the canine and two adjacent teeth are missing. These time-tested, traditional prosthodontic axioms indicate that posterior implants should not be placed without any anterior implant or natural tooth support.

SUMMARY

An Implant Dentistry Classification has been outlined that permits visualization of teeth and bone in partially edentulous arches. The foundation of this classification is the Kennedy-Applegate system, which is the most used classification in prosthodontics. Underlying the classification are the basic principles of available bone, which can be applied to outline implant treatment. Available bone is the most fundamental dental evaluation criterion for choosing and placing implants in dentistry. Similar treatment methods exist for similar classes and divisions of bone.

A classification for the completely edentulous arch based on available bone also has been developed. Once the patient has been evaluated and the final prosthesis designed to satisfy the patient's needs and desires, implants are considered when required to support the intended prosthesis. The most critical factor in selecting the type of implant is the available bone. The classification system of completely edentulous arches is based on the anatomic conditions of the edentulous ridge, and the implant treatment plan may be determined accordingly.

REFERENCES

1. Cummer WE: Possible combinations of teeth present and missing in partial restorations, *Oral Health* 10:421, 1920.

2. Kennedy E: *Partial denture construction,* Brooklyn, NY, 1928, Dental Items of Interest.

3. Bailyn M: Tissue support in partial denture construction, *Dent Cosmos* 70:998, 1928.

4. Neurohr F: *Partial dentures: a system of functional restoration,* Philadelphia, 1939, Lea & Febiger.

5. Mauk EH: Classification of mutilated dental arches requiring treatment by removable partial dentures, *J Am Dent Assoc* 29:2121, 1943.

6. Godfrey RJ: Classification of removable partial dentures, *J Am Coll Dent* 18:5, 1951.

7. Beckett LS: The influence of saddle classifications on the design of partial removable restoration, *J Prosthet Dent* 3:506, 1953.

8. Friedman J: The ABC classification of partial denture segments, *J Prosthet Dent* 3:517, 1953.

9. Austin KP, Lidge EF: *Partial dentures: a practical textbook,* St Louis, 1957, CV Mosby.

10. Skinner CNA: Classification of removable partial dentures based upon the principles of anatomy and physiology, *J Prosthet Dent* 9:240–246, 1959.

11. Applegate OC: *Essentials of removable partial denture prosthesis,* ed 3, Philadelphia, 1965, WB Saunders.

12. Avant WE: A universal classification for removable partial denture situations, *J Prosthet Dent* 16:533–539, 1966.

13. Misch CE, Judy WMK: Classifications of the partially edentulous arches for implant dentistry, *Int J Oral Implant* 4:7–12, 1987.

14. Kent JN: Correction of alveolar ridge deficiencies with non-resorbable hydroxylapatite, *J Am Dent Assoc* 105:99–100, 1982.

15. Misch CE: Available bone influences prosthodontic treatment, *Dent Today* 7:33–34, 1988.

16. Misch CE, Judy WMK: Classifications of the partially edentulous arches of implant dentistry, *Int J Oral Implant* 4:49–58, 1987.

Chapter 12

Treatment Options for Mandibular Implant Overdenture: An Organized Approach

Carl E. Misch

The dental profession and the public are well aware of the problems associated with a complete mandibular denture (see Chapter 1). The insertion of implants for support of an overdenture creates a more favorable environment for the restoration. This is also an ideal treatment to begin a learning curve in implant dentistry. There is more leeway in implant position or prosthesis fabrication with an implant overdenture. Hence, one of the most beneficial treatments rendered to patients is also the best introduction for a dentist into the discipline of implant dentistry. Maxillary overdentures are not required as often as mandibular and are also more difficult to place and to restore.

It has been estimated that only 15% of dental students receive any training in traditional overdentures, and fewer than 6% have any clinical exposure to attachment retained overdentures. As a result, treatment plans and overdenture concepts are attempted without proper understanding of the involved principles. Enquist at al. reported a 6% to 7% implant failure for mandibular implant-supported overdentures and 19% to 35% failure for maxillary implant overdenture.[6] Misch reports less than 2% failure in either arch when using the organized treatment option approach discussed in this chapter.[7]

This chapter presents five organized treatment options for implant-supported mandibular overdentures in the completely edentulous patient. In addition, a classification of prosthesis movement is proposed, as it relates to the five treatment plans. The options presented error on the side of safety, too reduce risk of failure or complications of bone loss, and/or superstructure loosening. The treatment is presented for completely edentulous patients with Division A anterior bone, and the anterior implants are Division A root forms. Modifications related to posterior ridge support and arch form are related to this anterior bone and implant type.

ADVANTAGES AND INDICATIONS

Advantages

Traditional overdentures must rely on the condition of the remaining natural teeth that are healthy enough to support the prosthesis. The location of these natural abutments is highly variable, and they are often compromised from past bone loss associated with periodontal disease. For a mandibular implant-supported overdenture, the implants may be placed in planned, specific sites and their number may be determined by the restoring doctor and patient. In addition, the overdenture implant abutments are healthy, rigid, and provide an excellent support system. As a result, the related benefits and disadvantages of each treatment option are predetermined.

The patient gains several advantages by investing additional time and money for an implant-supported prosthesis. Minimal bone resorption of the residual ridge occurs with the placement of implants. After the extraction of mandibular teeth, there is an average of 4 mm vertical bone loss during the 1st year following treatment. This bone loss continues over the next 25 years, with the mandible experiencing a fourfold greater vertical bone loss than the maxilla.[1] The bone under an overdenture may lose as little as 0.6 mm vertical bone over a 5-year period, and long-term resorption may remain at 0.1 mm per year.[2]

Bone loss dictates the appearance of the inferior third of the face. Once the lack of soft tissue support is evident, an overdenture provides greater support of the lips and soft tissues of the face than a fixed prosthesis. In addition, the denture tooth provides an esthetic replacement for natural dentition, which is more challenging for the technician creating porcelain to metal restorations.

A mandibular denture may move 10 mm during function. Under these conditions, designed occlusal contacts and the control of masticatory forces are near impossible. An implant overdenture provides stability of the prosthesis, and the patient is able to consistently reproduce a determined centric occlusion.[3] Soft tissue abrasions and accelerated bone loss are more symptomatic of horizontal movement of the prosthesis under lateral forces. An implant-supported overdenture may limit lateral movements and redirect forces more longitudinally.

The chewing efficiency with an overdenture is improved by 20% compared with a complete denture.[4] The maximum occlusal force of a denture patient may improve 300% with an implant-supported prosthesis.[5]

The stability of an overdenture is dramatically better than that of a traditional denture. If enough implant support is provided, the resulting prosthesis may be RP-4, completely implant supported. The retention of the restoration is also enhanced by the mechanical attachment of the implant support system. No longer is denture adhesive necessary to improve the retention of the prosthesis.

The mandibular complete denture often moves during mandibular movement and speech. The contraction of the mentalis, buccinator, and/or mylohyoid muscles may lift the denture off the soft tissue. As a consequence, the teeth may touch during speech and elicit clicking noises. The retentive implant overdenture remains in place during mandibular movement. The tongue and perioral musculature may resume a more normal position, because they are not required to limit mandibular denture movement.

The implant overdenture may reduce the amount of soft tissue coverage and extension of the prosthesis. This is especially important for new denture wearers or those who have low gagging thresholds. Also, the existence of a labial flange in a conventional denture may result in exaggerated facial contours for the patient with recent extractions. Implant-supported prostheses do not require labial extensions or extended soft tissue coverage.

Soft and hard tissue defects from tumor excision or trauma do not permit the successful rehabilitation of the patient with traditional denture support. Hemimandibulectomy patients and other maxillofacial patients may be restored with an implant overdenture.

The implant overdenture provides many practical advantages over the complete fixed partial denture. Fewer implants are required, because soft tissue areas may provide additional support. Regions of inadequate bone for implant placement may therefore be eliminated from the abutment treatment plan, rather than necessitating bone grafts or implants with poorer prognosis. Fewer prosthetic appointments and of shorter duration are necessary for removable restorations. Abutments do not require a specific location of placement since the prosthesis can completely cover the implant abutment.

The esthetics of an overdenture is improved compared with a fixed restoration. Soft tissue support to the facial features are often required for an implant patient, because bone loss is a common occurrence. The labial flange may be placed for optimal appearance, not related to hygiene conditions. In addition, a denture tooth is very esthetic and porcelain to metal restorations have difficulty routinely matching the natural teeth.

Hygiene conditions and home maintenance procedures are improved with an overdenture compared with a fixed prosthesis. Professional maintenance is also improved. Peri-implant probing is diagnostic, because a crown is not on the abutment, which prevents straight line access to the crest of the bone. The overdenture may be extended over the abutments to prevent food entrapment during function. Speech compromise is not present because the denture may extend to the soft tissue in the maxilla.

An overdenture may be removed at bedtime to reduce the effect of nocturnal parafunction and increased stresses on the implant support system. It may provide stress relief between the superstructure and prosthesis, and the soft tissue may share a portion of the occlusal load. The prosthesis is usually easier to repair than a fixed restoration. Shorter restorative appointments, reduced laboratory fees and fewer implants, allow the restoration of patients at reduced costs compared to a fixed prosthesis.

The major indications for a mandibular overdenture are therefore related to lack of retention or stability, function, speech, tissue sensitivity, and soft tissue abrasions. If an edentulous patient is willing to remain with a removable prosthesis, an overdenture is encouraged rather than a fixed restoration.

Disadvantages

The primary disadvantage of an overdenture is related to the patient's desire. Some patients want implants primarily because they do not want to be able to remove the prosthesis. An overdenture would not satisfy the psychologic need of these patients to feel the prosthesis is part of their body. On rare occasions, the lack of interarch space makes an overdenture system more difficult to fabricate than a porcelain to metal fixed prosthesis. Either an osteoplasty to increase interarch space or a fixed restoration is indicated.

Mandibular Implant Site Selection

The greatest height of available bone is located in the anterior mandible, between the mental foramina, or anterior loops of the mandibular canal when

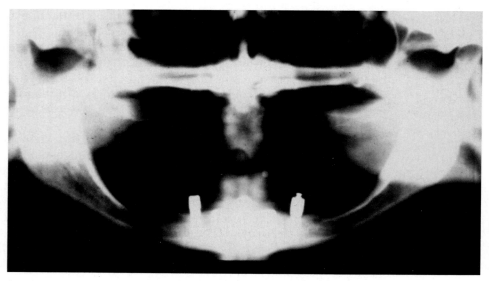

FIG 12–1.
Three implants were placed in the A, C, and E positions and an RP-5 restoration fabricated. Years later the patient desires a fixed restoration. Inasmuch as the B and D sites were left open, the additional implants can be inserted without compromise.

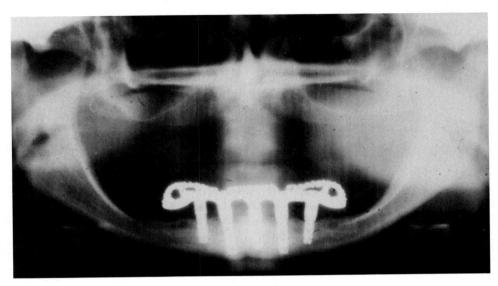

FIG 12–2.
Patient in Figure 12–1 after additional implants and fixed prosthesis.

present. This region usually presents the optimal density of bone for implant support. Anterior support for an overdenture has many advantages.[8] Therefore, the treatment options presented are designed for anterior implant placement.

The available bone of the anterior mandible is divided into five equal columns of bone serving as potential implant sites, labeled A, B, C, D, and E, starting from the patient's right. Regardless of the treatment option being executed, all five implant sites are designed at the time of surgery. In this way, the patient always has the option to obtain additional implant support in the future. For example, a patient may desire a fixed prosthesis but is unable to afford the treatment all at once. Three implants in the A, C, and E positions and an overdenture may be provided now, and in the future two implants may be added in the B and D locations and a completely implant supported overdenture or even a fixed restoration fabricated (Figs 12–1 and 12–2). Also, if an implant complication occurs, the preselected option sites permit corrective procedures. If implants were placed in the A, B, D, and E positions and an implant fails to achieve rigid fixation, the mobile implant may be removed and an additional implant placed in the C position at the same time. This saves an additional surgery and eliminates the time required for bone healing before an implant could be reinserted into the same location. Therefore, an organized pathway is provided for additional support or for the management of complications.

CLASSIFICATION OF OVERDENTURE MOVEMENT

Many types of precision attachments may be used in implant overdentures. Several authors have evaluated the range of motion of attachments.[9] The motion may occur in one to six directions: occlusal, gingival, facial, lingual, mesial, and/or distal. However, the actual overdenture movement may be completely different from the attachments when independent. In addition, prosthesis movement may vary from one to six directions even though the same type of attachments is used.

The author has sorted implant overdenture movement in six directions or range of movements, rather than attachment directions.[10] If the prosthesis is rigid while in place, but can be removed, the prosthesis movement (PM) is labeled PM-1, regardless of the attachments used. For example, O-rings have a range of motion of six different directions. But if the O-ring is placed on a complete arch bar in four different sites, and the prosthesis rests on the superstructure bar, it may be a PM-1 restoration movement. A hingelike prosthesis movement permits action in two planes and is therefore a PM-2 prosthesis. For example, the Hader bar and clip is a type 2 attachment. When this system is placed perpendicular to the axis of prosthesis rotation, the PM will also be in two planes (PM-2). However, if the Hader bar is at an angle or parallel to the direction of rotation, the prosthesis is rigid and a PM-1 system. An attachment system which permits vertical movement and a hinge motion is a Type 3 system; for example, a Dolder bar and clip. The bar and clip must also be perpendicular to the direction of prosthesis rotation for a PM-3 movement.

A PM-4 restoration is rarely available for an overdenture system. The type 5 attachment system allows a range of motion in an occlusal, mesial, distal, facial and lingual direction. A magnet is the most common implant attachment system illustrating a five-direction movement. However, the implants usually must be independent for this range of motion. If a superstructure connects the implants, the range of motion decreases. Independent magnets provide excellent retention, but often poor stability of the prosthesis.

An O-ring or ERA attachment corresponds to six directions of motion. However, the implants may need to remain independent to permit a PM-6 range of movement. A superstructure bar will limit this movement, depending on the design. A greater moment of the force is applied against the support system of an O-ring, since the vertical component of this attachment extends approximately 7 mm above the implant.

The classification system is used to evaluate the direction of movement of the implant-supported prosthesis not the overall range of motion for the individual attachment. The direction of movement is usually occlusal for PM-1 and the prosthesis is rigid while in place. A prosthesis with a hinge motion is PM-2, and a prosthesis with a vertical and hinge motion is PM-3. A PM-4 restoration is rarely observed for overdenture designs. A PM-5 allows movement in five directions, and the PM-6 has universal range of prosthesis movement. The prosthesis moment is often different than the attachment range of motion, especially when a superstructure connects the implants.

OVERDENTURE TREATMENT OPTIONS

The treatment options for mandibular overdentures range from primarily soft tissue support and implant retention (RP-5) prosthesis to a completely implant supported prosthesis (RP-4) with rigid retention. The patient's complaints, anatomy, desires, and financial commitment determine the amount of implant support required to predictably address these conditions. The amount of implant support designed in the restoration is related to the number and position of the implants (Table 12–1).

Overdenture Option One (OD-1)

The first treatment option for mandibular overdentures (OD-1) is rarely indicated. The patient's desires are minimal. The anatomic conditions of the

TABLE 12–1.

Mandibular Overdenture Treatment Options*

Option	Description†	Prosthesis Movement	Posterior Ridge
OD-1	Implants in the A, E positions, independent of each other	6	Good anatomy, stability, denture retention
OD-2	Implants in the B, D positions, joined rigidly by a bar	3–6	Good anatomic ridge form, good retention, denture stability
OD-3			
1	Implants in the A, C, E positions, rigidly joined by a bar if posterior ridge form is good	2–6	Moderate to good posterior anatomy; good lingual flange on the denture
2	Implants in the B, C, D positions, joined by a rigid bar when posterior ridge form is poor	3–6	Poor posterior anatomy; poor lateral stability in posterior region
OD-4	Implants in A, B, C, E positions, rigidly joined by a bar cantilevered to the distal about 10 mm	2 or 3	Poor posterior ridge anatomy and/or moderate patient desires
OD-5	Implants in the A, B, C, D, E positions, rigidly joined by a bar cantilevered to the distal about 15 mm	1	Poor ridge form and/or demanding patient desires

*From Misch 1984. Used by permission.

mandible are good to excellent for conventional denture retention and stability. The posterior ridge form is an inverted U shape, and lateral stability is good to excellent for the prosthesis. The problem associated with the existing denture relates only to the amount of retention. The financial commitment of the patient is low. Under these conditions, two implants may be inserted in the A and E position. The implants remain independent of each other, and are not connected with a superstructure. The most common type of attachment used in OD-1 is an O-ring or "ball and trailer hitch" design, and the prosthesis movement should be as much as practical (PM-6). The prosthesis splints these two implants together for additional support while it is in place. However, this support mechanism is poor, because stress relief is permitted in any plane (Fig 12–3).

The primary patient's advantage with OD-1 is cost. The existing restoration may often be adapted with a rebase procedure around the implants and attachment abutment sites.

The disadvantages of the OD-1 relate to its relatively poor implant support, compared with the other options because of the independent nature of the implants. There are many reasons why two implants placed in the A and E position should not be splinted together. Because these implants are placed just anterior to the mental foramina, they are usually in the first premolar positions. This results in a curved arch form anterior to the implant sites. The distance between these implants represents approximately a span of six teeth. The

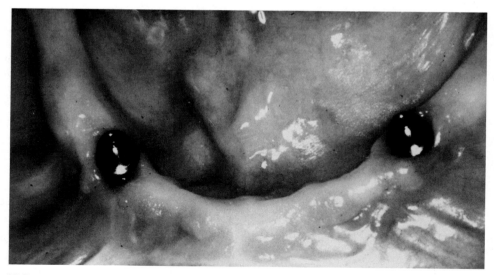

FIG 12–3.
Two implants in the A and E positions (OD-1) are in the premolar region. As a result, the implants should remain independent and permit retention of the prosthesis but little support (PM-6).

superstructure flexibility is related to the length. As a result, there is five times more flexure than if the implants were in the B and D locations.[11] The increase in superstructure movement may result in loosening of the coping screws. Once this occurs, the remaining attached implant receives a dramatic increase in moment of the forces from the long lever arm of the superstructure. This increase in force may result in bone loss, mobility of the implant, and possible fracture of an implant component.

The second problem of joining A and E implants is the position of the superstructure. If the bar is straight and not bent to follow the arch, it occupies a lingual position relative to the arch. The lingual flange of the denture then extends as much as 10 mm more lingual and 7 mm more vertical to accommodate the attachment, which is connected over the superstructure. In addition, because the teeth are set over or anterior to the crest of the ridge, anterior to the superstructure, rotation and tipping of the restoration are more prevalent. The moment of force on a straight bar connecting implants in the A and E positions is twice that for implants in the B and D locations.

The superstructure that follows the anterior curve of the arch results with an improved lingual contour of the restoration. However, because the shortest distance between two points is a straight line, the curve corresponds to an increased length and even greater flexibility of the superstructure. Because the bar is anterior to the implants, a greater moment of the force is also created. The prosthesis attachment system to the superstructure may also be compromised if clips are used for retention. If the prosthesis rests against the sides of the curved bar, the prosthesis movement is reduced and may even be rigid. This places a much greater lateral load on the implant system (Fig 12–4).

A common anatomic finding within the completely edentulous mandible is greater vertical bone height in the midline, which gradually decreases to the distal. As a result, implants placed in the A and E positions are often shorter than implants placed in the B and D locations. The surface area of the implant is reduced and shorter implants can not resist the moment of the force as well as longer implants.

The first premolar region illustrates minimal attached gingiva. Implants placed in this region often lack adequate attached gingiva on the facial aspect of the implant. Muscle attachments are also more common in this area, and soft tissue conditions may be compromised for long-term maintenance. Therefore, soft tissue corrections are common whenever implants are placed in the A or E position. Because the OD-1 is performed primarily to contain cost, additional procedures may increase the fee.

Because implants in the A and E positions are distal to the anterior curvature of the mandible, greater lateral stability is provided for the prosthesis. This may result with fewer degrees of freedom in the restoration, and increase in the lateral forces on the implants.

Implants splinted in the A and E positions have greater potential load per surface area compared with implants in the B and D regions when the bar is not

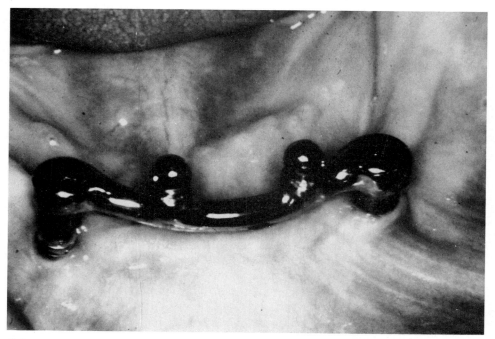

FIG 12–4.
Implants in the A and E positions splinted with a bar cause considerable force and flexure on the implants. Screw loosening is more common (right implant), which caused bone loss on the left implant and ultimately fractured the abutment.

cantilevered distal to implants. The bite force increases as it is measured to the posterior. As a result, a greater vertical load is also present, with increased stresses when implants are splinted in the A and E positions. In addition, there is twice as much moment of the force on the implants, than if the B, D position or A, C, E position was used.

As a result of these many disadvantages, the placement of two implants in the A, E position is strongly discouraged. If attempted, the anatomic ridge form should be good to excellent, and the overdenture should have excellent support and retention independent of the implants. The two implants should not be splinted to reduce complications because they are too far apart. A PM-6 range of movement is used in the restoration.

Overdenture Option Two (OD-2)

The second treatment option (OD-2) is selected only on occasion. The patient's anatomic conditions for a traditional denture are good to excellent. The posterior ridge form is an inverted "U" shape, and lateral stability is good to excellent. The patient's complaints are minimal, and relate primarily to retention. The patient requires a new prosthesis, and is willing to invest slightly more time and expense.

The implants are positioned in locations B and D and splinted together with a superstructure without any distal cantilever. The prosthesis should have a PM-3 or greater range of motion. The bar is often connected on the facial aspect of each implant coping. In this way, the lingual flange of the prosthesis remains within the contour of a traditional denture (Fig 12–5).

Overdenture Option Three (OD-3)

In the third option for a mandibular overdenture (OD-3), three root form implants are placed. A superstructure connects the implants, but is not cantilevered to the distal. This is the usual treatment for a patient with minor complications, concerned primarily with retention and anterior stability. If the posterior ridge form is good (Divisions A or B), the implants are placed in the A, C, and E area (Fig 12–6). If the posterior position is poor (Divisions C or D), the implants are placed in the B, C, and D region (Fig 12–7). The posterior ridge form determines the posterior lingual flange extension of the denture, which limits

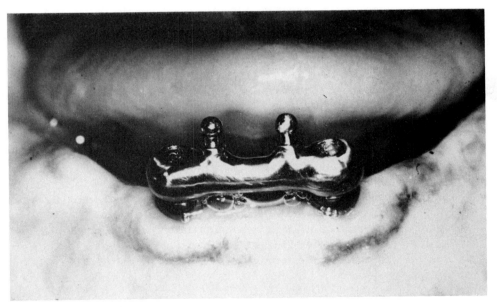

FIG 12–5.
Implants in the B and D positions (OD-2) may be splinted together. This reduces implant reaction forces and provides less stress to the implant at the crest of the bone.

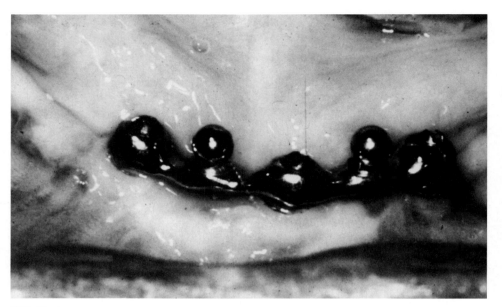

FIG 12–6.
Implants placed in the A, C, and E positions (OD-3) provide additional safety to the implants and retention of the superstructure. The attachments on the bar must permit movement of the prosthesis in several directions.

lateral movement of the restoration. Poor lateral stability places additional force on the anterior implants. Therefore, if the patient with poor posterior ridge form requires more stability, more than three implants are indicated. The prosthesis movement may be slightly more supportive in the A, C, E option, and a PM-2 to 6 range of motion is reasonable.

There are many advantages of splinting A, C, and E implants, over implants in the A and E or B and D positions. The additional C implant provides a sixfold reduction in superstructure flexure,[11] and limits the consequences previously discussed. In addition, screw loosening is less frequent because three coping screws retain the superstructure, rather than two.

Implant reaction forces are reduced with a third implant as compared to two implants.[11] The greater surface area of implant to bone allows better distribution of forces. Three permucosal sites distribute stresses more efficiently and minimize crestal bone loss. Because the crestal bone is the first region to be affected, this is a major advantage.

There is twice the reduction in maximum moment of the force with a three implant system than with two implants in the A and E regions.[11] The moment of the force may be reduced even more, when the "C" implant is often of greater length than the "A" and "E" implants.

The implants splinted in the A, C and E position should not form a straight line. The C implant is anterior to the more distal A and E implants and directly under the cingulum position of the teeth. The restoration benefits from vertical implant support in the anterior arch, and rotation of the prosthesis is limited, compared with OD-1 and OD-2. The greater the anterior-posterior distance of the A, E, and C implants, the greater the lateral stability of the system.

The prosthesis must not attach or contact angles formed by the superstructure. This would result with too rigid a system. If a clip attachment is designed for the prosthesis, the bar may connect the facial of the A and E implant copings to the lingual of the C coping. As a result, a straight bar perpendicular to the path of rotation may be fabricated. A PM-2 or greater prosthesis movement can be supported with three anterior implants. No cantilever should be designed within this system. Implants placed in the B, C, D regions are indicated with poor posterior ridge form. The increased horizontal movement of the restoration results with more lateral force on the implants. Because the A and E regions are eliminated, there is more freedom of the restoration, and less stress to the implants. The prosthesis movement should be PM-3 or greater to reduce the stress on the B, C, D implants.

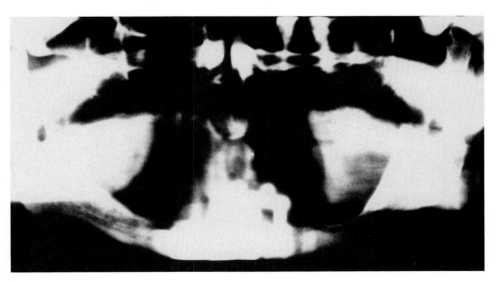

FIG 12–7.
Implants are placed in the B, C, and D positions (OD-3) when posterior ridge form is poor. This allows more movement in the prosthesis so the implants will not be overloaded. If more support is required, additional implants can be inserted.

Overdenture Option Four (OD-4)

In the fourth mandibular overdenture option (OD-4), four implants are placed in the A, B, D, and E positions. These implants provide enough support so that the superstructure may be cantilevered from the distal implant approximately 10 mm on each side (Fig 12–8). The cantilevered superstructure first makes its presence with 4 implants for two reasons. The first relates to the increase in implant support, compared with OD-1 to OD-3. The second is related to the additional retention system of the superstructure, which limits the risk of screw loosening and related complications.

The patient's indications for this treatment include poor posterior anatomy, which causes a lack of retention and stability; soft tissue abrasions; and difficulty with speech. The edentulous posterior mandible is often more resorbed than the anterior region. The buccal shelf may be covered with the buccinator muscle, and the mylohyoid ridge may correspond to the crest of the residual ridge. The patient's complaints and desires are more demanding than for the previous treatment options. The prosthesis may have more stability and a PM-2 range of motion is most common. The attachments are often placed in the distal cantilevers

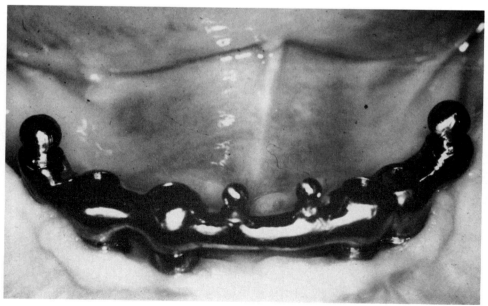

FIG 12–8.
Implants inserted in the A, B, D, and E positions (OD-4) permit a cantilever in the superstructure bar. The length of the cantilever is related to arch form, implant length, opposing arch density of bone, parafunction, and such. The average distance of the cantilever is < 10 mm, and the prosthesis is RP-5.

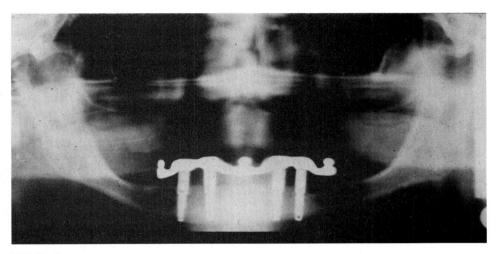

FIG 12–9.
Five-year postoperative radiograph of OD-4 treatment option.

and in the midline. The prosthesis is a RP-5, but has the least soft tissue support, than the other soft tissue–supported overdentures. The anterior attachment must be able to disengage from the bar, to permit rotation of the distal attachments.

The patient benefits from the four implants because there is greater vertical support and lateral stability. The prosthesis only loads the soft tissue over the second molar and retromolar pad regions. The amount of distal cantilever is related to the force factors previously discussed, and to the anterior-posterior distance from the center of the most anterior implants to the distal portions of the A and E implants. The arch form greatly affects this distance (Fig 12–9).

If the arch form is square and the anterior-posterior distance is reduced, the implants may be placed in the A, B, C, and E location for patients chewing primarily on the right side. The C implant is placed as far forward as practical, under the incisors of the restoration. This increases the anterior-posterior distance and increases the amount of distal cantilever to the 10-mm extent. If less than 4 mm is present between the distal portion of the A, E implants and the mid C position, no cantilever should be used in the superstructure and a PM-3 restoration is indicated.

Overdenture Option Five (OD-5)

A mandibular implant overdenture (OD-5) is designed for patients with moderate to severe problems related to a traditional restoration. The needs and desires of the patient are often most demanding. These may include limiting the

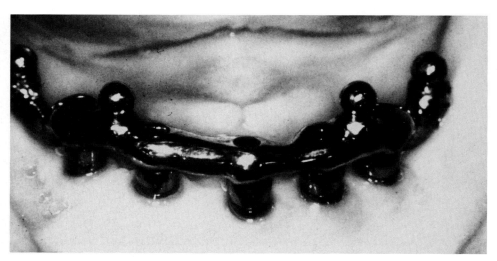

FIG 12–10.
Five implants in the A, B, C, D, and E positions may be splinted with a bar that is cantilevered as much as two and one-half times the anteroposterior distance of the implants (under ideal conditons).

bulk or amount of the prosthesis, major concerns regarding function or stability, sore spots, and inability to wear a mandibular denture.

In the OD-5 option, five implants are inserted in the A, B, C, D, and E positions. The superstructure is cantilevered distally approximately 15 mm, which places it under the first molar area. The restoration usually does not extend beyond the first molar, with either teeth or soft tissue covering. The restoration is RP-4, completely implant supported (Fig 12–10). The superstructure may be cantilevered an average of 15 mm for three reasons. The additional C implant increases the implant-bone surface area of the system and the additional implant adds another retentive element. In addition, the C position implant increases the anterior-posterior dimension of implant distance. This increases the support mechanism and helps counter the Class I lever action of the distal cantilever.

Five implants also allow the superstructure and prosthesis to be cantilevered forward from the anterior ridge. This is of particular benefit for Angle Skeletal Class II patients. The lower lip is supported by the maxillary teeth when the jaw is at rest. Traditional mandibular dentures reconstruct the horizontal overjet, so the lower anterior teeth position does not infringe on the neutral zone during rest or function. However, in a RP-4 restoration the teeth are set where they provide the best esthetic result in a skeletal Class I pattern. This also increases the amount of function in the anterior region. The distal cantilever is reduced to decrease the lever force. Because these patients are Class II, the forward tooth position also places the molars forward, and the need for distal cantilever is reduced.

DISCUSSION

The five treatment options proposed for mandibular implant supported overdentures provide an organized approach to solving a patient's complaints or anatomic limitations. The prosthesis support and range of motion should be part of the initial diagnosis. The treatment options proposed are designed for completely edentulous patients with Division A anterior bone. These options are modified if the anterior bone is Division C-h. The increase in crown-implant ratio and decrease in implant surface area support modification of these options. One additional implant is added to each option, and OD-1 is eliminated completely. Therefore, OD-2 has three implants (B, C, D position), OD-3 has four implants (A, B, D, E regions), OD-4 has five implants (A, B, C, D, E areas), and OD-5 has six implants. If six implants cannot be placed between the foramina, the cantilever length is reduced. Maxillary overdentures with Division A bone are treatment planned similar to mandibles with C-h bone. In addition, subantral augmentation is often performed to permit more distal implants and improve the anterior-posterior dimension of implant placement.

The doctor and staff can explain the amount of support each treatment option can provide by comparing them to the support system of a chair. Treatment options OD-2 or OD-3 are related to a two-legged chair. The prosthesis provides some vertical support, but can rock back and forth, like a two-legged chair. Option OD-4 with four implants is compared to a three-legged chair. This system provides further support but can be rocked one way or the other under lateral forces. A four-legged chair provides the greatest support and is similar to OD-5, which is a stable, retentive prosthesis and RP-4 in design.

CONCLUSION

Implant overdentures borrow several principles of tooth-supported overdentures. The advantages of implant overdentures relate to the ability to place rigid, healthy abutments in the anterior positions of choice. The number, location, superstructure design, and prosthetic range of motion can be predetermined and based upon patient's expressed needs and desires. A prosthesis movement (PM) classification relates the support of the restoration to each overdenture option. Two implants placed just anterior to the mental foramina should rarely be used.

The overdenture should be designed to predictably satisfy the patient's desires and anatomic limitations. A fixed prosthesis for the completely edentulous arch should be restricted to patients unable to be satisfied with a removable restoration.

REFERENCES

1. Tallgren A: The reduction in face height of edentulous and partially edentulous subjects during long-term denture wear: a longitudinal roentgenographic cephalometric study, *Acta Odontol Scand* 24:195–239, 1966.
2. Adell R: A 15-year study of osseointegrated implants in the treatment of the edentulous jaw, *Int J Oral Surg* 6:387, 1981.
3. Jamb T, Stallard PA: The effect of chewing movements on changing mandibular complete dentures to osseointegrated overdentures, *J Prosthet Dent* 55:357–361, 1986.
4. Rissin L et al: Clinical comparison of masticatory performance and electromyographic activity of patients with complete dentures, overdentures and natural teeth, *J Prosthet Dent* 39:508–511, 1978.
5. Sposetti VJ et al: Bite force and muscle activity in overdenture wearers before and after attachment placement, *J Prosthet Dent* 55:265–273, 1986.
6. Enquist B et al: A retrospective multicenter evaluation of osseointegrated implants supporting overdentures, *Int J Oral Maxillofac Implant* 3:129–134, 1988.
7. Misch C: Implant supported overdenture: a retrospective evaluation (in press).
8. Brewer AA, Morrow RM: *Overdentures,* St Louis, Mosby–Year Book, 1975.
9. Preiskel HW: *Precision attachments in prosthodontics: the applications of intracoronal and extracoronal attachments,* vol 1, Chicago, Quintessence, 1984.
10. Misch CE: Implantology basis of restorative work, *Dent Today* 7:26, 29, 1988.
11. Bidez M, Misch CE: Biomechanics of inter-implant spacing (abstract), *Int J Oral Implant* 7:76, 1990.

Chapter 13

Treatment Planning for Edentulous Maxillary Posterior Region

Carl E. Misch

The maxillary posterior edentulous region presents many challenging conditions in implant dentistry unique to this anatomic area of the jaws. However, treatment modalities exist that make treatment in this region as predictable as in any intraoral region. Most noteworthy are subantral augmentation to increase available bone height, modified surgical and treatment approaches related to bone density, and progressive bone loading during the prosthodontic phase of reconstruction. This chapter addresses the treatment options specific to the maxillary posterior edentulous region based on available bone.

ANATOMIC CONSIDERATIONS

Evolution of Posterior Maxilla With Loss of Teeth

Available alveolar bone height is lost in the posterior maxilla as a result of periodontal disease and bone resorption after tooth loss. The loss of maxillary posterior teeth results in an initial decrease in bone width at the expense of the labial bony plate. The width of the posterior maxilla decreases at a more rapid rate than in other regions of the jaws.[1] The resorption phenomenon is accelerated by the loss of vascularization of the alveolar bone and absence of muscle stimulation. The ridge width progressively decreases until the Division A bone volume is resorbed to Division B and the ridge crest shifts medially. The posterior maxilla may progressively remodel toward the midline, and as the bone division changes to Divisions C and D, medial inclination of the ridge crest continues.

The density of bone is dramatically decreased in the maxilla in the long-term edentulous patient, more than in any other region. Fewer trabeculae result, which decrease initial implant stability and force transfer to the bone. An absence of cortical plate on the crest of the ridge is often observed, which also decreases the initial stability of an implant at the time of insertion. The labial cortical plate becomes thin, and lateral cortical bone in contact along the height of the implant is observed less often. The occlusal forces in the posterior region are greater than in the anterior regions of the mouth.

Expansion of Maxillary Sinus

The maxillary sinus is the largest of the four paranasal sinuses and the first to develop in the human fetus. A primary pneumatization occurs at about 3 months of fetal development when the epithelium of the nasal floor is invaginated. At this time the maxillary sinus is a bud situated at the infralateral surface of the ethmoid infundibulum between the upper and middle meatus.[2] Prenatally, a secondary pneumatization occurs. At birth, the sinus is still an oblong grove on the mesial side of the maxilla just above the germ of the first deciduous molar.[3]

Postnatally and until the child is 3 months of age, the growth of the maxillary sinus is closely related to the pressure exerted by the eye on the orbit floor, the tension of the superficial musculature on the maxilla, and the forming dentition. As the skull matures, these three elements influence its three-dimensional development. At 5 months, the sinus appears as a triangular area medial to the infraorbital foramen.[3]

During the child's first year, the maxillary sinus expands laterally underneath the infraorbital canal, which is protected by a thin bony ridge. The height of the sinus antrum progressively replaces the space formerly occupied by the developing dentition. The growth in height is best reflected by the relative position of the sinus floor. At age 12 years pneumatization extends to the plane of the lateral orbital wall, and the sinus floor is level with the floor of the nose. Extension into the alveolar process lowers the floor of the sinus about 5 mm. The main development of the antrum occurs as the permanent dentition erupts and pneumatization extends throughout the body of the maxilla and the maxillary process of the zygomatic bone. Anteroposteriorly, the sinus expansion corresponds to the growth of the mid-face and is completed only with the eruption of the third permanent molars when the young person is about 16 to 18 years of age.[2–4]

In the adult, the sinus appears as a pyramid of four thin, bony walls, the base of which faces the lateral nasal wall and the apex of which extends toward the zygomatic bone. The maxillary sinus cavity is reinforced by bony septa joining the medial and/or lateral walls with buttress-like webs. These have the appearance of reinforcement webs in a wooden boat and rarely divide the antrum into separate compartments. These elements are present from the canine to the molar region and tend to disappear in the maxilla of the long-term edentulous patient.

The antrum is approximately 34 mm by 35 mm at its base, and the pyramidal apex extends 23 mm toward the zygomatic area. The average volume is

15 mL. [5] Individual variations in volume and measurements are common and also occur between the right and left sides of the individual. Variations may be inherited or acquired.

A fourth expansion phenomenon of the maxillary sinus occurs with the loss of posterior teeth. The antrum expands in both inferior and lateral aspects. In addition, the amount of available bone in the posterior maxilla decreases in height from the floor of the antrum. Maxillary antrum hypoplasia or aplasia (underdevelopment or absence of the maxillary sinus) may occur in about 8% of cases. This condition may not be clear on radiographs. As a result, the surgeon may be unable to explore or perform the sinus elevation, and the procedure is unnecessary in this condition.

As a result of periodontal disease, tooth loss, and sinus expansion, frequently less than 10 mm of vertical bone exists between the alveolar ridge crest and the maxillary sinus. This reduced vertical height of bone causes many endosteal implants in this region to be compromised in terms of basic bony support.

The intradental space should be evaluated prior to implant placement. The available space between the gingiva and the proper plane of occlusion should be greater than 5 mm. If less than this vertical space is present for prosthodontic reconstruction, a gingivectomy, osteoplasty, vertical osteotomy of the maxillary posterior alveolar process, and/or mandibular plane correction are indicated to restore the anatomy to the ideal occlusal plane.

TREATMENT HISTORY

In the past, oral surgeons avoided use of implants in the maxillary sinus. Small implants were often placed below the antrum. The decreased surface area provided poor implant stability, especially in the poor quality bone often present in this region. Attempts to place larger endosteal implants anterior and posterior to the antrum also resulted in complications. Rarely are third or fourth molar abutments indicated for proper prosthodontic support. This approach often requires three or more pontics between the implants. The typical spans result, with excessive flexibility of the prosthesis, unretained restorations, excess stresses, and implant failure. Subperiosteal implants have been used in the edentulous maxilla where bone height is inadequate. The thin, porous compacta often present on the crest of the ridge and on the lateral border of the maxilla serves as a poor foundation for this implant. Lack of adequate bone height often results in the implant being displaced laterally, off the bony ridge, from occlusal and parafunctional forces. Long-term success of maxillary subperiosteal implants is the most difficult to predict of any implant type.

In the late 1960s Linkow reported that the blade-vent implant could be blunted, and the maxillary sinus membrane could be slightly elevated to allow implant placement "into" the sinus in the posterior maxilla.[5] This technique required the presence of at least 7 mm of vertical bone height below the antrum. For long-term predictable results, vertical bone height of at least 10 mm in the posterior maxilla has been clinically determined to be necessary. Branemark et al. have shown that implants may be placed into the maxillary sinus without consequence if integration occurs between the implants and the bone below the sinus. Yet he also reports a higher failure rate (70%; 5 to 10 years) for this technique.[6] Ashkinazy[7] and others have reported on utilizing tomographic radiographs to determine whether adequate bone exists on the palatal aspect of the maxillary sinus for blade implants. Stoler[8] stated that after 25 consecutive computed tomographic scans of maxillae, adequate bone for implant support was not found on the medial aspect of the sinus. Thus, it seems that if sufficient bone is present medial to the sinus, it is the rare exception.

In the early 1970s, Tatum[9] began to augment the posterior maxilla with autogenous rib bone to produce adequate vertical bone for implant support. He found that onlay grafts below the existing alveolar crest would decrease the posterior intradental height significantly, yet very little bone for endosteal implants would be gained. Therefore Tatum developed a modified Caldwell-Luc procedure for sinus augmentation. The lateral wall of the maxilla was fractured and used to elevate the maxillary sinus membrane. Autogenous bone was then added in the area previously occupied by the inferior third of the sinus. Endosteal implants were inserted in this grafted bone after approximately 6 months. Implants would not be loaded with final prostheses for an additional 6 months.[9]

In 1975, Tatum developed a surgical technique that allowed the elevation of the sinus membrane and implant placement in the same surgical appointment. The implant system utilized was a one-piece ceramic implant, and a permucosal post was required during the healing period. Early ceramic implants were not designed adequately for this procedure, and results with the technique were unpredictable. In 1981, Tatum developed a submerged titanium implant, the Omni S, for use in the posterior maxilla.[9] The advantages of submerged healing, the use of titanium instead of aluminum oxide as a biomaterial, improved biomechanics, and improved surgical technique made this implant modality more predictable for the experienced practitioner.

In 1980, the application of the subantral augmentation (SA) technique with a lateral maxillary approach was further expanded by Tatum with the use of synthetic bone. The same year, Boyne and James reported on the use of autogenous bone for subantral grafts.[10] In 1984, Misch organized a treatment approach to the posterior maxilla based on the amount of bone below the antrum,[11] and in 1986 expanded the treatment approach to include the available bone width related to surgical approach and implant design. Since then minor modifications regarding the graft materials or surgical approach have also been proposed.[12] The procedure has proved highly predictable, provided proper case selection, adequate training, adequate experience, and patient cooperation are present.[13]

PATIENT EVALUATION

Clinical Assessment

Evaluation of the patient for maxillary posterior edentulous procedures is similar to evaluation for other implant procedures.[14] In addition, a thorough history and clinical examination of the posterior maxilla and maxillary sinus is conducted. Symptoms associated with the paranasal sinuses are one of the country's most common ailments, and affect over 31 million people each year. Approximately 16 million people will seek medical assistance related to sinusitis; yet sinusitis is one of the most frequently overlooked diseases in clinical practice. Potential consequences of surgery in the region of the sinuses include osteomyetites and, although rare, brain abscess.[15] In fact, paranasal sinus infection accounts for approximately 5% to 10% of all brain abscesses.[16] A past or present history of symptoms of sinusitis is important for implant treatment plans in which subantral augmentation is being considered. These symptoms are usually nonspecific and include the presence of a common cold or allergic rhinitis.

Acute and chronic maxillary sinusitis may be diagnosed by patient history and clinical examination. The usual cause of sinusitis is inhaled bacteria. The drainage through the ostium is then impaired by the swollen mucosa. A patient history often associated with acute sinusitis includes unilateral headaches and/or throbbing and constant pain in the maxillary sinus area, often radiating to the teeth or ears. The teeth are vital, but may be sore and painful to percussion. The skin overlying the canine region may also be swollen or red. In case of allergic sinusitis, sneezing and watering eyes may be observed. Vague headaches, fullness of the face, and mucopurulent hypersecretion are also associated with chronic sinusitis.

Sinusitis is observed most frequently related to maxillary or frontal sinus involvement.[17] A physical examination evaluates facial tenderness, nasal congestion, prevalent nasal discharge, anosmia, and halitosis. The clinical examination of the patient primarily concerns the regions surrounding the maxillary antrum. The patient may experience discomfort when the region over the infraorbital foramen is palpated. The nasal fluids may be evaluated by asking the patient to blow the nose in a waxed paper. The mucous should be clear and thin in nature. A yellow or greenish tint or thickened discharge indicates infection. The cause may be the existence of nasal polyps, cystic lesion, neoplasia, or cocaine abuse.[2, 15] A surgical intervention to establish a new sinus ostium may be indicated as treatment of acute or chronic sinusitis. This may include a nasoantrostomy in the inferior nasal meatus or Caldwell-Luc sinusotomy. If a Caldwell-Luc procedure is indicated, the ear, nose and throat specialist should be requested to approach the sinus from an anterior wall and to avoid the region of the future dental surgery so as not to conflict with a subantral augmentation procedure.

Less frequently encountered problems associated with the maxillary sinus include tumors or malignancies. Sixty percent of the squamous cell carcinomas of the paranasal sinuses are located in the maxillary sinus, usually in the lower half of the antrum. Clinical signs in the oral cavity illustrate the expansion of the tumor and increased mobility of the teeth involved. Invasion of the orbit or the infratemporal fossa are often also present.[2, 15] A negative history of symptoms and physical findings does not negate the presence of current sinusitis. However, known disease of the antrum should be treated before subantral augmentation.

Oroantral fistulas may exist as sequelae of tooth or implant extraction, trauma, or surgical entry into the maxillary sinus. Acute or chronic sinusitis contributes to their persistence. Clinically they may appear as a painless oral opening, often inflamed, with excess granulation tissue. Mucopurulent drainage may be observed. The patient may report exchange of food or air, and probing reveals a communication.

Radiographic Assessment

The clinical examination is accompanied by a careful evaluation by panoramic radiography. Although the maxillary sinus may be studied by a Waters' projection (face down, or modified), the contour of the sinus is better illustrated on a panoramic x-ray, and is also preferred to Waters' view for detection of cystlike densities.[16] However, the Waters' projection represents a better view than a panoramic film to illustrate cloudiness and sclerotic changes. Therefore, both may be used in sinus examinations, especially if history or clinical evaluation warrants.

The panoramic radiograph often demonstrates the maxillary sinus as multicompartmented, with radiopaque bony septa. The innominate line is a thin vertical radiopaque line in the posterior third of the antrum. It is an artifact corresponding in its lower half to the posterior surface of the zygomatic process of the maxilla and in its upper half to the posterior surface of the frontal process of the zygoma. It should be distinguished from the posterior wall of the antrum, which usually corresponds to the anterior portion of the pterygomaxillary fossa.

The hard palate or floor of the nose is usually present radiographically in the lower third of the maxillary sinus. The lower radiopaque line corresponds to its image, whereas the upper line represents the ghost image of the contralateral side. The distance between the palatal line and the floor of the antrum gives a good indication of the height of bone on the facial side below the zygoma for direct surgical access for the lateral approach to subantral augmentation. This is especially important in the Division D maxilla, where all other landmarks have disappeared. In these maxillae, the lateral access window may actually be prepared in the zygomatic arch.

To obtain a proper diagnostic image of the antrum, the patient's tongue must be kept in contact with the palate. Improper obturation of the airway results in a radiolucent region superimposed with the antrum image. Occasional radiopaque projections of the inferior and middle turbinates, or of the inferior, middle, or superior meati may also be present. Maxillary tori create a bilateral dense radiopaque image. The presence of oroantral fistulae may be occasionally detected on panoramic films, depending on their size and location.[16, 17] They are often associated with signs of acute or chronic sinusitis.

Computed tomography is currently the modality of choice in the evaluation of diseases of the nose and paranasal sinuses.[18] The images may enable one to evaluate the extent of mucoperiosteal thickening and details the regional anatomy. Mucoperiosteal thickening is most often found in the middle meatus and infundibular regions. The anterior ethmoid–middle meatal complex, the region through which the frontal and maxillary sinuses drain, is primarily responsible for mucocilary clearance of the sinus to the nasopharynx.[19] As a result, pathogenesis of sinusitis is usually the development of obstruction in one area of this complex.[20] Unfortunately, standard roentgenograms do not permit accurate evaluation of the anterior ethmoid sinus. Computed tomographic images are especially warranted if the patient's history, physical examination, or radiographic evaluation require further information. In addition, these views may provide the inexperienced surgeon an improved perspective on the entire surgical region.

Pathologic Assessment

Proper diagnosis, treatment planning, and surgical manipulation of the posterior maxilla require a knowledge of diseases and disorders of the maxillary sinus. Radiopaque images or the presence of fluid levels in the sinus regions often are signs of acute or allergic sinusitis. The fluid level, located in the lowest portion of the antrum, appears as a straight line parallel to the horizontal plane. A thickening of the membrane often indicates chronic sinusitis.

Because of the anatomic proximity of the sinus and the oral cavity, oral disease may extend into the sinus. Periapical, follicular, primordial, and odontogenic keratocysts may invade the antral cavity. A thin sclerotic border may sometimes delineate a cyst from the antrum. Fibrous dysplasia, ossifying fibromas, or giant cell lesions may also be diagnosed in the area.[21]

The pathologic conditions that involve the mucosa of the maxillary sinus include inflammatory conditions, neoplasms, and cysts. The terminology used to identify and characterize cysts is confusing, with numerous terms used interchangeably. These lesions are classified as either pseudocysts, retention cysts, or mucoceles.[22]

Pseudocysts are dome-shaped radiopacities frequently seen on the floor of the sinus. These lesions consist of an accumulation of inflammatory exudate which lifts the antral mucosa away from the underlying bone and requires no treatment. Retention cysts are caused by blockage and dilation of the ducts of the seromucinous glands of the sinus. They are small and are rarely evident radiographically. The pseudocyst and retention cyst do not require treatment, and subantral augmentation is not contraindicated.

Mucoceles are expansible, destructive lesions classified as primary and secondary.[21] Primary mucoceles result from blockage of the ostium, resulting in herniation of the mucosa through bony walls of the sinus. The secondary mucoceles are associated with trauma or surgical intervention into the sinus, usually the Caldwell-Luc procedure.[22, 23] In cases of destructive malignant lesions, the process usually destroys and perforates the thin, bony walls. An absence of a posterior wall image indicates a risk of a serious disorder and warrants further investigation. Tomograms are especially helpful to determine the extent of lesions or neoplasms in the area precisely. Computed tomography provides precise information on the extent of hard and soft tissue destruction by the progression of invasive lesions.

Any sign of acute sinusitis, root tips, cysts, or tumors complicate the procedure and mandate further evaluation. The surgery should be delayed, especially if the patient shows signs of nasal congestion, sinusitis, rhinitis, or upper respiratory tract disease. Referral to the appropriate medical or dental colleague is often indicated. In addition, it is recommended that the doctor develop a good referral relationship by joint evaluation of the patient after satisfactory completion of several subantral augmentations, to familiarize the physician with the procedure. The relationship established can prove beneficial in case of future complications or of other patients warranting referral.

TREATMENT SELECTION

The treatment plan approach to providing additional prosthodontic abutments in the maxillary posterior edentulous region has been organized by Misch into four alternative treatment options. The primary options are dependent on the available bone height between the floor of the antrum and the crest of the residual ridge in the region of the ideal implant location. Once the general height has been determined, the width of bone at the crest provides the key for implant design and the implant surgical approach.

A key to long-term success of posterior implants is adequate anterior teeth or implant placement. A treatment plan should include the presence of healthy anterior teeth or Division A bone in the premaxilla for implant placement. A minimum of a healthy abutment in the canine region or two abutments in the first premolar to central region are required before posterior implants are considered in the same quadrant.

Subantral Option One (SA-1): Conventional Implant Placement

The first treatment option, SA-1, occurs when there is sufficient available bone height (greater than 12 mm) to permit the placement of endosteal implants following the usual protocol. In the bone volume of Division A, root form implants are used for prosthetic support. Division B patients may be treated with osteoplasty or augmentation to increase the width to Division A or with the insertion of smaller surface area implants as plate form or small diameter root form implants (Fig 13–1). Osteoplasty may change the SA category if the height of the remaining bone is less than 12 mm. Augmentation for width with osteoinductive materials, osteoconductive materials, or both, is best accomplished with intrapositional grafts, leaving the lateral periosteum intact. Autogenous grafts may be onlay or oppositional in nature, under the periosteum. Smaller surface area implants require healthy abutment teeth or additional implants for adequate support. The Division A or B approach is similar for all four treatment options. If less than 2.5 mm of width is available in the edentulous region, the height of the ridge is reduced until a 2.5-mm width is obtained, or onlay autogenous bone grafts may be used to augment the width of available bone. The area is then reevaluated to determine the proper treatment plan classification. Augmentation in width of

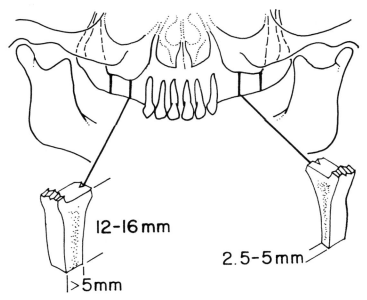

FIG 13–1.
The posterior maxilla, with greater than 12 mm height of bone placed in subantral option 1 (SA-1). When more than 5 mm width is present, the ridge is Division A *(left);* when 2.5 to 5 mm is present, the ridge is Division B *(right).*

the posterior maxilla is less often indicated, because this area is less involved with esthetics.

Although a common axiom in implant dentistry is to remain 2 mm or more from an opposing landmark, this is not indicated in this region. As long as the antrum is healthy and rotary instruments do not perforate the thin cortical plate lining the sinus, no contraindications exist to preparation or placement of implants at the level of or even through the cortical plate.

Endosteal implants in the SA-1 category are left to heal in a nonfunctional environment for approximately 4 to 8 months (depending on bone density) before the abutment post(s) is added for prosthodontic reconstruction. Care is taken to ensure that the implant is not traumatized in any way during the initial healing period.

Subantral Option Two (SA-2): Subantral Lift

The second subantral category, SA-2, is selected when 8 to 12 mm of vertical bone is present. To obtain the 12 mm of vertical bone necessary for improved implant survival, the antral floor is elevated from below. An implant osteotomy performed approximately 1 to 2 mm below the floor of the sinus is prepared as usual for the density of bone observed (see Chapter 21). A trial implant is inserted and tapped into position 2 to 4 mm beyond the prepared implant osteotomy. A greenstick fracture at the sinus floor usually elevates the bone and sinus membrane over the broad-based, flat-ended trial implant. The final implant may then be inserted into the implant osteotomy, and 2 mm to 4 mm new bone will form around the apical end of the implant. This approach may be used for root form or plate form endosteal implants. As in SA-1, root form implants are used in Division A. For Division B width, smaller diameter root forms or plate forms, osteoplasty, or augmentation may be used (Fig 13–2).

Worth and Stoneman have shown evidence of a relevant phenomena called "halo formation."[21] They observed that natural elevation of the sinus membrane will occasionally occur around teeth with periapical disease. The elevation of the sinus results in formation of new bone below it. The sinus membrane has properties similar to those of the periosteum, and bone generation is possible under a variety of circumstances.

The success of the sinus lift through the implant osteotomy cannot be confirmed at the time of implant placement. Six months after the surgical procedure, radiography is used to indicate the success of the 2 to 4 mm of increased vertical height. If sinus perforation occurs during placement of the trial or implant, bone formation is rare. Six to eight months are required to allow integration of bone with the implant and bone formation 0 to 4 mm below the elevated membrane. After this time interval, the patient's prosthodontic treatment is similar to that in the SA-1 category. If bone is not present around the apical

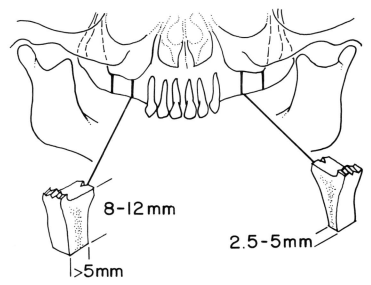

FIG 13–2.
A posterior maxilla with 8 to 12 mm of vertical height is placed into subantral option 2 (SA-2). When the width of bone is greater than 5 mm, treatment follows Division A *(left)* with a sinus lift. A width 2.5 to 5 mm is Division B *(right)*.

portion of the implant, the 8- to 11-mm implant portion in bone is treated in progressive loading as D-4 bone (see Chapter 30).

Subantral Option Three (SA-3): Sinus Membrane Elevation With Subantral Augmentation and Simultaneous Endosteal Implant Placement

The third approach to the maxillary posterior edentulous region, SA-3, is indicated when 5 to 8 mm of vertical bone and sufficient width are present between the antral floor and the crest of the residual ridge in the area of a needed prosthodontic abutment. A Tatum lateral maxillary wall approach is performed just superior to the residual alveolar bone. After the lateral access window and membrane are rotated in and upward to a superior position, a mixture of autogenous bone and alloplast and/or allograft material is placed in the space previously occupied by the sinus. This converts the posterior region to improved conditions for endosteal implants.

The implant design and surgical approach is similar to that used for other regions of the mouth. The division of bone, density of bone, and prosthetic option determine whether root form, plate form, or combinations are indicated. Therefore, if the crest of the ridge is Division A, root forms are indicated. For a

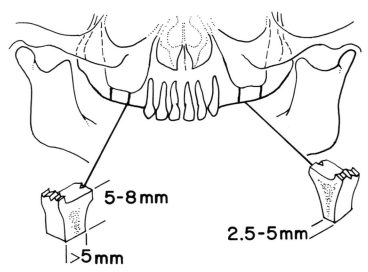

FIG 13–3.
The posterior maxilla with 5 to 8 mm between the crest of the ridge and the sinus floor is placed in subantral option 3 (SA-3). When more than 5 mm width is present the subantral augmentation converts the ridge to Division A *(left)*. When 2.5 to 5 mm width is present the subantral graft changes the ridge to Division B *(right)*.

ridge width of 2.5 to 5 mm, smaller diameter root forms, plate forms, or osteoplasty may be used until Division A root forms may be inserted (Fig 13–3). An osteoplasty may decrease the height of bone below 5 mm, in which case the treatment plan option is converted to SA-4 and implants should not be placed until the graft matures.

Six months to 10 months healing time is required before stage II uncovery and permucosal abutment placement, depending on the bone density below the original antrum, the amount of autogenous bone used in the subantral augmentation, and the gross amount of graft into the augmented region.

Subantral Option Four (SA-4): Sinus Elevation and Subantral Augmentation

The fourth option for treatment of the posterior maxilla, SA-4, serves to augment the region for future implant insertion. This therapy is indicated when less than 5 mm is present between the residual crest of bone and the floor of the maxillary sinus (Fig 13–4). There is not enough vertical host bone of dense quality in this region to permit predictable implant placement at the same time as augmentation under these conditions. In addition, these conditions usually result in less host bone surrounding the lateral, anterior, and distal areas of the graft, as well as the need for more graft material. The Tatum lateral wall approach is used to gain access to the maxillary sinus, elevate the sinus membrane, and allow placement of autogenous and alloplastic and/or allograft in the region.

The augmented region is allowed 6 to 10 months before reentry for endosteal implants. The design of the implant, as in any region, depends on the available bone and intended prosthesis. Typically, when less than 5 mm is present between the crest of the ridge and the floor of the antrum, the width of crestal bone is wide enough for root form implants after the subantral graft matures. As a result, the region is treated as Division A, because the graft permits endosteal implants with height enough for crown-implant ratios less than 1. However, the crest, although wide enough for root forms, is often more medial than the other SA treatment options. The implant is often placed in the region of a lingual cusp of the natural tooth originally in the region.

If the crest of the residual ridge is narrow and anterior teeth or root forms are available for support, a plate form or several small-diameter root form implants can be inserted in this Division B region. Regardless of endosteal implant design, 4 to 10 additional months elapse before prosthodontic reconstruction, depending on the bone density at the time of implant insertion.

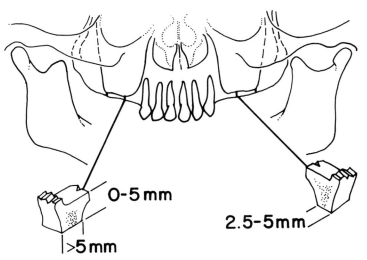

FIG 13–4.
A posterior maxilla with 0 to 5 mm between the crest of the ridge and the floor of the antrum is placed into subantral option 4 (SA-4). After the subantral augmentation, the width of bone 5 mm or greater is placed into Division A *(left)* and 2.5 to 5 mm is placed into Division B *(right)*.

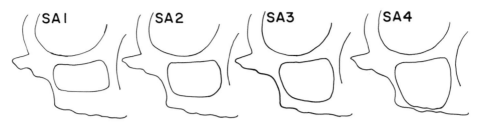

FIG 13–5.
Four subantral treatment options exist in the posterior maxilla. Options *SA-1* and *SA-2* use conventional methods of implant insertion, and sinus lift procedures as required based on the width of bone. Options *SA-3* and *SA-4* use a Tatum lateral wall approach for sinus elevation and subantral augmentation before implant insertion. These subantral options are based on height of available bone between the crest of the edentulous ridge and the floor of the sinus.

SUMMARY

The posterior maxilla has been reported as the least predictable area for implant survival. Causes cited include inadequate bone height, poor bone density, and high occlusal forces. Past implant approaches to this region attempt to avoid the maxillary sinus. This results in excessive cantilevers when posterior implants are not inserted, or excess numbers of pontics when implants are placed posterior to the antrum.

The maxillary sinus may be elevated and subantral bone formed to improve implant height. Tatum began to develop these techniques as early as mid-1970s. Misch developed four options for treatment of the posterior maxilla in 1984 based on the height of bone between the floor of the antrum and the crest of the residual bone. These options were further modified to reflect the width of available bone, once adequate height was obtained (Fig 13–5). The Division A edentulous site is 5 mm or more wide, 5 mm or more long, 12 mm or more high, and has an angulation of 30 degrees or less between load and implant body and a crown-implant ratio less than 1. Root form implants are indicated under these conditions. When the ridge anatomy is 2.5 to 5 mm in width and the length is 15 mm or more, while the remaining factors remain similar, a Division B anatomy is present. These ridges may be treated by osteoplasty or with endosteal implants having narrow, smaller surface areas (plate forms or narrow root forms).

REFERENCES

1. Pietrokovski J: The bony residual ridge in man, *J Prosthet Dent* 34:456–462, 1975.
2. Blitzer A, Lawson W, Friedman WH, editors: *Surgery of the paranasal sinuses,* Philadelphia, WB Saunders, 1985.

3. Lang J, editor: *Clinical anatomy of the nose, nasal cavity and paranasal sinuses,* New York, Medical Publishers, 1989.
4. Pederson GW: *Oral surgery,* Philadelphia, WB Saunders, 1988.
5. Linkow LI: *Maxillary implants: a dynamic approach to oral implantology,* North Haven, Connecticut, Glarus Publishing, 1977.
6. Branemark PI et al: An experimental and clinical study of osseointegrated implants penetrating the nasal cavity, *Maxillofac Surg* 42:497, 1984.
7. Ashkinazy LR: Tomography on implantology, *J Oral Implant* 10:100–118, 1982.
8. Stoler A: The CAT-scan subperiosteal implant, International Congress of Oral Implantologist World Meeting, Hong Kong, 1986.
9. Tatum H Jr: Maxillary and sinus implant reconstruction, *Dent Clin North Am* 30:207–229, 1986.
10. Boyne PJ, James RA: Grafting of the maxillary sinus floor with autogenous marrow and bone, *J Oral Surg* 38:613–616, 1980.
11. Misch CE: Maxillary sinus augmentation for endosteal implants: organized alternative treatment plans, *Int J Oral Implant* 4:49–58, 1987.
12. Misch CE: Subantral augmentation (abstract 16), UCLA Symposium on Implants and the Partially Edentulous Patient, Los Angeles, Calif, April 19, 1990.
13. Chanavaz M: Maxillary sinus: anatomy, physiology, surgery, and bone grafting related to implantology—seven years of surgical experience (1979–1990), *J Oral Implant* 16:199–210, 1990.
14. Misch CE: Medical evaluation of the implant candidate, Part II, *Int J Oral Implant* 2:11–18, 1982.
15. Harter DH: Infections and inflammatory disorders of nervous system, in Wyngarden JB, Smith LH, Jr, editors: *Cecil textbook of medicine,* ed 16, Philadelphia, WB Saunders, 1982, pp 2073–2074.
16. Worth HM: *Principles and practice of oral radiologic interpretation,* Chicago, Year Book, 1963.
17. Juhl JM: The sinuses and mastoids, in Juhl JH, editor: *Paul and Juhl's: essentials of roentgen interpretation,* ed 4, Philadelphia, Harper & Row, 1981, pp 1132–1153.
18. Zinreich SJ et al: Paranasal sinuses: CT imaging requirements for endoscopic surgery, *Radiology* 163:769–775, 1987.
19. Meserklinger W: *Endoscopy of the nose,* Baltimore, Urban and Schwartzenberg, 1978.
20. Zinreich, Messerklizer, Drettner B: The obstruction of the maxillary ostium, *Rhinology* 5:100–104, 1967.
21. Worth HM, Stoneman DW: Radiographic interpretation of antral mucosal changes due to localized dental infection, *J Can Dent Assoc* 38:111, 1972.
22. Kudo K et al: Clinicopathological study of post operative maxillary cysts, *J Jpn Stomatol Soc* 21:250–257, 1972.
23. Kubo I: A buccal cyst occurring after a radical operation of the maxillary sinus, *Z Otol* (Tokyo) 33:896, 1927.

Part II

Fundamental Sciences

Chapter *14*

Biomaterials for Dental Implants

Jack E. Lemons
Ralph W. Phillips

COMPATIBILITY OF SURGICAL BIOMATERIALS

The biocompatibility profiles of synthetic substances (biomaterials) used for the replacement or augmentation of biological tissues have been a critical concern within the health care disciplines throughout the histories of medicine and dentistry. Special circumstances are associated with dental implant prosthetic reconstruction of the oral-maxillofacial areas because the devices extend from the mouth, across the protective epithelial zones, and onto or into the underlying bone. The functional aspects of use also include the transfer of force from the occlusal surfaces of the teeth through the crown and bridge and neck-connector region of the implant and into the implant for interfacial transfer to the supporting soft and hard tissues. This situation represents a very complex series of chemical and mechanical environmental conditions.

It has long been recognized that synthetic biomaterials should be mechanically and chemically clean at the time of surgical placement. This most critical aspect of biocompatibility is, of course, dependent on the basic bulk and surface properties of the biomaterial. All aspects of basic manufacturing, finishing, packaging and delivering, sterilizing, and placing (including surgical) must be adequately controlled to assure clean conditions. The importance of these considerations has been reemphasized through the concept and practice of osteointegration of endosteal root form implant systems.

The disciplines of biomaterials and biomechanics are complementary to the understanding of device-based function. The physical, mechanical, chemical, and electrical properties of the basic material components must always be fully evaluated for any biomaterial application, as these properties provide key inputs into the interrelated biomechanical analyses of function. It is important to separate the roles of macroscopic implant shape from the microscopic transfer of stress and strain along biomaterial-to-tissue interfaces. The macroscopic distribution of mechanical stress and strain is predominantly controlled by the shape and form of the implant device. One important material property related to design (shape and form) optimization is the elastic strain (one component of the elastic modulus) of the material. The localized microscopic strain distribution is controlled more by the basic properties of the biomaterial (e.g., surface chemistry, microtopography, and modulus of elasticity) and by whether the biomaterial surface is chemically bonded to the adjacent tissues. Engineering analyses of implant systems include optimization considerations related both to the design and to the biomaterial used for construction. Therefore, the desire to control tissue responses and biodegradation often places restrictions on which materials can be safely used within the oral and tissue environments. Designs are often evolved for specific biomaterials because of the imposed environmental or restorative conditions.

HISTORY OF MATERIALS AND DESIGNS

Over the past 3 decades, definitions of material biocompatibilities have evolved and reflect an ever-changing opinion related to philosophies of surgical implant treatment. In the 1960s, emphasis focused on making the biomaterials more inert and chemically stable within biological environments. The high-purity ceramics of aluminum oxide, carbon, and carbon-silicon compounds, and extra-low-interstitial (ELI) grade alloys are classic examples of these trends. In the 1970s, biocompatibility was defined in terms of minimal harm, to the host or to the biomaterial. The importance of a stable interaction then moved into central focus for both the research and clinical communities. Now, many biomaterials are being constituted, fabricated, and surface-modified to directly influence short- and long-term tissue responses. Bioactive coatings on most classes of biomaterials are within stages of human clinical trials.

Of interest, dental implants have significantly influenced these trends. In the 1960s, dental devices were recognized as being in a research and development phase, and critical longitudinal reviews of clinical applications were strongly recommended.[1] During this time, longevity studies of various devices demonstrated that the longest duration of clinical applications were for orthopedic prostheses. In the 1980s, controlled clinical trials have shown that dental implants can provide functional longevities that exceed most other types of functional tissue replacement modalities.[2, 3] Clearly, these clinical studies have strongly influenced both the research and development and the clinical application processes.

The evolution of any implant modality is a multicomponent story in which significant roles have been played by biomaterials; biomechanical analyses of designs, tissues, and function; wound healing along interfaces; surgical methods to minimize mechanical, chemical, and thermal trauma; prosthodontic and periodontal treatment modalities; and protocols for controlled multidisciplinary clinical trials. The interdependence of all phases of basic and applied research should be recognized. All interrelate and must evolve to provide a level of better understanding of the basic physical and biological phenomena associated with the implant systems before the best system can be fully described.

Evaluations of endosteal and subperiosteal dental implants raise interesting questions with respect to the interrelationships among material and design selection. One now has the opportunity to select a material from a number of systems, such as ceramics, carbons, polymers, or composites. Also, implant shape and form (design) are limited only by the available anatomic dimensions and the requirement to interconnect to some form of intraoral restorative device. Because of the wide range of biomaterial properties demonstrated by the classes of materials available, it is not advisable to fabricate any new implant design without a thorough biomechanical analysis. Another approach now often utilized is to determine a specific design based on clinical considerations and then to select the biomaterial of choice from computer-based analyses. The safety of these combinations can then be demonstrated through laboratory and laboratory animal investigations. Controlled clinical trials following prospective protocols, of course, provide the final evaluation for both safety and effectiveness.

RESEARCH AND DEVELOPMENT

Basic studies within the physical and biological sciences have been supportive of the development of surgical implant systems. One example is the continued progress from materials that have been available for industrial applications to the new classes of composites that have evolved for biomedical applications. This same situation exists within a broad area, for example, surface science and technology, mechanics and biomechanics of three-dimensional structures, pathways and processes of wound healing along biomaterial interfaces, and the description of the first biofilms that evolve upon contact with blood or tissue fluids.[4] The progressive move from materials to quantitatively characterized biomaterials has been extremely important to the biomedical applications of surgical implants. Dental implant investigations now play a leadership role within selected areas of this overall process, and all phases of medicine and dentistry should be benefactors.

The basic disciplines of biomaterials and biomechanics now include established professional societies, annual meetings with large numbers of scientific and applied papers, referred journals, and active collaborations with affiliated disciplines. This situation has existed within the dental materials field for many years. Merging of the technologies involved in general medical implant biomaterials and dental materials is anticipated, is to be encouraged, and should be complementary to all involved as both the medical and dental disciplines expand throughout the world.

It has often been suggested that dental implant treatment modalities will eventually become a conservative phase of dental care. The basic proposal is that when a tooth is lost, a root form implant will preserve the adjacent tissues; provide normal function through a fixed, single root-crown–based system; and thereby avoid the need to prepare adjacent teeth for bridges. This type of philosophy is driving investigations on single root form and crown replacement systems. Bonding of soft and hard tissue components along biomaterial interfaces and designs that functionally distribute interfacial stresses are critical to this process.

METALS AND ALLOYS

Most of the dental implant systems available within the United States in 1989 were constructed from metals or alloys. These materials are reviewed in this chapter by separating the metals and alloys according to their elemental compositions and the primary dental implant components.

Titanium and Titanium-6 Aluminum-4 Vanadium

The reactive group metals and alloys (with primary elements from this reactive group) form oxides in air or oxygenated solutions. Titanium oxidizes (passivates) upon contact with room temperature air or normal tissue fluids. This reactivity is favorable for dental implant devices. In the absence of interfacial motion or adverse tissue conditions, this passivated surface condition minimizes biocorrosion phenomena. In situations where the implant would be placed within a closely fitting receptor site in bone, areas scratched or abraded during placement would repassivate in vivo. This characteristic is one important property consideration related to the use of titanium for dental implants.

The general engineering properties of the metals and alloys used for dental implants are summarized in Table 14–1. Titanium shows a relatively low modulus of elasticity and tensile strength when compared with the alloys. The strength values for the wrought soft and ductile metallurgical condition (normal for root forms and blades) are approximately 1.5 times greater than the strength of compact bone. In most designs where the bulk dimensions and shapes are simple, strength of this magnitude is adequate. Because fatigue strengths are normally half or less than the corresponding tensile strengths, implant design criteria are decidedly important. Sharp corners or thin sections must be avoided for regions loaded under tension or shear conditions. The modulus of elasticity is 5 times greater than that of compact bone, which emphasizes the importance of design

TABLE 14–1.

Engineering Properties of Metals and Alloys Used for Surgical Implants*

Material	Nominal Analysis (w/o)	Modulus of Elasticity GN/m^2 (psi $\times$ 10^6)	Ultimate Tensile Strength MN/m^2 (ksi)	Elongation to Fracture (%)	Surface
Titanium (Ti)	99$^+$Ti	97 (14)	240–550 (25–70)	>15	Ti oxide
Titanium-aluminum-vanadium (Ti-Al-V)	90Ti-6Al-4V	117 (17)	860–896 (125–130)	>12	Ti oxide
Cobalt-chromium-molybdenum (casting) (Co-Cr-Mo)	66Co-27Cr-7Mo	235 (34)	655 (95)	> 8	Cr oxide
Stainless steel (316L)	70Fe-18Cr-12Ni	193 (28)	480–1,000 (70–145)	>30	Cr oxide
Zirconium (Zr)	99$^+$Zr	97 (14)	552 (80)	20	Zr oxide
Tantalum (Ta)	99$^+$Ta	—	690 (100)	11	Ta oxide
Gold (Au)	99$^+$Au	97 (14)	207–310 (30–45)	>30	Au
Platinum (Pt)	99$^+$Pt	166 (24)	131 (19)	40	Pt

*Minimum values from the American Society for Testing and Materials Committee F4 documents are provided. Selected products provide a range of properties. GN/m^2 = giganewton per meter squared. MN/m^2 = meganewton per meter squared; ksi = thousand pounds per inch squared; psi = pounds per inch squared; w/o = weight percent.

in the proper distribution of mechanical stress transfer. Surface areas that are loaded in compression have been maximized for some of the newer implant designs.

The alloy of titanium most often used is titanium-aluminum-vanadium. The wrought alloy condition is 6 times stronger than compact bone and thereby affords more opportunities for designs with thinner sections (e.g., plateaus, thin interconnecting regions, rectangular scaffolds, porosities). The modulus of elasticity of the alloy is slightly greater than that of titanium, being about 5.6 times that of compact bone. The alloy and the primary element (Ti) both have titanium oxide (passivated) surfaces. Information has been developed on the oxide thickness, purity, and stability as related to implant biocompatibilities.[2] In general, titanium and alloys of titanium have demonstrated interfaces described as osteointegration for implants in humans. Also, surface conditions where the oxide thickness has varied from hundreds of angstroms to 100% titania (TiO_2 ceramic) have demonstrated osteointegration.

The possible influences of aluminum and vanadium biodegradation products on local and systemic tissue responses have been reviewed from the perspectives of basic science and clinical applications.[5] Although many basic science questions remain, clinical applications of these alloys in orthopedic and dental surgical systems have not demonstrated significant numbers of identifiable associated sequelae.

Electrochemical studies support the selection of conditions where elemental concentrations would be relatively low in magnitude.[4] Electrochemically, Ti and Ti-alloy are different with regard to electromotive and galvanic potentials when compared to other electrically conductive dental materials. Some data on these electrochemical potentials have been published previously.[2] In general, titanium- and cobalt-based systems are electrochemically similar; gold-, platinum-, and palladium-based systems are noble; and nickel-, iron-, copper-, and silver-based systems are significantly different (subject to galvanic coupling and preferential in vivo corrosion).

Critical to the use of titanium, or any other implant biomaterial, is the necessity to retain mechanically and chemically clean conditions. Mechanically, Ti is much more ductile (bendable) than Ti-alloy. This feature has been a very favorable aspect related to the use of endosteal blades. The need for adjustment or bending to provide parallel abutments for prosthetic treatments has caused manufacturers to control microstructures and residual strain conditions. Coining, stamping, or forging followed by controlled annealing is routinely used during metallurgical processing. If an implant abutment is bent, the metal is strained locally at the neck region and the local strain is cumulative and dependent on the amount of deformation. This is one reason, other than fatigue cycling, why reuse of implants is not recommended. Sometimes, mechanical processes can contaminate implant surfaces. Any residues of surface changes must be removed prior to implantation to assure clean conditions.

Cobalt-Chromium-Molybdenum–Based Alloy

The cobalt-based alloys are most often used in an as-cast or cast-and-annealed metallurgical condition. This permits the fabrication of implants as custom designs such as subperiosteal frames. The elemental composition of this alloy includes cobalt, chromium, and molybdenum as the major elements. Cobalt provides the continuous phase for basic properties; secondary phases based on cobalt, chromium, molybdenum, nickel, and carbon provide strength (4 times that of compact bone) and surface abrasion resistance; chromium provides corrosion resistance through the oxide surface; while molybdenum provides strength and bulk corrosion resistance. All of these elements are critical, as is their concentration, which emphasizes the importance of casting and fabrication technologies. Also included in this alloy are minor concentrations of nickel, manganese, and carbon. Nickel has been identified in biocorrosion products, and carbon must be precisely controlled to maintain mechanical properties such as ductility. Surgical alloys of cobalt are not the same as those used for partial dentures, and substitutions should be avoided.

In general, the cobalt alloys are the least ductile of the alloy systems used for dental surgical implants, and bending should be avoided. Because many of these alloy devices are fabricated by dental laboratories, all aspects of quality control and analysis for surgical implants must be followed during alloy selection, casting, and finishing. Critical considerations include the chemical analysis, mechanical properties, and surface finish as specified by the American Society for Testing and

Materials (ASTM) committee F-4 on surgical implants[6] and the American Dental Association.[7] When properly fabricated, implants from this alloy group have shown excellent biocompatibility profiles.

Iron-Chromium-Nickel–Based Alloys

The surgical stainless steel alloys (e.g., 316 low carbon) have a long history of use for orthopedic and dental implant devices. This alloy, as with titanium systems, is used most often in a wrought and heat-treated metallurgical condition, which results in a high-strength and high-ductility alloy. The ramus blade, ramus frame, stabilizer pins (old), and some mucosal insert systems have been made from the iron-based alloy.

The ASTM F-4 specification for surface passivation[6] was first written and applied to the stainless steel alloys. In part, this was done to maximize corrosion-biocorrosion resistance. Of the implant alloys, this alloy is most subject to crevice and pitting biocorrosion and care must be taken to utilize and retain the passivated (oxide) surface condition. Because this alloy contains nickel as a major element, use in patients allergic to nickel should be avoided. Also, if a stainless steel implant is modified prior to surgery, recommended procedures call for repassivation to obtain a surface condition to minimize in vivo biodegradation.

The iron-based alloys have galvanic potentials and corrosion characteristics that make them subject to galvanic coupling biocorrosion if interconnected with titanium, cobalt, zirconium, or carbon implant biomaterials. In some clinical conditions more than one alloy may be present within the same dental arch of a patient. For example, if a bridge of a noble or a base metal alloy touches the abutment heads of a stainless steel and titanium implant simultaneously, an electrical circuit would be formed through the tissues. If used independently, where the alloys are not in contact or not electrically interconnected, the galvanic couple would not exist and each device could function independently.

As with the other metal and alloy systems discussed, the iron-based alloys have a long history of clinical applications. Long-term device retrievals have demonstrated that, when used properly, the alloy can function without significant in vivo breakdown. Clearly, the mechanical properties and cost characteristics of this alloy offer advantages with respect to clinical applications.

Other Metals and Alloys

Many other metals and alloys have been used for dental implant device fabrication. Early spirals and cages included tantalum, platinum, irridium, gold, palladium, and alloys of these metals. More recently, devices made from zirconium, hafnium, and tungsten have been evaluated.[8, 9] Some significant advantages of these reactive group metals and their alloys have been reported, although large numbers of such devices have not been fabricated in the United States.

Gold, platinum, and palladium are metals of relatively low strength, which places limits on design. Also, cost per-unit-weight and the weight of the device along the upper arch have been suggested as possible limitations for gold and platinum. These metals, especially gold, because of mobility and availability, have been used as surgical implant materials. Current use for dental implants is minimal.

Ceramics and Carbon

Oxide ceramics were introduced for surgical implant devices because of inertness to biodegradation, high strength, and physical characteristics such as color and minimal thermal and electrical conductivity and a wide range of elastic properties.[10, 11] In many cases, however, the low ductility or inherent brittleness has resulted in limitations. Ceramics have been used in bulk forms and more recently as coatings on metals and alloys.

Aluminum, Titanium, and Zirconium Oxides

High ceramics from aluminum, titanium, and zirconium oxides have been utilized for root form, endosteal blade, and pin-type dental implants. The overall characteristics of these ceramics are summarized in Table 14–2. The compressive, tensile, and bending strengths exceed the strength of compact bone by 3 to 5 times. These properties, combined with high moduli of elasticity and especially with fatigue and fracture strengths, have resulted in specialized design requirements for these classes of biomaterials. For example, the fabrication of a subperiosteal device from a high ceramic could not be done because of fracture resistance and the relative cost for manufacturing.

TABLE 14–2.

Engineering Properties of Some Inert Ceramics Used as Biomaterials*

Material	Modulus of Elasticity GN/m^2 (psi $\times 10^6$)	Ultimate Bending Strength MPa (ksi)	Surface
Aluminum oxide			
Polycrystalline	372 (54)	300–550 (43–80)	Al_2O_3
Single crystal (sapphire)	392 (56)	640 (93)	Al_2O_3
Zirconium oxide zirconia (PSZ)	195–210 (28–30)	500–650 (72–94)	ZrO_2
Titanium oxide (titania)	283 (41)	69–103 (10–15)	TiO_2

*These high ceramics have 0% permanent elongation at fracture. GN/m^2 = giganewton per meter squared; psi = pounds per inch squared; MPa = megaPascal; ksi = thousand pounds per inch squared.

The aluminum, titanium, and zirconium oxide ceramics have a clear, white, cream, or light grey color, which is beneficial for applications such as anterior root form devices. Minimal thermal and electrical conductivity, minimal biodegradation, and minimal reactions with bone, soft tissue, and the oral environment are also recognized as beneficial when compared with other biomaterials. In early studies of dental and orthopedic devices in laboratory animals and humans they have exhibited direct interfaces with bone, now called an osteointegrated condition. Also, characterization of gingival attachment zones along sapphire root form devices in laboratory animal models have demonstrated regions of localized bonding.[2]

Although the ceramics are chemically inert, care must be taken in the handling or placement of these biomaterials. Exposure to steam sterilization results in a measurable decrease in strength for some ceramics; scratches or notches may introduce fracture-initiation sites; chemical solutions leave residues; and the hard and sometimes rough surfaces may readily abrade other materials upon contact. Dry heat sterilization within a clean atmosphere is recommended for most ceramics.

One series of root form and blade devices utilized during the 1970s resulted in intraoral fractures after several years of function.[12, 13] The fractures were initiated by fatigue cycling along regions of localized bending and tensile strain. Although initial testing showed adequate mechanical strengths for these polycrystalline alumina materials, the long-term clinical results clearly demonstrated a functional design-related and material-related limitation. This illustrates the need for controlled clinical investigation to relate basic properties to in vivo performance. The established chemical biocompatibilities, improved strength and toughness capabilities of sapphire and zirconia, and the basic property characteristics of high ceramics continue to make them excellent candidates for dental implants.

BIOACTIVE AND BIODEGRADABLE CERAMICS BASED ON CALCIUM PHOSPHATES

Bone Augmentation and Replacement

The calcium phosphate ($Ca \cdot PO_4$) ceramics used in dental reconstructive surgery include a wide range of implant types and thereby a wide range of clinical applications. Early investigations emphasized solid and porous particulates with nominal compositions that were relatively similar to the mineral phase of bone. Microstructural and chemical properties of these particulates were controlled to provide forms that would either dissolve or remain intact for structural purposes after implantation. The laboratory and clinical results for these particulates were most promising and led to implant expansions, including larger implant shapes (such as rods, cones, blocks, H-bars) for structural support under relatively high magnitude loading conditions.[14, 15] Also, the particulate size range for bone replacements was expanded to both smaller and larger sizes for combined applications with organic compounds. Mixtures of particulates with collagen, and subsequently with drugs and active organic compounds such as Bone Morphogenic Protein (BMP), increased the range of applications. Over the past 15 years, these types of products and their uses have continued to expand significantly.[15–18]

Endosteal and Subperiosteal Implants

The first series of structural forms for dental implants included rods and cones for filling tooth root extraction sites (ridge retainers)[19] and, in some cases, load-bearing endosteal implants.[20] Limitations in mechanical property characteristics soon resulted in internal reinforcement of the $Ca \cdot PO_4$ ceramic implants through mechanical (central metallic rods) or physicochemical (coating over another substrate) techniques.[21]

The coatings of metallic surfaces using flame or plasma spraying (or other techniques) increased rapidly for the $Ca \cdot PO_4$ ceramics.[15] The coatings have been applied to a wide range of endosteal and subperiosteal dental implant designs with an overall intent of improving implant surface biocompatibility profiles and implant longevities.

Advantages and Disadvantages[22]

The recognized advantages associated with the $Ca \cdot PO_4$ ceramic biomaterials are:

1. Chemical compositions of high purity and of substances that are similar to constituents of normal biological tissue (calcium, phosphorus, oxygen, and hydrogen)
2. Excellent biocompatibility profiles within a variety of tissues when used as intended
3. Opportunities to provide attachments between selected $Ca \cdot PO_4$ ceramics and hard and soft tissues
4. Minimal thermal and electrical conductivity plus capabilities to provide a physical and chemical barrier to ion transport (e.g., metallic ions)
5. Moduli of elasticity more similar to bone than many other implant materials used for load-bearing implants
6. Color similar to bone, dentin, and enamel
7. An evolving and extensive base of information related to science, technology, and application

Some of the possible disadvantages associated with these types of biomaterials are:

1. Variations in chemical and structural characteristics for some currently available implant products
2. Relatively low mechanical tensile and shear strengths under condition of fatigue loading
3. Relatively low attachment strengths for some coating-to-substrate interfaces
4. Variable solubilities depending on the product and the clinical application
5. Limited information about the structural and mechanical stabilities of coatings under in vivo load-bearing conditions (especially tension and shear)
6. Alterations of substrate chemical and structural properties related to some available coating technologies
7. Expansion of applications that sometimes exceed the evolving laboratory information on properties

Critical to applications are the basic properties of these substances. Table 14–3 provides a summary of some properties of bioactive and biodegradable ceramics. In general, these classes of bioceramics have lower strengths, hardnesses, and moduli of elasticity than the more chemically inert forms previously discussed. Fatigue strengths, especially for porous materials, have imposed limitations with regard to some dental implant designs. In certain instances, these characteristics have been used to provide improved implant conditions (e.g., biodegradation of particulates).

Calcium aluminates, sodium-lithium invert glasses with calcium phosphate additions (Bioglass or Ceravital), and glass ceramics (AW glass-ceramic) provide a wide range of properties.

TABLE 14–3.

Properties of Bioactive and Biodegradable Ceramics*

Material	Modulus of Elasticity GPa (psi × 10^6)	Ultimate Bending Strength MPa (ksi)	Surface
Hydroxylapatite	40–120 (6–17)	40–300 (6–43)	$Ca_{10}(PO_4)_6(OH)_2$
Tricalcium phosphate	30–120 (4–17)	15–120 (2–17)	$Ca_3(PO_4)_2$
Bioglass or Ceravital	40–140 (6–20)	20–350 (3–51)	$Ca \cdot PO_4$
AW ceramic	124 (18)	213 (31)	$Ca \cdot PO_4 + F$
Carbon	25–40 (4–6)	150–250 (22–36)	C
Carbon-silicon (LTI)	25–40 (4–6)	200–700 (29–101)	$C \cdot Si$

*These ceramics and carbons have 0% permanent elongation at fracture. GPa = gigaPascal; psi = pounds per inch squared; MPa = megaPascal; ksi = thousand pounds per inch squared; LTI = low temperature isotropic.

Ca•PO$_4$ Ceramic Properties

Chemical Analysis

The atomic relationships of the basic elements, stoichiometric ratios, and the normal chemical names for several characterized calcium phosphate ceramics are provided in Table 14–4. The general family of apatites has a formula of $M_{10}^{2+}(XO_4^{3-})_6Z_2^{1-}$. Very often apatite atomic ratios are nonstoichiometric, that is, 1 mole of apatite may contain less than 10 moles of metallic ions (M^{2+}) and less than 2 moles of anions (Z^{1-}).[23] The number of (XO_4^{3-}) retains a number of 6. Multiple metals and anions can be substituted within this formulation. Most importantly, the relative physical, mechanical, and chemical properties of each final calcium phosphate material, including each of the apatites, are different from one another.[17] Additionally, the microstructure of any final product (solid structural form or coating) is equally important to the basic properties of the substance alone. The crystalline monolytic hydroxylapatite (HA) [fired ceramic $Ca_{10}(PO_4)_6(OH)_2$] of high density and purity (< 50 ppm impurities) has provided one standard for comparison related to implant applications. The ratio of calcium to phosphorus of $Ca_{10}(PO_4)_6(OH)_2$ is 1.67, and the ceramic can be fully crystalline. Considerable differences exist between the synthetic HA ceramics (hydroxylapatites) that are produced by elevated temperature processing and biological apatites (hydroxyapatites). Biological apatites contain trace amounts of CO_3^{2-}, sodium, magnesium, fluorine, and chlorine ions. These exist in varying ratios and distributions and of course are only one phase of calcified tissues.

The crystalline tricalcium phosphate [β $Ca_3(PO_4)_2$] (TCP) ceramic has also provided a high-purity (< 50 ppm impurities) biomaterial for comparison with other products. National standard specifications related to the basic properties and characteristics of both HA and TCP now have been published.[6] These two

TABLE 14–4.

Names, Formulae, and Atomic Ratios for Some Calcium Phosphate Materials

Mineral or General Name	Formula	Ca:P Ratio	Applications
Monetite (DCP)	$CaHPO_4$	1	Nonceramic bone substitute particulate
Brushite (DCPD)	$CaHPO_4 \cdot 2H_2O$	1	Phase of some Ca·PO$_4$ biomaterials
Octa calcium phosphate (OCP)	$Ca_8(HPO_4)_2(PO_4) \cdot 5H_2O$	1.33	Phase of some Ca·PO$_4$ biomaterials
Whitlockite (WH)	$Ca_{10}(HPO_4)(PO_4)_6$	1.43	Phase of some Ca·PO$_4$ biomaterials
β Whitlockite (βTCP)	$Ca_3(PO_4)_2$	1.48	Biodegradable Ca·PO$_4$ ceramic for bone substitute and coatings; also a phase of some Ca·PO$_4$ biomaterials
Defective hydroxyapatite (DOHA)	$Ca_9(HPO_4)(PO_4)_5(OH)$	1.5	Component of some Ca·PO$_4$ biomaterials
Hydroxyapatite (OHA)	$Ca_{10}(PO_4)_6(OH)_2$	1.67	Major mineral phase of bone; when fired as a ceramic, named hydroxylapatite (HA)

compositions have been used most extensively as particulates for bone augmentation and replacement, carriers for organic products, and as coatings for endosteal and subperiosteal implants.

One of the more important aspects of the $Ca\bullet PO_4$ ceramics relates to the possible reactions with water. For example, hydration can convert TCP to HA; also, phase transitions among the various structural forms can exist with any exposure to water. This has caused some confusion in the literature in that some $Ca\cdot PO_4$ ceramics have been steam autoclaved for sterilization purposes prior to surgical implantation. Steam or water autoclaving could significantly change the basic structure and properties of $Ca\cdot PO_4$ (or any bioactive surface) and thereby provide an unknown biomaterial condition at the time of implantation. This is to be avoided through the use of presterilized or clean, dry, heat-sterilization conditions.

Forms, Microstructures, and Mechanical Properties

Particulate HA, provided in a nonporous ($<5\%$ porosity) form as angular or spherically shaped particles, is an example of a crystalline, high-purity HA biomaterial.[24] These particles can have relatively high compressive strengths (>500 MPa), with tensile strengths in the range of 50 to 70 MPa. These same mechanical characteristics exist for the solid portions of several porous HA particulates and blocks. The macro- ($\bar{l} > 50$ μm), or micro- ($\bar{l} < 50$ μm) porous particulates have an increased surface area per unit volume. This provides more surface area for dissolution under static conditions and a significant reduction in compressive and tensile strengths. The porous materials also provide additional regions for tissue ingrowth and integration (mechanical stabilization) and thereby a minimization of interfacial motion and dynamic (wear-associated) interfacial breakdown. The strength characteristics after tissue ingrowth would then become a combination of the ceramic and the investing tissues.[25]

A number of the $Ca\cdot PO_4$ ceramics are phase mixtures of HA and TCP, while some compounds are composites or mechanical mixtures with other materials.[15] These classes of bioactive ceramics, including glasses, glass-ceramics, mixtures of ceramics, combinations of metals and ceramics, or polymers and ceramics, exhibit a wide range of properties. In general, these biomaterials have shown acceptable biocompatibility profiles from laboratory and clinical investigations. These various compositions and applications have been summarized in a recently published 2-volume book, and the reader is referred to this reference.[18]

The coatings of $Ca\cdot PO_4$ ceramics onto metallic (cobalt- and Ti-based) biomaterials have become a routine application for dental implants. These coatings, for the most part, are applied by flame or plasma spraying; have average thicknesses between 20 and 100 μm; are mixtures of crystalline and amorphous phases; and have variable microstructures (phases and porosities) compared with the solid portions of the particulate forms of HA and TCP biomaterials.[15] At this time, coating characteristics are relatively consistent, and the quality control and quality assurance programs from the manufacturers have greatly improved the consistency of coated implant systems.

Concerns continue to exist about the fatigue strengths of the $Ca \cdot PO_4$ coatings and coating-to-substrate interfaces under tensile and shear loading conditions. There have been some reports of coating loss as a result of mechanical fracture, although the number reported is small. This has caused some clinicians and manufacturers to introduce designs in which the coatings are applied to shapes (geometrical designs) that minimize implant interface shear or tensile loading conditions (such as porosities, screws, spirals, plateaus, vents). From theoretical considerations, the coating of mechanically protected areas seems most desirable.

Density, Conductivity, and Solubility

The relative densities of $Ca \cdot PO_4$ coatings on implants are lower than the solid particulate forms. This is because most of the coatings exhibit inclusive porosities, combinations of phases, and irregular microstructural features. Some reports have suggested that coatings have a density gradient, becoming more dense under the outer surface. This gradient has been associated with early biodegradation profiles.

The $Ca \cdot PO_4$ coatings are nonconductors of heat and electricity. This can provide a relative benefit for dental implants on which mixtures of materials are often included in the overall prosthetic reconstruction. In combination with color (off-white), these properties are considered to be advantageous.

Relative solubilities of the $Ca \cdot PO_4$ ceramics have been determined for both particulates and coatings.[26, 27] In general, solubility is greater for TCP than for HA. Each increases relative to increasing surface area per unit volume (porosity), and the $Ca \cdot PO_4$ ceramic solubility profiles depend on the environment (pH, mechanical motion, and so forth). In most applications within bone, solubilities are higher over the first few weeks, then decrease with continued in vivo exposure and the apposition of mineralized structures. However, some investigators have shown situations where osteoclastic resorption has removed localized zones of $Ca \cdot PO_4$ coatings.[28] This raises interesting questions about long-term in vivo stabilities. At this time, clinical results have been acceptable, and expanded applications continue.

CURRENT STATUS AND FUTURE CONSIDERATIONS

The $Ca \cdot PO_4$ ceramics have proved to be one of the more successful high technology–based biomaterials that has evolved within the past 2 decades. Their advantageous properties strongly support the expanding clinical applications and the enhancement of the biocompatibility profiles for surgical implant uses.

It is anticipated that the calcium phosphate ceramics will be among the major biomaterials for providing the intended chemical-biochemical reactions along tissue interfaces. Within the overall theme for new generation biomaterials to be chemically (bonding to tissue) and mechanically (nonuniform multidirectional properties) anisotropic, the Ca•PO$_4$ ceramics could be the biomaterial surfaces of choice for many device applications.

Carbon and Carbon Silicon Compounds

Carbon compounds are often classified as ceramics because of their chemical inertness and absence of ductility; however, they are conductors of heat and electricity. Extensive applications for cardiovascular devices, excellent biocompatibility profiles, and moduli of elasticity close to that of bone have resulted in clinical trials of these compounds in dental and orthopedic prostheses. One two-stage root replacement system (Vitredent) was quite popular in the early 1970s.[3] Design, material, and application limitations resulted in a significant number of clinical failures and the subsequent withdrawal of this device from clinical use.

Ceramic and carbon substances continue to be used as coatings on metallic and ceramic materials. These biomaterial characteristics have been reviewed in recent publications[15] and therefore are not discussed in detail here. Advantages of coatings include tissue bonding; components that are normal to physiological environments; regions that serve as barriers to elemental transfer, heat, or electrical current flow; control of color; and opportunities for the attachment of active biomolecules or synthetic compounds. Possible limitations relate to mechanical strength properties along the substrate-to-coating interface; biodegradation that could adversely influence tissue stabilities; time-dependent changes in physical characteristics; minimal resistance to scratching or scraping procedures associated with oral hygiene; and susceptibility to standard handling, sterilizing, or placing methodologies. Because coatings are experimental (limited 5-year clinical data) at this time, readers are cautioned to read manufacturers' instructions and the evolving literature in this area carefully. Expanded utilizations of surface-coated dental implants are anticipated by the research and development communities.

Critical consideration with respect to the maintenance of chemically and mechanically clean biomaterial conditions are equally important for the surface-coated implants. Most systems are now provided in a presterilized container with a holding and transfer attachment to be used for clinical placement. These materials tend to optimize the manipulative consideration with respect to the various dental implant designs.

Polymers and Composites

The utilization of synthetic polymers and composites continues to expand for biomaterial applications. Fiber-reinforced polymers offer advantages in that they can be designed to match tissue properties, can be anisotropic with respect to mechanical characteristics, can be coated for tissue attachment, and can be fabricated at relatively low cost. Expanded future applications for dental implant systems, beyond force transfer inserts such as those used in the IMZ (Interpore Inc.) and Flexiroot (Interdent Corp.) systems, are anticipated.

Structural Biomedical Polymers

The more inert polymeric biomaterials include polytetrafluoroethylene (PTFE), polyethylene terephthalate (PET), polymethylmethacrylate (PMMA), ultrahigh molecular weight polyethylene (UHMW-PE), polypropylene (PP), polysulfone (PSF), and polydimethylsiloxane (PDS or silicone rubber, SR). These are summarized in Table 14–5. In general, the polymers have lower strengths and elastic moduli and higher elongations to fracture compared with other classes of biomaterials. They are thermal and electrical insulators, and, when constituted as a high molecular weight system without plasticizers, are relatively resistant to biodegradation. Compared with bone, most polymers have lower elastic moduli, with magnitudes closer to soft tissues.

Polymers have been fabricated in porous and solid forms for tissue attachment, replacement, and augmentation and as coatings for force transfer to soft tissue and hard tissue regions. Cold flow characteristics and creep and fatigue strengths are relatively low for some classes of polymers (e.g., PMMA) and have resulted in some limitations. In contrast, some are extremely tough and fatigue cycle resistant (PP, UHMW-PE, PTFE) and afford opportunities for mechanical force transfer in selected implant designs. Most utilizations have been for internal

TABLE 14–5.

Engineering Properties of Polymers (Some Medical Grades)*

Material†	Modulus of Elasticity GPa (psi × 10^5)	Ultimate Tensile Strength MPa (ksi)	Elongation to Fracture (%)
PTFE	0.5–3 (0.07–4.3)	17–28 (2.5–4)	200–600
PET	3 (4.3)	55 (8)	50–300
PMMA	3 (4.3)	69 (10)	2–15
PE	8 (1.2)	48 (7)	400–500
PP	9 (1.3)	35 (5)	500–700
PSF	3.5 (5)	69 (10)	20–100
SR	0.1 (0.014)	5 (1.1)	300–900
POM	3 (4.3)	70 (10.1)	10–75

*Polymer properties exhibit a wide range depending on processing and structure. These values have been taken from general tables. GPa = gigaPascal; psi = pounds per inch squared; MPa = megaPascal; ksi = thousand pounds per inch squared.
†PTFE = polytetrafluorethylene; PET = polyethylene terephthalate; PMMA = polymethylmethacrylate; PE = polyethylene; PP = polypropylene; PSF = polysulfone; SR = silicone rubber; POM = polyoxymethylene (IME insert).

force distribution connectors for osteointegrated implants where the connector is intended to better simulate biomechanical conditions for normal tooth functions.

Composites

Combinations of polymers and other categories of synthetic biomaterials continue to be introduced. Several of the more inert polymers have been combined with particulate or fibers of carbon, aluminum oxide, hydroxylapatite, and glass ceramics. Some are porous, while others are constituted as solid composite structural forms.[29]

In some cases, biodegradable polymers, such as polyvinyl alcohol (PVA), polylactides or glycolides, cyanoacrylates, or other hydratable forms, have been combined with biodegradable $Ca \cdot PO_4$ particulate or fibers.[30] These are intended as structural scaffolds, plates, screws, or other such applications. Biodegradation of the entire system, after tissues have adequately reformed and remodeled, is proposed to be significantly advantageous.

In general, polymers and composites of polymers are especially sensitive to sterilization and handling techniques. If intended for implant use, most cannot be sterilized by steam or ethylene oxide. Most are electrostatic and tend to gather dust or other particulate if exposed to semi-clean air environments. Since many can be shaped by cutting or autopolymerizing in vivo (PMMA), extreme care must be taken to maintain quality surface conditions of the implant. Porous polymers can be elastically deformed to close open regions intended for tissue ingrowth. Also, cleaning of contaminated porous polymers is not possible without a chemical laboratory environment. Talc or starch on surgical gloves, contact with a towel or gauze pad, or the touching of any contaminated area must be avoided for all biomaterials.

Long-term experience, excellent biocompatibility profiles, ability to control properties through composite structures, and properties that can be altered to suit the clinical application make polymers and composites excellent candidates for biomaterial applications. Further expansion of applications of this class of biomaterial may be expected.

Inserts and Intramobile Elements

Relatively low moduli of elasticity (compared to metals and ceramics), high elongations to fracture, and inherent toughnesses have resulted in use of selected polymers for connectors or interpositional spacers for dental implants. One popular polymer insert system was included in Table 14–5 for general reference purposes. The most significant limitation has been the polymeric materials resistance to cyclic-load creep and fatigue phenomena. Retrieved transfer systems, in some clinical retrievals, have shown significant plastic deformation and fracture.[31] However, within design limits, these systems tend to provide improvements in flexibility and have biomechanical movement profiles more similar to soft tissues, such as periodontal ligaments. This area has been reviewed recently, and the reader is directed to the referenced publications for more details.[32]

FUTURE TRENDS

Synthetic substances for tissue replacement have evolved from selected industrial grade materials such as metals, ceramics, polymers, and composites. In the 1990s, these classes of materials will be constituted and fabricated for biomaterial applications. This situation offers opportunities for improved control of basic properties. The simultaneous evolution of the biomechanical sciences also provides optimization of design and material concepts for surgical implants. Knowledge of tissue properties and computer-assisted modeling and analyses also support future developments. The introduction of anisotrophy with respect to mechanical properties; chemical gradients from device surface-to-center, with bonding along the tissue interfaces; and control of all aspects of manufacturing, packaging, delivering, placing, and restoring enhance the opportunities for optimal application and, it is hoped, device treatment longevities. Health care delivery would benefit from better availability and decreased per-unit costs.

Combinations for composition of bioactive surfaces, the addition of active biomolecules of tissue inductive substances, and a stable transgingival attachment mechanism should improve device systems. An integrated chemical and physical barrier at the soft tissue transition region would enhance clinical longevities. Devices that function through bone or soft tissue interfaces along the force transfer regions could be systems of choice, depending on the clinical situation.[2] Osseous or fibro-osseous integration might be valuable, depending on the system utilized.

Unquestionably, the trend for conservative treatment of oral diseases will continue to accelerate. Thus, it can be anticipated that dental implants will frequently be a first-treatment option. Therefore, increased usage of root form systems is to be expected. Clearly the true efficacy of the various systems will be determined by controlled clinical studies with 10- to 20-year follow-up periods for quantitative analyses.

Acknowledgment

In 1970, while attending my first American and International Associations for Dental Research (AADR/IADR) meeting, I was introduced to Ralph Phillips within a group discussion on dental materials. He quickly determined that I knew little about the "dental" and some about the "materials." He brought me into the interactions with carefully placed and directed questions and comments so that I was not excluded. This happened repeatedly over the years, until I had the opportunity to reverse the exchange after making a presentation in behalf of the AADR/IADR Dental Materials Group on basic biocompatibility testing, with Ralph as my overview discussant. My opportunity was to coordinate and help direct some of the emerging exchanges among those experienced in the material and biologic sciences. Subsequently our ongoing interactions fostered many wonderful times with colleagues, students, and friends throughout the world.

This chapter represents a later stage, in which Ralph provided written comments and opinions about implant biomaterials as one extension of "dental" biomaterials. I dedicate this chapter to his memory, and most especially to our long-term friendship. I also extend a bon voyage from another close friend as I have been afforded the opportunity to provide material- and biomaterial-based information for Dr. Misch. The dental implant field, in my opinion, will benefit from a continuation of a multidisciplinary approach to the science, technology, and applications. I wish that Ralph could have continued, and we certainly will miss his counsel.

REFERENCES

1. Natiella J et al: Current evaluation of dental implants, *J Am Dent Assoc* 84:1358, 1972.
2. Rizzo A, editor: Proceedings of the consensus development conference on dental implants, *J Dent Educ* 52:678, 1988.
3. Schnitman PA, Shulman LB, editors: Dental implants: benefit and risk, PHS No 81–1531, Proceedings of the Harvard–National Institute of Dental Research Conference, 1980.
4. VonRecum A, editor: *Handbook of biomaterials evaluation*, New York, 1986, Macmillan.
5. Lang B, Mossie H, Razzoog M: *International workshop: biocompatibility, toxicity and hypersensitivity to alloy systems used in dentistry*, Ann Arbor, 1985, University of Michigan Press.
6. *Annual book of standards*, 13.01, medical devices, Philadelphia, 1990, American Society for Testing and Materials.
7. *Dentists' desk reference: materials, instruments and equipment*, Chicago, 1988, American Dental Association.
8. Proceedings of the Third World Biomaterials Congress 11, Society for Biomaterials, Kyoto, Japan, 1988.
9. Symposium on Retrieval and Analysis of Surgical Implants and Biomaterials, Society for Biomaterials, Snowbird, Utah, 1988.
10. Hench LL, Ethridge EC: *Biomaterials, an interfacial approach*, New York, 1982, Academic Press.
11. Vincenzini P, editor: *Ceramics in surgery*, Amsterdam, 1983, Elsevier.
12. Brose M et al: Six year evaluation of submerged alumina dental root implants in humans (IADR abstract 56), *J Dent Res* 66:113, 1987.
13. Driskell TD: History of implants, *J Calif Dent Assoc* 16–25, 1987.
14. deGroot K, editor: *Bioceramics of calcium phosphate*, Boca Raton, Fla, 1983, CRC Press.

15. Ducheyne P, Lemons JE, editors: *Bioceramics: material characteristics versus in vivo behavior,* New York, 1988, New York Academy of Science.
16. Koeneman J: Workshop on characterization of calcium phosphate materials, *J Appl Biomater* 1:79, 1990.
17. LeGeros RZ: Calcium phosphate materials in restorative dentistry: a review, *J Dent Res* 2:164–180, 1988.
18. Yamamuro T, Hench L, Wilson J, editors: *Handbooks of bioactive ceramics,* vols I and II, Boca Raton, Fla, 1990, CRC Press.
19. Kent J et al: Augmentation of deficient edentulous alveolar ridges with dense polycrystalline hydroxylapatite (abstract 3.8.2), Final Programme and Book of Abstracts, First World Biomaterials Congress, Society for Biomaterials, Vienna, Austria, 1980.
20. dePutter C, deGroot K, Sillevis-Smitt P: Transmucosal apatite implants in dogs, *Trans Soc Biomater* 9:115, 1981.
21. English C: Cylindrical implants, *J Calif Dent Assoc* 16:17–40, 1988.
22. Lemons JE: Hydroxylapatite coatings, *Clin Orthop Rel Res* 235:220, 1988.
23. Driessens F: Formation and stability of calcium phosphates in relation to phase composition of the mineral in calcified tissues. In deGroot K, editor: *Bioceramics of calcium phosphates,* Boca Raton, Fla, 1983, CRC Press.
24. Jarcho M: Calcium phosphate ceramics as hard tissue prostheses, *Clin Orthop Rel Res* 157:259–278, 1981.
25. Hjørting-Hansen E, Worsaae N, Lemons JE: Histological response after implantation of porous hydroxylapatite ceramics in humans, *Int J Oral Maxillofac Implant* 5:255, 1990.
26. Cook SD et al: Variables affecting the interface strength and histology of hydroxylapatite coated implant surfaces, *Trans Soc Biomater* 9:14, 1986.
27. Lee DR, Lemons J, LeGeros RZ: Dissolution characterization of commercially available hydroxylapatite particulate, *Trans Soc Biomater* 12:161, 1989.
28. Gross U et al: Biomechanically optimized surface profiles by coupled bone development and resorption at hydroxylapatite surfaces, *Trans Soc Biomater* 13:83, 1990.
29. Hollinger JO, Battistone GC: Biodegradable bone repair materials, *Clin Orthop Rel Res* 20:290–305, 1986.
30. Andrade JD: The interface between physics, materials, science and biology, Keynote session, *Trans Soc Biomater* 12:6, 1989.
31. Kirsch A, Mentag P: The IMZ endosseous two phase implant system, *J Oral Implant* 12:494–498, 1986.
32. Brunski JB: Biomechanics of oral implants: future research directions, *J Dent Educ* 52:775–788, 1988.

Chapter 15

Clinical Biomechanics

Martha Warren Bidez
Carl E. Misch

Bioengineering, a marriage of engineering with the medical and dental fields, has unfolded a new era in diagnosis, treatment, and rehabilitation in patient care. One aspect of this discipline, biomechanics, concerns the response of biological tissues to applied loads. In biomechanics, the tools and methods of applied engineering mechanics are employed in search of structure-function relationships in living materials.[1] Advancements in prosthesis and instrumentation design have been realized as a consequence of mechanical design criteria.[2] This design process is dynamically at work in implant dentistry. The purpose of this chapter is to provide fundamental concepts and principles of dental biomechanics as they relate to the long-term success of dental implants and restorative procedures. In addition, a discussion of bone as a structural foundation for implants and its biological response under functional load is presented.

BASIC CONCEPTS AND PRINCIPLES OF BIOMECHANICS

Loads Applied to Dental Implants

Dental implants are subjected to a variety of loads when placed in function. Basic units of mechanics are used to provide the tools for the consistent description and understanding of such physiologic loads.

Mass, Force, and Weight

Mass, a property of matter, is the degree of gravitational attraction the body of matter experiences. Consider two cubes composed, respectively, of hydroxylapatite and commercially pure–titanium (Fig 15–1). If the two cubes are restrained by identical springs, each spring will deflect by a certain amount relative to the attraction of gravity for the two cubes. The two spring deflections

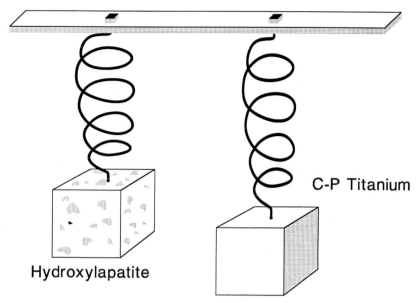

C-P Titanium

Hydroxylapatite

FIG 15–1.
Two cubes made of different materials, when restrained by identical springs, will deflect by differing amounts, relative to the attraction of gravity for the two cubes.

in this example can be made equal by removing part of the material from the titanium cube. Thus, even though the cubes are of completely different composition and size, they can be made equivalent with respect to their response to the pull of gravity. This innate property of each cube that is related to the amount of matter in physical objects is referred to as "mass." The unit of mass in the metric (SI) system is the kilogram (kg); in the English system, it is the pound mass (lbm).

A force was described by Sir Isaac Newton in 1687 in what is now referred to as Newton's Laws of Motion.[3] In his second law, Newton stated that the acceleration of a body is inversely proportional to its mass and directly proportional to the force that caused the acceleration. This is expressed in the familiar relation

$$F = m \cdot a \qquad (1)$$

where F = force (newtons), m = mass (kg), and a = acceleration (meters per second squared; m/s^2).* In the dental implant literature, force frequently is

---

* To convert kilograms of force to newtons of force, multiply kilograms by 9.8. The SI term newton is comparable to the term pound force (lbf) used in the English system of scientific terminology (see conversion table on p. 281).

expressed as kilograms of force. The gravitational constant ($a = 9.8$ m/s^2) in Equation 1 is approximately the same as at every location on Earth; therefore, mass (kilograms) is the determining factor in establishing the magnitude of a static load.

Weight is simply a term for the gravitational force acting on an object at a specified location. Weight and force therefore can be expressed by the same units, newtons or pound force. If one considers a titanium cube placed on the moon, its weight (force due to gravity) is different from its weight on the earth. The mass in the cube has not changed, but the *acceleration due to gravity* has changed. Recalling Sir Isaac Newton, it is useful to remember that an apple weighs approximately 1 newton. The following conversion factors also are useful[4]:

Mass

$$1 \text{ kg} = 2.205 \text{ lbm}$$
$$1 \text{ lbm} = 0.45 \text{ kg}$$

Force

$$1 \text{ newton} = 1 \text{ kg} \cdot \text{m/s}^2 = 0.225 \text{ lbf}$$
$$1 \text{ lbf} = 4.448 \text{ newtons}$$

Area

$$1 \text{ m}^2 = 10.764 \text{ ft}^2$$
$$1 \text{ ft}^2 = 0.093 \text{ m}^2$$
$$1 \text{ in}^2 = 6.452 \times 10^{-4} \text{ m}^2$$

Pressure

$$1 \text{ Pa} = 1 \text{ newton/m}^2 = 1.450 \times 10^{-4} \text{ psia} = 0.021 \text{ lbf/ft}^2$$
$$1 \text{ lbf/in}^2 \text{ (psia)} = 144 \text{ lbf/ft}^2 = 6894.8 \text{ Pa}$$

Force and Moment

Force

Forces acting on dental implants are referred to as vector quantities; that is, they possess both magnitude and direction. Implants are subjected to a broad range of bite force magnitudes (see Chapter 8). These forces typically are three-dimensional, with components directed along one or more of the clinical coordinate axes (Fig 15–2). Such force components may be described within two general categories: normal (i.e., compression or tension) and shear forces.

Normal forces act perpendicular to the surface or plane of interest (Fig 15–3). Compressive forces tend to maintain the integrity of a bone-to-implant interface, whereas tensile forces tend to disrupt or distract such an interface. Shear forces typically act parallel to the surface or plane of interest and also are destructive with respect to maintaining a contiguous bone-to-implant interface. Table 15–1 provides data on cortical bone strengths in human femoral specimens under compression, tension, and shear loading conditions. Note that cortical bone is strongest in compression and weakest in shear.

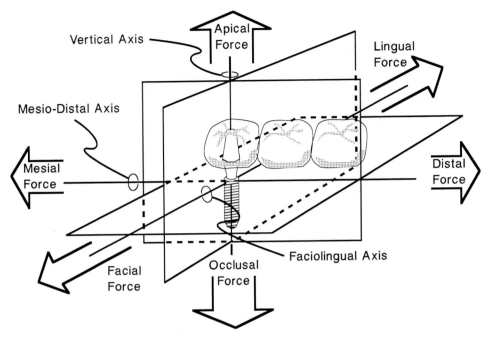

FIG 15–2.
Forces are three dimensional, with components directed along one or more of the clinical coordinate axes.

Any force can be resolved into a combination of normal and shear force components in a given plane. Referring to Figure 15–4, the same magnitude of force may have quite different effects on the implant-to-tissue interface, simply as a function of the *direction* of load application. In those load directions where a high shear component exists, the interface is clearly at risk for mechanical failure. This type of force is applied to an implant body when the abutment is screwed into position. This is a concern because the interface is still composed of woven bone and weaker in design than mature lamellar bone. Occlusion obviously serves as an important determinant in establishing load direction. The position of occlusal contacts on the prosthesis is directly related to the type of force components distributed throughout the implant system. Offset loading results in combination vectors of force. As a result, an increase in tensile and shear force components is often found. Compressive forces should typically be dominant in implant prosthetic occlusion.

In general, the greater the magnitude of force applied to a prosthesis, the greater the resultant force applied to the bone-implant interface. Thus, the range of forces applied to implant interfaces are highly dependent on both the location and magnitude of the applied force. Compressive forces, in general, are best

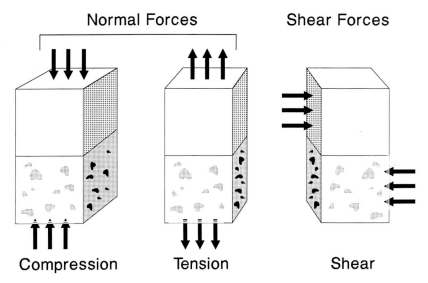

FIG 15–3.
Normal forces act perpendicular to the surface or plane of interest. Shear forces act parallel
to the surface or plane of interest and are destructive to the bone-implant interface.

accommodated by the complete implant-prosthesis system. Cortical bone is
strongest in compression. Additionally, cements and retention screws, implant
components, and bone-implant interfaces all accommodate greater compressive
forces than tensile or shear. For example, whereas the compressive strength of an

TABLE 15–1.

Cortical Bone Strengths in Human Femur Specimens*

Type of Force Applied	Strength (MPa)†	Load Direction/ Comments
Tensile	133.0 (11.7)	Longitudinal
	100.0 (8.6)	30° off axis
	60.5 (4.8)	60° off axis
	51.0 (4.4)	Transverse
Compressive	193.0 (13.9)	Longitudinal
	173.0 (13.8)	30° off axis
	133.0 (15.0)	60° off axis
	133.0 (10.0)	Transverse
Shear	68.0 (3.7)	Torsion

*From Reilly DT, Burstein AH: *J Biomech* 8:393, 1975. Used by permission.
†Standard deviations are given in parentheses.

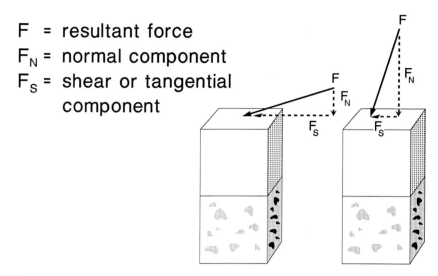

F = resultant force

F_N = normal component

F_S = shear or tangential component

FIG 15–4.
Force can be resolved into a combination of normal and shear force components in a given plane. Depending on the direction of load application, the same magnitude of force has different effects.

average zinc-phosphate dental cement is approximately 83 to 103 MPa (12,000 to 15,000 psi), the resistance to tension and shear is significantly less.[6]

Moment

The moment of a force about a point tends to produce rotation or bending about that point. In Figure 15–5, the moment is defined as a vector, *M*, whose magnitude equals the product of the force magnitude multiplied by the perpendicular distance (also called the "moment arm") from the point of interest to the line of action of the force. This imposed moment load is also referred to as a torque or torsional load and may be quite destructive with respect to implant systems. Torques or bending moments imposed on implants as a consequence of, for example, excessively long cantilever bridge or bar sections, may result in interface breakdown, bone resorption, prosthetic screw loosening, and/or bar/bridge fracture. Proper restorative design must necessarily include consideration of both forces and moments due to those loads.

Large moments may develop in prosthetic environments designed with cantilever extensions from rigidly fixed implants. An implant with a cantilevered mesobar extending 10 mm, 20 mm, and 30 mm has significant ranges of moment loads. A 100-newton force applied directly over the implant does not induce a moment load or torque because no rotational forces are applied through an offset distance. This same 100-newton force applied 10 mm from the implant results in an approximate 1,000 newton/mm moment load. Similarly, if the load is applied 20 mm from the implant, a 2,000 newton/mm torque is applied to the implant-bone region, and 30 mm results in an approximate 3,000 newton/mm moment load.

Moments may develop about all three clinical coordinate axes previously described (vertical, faciolingual, and mesiodistal axes). Referring to Figure 15–6 such moments tend to induce rotations in three planes (transverse, faciolingual, and mesiodistal). Clockwise and counterclockwise rotations of the implant, and/or restoration in each of these three planes, results from six moment loads: lingual-transverse and facial-transverse moments (in the transverse plane), occlusal and apical moments (in the mesiodistal plane), and facial and lingual moments (in the faciolingual plane). Clearly, dental implants are subjected to a complex, three-dimensional system of forces and moments in vivo.

The occlusal height of the prosthesis may affect the resultant moment load on the implant and/or biological tissues in one or more planes. Referring to Figure 15–7,A, note that the occlusal height serves as the moment arm for force components directed along the faciolingual axis (e.g., in tongue thrusts, or in "passive" loading by cheek and oral musculature (Fig 15–7,B), as well as force components directed along the mesiodistal axis (Fig 15–7,C). Clearly a lingual force component may also induce a twisting (lingual-transverse) moment about the implant neck axis if applied through a cantilever length (Fig 15–7,D). Note that the moment contribution of a force component directed along the vertical axis is

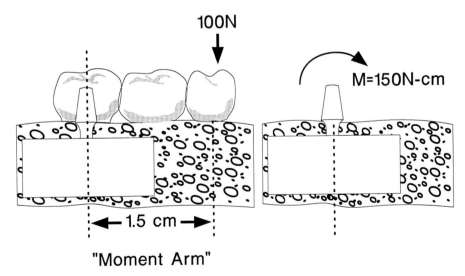

FIG 15–5.
Moment is defined as a vector, M, the magnitude of which equals the product of the force magnitude multiplied by the perpendicular distance ("Moment arm") from the point of interest to the line of action of the force.

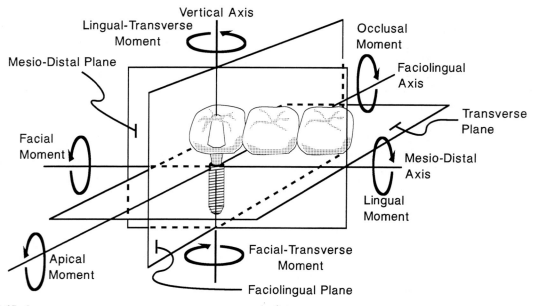

FIG 15–6.
Moment loads tend to induce rotations in three planes. Clockwise and counterclockwise rotations in these three planes result in six moments : lingual-transverse, facial- transverse, occlusal, apical, facial, and lingual.

not affected by the occlusal height because its effective moment arm is the cantilever length if positioned centrically (Fig 15–7,E). Therefore, occlusal height, which is exacerbated by bone loss, has a direct bearing on the amount of moment load imposed on the implant system, applied either with or without a cantilevered extension force. For a given force, Division A bone (see Chapter 7) has less moment load at the crest as compared with, for example, Division C or D bone, because the crown height is adversely affected (Fig 15–8, Table 15–2).

Cantilever prostheses attached to splinted implants result in a complex load reaction. In its simplest form, a Class I lever action may be expressed. If two implants 10 mm apart are splinted together, and a 20-mm distal cantilever is designed with a 100-newton load, the following forces result. Referring to Figure 15–9,A), the 100-newton load is resisted with a 200-newton force by the mesial implant, and the distal implant acts as a fulcrum with a 300-newton load. If the position and amount of distal load remain the same, but the distal implant is positioned 5 mm anterior, the resultant loads on the implants change (Fig 15–9,B). The anterior implant must resist a 500-newton force and the distal, fulcrum implant receives 600-newton force. Therefore, the tensile force is increased 2.5 times on the anterior implant, while the compressive force is increased twofold.

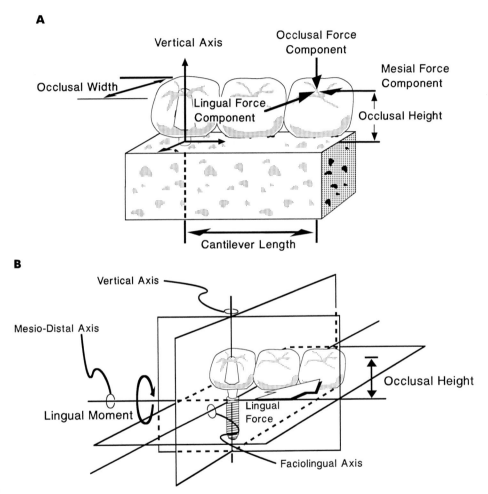

FIG 15–7.
Occlusal height may affect the resultant moment load **(A).** Occlusal height serves as the moment arm for force components directed along the faciolingual axis **(B),** and the force components directed along the mesiodistal axis **(C).** A lingual force component may also induce a twisting moment about the implant neck if applied through a cantilever length.

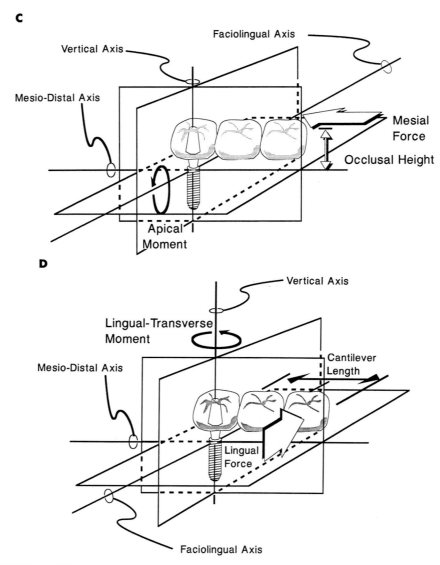

FIG 15-7, cont'd.
(D). The moment of a force along the vertical axis is not affected by the occlusal height, because its effective moment arm is the cantilever length if positioned centrically **(E).**

Continued.

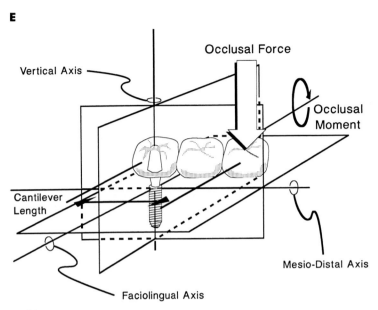

E

FIG 15-7, cont'd.

Because bones and screws are weaker under the action of tensile forces, the anterior implant becomes more at risk for complications.

Similar principles regarding Class I lever forces apply to cantilever loads with anterior splinted implants placed on a curve with distal extended prostheses. The greater the anterior-posterior distance between the center of the most anterior implant(s) to the most distal aspect of the posterior implants, the smaller the resultant loads on the implant system from cantilevered forces due to the stabilizing effect of the anterior-posterior distance. Clinical experiences suggest that the distal cantilever should not extend 2.5 times the anterior-posterior distance under ideal conditions. This guideline is also determined by the implant length, bone density, and the amount and frequency of the distal load. This is why the arch form relates to the number of implants and to the design of the prosthesis. A square arch form involves smaller anterior-posterior distances between the splinted implants, and should have smaller length cantilevers. A tapered arch form has the largest distance between anterior and posterior implants, and may have the longest cantilever design. The maxilla has less dense bone than the mandible, and more often has an anterior cantilever with the prosthesis. As a result, more distal implants may be required in the maxilla than in the mandible, and sinus augmentation may be required in order to permit ideal placement of the implant. A need exists for research in the quantitative assessment of each of these variables to determine their relative contributions in system stability.

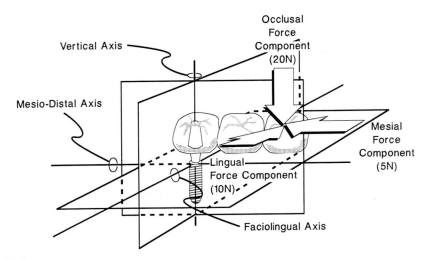

FIG 15–8.
For a given force, Division A bone has less moment load at the crest than divisions C or D because the crown height is adversely affected in those two divisions.

Force Transfer

Stress

One manifestation of force imposed on a dental implant is referred to as stress. In the simplest sense, stress is a representation of the force magnitude distributed over the area over which the force acts. The internal stresses that develop in an implant and surrounding biological tissues under an imposed load may have a significant influence on the long-term longevity of the implants in vivo.

TABLE 15–2.

Moment Load at Crest, Division A Bone When Subjected to Forces Shown in Figure 15–8

Influences on Moment		Imposed Moments (newton/mm) at Implant Crown-to-Crest Interface					
Occlusal Height (mm)	Cantilever Length (mm)	Lingual	Facial	Apical	Occlusal	Facial-Transverse	Lingual-Transverse
10	10	100	0	50	200	0	100
	20	100	0	50	400	0	200
	30	100	0	50	600	0	300
20	10	200	0	100	200	0	100
	20	200	0	100	400	0	200
	30	200	0	100	600	0	300

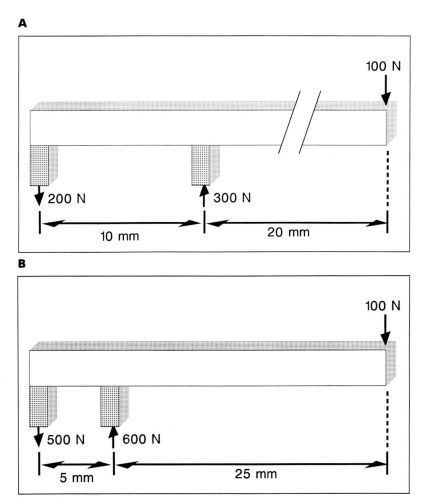

FIG 15–9.
If two implants are designed 10 mm apart and splinted together with a 20-mm distal cantilever, a 100-newton load is resisted by a 200-newton force by the mesial implant and the distal implant acts as a fulcrum with a 300-newton load **(A).** If the implants are 5 mm apart, the anterior implant must resist a 500-newton force, and the distal fulcrum implant receives a 600-newton force **(B).**

Like force components, stress components may be both normal (given the symbol, σ) and shear (given the symbol, τ). A three-dimensional stress element (e.g., a cube of trabecular bone) is illustrated in Figure 15–10. Note there is one normal stress and two shear stresses acting on each (x,y,z) plane. It may be shown that $\tau_{xy} = \tau_{yx}$, $\tau_{yz} = \tau_{zy}$, and $\tau_{xz} = \tau_{zx}$. Thus, any three-dimensional element may

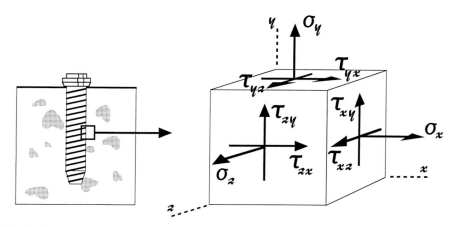

FIG 15–10.
Three-dimensional stress element. There is one normal stress and two shear stresses acting on each (x,y,z) plane. $\tau_{xy} = \tau_{yx}$, $\tau_{yz} = \tau_{zy}$, and $\tau_{xz} = \tau_{zx}$. Any three-dimensional element may have its stress state completely described by three normal stress components and three shear components.

have its stress state completely described by three normal stress components and three shear components.

The question arises as to what are the peak stresses or maximum stresses that an implant and the surrounding interfacial tissues experience. Peak stresses occur when the stress element is positioned in a particular orientation (or geometric configuration) in which all shear stress components are zero. When an element is in this configuration, the normal stresses are given a particular name, principal stresses, and indicated as σ_1, σ_2, and σ_3. By convention, sigma 1 (σ_1) stresses represent the most positive stresses (typically peak tensile stresses) in an implant or tissue region and sigma 3 (σ_3) stresses, the most negative stresses (typically peak compressive stresses). Sigma 2 (σ_2) represents a value intermediate between σ_1 and σ_3. Determination of these peak normal stresses in a dental implant system and tissues may give valuable insights regarding sites of potential implant fracture and bony atrophy.

Deformation and Strain

A load applied to a dental implant may induce deformation of both the implant and surrounding tissues. As will be described later in this chapter, biological tissues may be able to interpret deformation or a manifestation thereof and respond with the initiation of remodeling activity.

The deformation and stiffness characteristics of the materials used in implant dentistry, particularly the implant materials, may influence interfacial tissues, ease of implant manufacture, and clinical longevities. Referring to Table 15–3 elongation (deformation) of biomaterials used for surgical dental implants range from 0% for aluminum oxide (Al_2O_3) ceramics to up to 55% for annealed 316-L stainless steel. Related to deformation is the concept of strain.

Referring to Figure 15–11 under the action of a tensile force, F, the straight bar (of original gage length, 1_o) undergoes elongation to a final length $1_0 + \Delta l$. Engineering strain, which is unitless, is defined as elongation per unit length and is given the symbol, ϵ.

$$\epsilon = \frac{\Delta l}{1_o} \qquad (2)$$

where Δl = elongation, and 1_o = original gage length. Shear strain, γ, describes the change in a right angle of a body or stress element under the action of a pure shearing load. All materials (both biologic and nonbiologic) are characterized by a maximum elongation possible before permanent deformation or fracture results. Further, biologic materials exhibit strain rate dependence in that their material properties (such as modulus of elasticity, ultimate tensile strength) are altered as a function of the rate of loading (and subsequent deformation rate).

Experimental observation has also demonstrated that lateral strain also accompanies axial strain under the action of an axial load. Within an elastic range (to be defined later in this section), these two strains are proportional to one another as described by *Poisson's ratio, μ.* For tensile loading,

$$\mu = \frac{\text{Lateral strain}}{-\text{Axial strain}} \qquad (3)$$

The material/mechanical properties described provide for the determination of implant-tissue stress-strain behavior according to established relationships in solid mechanics theory.[8]

Stress-Strain Relationship

A relationship is needed between the applied force (and stress) that are imposed on the implant and surrounding tissues and the subsequent deformation (and strain) experienced throughout the system. If any elastic body is experimentally subjected to an applied load, a load-vs.-deformation curve may be generated (Fig 15–12,A). If the load (force) values are divided by the surface area over which they act and the change in the length by the original length, a classic engineering stress-strain curve is produced (Fig 15–12,B). Such a curve provides for the prediction of how much strain will be experienced in a given material under the action of an applied load. The slope of the linear (elastic) portion of this curve is referred to as the modulus of elasticity, E, and its value is indicative of the stiffness of the material under study.

The closer the modulus of elasticity of the implant resembles that of the contiguous biological tissues, the smaller the likelihood of relative motion at the

TABLE 15-3.

Mechanical Properties of Selected Surgical Implant Biomaterials

| | | | | Co Alloy (wrought) | |
| | Biomaterial | | | | |
Property	Ti (wrought)	Ti-Al-V (wrought)	Co-Cr-Mo (cast)	Annealed	Cold Worked
Density (g/cc)		4.5	8.3	9.2	9.2
Hardness (Vickers)	$R_b 100$	—	300	240	450
Yield strength					
MPa	170–485	795–827	490	450	1,050
(ksi)	(25–70)	(115–120)	(71)	(62)	(152)
Ultimate tensile					
strength MPa	240–550	860–896	690	950	1,540
(ksi)	(35–80)	(125–130)	(100)	(138)	(223)
Elastic modulus					
GPa	96	105–117	200	230	230
(ksi $\times$ 10^3)	(14)	(15–17)	(29)	(34)	(34)
Endurance limit (fatigue)					
MPa	—	170–240	300	—	240–490
(ksi $\times$ 10^3)		(24.6–35)	(43)		(35–71)
Elongation%	15–24	10–15	8	30–45	9

From Lemons JE, Bidez MW, Biomaterials and biomechanics in implant dentistry. In McKinney editor: *Implant Dentistry,* St Louis, 1991, CV Mosby.

tissue-to-implant interface. In terms of full arch kinematics, consider that the mandible flexes toward the midline upon opening. A prosthesis and implant support system that is splinted from molar to molar must provide similar movement.

Referring to Figure 15–13, once a particular implant system (that is, a specific material) is selected, the only way for an operator to control the strain experienced by the tissues is to control the applied stress. Such stress (recall: force/area) may be influenced by the implant design, surgery, and the restoration. The macrogeometry of the implant (that is, the amount and orientation of surface area available to transmit loads) has a very strong influence on the nature of the force transfer at the tissue-implant interface. Surgical grafting procedures may be used to increase both the quantity and quality of bone contiguous to the implant. The applied stress is also influenced by the restoration of the size of occlusal tables, stress breakers, overdenture vs. fixed prosthesis, and occlusal design. Generally the greater the magnitude of stress applied to a dental implant system (refer to Fig 15–13), the greater the difference in strain between the implant material and bone. In such cases, the implant is less likely to stay attached to the bone, and the probability of fibrous tissue ingrowth into the interfacial region to accommodate the range of difference becomes greater.

Biomaterial							
Fe-Cr-Ni 316-L		C-Si	Al_2O_3		UHMW	PMMA	PTFE
Annealed	Cold Worked		Sapphire	Alumna	Polyethylene		
7.9	7.9	1.5–2.0	3.99	3.9	0.94	1.2	2.2
170–200	300–350	—	—	HV23.000	D65	M60–100	D50–65
240–300 (35–44)	700–800 (102–116)	—	—	—	—	—	—
600–700 (87–102)	1,000 (145)	350–517 (51–75)	480 (70)	400 (58)	21–44 (3.0–6.4)	55–85 (8.0–12.3)	14–34 (2–5)
200 (29)	200 (29)	28–34 (4.0–4.9)	414 (60)	380 (55.1)	1 (0.145)	2.4–3.3 (0.348–0.479)	0.4 (0.058)
300 (43) 35–55	230–280 (33.3–40.6) 7–22	— 0	— 0	— 0	— 400	— 2–7	— 200–400

Hooke's Law is the name given to the relationship between stress and strain; in its simplest form, it is described mathematically as

$$\sigma = E\,\epsilon \qquad (4)$$

where σ = normal stress (Pa or psi), E = modulus of elasticity (Pa or psi), and ϵ = normal strain (unitless). A similar relationship may be generated for shear stress and shear strain, where the constant of proportionality is the modulus of rigidity, G, expressed by

$$\tau = G\gamma \qquad (5)$$

where τ = shear stress (Pa or psi), G = modulus of rigidity (Pa or psi), and γ = shear strain (unitless).

Impact Load and Impulse

When two bodies collide in a very small interval of time, relatively large reaction forces develop. Such a collision is described as impact. Upon impact, the two elastic bodies are compressed until their mass centers attain the same velocity; they then move apart at characteristic speeds and velocities. The resultant behavior of these colliding bodies is dependent upon many factors, including the material properties of the bodies themselves.[3]

For a perfectly elastic collision, the velocity of the collided bodies upon separation is equal to their initial approach velocity, whereas for a perfectly plastic impact, the bodies remain in contact. In such cases, there is always a dissipation of mechanical energy into heat and permanent deformation.

Such plastic impact is illustrated in Figure 15–14, which is analogous to the dental situation. In dental implant systems subjected to occlusal impact loads, deformation may occur in the prosthodontic restoration, in the implant itself, and/or in the contiguous interfacial tissues. The nature of the relative stiffness of these components in the overall implant system largely controls the response of the system to the impact load.

To explain this further, let us define linear momentum as the product of mass and velocity. Impulse of a force, I, over a time interval is equal to the change in momentum of a body (particle) during that time interval.[3]

$$I = m \, V_f - m \, V_i$$

where I = impulse of a force, m = mass, V_f = velocity, final, and V_i = velocity, initial. The stiffer any of the individual components of a system, the smaller the final velocity and the greater the impulse load. The greater the impulse (that is,

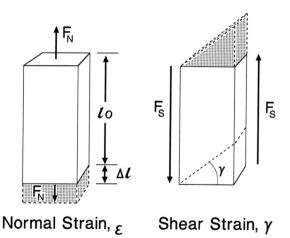

Normal Strain, ϵ   **Shear Strain, γ**

FIG 15–11.
Under the action of a tensile force, F, the straight bar originally, l_o, undergoes elongation to the final length, l_o, + 1. Engineering strain ϵ is the deformation per unit length. Shear strain γ is the change in a right angle of a body or stress element under the action of a pure shearing load.

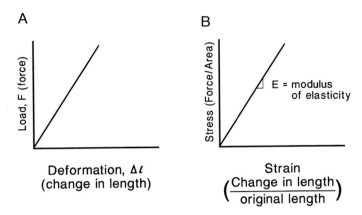

FIG 15–12.
Load vs. deformation curve may be generated for any elastic body experimentally subjected to a load **(A)**. If the load values are divided by the surface area, and the deformation by the specimen's original gage length, a stress-strain curve is produced **(B)**.

the force acting over a short time interval), the greater the risk of implant and bridge failure and bone fracture.

Various methods have been proposed to address the issue of reducing impact loads. Skalak[9] has suggested the need for using acrylic teeth in conjunction with osteointegrated fixtures to partially mitigate high impact loads which might damage bony tissues adjacent to the implant. Weiss[10] has proposed that a fibrous tissue-to-implant interface provides for physiologic shock absorption in a similar fashion to that exhibited by a functioning periodontal ligament. At least one implant has attempted to incorporate shock absorption capability in the design itself, by the use of an "intramobile element" of lower stiffness as compared to the rest of the implant.[11] Misch advocates an acrylic provisional restoration with a progressive occlusal loading to improve the bone-implant interface before the final restoration, occlusal design, and masticatory loads are distributed to the system.[12] Quantitative measurements of the reduction in impact loads to biologic tissues adjacent to dental implants using these or other methods have not been performed to date. Only limited data exist with respect to impact forces on natural dentition and tooth-supported bridgework.[13, 14]

BONE AS A STRUCTURAL FOUNDATION

The current state of understanding regarding the mechanical properties of both cortical and cancellous bone has recently been comprehensively reported in

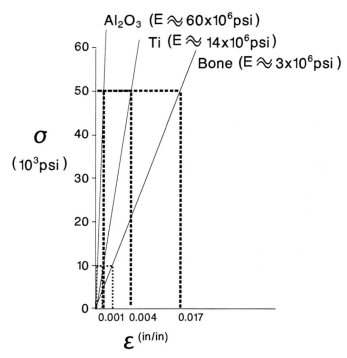

FIG 15–13.
Once a particular implant system is selected, the only way to control the strain on the tissues is to control the applied stress. The greater the magnitude of stress applied to the system, the greater the difference in strain between the implant material and bone.

a book by Cowin.[15] A brief summary of bone properties related to its role as a structural foundation for dental implant devices is presented in the following section.

Cortical Bone

Dependence on Direction of Loading

The structure of cortical bone is described in Chapter 16. The degree to which the mechanical properties of cortical bone are dependent on its structure is referred to as anisotropy. This concept is presented graphically in Figure 15–15, which illustrates how a material may exhibit directionally dependent mechanical properties (for example, modulus of elasticity). A material is said to be orthotropic if it exhibits *different* properties in all three directions and isotropic if the properties are the *same* in all three directions. Transversely isotropic describes a material in which two of the three directions exhibit the same mechanical properties.

Bone has been reported to be transversely isotropic by Reilly and Burstein[5] and by Yoon and Katz[16] (referring to Fig 15–15, E_1 and E_2 are the same). Knets and Malmeisters[17] and Ashman et al.[18] have described bone as orthotropic (that is, $E_1 \neq E_2 \neq E_3$). The mandible has been reported as transversely isotropic with the stiffest direction oriented around the arch of the mandible[19] (see Fig 15–15). These authors suggest that the cortical bone of the mandible functions as a long bone which has been molded into a curved beam geometry. The stiffest direction (around the arch) thus corresponds to the long axis of the tibia or femur. Such data raise interesting questions regarding the primary loads that the mandible experiences: occlusal loads or flexural loads imposed during opening and closing of the mouth. Clinical experience has qualitatively revealed that the actual mandible has a more compact bone at the inferior border, less compact bone on the superior aspect, and greater quality of trabecular bone, especially between the mental foramenae. In addition, the presence of teeth and/or implants significantly increases the trabecular bone amount and density within the residual alveolar bone. Further studies are indicated to quantitatively determine the variation of

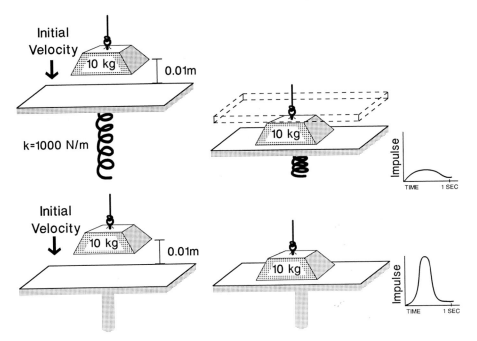

FIG 15–14.
Impact loads. The stiffer the components of the system, the smaller the final velocity and the greater the impulse load. The greater the impulse (the force acting over a short time interval), the greater the risk of implant and bridge failure and bone fracture.

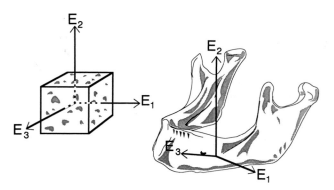

FIG 15–15.
Cortical bone of the human mandible has been reported as transversely isotropic, with the stiffest direction oriented around the arch of the mandible (E_3).[19]

bone material properties as a function of location within the mandibular and maxillary arches.

Dependence on Rate of Loading

A material is said to be viscoelastic if its mechanical behavior is dependent on the rate of load application. The strain rate dependence of bone was investigated by McElhaney[20] and is graphically illustrated in Figure 15–16. A significant difference can be noted in both ultimate tensile strength and modulus of elasticity over a wide range of strain rates, with bone acting both stiffer and stronger at higher strain rates. Restated, bone fails at a higher load, but with less allowable elongation (deformation) at higher as compared to lower strain rates. Thus, bone behaves in a more brittle fashion at higher strain rates.

Carter and Hayes[21] have reported both strength and elastic modulus of human bone to be proportional to strain rate raised to the 0.06 power. Strain rate to which bone is normally exposed varies from $0.001s^{-1}$ for slow walking to $0.01s^{-1}$ for higher levels of activity. While closure speeds of the human mouth have been reported by one author,[22] no data is available regarding human mandibular or maxillary bone strain rates in vivo.

Dependence on Duration of Loading

Carter and Caler[23] have described bone damage or fracture due to mechanical stress as the sum of both the damage due to creep or time-dependent loading and cyclic or fatigue loading, and the relative interaction of these two types of damage.

Creep refers to the phenomenon whereby a material continues to exhibit increasing deformation as a function of time when subjected to a constant load. Carter and Caler[24] have reported the creep-fracture curve for adult human bone at a constant stress of 60 MPa (Fig 15–17). Over a time period of approximately

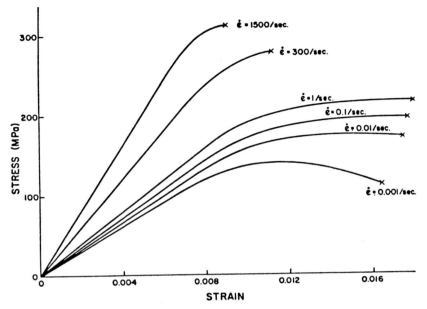

FIG 15–16.
Strain rate dependence of bone. (From McElhaney JH: *J Appl Physiol* 1966; 21:1231. Used by permission.)

6 hours, a threefold increase in strain was observed. Such data raise the question of whether resorption and/or failure in the dental bruxer or "clencher" patient may be partially (or wholly) the result of an accumulation of creep damage.

Fatigue strength of a material refers to an ultimate strength below which the material may be repetitively subjected for an infinite number of cycles without failure. Carter et al.[25, 26] have investigated the fatigue properties of human cortical bone. Fatigue failure has been reported for in vivo bone by Carter and associates and by others[27–29] at relatively low cycles (10^4 to 10^8 cycles). Given the high magnitude of cycles encountered in oral function, the relatively low in vivo fatigue life reported in bone (that is, accumulated fatigue damage) is likely accommodated in vivo through the normal process of bone remodeling.

Cancellous Bone

Cancellous bone is a porous, structurally anisotropic, inhomogeneous material. Current research efforts attempt to describe and quantify the structure of cancellous bone, and strength and modulus of elasticity. If noninvasive imaging techniques can provide quantitative information regarding the structure of

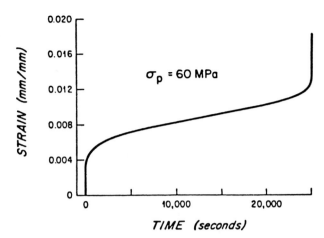

FIG 15–17.
Creep curve for adult human cortical bone at a constant stress of 60 MPa. (From Carter DR, Caler WE: *J Biomech Engr* 1983; 105. Used by permission.)

cancellous bone, mathematical relationships may be used to predict corresponding bone strength and stiffness properties. Ultimately, diagnostic imaging techniques may provide a *quantitative* assessment of cancellous bone as a structural foundation for dental implant placement.

Dependence of Elastic Modulus on Structural Density

A 25-year literature base documents the work of numerous investigators[30–48] who have reported in vitro data used in the development of a mathematical relationship between elastic modulus and structural density of cancellous bone. Most recently, Rice et al.[48] found that the axial (longitudinal) modulus of elasticity was proportional to the square of the structural density in tests conducted at a strain rate of 0.01 s^{-1}. Differences in their results were noted as a function of species (bovine vs. human), direction (longitudinal, medial/lateral, and anterior-posterior) and axial stress conditions (compression vs. tension).

Dependence of Strength on Structural Density

As was the case with elastic modulus, axial compressive strength has been found to exhibit a quadratic dependence (that is, proportional to the second power) on structural density.[37, 38, 48]

Rice et al.[48] again reported differences in strength values as a function of species, direction, and stress type. No differences were noted between compressive strength and tensile strength. This finding is consistent with that reported by other groups.[40, 42] Also noteworthy is their observation of higher structural density coefficients in the longitudinal as compared with transverse directions. These data are expected, because the specimens tested were taken from long bones whose primary load-bearing direction was along the longitudinal axis of the shaft.

While the empirical relationships presented in this subsection have been derived on the basis of experimental data from long bones in the human and bovine models, extrapolations to mandibular and maxillary bone seem plausible. Additional research is indicated to confirm these findings in the mandible and explore the mechanical characterization of the maxilla.

Role of External and Internal Geometry in Edentulous Mandible in Force Transfer

The finite element method (FEM) is a numerical technique commonly used in engineering disciplines for the solution of problems in continuum mechanics.[49] For more than a decade, multiple investigators have applied the FEM in implant dentistry in an attempt to gain insights into the stress distributions throughout a dental implant and into the surrounding tissues (under functional loading conditions).[50–62] The technique may also be used to gain preliminary insights into the role of external and internal geometry in force transfer through an edentulous human mandible.

Three-dimensional finite element models of molar mandibular regions were constructed by the authors to simulate Division A, B, and C bone. The models included cortical and cancellous bone regions of varying densities. Rigid constraints were imposed along the inferior border of each of the mandibular sections and a vertically oriented (occlusal-apical) force of 450 newtons was imposed on the crest. Two questions were addressed: (1) What is the effect of variations in external geometry on force transfer through an edentulous mandibular section with structural density held constant and (2) What is the effect of internal geometry variations (changes in structural density) with external geometry held constant?

Utilizing the quadratic relationship of Rice and colleagues,[48] values for modulus of elasticity and ultimate compressive strength were calculated for four cancellous bone densities (Table 15–4). Static analyses were performed and

TABLE 15-4.

Material Properties Used in FEA Models

Density (g/mm^3)	Modulus of Elasticity (GPa)	Ultimate Compressive Strength (MPa)
$\rho_{100\%} = 1.00$	$E_{100\%} = 0.96$	$S_{100\%} = 22.57$
$\rho_{75\%} = 0.75$	$E_{75\%} = 0.57$	$S_{75\%} = 13.76$
$\rho_{50\%} = 0.50$	$E_{50\%} = 0.29$	$S_{50\%} = 7.48$
$\rho_{25\%} = 0.25$	$E_{25\%} = 0.12$	$S_{25\%} = 3.71$

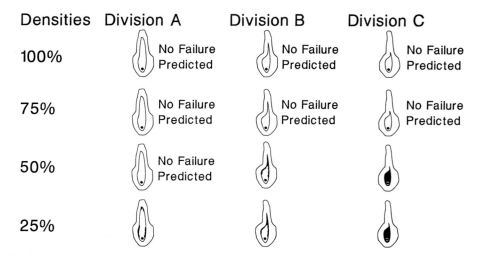

FIG 15–18.
Internal stresses predicted by FEA exceed maximum compressive strength in bone models exhibiting compromised internal and external geometry *(darkened regions).*

resultant internal stresses were compared with the respective ultimate strength values of each section, to assess likelihood of trabecular fracture under the applied load of 450 newtons.

Figure 15–18 shows areas where internal compressive stresses exceeded the maximum compressive strength of the bone for each of the three external geometries and four internal geometries evaluated. Clearly, both external and internal geometries are important variables in force transfer through mandibular bone and warrant further study.

BIOLOGICAL RESPONSE TO LOADED DENTAL IMPLANTS

Bone Remodeling Theories

Current research efforts in the area of bone remodeling focus on the understanding and quantitative delineation of bone adaptation to functional loads. A thorough comprehension of the mechanisms of such remodeling activity may ultimately lead to the prediction of the biologic response to a given mechanical environment. In a recent review of bone modeling and remodeling theories, Hart and Davy[63] describe two fundamental modeling assumptions relative to current theories. The first assumption is that strain history is the likely catalyst for remodeling activity, as numerous potential mechanisms by which bone may transduce mechanical strain have been described.[64] The immediate strain environment appears to have a more direct impact on adaptive activity compared to remote events in the strain history of the tissue. This appears evident when implants are placed into bone regions which have reduced density, presumably from decreased loads to the area. Clinical experience has shown that the implanted region will increase in amount and density of trabecular and cortical bone if physiologic factors are maintained.

A second concept characteristic of remodeling theories is that of a "remodeling equilibrium." This describes the mechanical environment whereby bone is simultaneously resorbed and deposited with no net change in the macrogeometry of the tissue or its mechanical properties. All adaptive remodeling activity subsequent to an applied load or altered mechanical environment is postulated to be driven to approach such a state of remodeling equilibrium. This phenomena is present after the equilibrium of force and implant system is established.

The range of remodeling equilibrium related to adaptive behavior may be necessarily broad, as the bones of the human skeleton serve many different functions. Published studies of the functional adaptation of bone exist in the orthopedic biomechanics literature (particularly for long bone models). No data are available relating the functional adaptation of mandibular or maxillary bone to its mechanical environment, and only limited theoretical dental models have been correlated with in vivo human or animal data.

One of the earliest remodeling theories was postulated by Kummer,[65] in which a relationship was sought between stress and the magnitude of bone remodeling (positive deposition or negative resorption).

Gjelsvik[66, 67] proposed a piezoelectric model for bone remodeling activity in which adaptive behavior was activated by a stress-induced polarization vector. More recent studies[68] suggest that streaming potentials may provide a significantly more important role than piezoelectric phenomena in adaptive activity.

The earliest attempt to describe adaptive behavior is attributed to Wolff,[69] whose qualitative observations in 1869 have become widely known as "Wolff's Law." Wolff stated that bony architecture is influenced by principal stress orientation (that is, the trajectoral hypothesis) and that cortical and trabecular bone were essentially the same material, differing only in the relative porosity. Fyhrie and Carter[70] in 1986 postulated two objective functions (aligning trabecular architecture with principal stress direction and maximizing material strength while minimizing the amount of material) which were optimized by remodeling phenomena. In this theory, the material's apparent density is said to adapt to an "effective stress." The trabecular bone remodeling model of Fyhrie and Carter agrees with the two-dimensional analytical results of Hayes and Snyder,[71] in which a significant correlation was identified between the von Mises effective stress and density. In a later, three-dimensional model by Stone et al.,[72] only a very weak correlation was observed between the von Mises stress and density.

The theory of adaptive elasticity[73–76] differs from the self-optimization theory of Fyhrie and Carter in that it describes the remodeling activity of bone as a function of changing mechanical environments rather than predicting the optimal configuration of normal bone. More specifically, adaptive elasticity predicts that bone (cortical) will adapt under load to achieve an equilibrium strain state and that the remodeling rate is determined by the difference between the equilibrium and the actual strain states. The theory predicts changes in both elastic modulus of the bone tissue and external geometry. Agreement between experimental results and theoretical predictions from "adaptive elasticity" have been reported.[77] Cowin's phenomenological model has been modified and broadened by Hart and Davy.[63] In their writings, the remodeling rate constants are described in terms of such biological parameters as the number of different cells present and their average activity.

Huiskes et al.[78, 79] have proposed an alternative form of Cowin's adaptive elasticity model replacing strain with strain energy density as the feedback control variable for adaptive activity. Strain energy density (SED) is defined as the amount of work done by all the forces (on an implant) per unit volume.[8] The driving force for remodeling behavior is the difference between an actual and homeostatic equilibrium SED state. The adaptive remodeling formulation of Huiskes has been applied to the classic problem of density distribution in the femur and in the case of stress shielding around an intramedullary rod model and demonstrated reasonable agreement with clinical results.

Effect of Implant-to-Tissue Relative Motion

Many studies throughout the orthopedic and dental literature have cited a strong correlation between tissue-to-implant relative motion and the development of specific interfacial tissue types.

Brunski et al.[80] reported results of interfacial development surrounding smooth-surfaced, titanium dental implants placed in dog mandibles. Two implants per dog were placed; one implant was placed in function following implantation, whereas the contralateral implant was shielded from direct occlusal loads. A "fibrous capsule" was observed around implants placed in early function as compared with mineralized tissue in the shielded implants. Brunski and associates postulated that relative movement between the implant and the interface resulted in the formation of fibrous tissue.

Branemark and colleagues[81, 82] have observed direct bone at the light microscopic level at the implant interface in implants subjected to a submerged (nonactive loading) healing period of 4 to 6 months' duration.

Controlled laboratory studies as well as clinical observation suggest that the development of implant-to-tissue interfaces may be strongly influenced by the mechanical environment. The biological response to loaded dental implants is influenced by a multitude of factors, including surgically related thermal injury of bone,[83] biocorrosion phenomenon,[84] and implant surface conditions.[85] The long-term determinant of interface type and stability is also clearly force-related.

REFERENCES

1. Schmid-Schonbein GW, Woo SL-Y, Zweifack BW, editors: *Frontiers in biomechanics,* New York, 1986, Springer-Verlag.
2. National Institutes of Health Consensus Development Conference Statement on Dental Implants, June 13–15, 1988. *J Dent Educ* 52:824–827, 1988.
3. Higdon A et al: *Engineering mechanics*—volume II, *Dynamics,* Englewood Cliffs, NJ, 1976, Prentice-Hall.
4. Baumeister T, Avallone EA, Baumeister T, editors: *Marks standard handbook for mechanical engineers,* ed 8, New York, 1978, McGraw-Hill.
5. Reilly DT, Burstein AH: The elastic and ultimate properties of compact bone tissue, *J Biomech* 8:393, 1975.
6. Leinfelder KF, Lemons JE: *Clinical restorative materials and techniques,* Philadelphia, 1988, Lea & Febiger.
7. *Annual Book of ASTM Standards,* Philadelphia, 1976. American Society for Testing and Materials, Part 46, pp 381, 398.
8. Timoshenko SP, Goodier JN: *Theory of elasticity,* ed 3, New York, 1970, McGraw-Hill.
9. Skalak R: Biomechanical considerations in osseointegrated prostheses, *J Prosth Dent* 49:843–848, 1983.
10. Weiss CM: Fibro-osteal and osteal integration: a comparative analysis of blade and fixture type dental implants supported by clinical trials, *J Dent Educ* 52:706–711, 1988.
11. Kirsch A: The two-phase implantation method using IMZ intramobile cylinder implants, *J Oral Implant* 11:197–210, 1983.
12. Misch CE: *Periodont Prosthodont.*
13. Salis SG, Hood JA, Stokes AN, et al: Impact-fracture energy of human pre-molar teeth, *J Prosth Dent* 58(1):43–48, 1987.
14. Saunders WP: The effects of fatigue impact forces upon the retention of various designs of resin-retained bridgework, *Dent Mater* 3:85–89, 1986.
15. Cowin SC: *Bone mechanics,* Boca Raton, Fla, 1989, CRP Press.
16. Yoon HS, Katz JL: Ultrasonic wave propagation in human cortical bone. II: measurements of elastic properties and micro-hardness, *J Biomech* 9:459, 1976.
17. Knets I, Malmeister A: Deformability and strength of human compact bone tissue. In Brankov G, editor: *Mechanics of biological solids,* Proceedings of the Euromechanic Colloquium 68, Sofia, 1977, Bulgarian Academy of Sciences, p 133.
18. Ashman RB et al: A continuous wave technique for the measurement of the elastic properties of bone, *J Biomech* 17:349, 1984.
19. Ashman RB, Van Buskirk WC: The elastic properties of a human mandible, *Adv Dent Res* 1:64–67, 1987.

20. McElhaney JH: Dynamic response of bone and muscle tissue, *J Appl Physiol* 21:1231, 1966.
21. Carter DR, Hayes WC: The compressive behavior of bone as a two-phase porous structure, *J Bone Joint Surg [Am]* 59(A):954, 1977.
22. Harrison A, Lewis TT: The development of abrasion testing machine, *J Biomed Mater Res,* 9:341, 1975.
23. Carter DR, Caler WE: A cumulative damage model for bone fracture, *J Orthop Res* 3:84, 1985.
24. Carter DR, Caler WE: Cycle dependent and time dependent bone fracture with repeated loading, *J Biomech Eng* 105:166, 1983.
25. Carter DR et al: Fracture behavior of adult cortical bone—the influence of mean strain and strain range, *Acta Orthop Scand* 52:481, 1981.
26. Carter DR et al: Uniaxial fatigue of human cortical bone—the influence of tissue physical characteristics, *J Biomech* 14:461, 1981.
27. Gray RJ, Korbacher GK: Compressive fatigue behavior of bovine compact bone, *J Biomech* 14:461, 1981.
28. Swanson SAV, Freeman MAR, Day WH: The fatigue properties of human cortical bone, *Med Biol Eng* 9:23, 1971.
29. Lafferty JF, Raju PVV: The influence of stress frequency on fatigue strength of cortical bone, *J Biomed Eng* 101:112, 1979.
30. McElhaney JH: Dynamic response of bone and muscle tissue, *J Appl Physiol* 21:1231, 1966.
31. Currey JD: The mechanical consequences of variation in the mineral content of bone, *J Biomech* 2:1, 1969.
32. Pugh JW, Rose RM, Radin EL: Elastic and viscoelastic properties of trabecular bone: dependence on structure, *J Biomech* 6:475, 1973.
33. Crowninshield RD, Pope MH: The response of compact bone in tension at various strain rates, *Ann Biomed Eng* 2:217, 1974.
34. Townsend PR, Rose RM, Radin EL: Buckling studies of single human trabeculae, *J Biomech* 2:217, 1974.
35. Runkle, JC, Pugh JW: The micromechanics of cancellous bone. II: determination of the elastic modulus of individual trabeculae by a buckling analysis, *Bull Hosp Jt Dis,* Orthop Inst 36:2, 1975.
36. Wright TM, Hayes WC: Tensile testing of bone over a wide range of strain rates: effects of strain rate, microstructure and density, *Med Biol Eng* 14:671, 1976.
37. Carter DR, Hayes WC: Bone compressive strength: the influence of density and strain rate, *Science,* 194:1174, 1976.
38. Carter DR, Hayes WC: The compressive behavior of bone as a two-phase porous structure, *J Bone Joint Surg [Am]* 59:954, 1977.
39. Brown TD, Ferguson AB: Mechanical property distributions in the cancellous bone of the human proximal femur, *Acta Orthop Scand* 51:429, 1980.
40. Carter DR, Schwab GH, Spengler DM: Tensile fracture of cancellous bone, *Acta Orthop Scand* 5:733, 1980.
41. Williams JL, Lewis JL: Properties and an anisotropic model of cancellous bone from the proximal tibial epiphysis, *J Biomech Eng* 104:50, 1982.

42. Bensusan JS et al: Tensile, compressive and torsional testing of cancellous bone, *Transactions of the 29th Annual Meeting of the Orthopedic Research Society* 8:132, 1983.

43. Stone JL, Beaupre GS, Hayes WC: Multiaxial strength characteristics of trabecular bone, *J Biomech* 16:743, 1983.

44. Goldstein SA et al: The mechanical properties of human tibial trabecular bone as a function of metaphyseal location, *J Biomech* 16:965, 1983.

45. Ryand SD, Williams JL: Tensile testing of individual bovine trabeculae, *Proceedings of the 12th NE Bio-Engineering Conference*, 1986, p 35.

46. Kuhn JL et al: The mechanical properties of single trabeculae, *Transactions of the 33rd Annual Meeting of the Orthopedic Research Society,* 12:48, 1987.

47. Mente PL, Lewis JL: Young's modulus of trabecular bone tissue, *Transactions of the 33rd Annual Meeting of the Orthopedic Research Society,* 12:49, 1987.

48. Rice JC, Cowin SC, Bowman JA: On the dependence of the elasticity and strength of cancellous bone on apparent density, *J Biomech* 21:155, 1988.

49. Cook RD: *Concepts and applications of finite element analysis,* New York, 1981, John Wiley & Sons.

50. Privitzer E, Widera GE, Tesk JA: Some factors affecting dental implant design, *J Biomed Mater Res Symp* 6:251–255, 1975.

51. Lavernia CJ et al: An analysis of stresses in a dental implant system, *J Biomech* 14:555–560, 1981.

52. Knoell AC: A mathematical model of an in vitro human mandible, *J Biomech* 10:159–166, 1977.

53. Cook SD, Weinstein AM, Klawitter JJ: Parameters affecting the stress distribution around LTI carbon and aluminum oxide dental implants, *J Biomed Mater Res* 6:875–885, 1982.

54. Buch JD, Crose JG, Bechtol CE: Biomechanical and biomaterial considerations of natural teeth, tooth replacements, and skeletal fixation, *Biomater Med Devices Artif Organs* 2:171–186, 1977.

55. Borchers L, Reichart P: Three-dimensional distribution around a dental implant at different stages of interfacial development, *J Dent Res* 62:155–159, 1983.

56. Widera GE, Tesk JA, Privitzer E: Interaction effects among cortical bone, cancellous bone, and periodontal membrane of natural teeth and implants, *J Biomed Mater Res Symp* 7:613–623, 1976.

57. Bidez MW, Stephens BJ, Lemons JE: Investigations into the effect of body length of blade dental implants on interfacial tissue stress profiles, American Society of Mechanical Engineers Winter Annual Meeting, Computational Biomechanics Symposium, Chicago, 1988.

58. Bidez MW, Stephens BJ, Lemons JE: Stress distributions within a CP-Ti dental implant system as a function of interfacial boundary conditions, *Proceedings of Society for Biomaterials World Congress Meeting,* Kyoto, Japan, 1988.

59. Bidez MW, McLoughlin S, Lemons JE: Finite element analyses of blade implant design and interfacial tissue stress profiles. I: the effect of implant height, *Proceedings of the 1989 ASME Winter Annual Meeting,* San Francisco, Calif.

60. McLoughlin S, Bidez MW, Lemons JE: Finite element analyses of blade implant de-

sign and interfacial tissue stress profiles. II: the effect of implant neck width, *Proceedings of the 1989 ASME Winter Annual Meeting,* San Francisco, Calif.

61. Bidez MW et al: Finite element analysis of an edentulous human mandible, *Proceedings of The First World Congress of Biomechanics,* San Diego, Calif, 1990.

62. Bidez MW, McLoughlin S, Lemons JE: FEA investigations in plate-form dental implant design, *Proceedings of The First World Congress of Biomechanics,* San Diego, Calif, 1990.

63. Hart RT, Davy DT: Theories of bone modeling and remodeling. In Cowin SC, editor: *Bone Mechanics,* Boca Raton, Fla, 1989, CRC Press, p 253.

64. Treharne RW: Review of Wolff's law and its proposed means of operation, *Orthop Rev* 10:35, 1981.

65. Kummer BKF: Biomechanics of bone: mechanical properties, functional structure, functional adaptation. In Fung YC, Perrone N, Anliker M, editors: *Biomechanics: its foundations and objectives,* Englewood Cliffs, NJ, Prentice-Hall, 1972, p 237.

66. Gjelsvik A: Bone remodeling and piezoelectricity—I, *J Biomech* 6:69, 1973.

67. Gjelsvik A: Bone remodeling and piezoelectricity—II, *J Biomech* 6:187, 1973.

68. Pollack SR, Salzstein R, Pienkowiski D: The electric double layer in bone and its influence on stress-generated potential, *Calcif Tissue Int* 36:77, 1984.

69. Wolff J: Ueber Die, Bebeutung der Architektur der Spongiosen Substanz, *Zentralbl Bl Med Wiss* 6:223, 1869.

70. Fyhrie DP, Carter DR: A unifying principle relating stress to trabecular bone morphology, *J Orthop Res* 4:304, 1986.

71. Hayes WC, Snyder B: Toward a quantitative formulation of Wolff's law in trabecular bone. In Cowin SC editor: *Mechanical properties of bone,* New York, 1981, American Society of Mechanical Engineers, p 43.

72. Stone JL, Beaupre GS, Hayes WC: Multiple strength characteristics of trabecular bone, *J Biomech* 16:743, 1983.

73. Cowin SC, Hegedus DH: Bone remodeling. I: theory of adaptive elasticity, *J Elasticity* 6:313, 1976.

74. Hegedus DH, Cowin SC: Bone remodeling. II: small strain adaptive elasticity, *J Elasticity* 6:337, 1976.

75. Firoozbakhsh K, Cowin SC: Devolution of inhomogeneities in bone structure—predictions of adaptive elasticity theory, *J Biomech Eng,* 102:287, 1980.

76. Cowin SC, Firoozbakhsh K: Bone remodeling of diaphyseal surfaces under constant load: theoretical predictions, *J Biomech* 14:471, 1981.

77. Cowin SC et al: Functional adaptation in long bones: establishing in vivo values for surface remodeling rate coefficients, *J Biomech* 18:665, 1985.

78. Huiskes R et al: Adaptive bone remodeling theory applied to prosthetic-design analysis, *J Biomech* 20:1135, 1987.

79. Huiskes R, Blankevoort L: Computational methods in orthopaedics. In Spilker RL, Simon BR, editors: *Computational methods in bioengineering,* New York, 1988, American Society of Mechanical Engineers, p 15.

80. Brunski JB et al: The influence of functional use of endosseous dental implants on the tissue-implant interface. I: histological aspects, *J Dent Res* 58:1953–1969, 1979.

81. Branemark P-I, Zarb G, Albrektsson T, editors: *Tissue integrated prostheses,* Chicago, 1985, Quintessence.

82. Albrektsson T et al: The long-term efficacy of currently used dental implants: a review and proposed criteria of success, *Int J Oral Maxillofac Implants* 1:11, 1986.
83. Eriksson RA, Albrektsson T: Temperature threshold levels for heat-induced bone tissue injury, *J Prosthet Dent* 50:101–107, 1983.
84. Lemons JE: Corrosion and biodegradation. In Von Recum A, editor: *Biomaterials: characterization handbook for foro biomaterials evaluation,* 1986, Collamore Press, pp 109–114.
85. Lemons JE: Dental implant tissue interfaces. In Lewis JL, Galante JO, editors: *The Bone-implant interface.*

Chapter 16

Applied Anatomy and Physiology for Dental Implants

APPLIED ANATOMY

Mohamed Sharawy
Carl E. Misch

MUSCLE ATTACHMENT TO MANDIBLE AND MAXILLA [1–7]

Mandible

As the mandibular alveolar bone resorbs, the residual ridge migrates toward many of the muscles that originate or insert on the mandible. The origin, insertion, innervation, and function of the muscles of surgical importance to the implant dentist are discussed (Fig 16–1).

Lingual or Medial Attachments

Mylohyoid Muscle—The mylohyoid muscle is the main muscle of the floor of the mouth. It takes origin from the whole lengths of the mylohyoid lines on the medial aspect of the mandible bilaterally (Fig 16–2). The most posterior fibers of the mylohyoid insert into the body of the hyoid bone, while the other fibers meet in the midline to form a median raphe, which extends from the mandible to the hyoid bone. The structures above the mylohyoid muscle are sublingual or intraoral in location, while the structures below the mylohyoid muscles are extraoral or subcutaneous. With a severely resorbed residual ridge, the origin of the mylohyoid muscle approximates the crest of the ridge. In these cases, surgical manipulation at the crest of the ridge may injure the mylohyoid muscle. A mandibular periosteal reflection for subperiosteal implant often reflects this

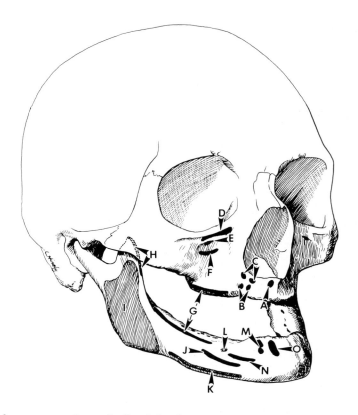

FIG 16–1.
A, origin of depressor septi muscle; *B,* origin of superior incisivus muscle; *C,* origin of nasalis muscle; *D,* origin of levator labii superioris muscle; *E,* infraorbital foramen; *F,* origin of levator anguli oris (canius) muscle; *G,* origin of buccinator muscle; *H,* insertion of lateral tendon of temporalis muscle; *I,* insertion of masseter muscle; *J,* origin of depressor anguli oris (triangularis) muscle; *K,* insertion of platysma muscle; *L,* mental foramen; *M,*origin of inferior incisivus muscle; *N,* origin of depressor labii inferioris muscle; *O,* origin of mentalis muscle.

muscle to the second molar region. The substructure of the implant then has a permucosal site in the first molar area and a lingual primary strut above and below the mylohyoid muscle. Surgical manipulation of the tissue of the floor of the mouth may lead to edematous swelling of the sublingual space (above the mylohyoid muscle) and/or the submandibular space (below the mylohyoid muscle). Ecchymosis resulting from blood accumulation may occur subcutaneously and/or submucosally. In some cases, infection may start and spread lingually and lead to an abscess or cellulitis either sublingually (intraoral) or submandibularly (extraoral), depending on the site of origin of the infection in relation to the origin of the mylohyoid muscle. Extensive bilateral cellulitis of the sublingual spaces may push the tongue backward or compress the pharynx, which may result in airway obstruction and necessitate a tracheotomy or cricothyroidotomy to maintain the airway. Functionally, the mylohyoid muscle raises the hyoid bone and floor of the mouth, or it can depress the mandible if the hyoid bone is fixed. The muscle is innervated by the mylohyoid nerve, which is a motor branch of the inferior alveolar nerve.

Genioglossus—The genioglossus muscle forms the bulk of the tongue. It takes origin from the superior genial tubercle. The anterior fibers insert into the dorsal surface of the tongue from the root to its tip, while the posterior fibers insert into the body of the hyoid bone. The genioglossus muscle is the main protruder of the tongue. The genial tubercles, particularly the superior pair, may be located near the crest of the alveolar ridge in the atrophic mandible. During the elevation of the lingual mucosa prior to making an impression for a subperiosteal implant, one should be aware of the origin of this structure to prevent its injury during the procedure. A portion of this muscle may be reflected from the genial tubercle. However, the muscle should not be completely detached from the tubercle, because this may result in retrusion of the tongue and possible airway obstruction. The genioglossus is supplied by the hypoglossal nerve (cranial nerve XII).

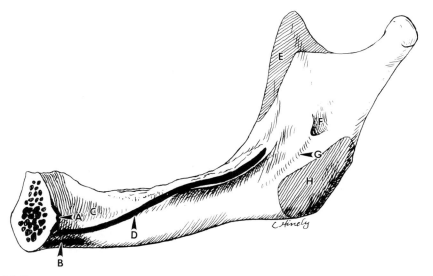

FIG 16–2.
A, genial tubercles, site of origin of genioglossus (superior tubercle) and geniohyoid (inferior tubercle) muscles; *B,* digastric fossa, site of origin of anterior belly of digastric muscle; *C,* sublingual fossa, location of sublingual gland; *D,* mylohyoid line, site of origin of mylohyoid muscle; *E,* insertion of medial tendon of temporalis muscle; *F,* mandibular foramen; *G,* mylohyoid groove, formed by mylohyoid nerve; *H,* site of insertion of medial pterygoid muscle.

Medial Pterygoid—The majority of the fibers of the medial pterygoid muscle take origin from the medial surface of the lateral pterygoid plate of the sphenoid bone. A small slip of muscle originates from the tuberosity of the maxilla. The muscle inserts on the medial surface of the angle of the mandible. The medial pterygoid muscle bounds the pterygomandibular space medially. This space is entered when an inferior dental nerve block is administered. Furthermore, during surgical procedures medial to the medial tendon of the temporalis muscle, such as in preparation for the insertion of unilateral subperiosteal implant, the pterygomandibular space is usually involved. Infection of this space is dangerous because of its proximity to the parapharyngeal space and the potential for spread of the infection to the mediastinum. Surgical exposure of tissue posterior to the maxillary tuberosity may also involve the medial pterygoid muscle, because a portion of the muscle takes origin from the maxillary tuberosity. However, the number of fibers originating from the tuberosity are few in comparison to the fibers from the medial surface of the lateral pterygoid plate. The muscle is innervated by a branch of the mandibular division (V3) of the trigeminal nerve.

Lateral Pterygoid—Although the lateral pterygoid muscles rarely are involved in surgery for implants, their possible action in mandibular flexure or adduction during opening, and the effect of this phenomenon on subperiosteal implants or prosthetic full arch splitting of mandibular implants in the molar region warrant its consideration. The lateral pterygoid muscle consists of superior and inferior heads. The superior head takes origin from the infratemporal surface and crest of the greater wing of the sphenoid bone (roof of the infratemporal fossa), while the inferior head takes origin from the lateral surface of the lateral plate of the pterygoid process of the sphenoid bone. The fibers of the superior head run downward to insert on the anterior band of the temporomandibular joint disc (~15% of its fibers) and the pterygoid fovea on the neck of the mandible. The fibers of the inferior head run upward to insert on the pterygoid fovea and also on the medial pole of the condyle, median capsule and median collateral ligament of the TMJ disc. Because of the angulation of the lateral pterygoid muscles, many authors believe that the mandibular flexure causing alteration in the mandibular arch width, and sometimes pain in patients with a full arch subperiosteal implant or prosthetic splint may be caused by contraction of the lateral pterygoid muscles. The muscles normally function in protraction of the mandible. It is innervated by a branch of the mandibular nerve (V3).

Temporalis—The temporalis is a fan-shaped muscle of mastication. It takes origin from the temporal fossa and inserts into the coronoid process of the mandible and the anterior border of the ramus as far inferiorly as the last molar at the site of the retromolar fossa. The muscle has two tendons, which insert into the mandible. The superficial tendon is located laterally, while the deep tendon is inserted medially. The temporalis tendons and their associated fascia project anteromedially and inferiorly and serve as a common point for attachment for the temporalis, masseter, and medial pterygoid muscles as well as for the buccinator and superior pharyngeal constrictor muscles. The long buccal nerve and vessels are also located in this area. This temporalis tendon-fascial complex extends into what is traditionally called the retromolar triangle. Surgical exposure of the mandibular ramus medially would involve this tendon-fascial complex with its contents of muscle fibers, nerves, and vessels. Incisions placed on the anterior ascending ramus for subperiosteal or blade implants should be inferior to the insertion of the two tendons of the temporalis muscle. The temporalis muscle, like all the major muscles of mastication, is innervated by a branch of V3.

Buccal or Facial Attachments

Mentalis Muscle—The external surface of the mandible in the midline presents a ridge indicative of the location of the symphysis menti. The ridge leads inferiorly to a triangular elevation known as the mental protuberance. The base of the triangle is raised on either side into the mental tubercles. The mentalis muscles take origin from the periosteum of the mental tubercles. Above the mentalis origin, the incisivus muscles take origin from small fossae called the incisivus fossae. Complete reflection of the mentalis muscles for the purpose of extension of a subperiosteal implant or symphyseal intraoral graft may result in "witch's chin," probably caused by the failure of muscle reattachment. Therefore the inferior portion of the mental protuberance should not be interfered with. The mentalis muscle receives its nerve supply from the marginal (mandibular) branch of the facial nerve.

Buccinator—The fibers of the buccinator muscle (cheek muscle) take origin from the lateral surfaces of the alveolar processes of the maxilla and the mandible in the area of the molars, the maxillary tuberosity, the pterygoid hamulus, pterygomandibular raphe, and the retromolar fossa of the mandible. The insertion of the muscle is complex. The upper and lower fibers of the buccinator blend with the fibers of the orbicularis oris at the upper and lower lips. The central fibers decussate at the modiolus before they insert into the orbicularis oris. The modiolus is the site of crossing and intermingling of fibers from the buccinator muscle with fibers from the elevator and depressor muscles of the angle of the mouth. The modiolus forms a palpable node inside the angle of the mouth opposite to the upper first premolar tooth. The buccinator muscle is pierced by the parotid duct opposite the maxillary second molar.

Some patients wearing lower subperiosteal implants complain of episodic swelling and pain at the site of origin of the buccinator muscle, particularly following periods of heavy mastication or bruxism. Incision of these swellings do not usually yield exudate or purulance. The condition responds well to heat application, anti-inflammatory drugs, and rest. Although the cause for this condition is not known, one may speculate that myositis of a detached buccinator muscle may cause it. The process of muscle reattachment to the implant surface or to a new site should be investigated. The muscle is innervated by the buccal branch of the facial nerve.

Masseter—This strong muscle of mastication covers the lateral surface of the ramus and angle of the mandible. The masseter has a dual origin from superficial and deep heads. The superficial head takes origin from the anterior two thirds of the lower border of the zygomatic arch. The deep head originates from the posterior one third of the zygomatic arch and the entire deep surface of the arch. The muscle inserts into the outer surface of the ramus of the mandible from the sigmoid notch to the angle. However, the muscle can be easily deflected during surgery to expose the bone for the ramus extension needed for lateral support of a subperiosteal implant. The space between the masseteric fascia and the muscle is a potential surgical space, known as the masseteric space, into which an infection may spread, causing myositis and trismus. The masseter is one of the main elevators of the jaw. The innervation of the muscle is provided by the masseteric nerve, which is a branch of the mandibular division (V3) of the trigeminal nerve.

Maxilla

As the maxillary alveolar bone resorbs, the crest of the residual ridge migrates toward the muscles that take their origin from the basal bone of the maxilla. Muscles of surgical importance to oral implantologists are as follows.

Buccinator

The buccinator muscle originates from the base of the alveolar process opposite the first, second, and third molar of both jaws. This muscle also takes origin from the pterygoid hamulus of the medial pterygoid plate of the sphenoid bone and therefore bridges the gap between the maxillary tuberosity anteriorly and the hamulus posteriorly. The extension of a subperiosteal frame design into the pterygoid plates will run the risk of interfering with the fibers of these muscles without adding too much to the retention of the implant. When incising and reflecting the mucosa overlying the areas of the maxillary tuberosity and hamular notch prior to taking impressions for maxillary subperiosteal implants, one must avoid injury to the tendon of the tensor velli palatini muscle, which passes around the pterygoid hamulus. The tendon moves every time the soft palate moves and therefore may become irritated by the subperiosteal frame and result in inflammation and pain. Fibers of the buccinator and medial pterygoid muscles are also found in the area of reflection. The majority of the fibers of the medial pterygoid muscle originate from the medial surface of the lateral pterygoid plate of the sphenoid bone, which is in close proximity to the maxillary tuberosity. Near the pterygoid hamulus a fibrous tissue raphe is found between the buccinator and the superior pharyngeal constrictor muscles. Injury to the latter muscle should be avoided during reflection of the mucosa, particularly on the palatal aspect of the area of the hamulus.

Levator Labii Superioris

The levator superioris muscle takes origin from the infraorbital margin above the infraorbital foramen and therefore is rarely of concern to the implant surgeon. It is innervated by the zygomatic branch of the facial nerve.

Levator Anguli Oris (Caninus)

The levator anguli oris muscle originates in the maxilla below the infraorbital foramen. The infraorbital nerve and vessels arise between this muscle and the levator labii superioris. In subperiosteal implant cases that require extensive framework extension for retention, the operator should be aware of the location of the infraorbital neurovascular bundle in relation to the caninus and levator labii superioris muscles. The caninus muscle is innervated by the zygomatic branch of the facial nerve.

INNERVATION OF JAWS[1]

Sensory innervation to the mandible is supplied by the mandibular division of the trigeminal nerve (V3), while the maxilla is supplied by the maxillary division of the trigeminal nerve (V2). The skin overlying the angle of the mandible is usually innervated by the greater auricular nerve, which is a branch of the anterior primary rami of cervical nerves two and three (C2, C3). This nerve can give rise to branches that enter the mandible and provide accessory innervation to the region of the third molars. The muscles of mastication receive their innervation by way of the motor branch of the mandibular nerve (V3). All of the muscles of facial expression, including those that attach to the jaws, receive their innervation by way of the various branches of the facial nerve (cranial nerve VII). The sensory nerves of the upper and lower jaws remain after the teeth are extracted. They are reviewed here because they may be involved during various implant surgical procedures.

Innervation of Lower Jaw and Associated Structures

Inferior Alveolar (Dental) Nerve—This nerve arises as a branch of the mandibular nerve (V3) in the infratemporal fossa. It appears at the inferior border of the inferior head of the lateral pterygoid muscle, courses downward, and enters the mandibular foramen on the medial aspect of the ramus. Before the nerve enters the mandibular foramen it gives numerous sensory branches that innervate the mandibular bone. These small nerves are in association with small vessels in neurovascular channels. The inferior dental nerve can run as one unit through the mandibular canal until it reaches the premolar region, where it divides into the mental and the incisive nerves. The mental nerve exits the canal through the mental foramen. In an excessively resorbed ridge the mental foramen, with its contents of mental nerve and vessels, can be found on the crest of the ridge. An incision or reflection of the mucosa in this area must avoid injury to these vital structures. A knowledge of the position of the inferior dental canal in vertical as well as in buccolingual dimensions is of paramount importance during site preparation for implants. The potential use of reconstruction techniques on computed tomographic scans and magnetic resonance imaging may increase our ability to locate the inferior dental canal precisely within the jaw bone. In some cases the inferior dental nerve may divide into two or three rami that occupy separate canals as the nerve travels in the mandible to supply the bone. These variations can be determined by conventional x-ray techniques, and the operator should modify the surgical approach and type of implant in order to avoid injury to the portion of the nerve that exits the foramen. Injury to the portion of the inferior alveolar nerve that remains in the atrophied bone and does not innervate soft tissues is of far less consequences. The fibrous tissue around these nerves, however, may cause an increase in the amount of fibrous tissue around an implant that is inserted in contact with these structures.

Lingual Nerve—The lingual nerve is a branch of the mandibular nerve that is given off in the infratemporal fossa. It appears at the inferior border of the inferior head of the lateral pterygoid muscle anterior to the inferior alveolar nerve. It passes downward and forward between the ramus of the mandible and the medial pterygoid muscle. The nerve enters the oral cavity above the posterior edge of the mylohyoid muscle close to its origin at the third molar region. Because the nerve lies just medial to the retromolar pad, incision in this region should remain lateral to the pad, and the mucosal reflection should be done with the periosteal elevator in constant contact with bone to avoid injury to the nerve. The nerve proceeds on the surface of the hyoglossus muscle and then crosses the duct of the submandibular gland medially to enter the floor of the mouth and the tongue. While in the infratemporal fossa the nerve is joined by the chorda tympani nerve, which is a branch of cranial nerve VII. The chorda tympani nerve carries taste fibers from the anterior two thirds of the tongue and parasympathetic preganglionic fibers to the submandibular autonomic ganglion. The ganglion is connected to the lingual nerve on the surface of the hyoglossus muscle. The postganglionic neurons from the submandibular ganglion supply the submandibular and sublingual salivary glands. The branches of the lingual nerve in the oral cavity carry sensory information from the lingual mucosa, the mucosa of the floor of the mouth, and the anterior two thirds of the tongue. Improper reflection of a lingual mucoperiosteal flap may injure the lingual nerve and produce paresthesia or anesthesia of the area. The extent of involvement depends on the degree of injury to the nerve.

Nerve to Mylohyoid—The mylohyoid motor branch of the inferior dental nerve is given off just before the nerve enters the mandibular foramen. This branch descends in a groove on the medial surface of the mandibular ramus and then appears in the submandibular triangle at the posterior border of the mylohyoid muscle. The nerve supplies the mylohyoid muscle and then proceeds on its surface with the submental artery (branch of the facial artery) until it reaches the anterior belly of the digastric muscle, which it also supplies. Because the nerve is so closely related to the ramus of the mandible, surgical intervention in this area may lead to injury of this important motor nerve.

Long Buccal Nerve—This nerve is a sensory branch of the mandibular division of the trigeminal nerve. It is distributed to the skin and mucous membrane of the cheek as well as the buccal gingiva opposite the mandibular molar region. The nerve courses between the two heads of the lateral pterygoid muscle, then proceeds medial to, or sometimes within the medial temporalis tendon, to gain access to the surface of the buccinator muscle. Surgical manipulation in this area, for example, during insertion of a subperiosteal implant, may injure this nerve.

Innervation of Upper Jaw and Associated Structures

The sensory innervation to the upper jaw and associated structures is from the maxillary division (V2) of the trigeminal nerve (cranial nerve V).

Posterior Superior Alveolar (Dental) Nerve—The nerve arises within the pterygopalatine fossa, courses downward and forward passing through the pterygomaxillary fissure, and enters the posterior aspect of the maxilla. It runs between the bone and the lining of the maxillary sinus. This nerve supplies the sinus, the molars, the buccal gingiva, and the adjoining portion of the cheek. This nerve may be injured during a sinus augmentation with a lateral approach. Clinically, this does not appear to be of major consequences.

Infraorbital Nerve—This nerve is a continuation of the main trunk of the maxillary division. It leaves the pterygopalatine fossa by passing through the inferior orbital fissure to enter the floor of the orbit. It runs in the infraorbital groove and then in the infraorbital canal. The nerve exits the orbit through the infraorbital foramen to give cutaneous branches to the lower eyelid, the ala of the nose and the skin, and the mucous membrane of the lip and cheek. The infraorbital foramen is located between the levator labii superioris muscle, which takes origin above the foramen, and the levator anguli oris or caninus muscle, which takes origin below the foramen. Subperiosteal implants designed for an atrophied maxilla should not extend into the site of the infraorbital nerve and vessels. In some cases of maxillary sinus disorder, the site of the infraorbital foramen becomes tender, probably as a result of inflammation of the infraorbital nerve. This is an important diagnostic test for possible postoperative involvement following sinus augmentation procedures.

Middle Superior Alveolar (Dental) Nerve—This branch of the infraorbital nerve is given off as the infraorbital nerve passes through the infraorbital groove. The middle superior alveolar nerve runs downward and forward in the lateral wall of the sinus to supply the maxillary premolars.

Anterior Superior Alveolar (Dental) Nerve—This branch of the infraorbital nerve arises within the infraorbital canal. It initially runs laterally within the sinus wall then curves medially to pass beneath the infraorbital foramen. It turns downward to supply the maxillary anterior teeth. A nasal branch passes into the nasal cavity to supply the mucosal lining of a portion of the nasal cavity. Implant dentists must anesthetize this branch prior to placement of implants in the incisor region.

The anterior, middle, and posterior superior alveolar nerves intermingle to form the superior dental plexus. The posterior, middle, and anterior superior alveolar nerves run in the facial wall of the maxillary sinus between its lining membrane and the bone. During antrostomy procedures to augment the floor of the sinus, the operator should be aware of these structures, which are present even in the absence of teeth.

Palatine Nerve—The greater (anterior) and lesser (posterior) palatine nerves supply the hard and soft palate, respectively. They exit the pterygopalatine fossa through the superior opening of the descending palatine canal, travel downward, and enter the oral cavity by way of the greater and lesser palatine foramina. The greater palatine nerve runs forward in a groove on the inferior surface of the hard palate to supply the palatal mucosa as far forward as the incisor teeth. Here, the nerve communicates with the nasopalatine nerve. The nerve supplies the gingiva, mucous membrane, and glands of the hard palate.

The greater palatine artery and vein accompany the nerve during its course in the hard palate. As the maxillary alveolar process atrophies, it brings the crest of the ridge closer to the groove where the greater palatine neurovascular bundle is found. The implant dentist should be aware that an incision too palatal to the crest of the ridge may injure these vital structures.

Nasopalatine (Sphenopalatine) Nerve—This nerve leaves the pterygopalatine fossa through the sphenopalatine foramen located in the medial wall of the fossa. It enters the nasal cavity and supplies portions of the lateral and superior aspects of the nasal cavity. The longest branch reaches the nasal septum, where it turns downward and forward, traveling on the surface of the septum. While on the septum it forms a groove on the vomer bone. It supplies the nasal mucosa and descends to the floor of the nose near the septum, passes through the nasopalatine canal, and then exits onto the hard palate through the incisive foramen. The latter opening is deep to the incisive papilla. The nerve communicates with the greater palatine nerve. The incisive nerve should be anesthetized prior to elevation of the mucosa of the floor of the nose in the incisor region.

BLOOD SUPPLY TO MAXILLA AND MANDIBLE

The head and neck region has an abundant blood supply with many anastomoses. The upper and lower jaws are no exception. The blood supply to both the mandible and maxilla is derived from a common source, the external carotid artery. The external carotid artery is a branch of the common carotid artery, which is a direct branch off the arch of the aorta on the left side and a branch of the brachiocephalic artery on the right side of the body.

The main artery supplying the mandible is the inferior alveolar (dental) artery, which serves as the nutrient artery to the bone and other tissues within the lower jaw. The bone tissue of the maxillae is supplied by branches of two major vessels, the posterior superior alveolar (dental) artery, and the infraorbital artery. The major branch of the infraorbital artery that supplies the maxilla is the anterior superior alveolar (dental) artery. The posterior superior alveolar and infraorbital arteries are branches of the maxillary artery, which is one of the two terminal branches of the external carotid artery.

General Concepts

The circulation of blood within long bones is centrifugal; that is, the blood circulates from the marrow (medullary) region outward through the cortical bone to end in vessels located in the periosteum and soft tissues associated with the bone.[8, 9] The blood supply to the medullary region is by way of nutrient arteries, which are relatively large vessels that pass through the bone by way of nutrient canals to enter the marrow spaces. Within the marrow spaces the nutrient artery forms a network of vessels called the endosteal or medullary plexus. Vessels from this plexus enter the cortical bone through Volkmann's canals and eventually reach the surface of the bone. While blood is passing through the cortical bone, numerous vessels are given off at right angles to these intraosseous vessels within the Volkmann's canals. These branches are the vessels that are found within the haversian canals of the osteons.[8, 9] Osteonal bone is the major type of bone found in the cortical bone of the jaws. Once the intraosseous vessels reach the outer surface of the bone they anastomose with vessels within the fibrous layer of the periosteum or with arteries supplying the soft tissues. The network of vessels associated with the periosteum is called the periosteal plexus. The periosteal plexus in turn communicates with vessels that are supplying arterial blood to muscles and other soft tissues in the area.

The mandible and maxilla are membrane bones and as such do not develop in the same manner as long bones. It is generally agreed, however, that the circulation of blood within the body of the mandible[10] and in the maxilla[11, 12] is centrifugal under normal conditions. As in the long bones, there are endosteal and periosteal plexuses that are connected with one another.[12, 13] In addition to these vascular networks, a periodontal plexus is found associated with the teeth.[12, 13] When teeth are present, intraosseous vessels send branches into the alveolar processes (intra-alveolar arteries), to the teeth (apical arteries), and to branches of the periodontal plexus. The intra-alveolar arteries and periodontal plexus in turn connect with vessels of the periosteal plexus as well as with vessels within the soft tissues surrounding the bone. Once a tooth is removed, its periodontal plexus is lost. When abnormal circulatory conditions exist within the mandible or maxilla, such as occlusion of the nutrient artery, the blood supply to the bone is reversed so that the direction of flow is from the outside to the inside of the bone.[10, 11, 14] This is called centripetal circulation.

Maxilla

The vessels that supply the maxilla are branches of the third part of the maxillary artery. The posterior superior alveolar artery leaves the maxillary artery and travels on the infratemporal portion of the maxilla where it divides into several branches. Some of the branches enter alveolar canals within the posterior aspect of the maxilla to become intraosseous arteries, which supply the molar and premolar teeth as well as the lining of the maxillary sinus. Other branches of the posterior superior alveolar artery travel on the surface of the maxilla to supply the gingiva of the posterior maxillary teeth. Injury to this artery within the bone during lateral approach sinus-elevation procedures may cause hemorrhage, which requires coagulation or the use of bone wax to control the bone bleeding.

The infraorbital artery leaves the maxillary artery and enters the orbital cavity by way of the inferior orbital fissure. The artery runs in the infraorbital groove and later in the infraorbital canal. Both of these structures are located in the floor of the orbit. The infraorbital canal opens on the face as the infraorbital foramen. Within the canal the artery gives off the anterior superior alveolar artery, which descends through anterior alveolar canals to supply the maxillary anterior teeth as well as the mucous membrane of the maxillary sinus. The anterior and posterior superior alveolar arteries join together to form an arterial loop. The middle superior alveolar artery is rarely a separate branch.[15] The infraorbital artery also supplies branches to the maxillary sinus.[16]

Gingival, buccal, labial, palatal, nasal, and maxillary sinus blood vessels anastomose with the arterial networks associated with the maxilla. These vessels not only join with the periosteal plexus but also penetrate the bone to connect with vessels of the endosteal and periodontal plexuses. In addition, abundant midline crossover is possible in the soft tissues of the palate and face.[13]

The mucoperiosteum of the anterior maxilla is supplied by branches of the infraorbital as well as branches of the superior labial artery, which is a major branch of the facial artery.[13] The buccal mucoperiosteum of the maxilla is supplied by vessels of the posterior superior alveolar, anterior superior alveolar, and buccal arteries. The mucoperiosteum of the hard palate is supplied by branches from the greater (anterior) palatine and the nasopalatine arteries. The soft palate is supplied by the lesser (posterior) palatine artery. Communications of the lesser palatine arteries with the ascending pharyngeal branch of the external carotid artery and the ascending palatine branch of the facial artery are critical in many of the surgical orthognathic procedures that are performed on the maxilla.[12] In these surgical procedures, the major nutrient arteries to the maxilla are sometimes severed, but the blood supply is maintained by means of the anastomoses present in the soft palate. The vessels of the soft palate unite with vessels of the hard palate, which in turn communicate with the periosteal, periodontal, and endosteal plexuses of the upper jaw. Thus, the vitality of the tissues of the maxilla is maintained through an arterial supply derived entirely from vessels that normally supply the soft palate.

Mandible

The major artery supplying the blood of the mandible is the inferior alveolar artery. The artery enters the medial aspect of the ramus of the mandible, and courses downward and forward within the mandibular canal to enter the body of the mandible. The artery branches in the premolar region to give rise to two terminal branches: the mental and incisive arteries. The incisive artery continues medially within the body to anastomose with the artery of the opposite side. The mental artery exits the body of the mandible through the mental foramen and supplies the region of the chin and anastomoses with the submental and inferior labial arteries. Near its origin, the inferior alveolar artery gives off a lingual branch, which supplies blood to the oral mucosa.[16]

Studies in animals have demonstrated that the coronoid process, the condylar process, and the angle of the mandible are supplied by arteries which provide blood to the muscles that attach to these sites.[16] Studies of human cadaver material show that the condylar process is supplied by the vascular network of the temporomandibular joint capsule and the lateral pterygoid muscle. The coronoid process was shown to be supplied exclusively by vessels from the temporalis muscle, while the angle of the mandible is supplied by the inferior alveolar artery as well as the muscles attached to the area. In addition, the anterior portion of the ramus is thought to be supplied by vessels that supply the pterygomasseteric sling, namely, the medial pterygoid and masseter muscles.[18] Empirical findings from mandibular osteotomy procedures in humans support many of these findings.[17] Thus, the repositioning of the inferior alveolar artery laterally, a procedure that may be needed in some cases prior to implant insertion, should not eliminate the blood supply to the bone in this region (see the discussion that follows).

Changes in Blood Supply to Mandible With Age

Although the normal circulation within the body of the mandible is centrifugal in young individuals, the direction of blood flow may reverse with aging. It has been shown that the inferior alveolar artery is very susceptible to arteriosclerotic changes and tends to become tortuous and narrow with age.[19, 20] Blockage of the inferior alveolar artery occurs years prior to any clinical evidence of blockage in the carotid vessels. Angiographic studies of living human subjects of all ages demonstrated blockage of the inferior alveolar artery in 79% of all individuals studied, and in 33% of the patients arterial flow was absent.[20] The incidence of absence of flow in the inferior alveolar artery increased with age. The reduction or absence in flow within the inferior alveolar artery may be associated with tooth extraction.[20] Studies in completely edentulous humans indicate that the inferior alveolar artery degenerates to such an extent as to be negligible in the supply of blood to the mandible.[19] In these cases, the blood supply to the bone and internal structures was dependent on the connections with the external blood supply located within the periosteum and soft tissues associated with the mandible.[19, 20] Major arteries which probably supply blood to the mandible following the interruption of the inferior alveolar artery blood flow include the mental artery,[14] the mandibular branch of the sublingual artery,[14] the facial artery,[10] and muscular branches of the maxillary artery. These anastomoses are critical in surgical procedures in which mucoperiosteal flaps are created in the mandible. The changes in pattern of blood flow to the atrophic mandible are of special importance to implant dentistry. Mucoperiosteal flap reflection for subperiosteal implant usually exposes 75% of the body of the mandible and approximately 50% of the inferior third of the ramii. Dehesence of the mucosa at the incision lines has been reported. The reduction in atrophied bone blood supply may be a contributing factor. In addition, endosteal implants placed in an atrophied anterior mandible may have less blood supply to the interface, and may require longer time for load-bearing bone to develop. These speculations, of course, require experimental verification. Similar blood flow reversal with age has not been reported in the maxilla, but final comment concerning blood flow in the aged edentulous maxilla awaits further investigation.*

Acknowledgment

We thank Dr. Francis T. Lake for contributing to the section on blood supply of edentulous jaws, and Mr. Lewis Hinley for skillful medical illustration.

* For references 1 through 20, see pp. 351–352.

BONE PHYSIOLOGY AND METABOLISM

W. Eugene Roberts
Lawrence P. Garetto
Naphthali Brezniak

Rigid intraosseous implants are viable treatment options for a wide variety of clinical problems. There are few definitive data establishing many of the devices on the market and clinical applications currently in vogue. It is essential for a contemporary clinician to have a firm grasp of the modern concepts of bone physiology, metabolism, and biomechanics. This is often the only objective means for designing and implementing an innovative treatment plan.

METABOLISM

Bone mineral is the primary metabolic store of the essential element calcium.[21] In addition to its obvious structural role, bone has a more primitive and essential function — that of calcium metabolism (Fig 16–3).[22] Phylogenetically, the original purpose of internal stores of mineralized tissue was to serve as a physiologic reservoir of calcium. Calcium metabolism remains a critical life-sustaining function. Secondarily, mineralized tissues developed support capabilities.[23] The masticatory apparatus is one of the most highly refined mechanical structures in the body. However, the jaws are susceptible to metabolic attack,[24] particularly when mechanical protection is compromised by an atrophic, mutilated dentition.

Bone physiology is controlled by an interaction of mechanical and metabolic factors. Under most physiologic circumstances, bone formation is regulated primarily by functional loading (peak strains).[25] On the other hand, biochemical mediators of calcium metabolism (such as parathyroid hormone, estrogen, vitamin D) predominate in control of bone resorption.[26] Clinicians must appreciate the primary metabolic role of osseous tissue. Complex structural deficits, compromised healing responses, and suboptimal resistance to loading may be metabolically related.[27]

CALCIUM METABOLISM

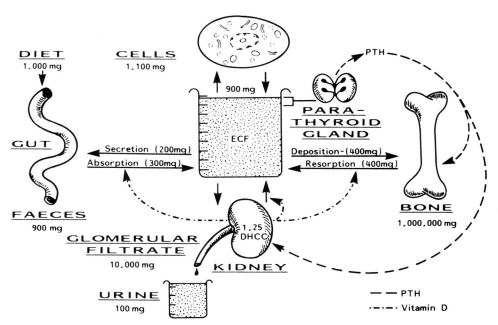

FIG 16–3.
Under conditions of zero calcium balance (stable bone volume), 300 mg of calcium is lost daily through gut secretion (200 mg) and kidney excretion (100 mg). To maintain bone volume, this loss must be offset by 300 mg of calcium absorption from the gut. The latter requires abundant calcium in the diet (at least 800 mg/day, preferably 1,000 mg/day in older adults) and adequate levels of the active metabolite of vitamin D (1,25-DHCC). ECF = extracellular fluid; PTH = parathyroid hormone. (From Roberts WE, et al: *J Am Dent Assoc* 122:55, 1991. Used by permission.)

STRUCTURE

Bone is a highly ordered composite of organic matrix and inorganic mineral. Osseous matrix, referred to as osteoid before mineralization, is primarily collagen fibers embedded in ground substance. The latter is a viscous gel of water and polysaccharide/protein complexes. Ground substance also contains numerous organic factors (cytokines, growth factors, and so forth) that help control cell activation, matrix maturation, and mineralization. During mineralization, small crystals of hydroxyapatite are densely packed in an ordered array according to collagen fiber orientation.[23] Depending on environmental conditions, bone forms as a remarkably ordered biomaterial at both the molecular and macroscopic levels.[28]

Bone structural deficits (mass, quality, and distribution) at the desired implantation site may result in serious limitations for many prospective patients. The principal factors determining the potential of bone to support an implant are: (1) the metabolic status of the host; (2) functional loading history of the implantation site; (3) surgical trauma during implant placement; (4) response to local cytokines and growth factors during the healing phase[29]; and (5) biomechanics during the functional phase.[25]

CLASSIFICATION

Bones are organs because they are functionally related groups of tissues. Each bone has a unique form and function. Specific combinations of mineralized tissue types, periosteum, cartilage, marrow, vascularity, nerves, tendons, and ligaments fulfill a particular role in mechanical support and metabolism. Macroscopically, osseous structure is classified according to density as compact or trabecular bone. However, bone density is actually a continuum including fine trabeculae, coarse trabeculae, porous compacta, and dense compacta (Fig 16–4). Precise classification can be difficult. For instance very coarse trabeculae may be similar to markedly porous compacta.[23]

The fundamental architecture of bone is a mechanically efficient distribution of compact and cancellous bone. Bone size and shape are dictated by an interaction of genetic and environmental factors. Contralateral bones or adjacent sections of the same bone vary considerably, depending on the functional loading history.[30]

Differential analysis of cortical bone is best assessed in sawed sections of fully mineralized bone. Brightfield microscopy is of limited value in critically assessing mineralized sections. However, with more modern methods of quantitative analysis, a bone section becomes a historical record of physiologic activity (Figure 16–5). Because of the birefringence of collagen, polarized light microscopy yields information on the fiber orientation of the mineralized matrix (Figure 16–6). Microradiography (high resolution x-ray with fine-grain film) of the same bone section provides a microscopic view of tissue mineralization patterns.

Osseous tissue is formed in a number of configurations. Depending on the organism's age, function, and physiologic history, bones are composed of four microscopic tissue types: woven, lamellar, bundle, and composite bone.

Woven bone is a highly cellular osseous tissue that is formed rapidly (30 to 50 μm/day or more) in response to growth or injury (Figure 16–7). Compared with mature bone, it has relatively low mineral content, a more random fiber orientation, and minimal strength. Woven bone serves an important stabilization

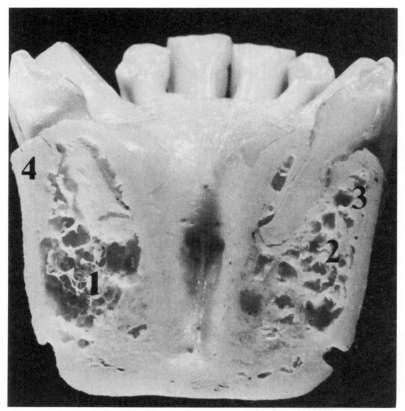

FIG 16–4.
Cross-section through a monkey mandible showing variable cortical and trabecular bone patterns: *(1)* fine trabeculae, *(2)* coarse trabeculae, *(3)* porous compacta, and *(4)* dense compacta. (From Roberts WE, et al: *Calif Dent Assoc J* 15:54, 1987. Used by permission.)

role in the initial healing of endosseous implants. Because woven bone is more pliable than mature lamellar bone, it is more forgiving of the relative micromotion associated with interface healing. Although it is capable of stabilizing an unloaded implant, woven bone lacks the strength to resist functional loads.

Lamellar bone is the principal load-bearing tissue of the adult skeleton. It is the predominant component of mature cortical and trabecular bone. In adults lamellae form relatively slowly (<1.0 μm/day), have a highly organized matrix, and are densely mineralized (Fig 16–8). Lamellar bone is histologically similar regardless of the age at which it forms.[31]

Bundle bone is characteristic of ligament and tendon attachments along bone-forming surfaces (Fig 16–9). Striations are oriented across the underlying lamellar pattern. These striations are extensions of Sharpey's fibers composed of collagen bundles from adjacent connective tissue that insert directly into bone. Bundle bone is well known in dentistry because it is formed adjacent to the periodontal ligament of physiologically drifting teeth (*P* in Fig 16–9). "Pseudo-periodontium" and "fibro-osseous integration" mechanisms have been proposed for some types of mobile "endosteal" implants.[32, 33] However, true bundle bone, the osseous hallmark of a ligamentous attachment, has never been demonstrated in a physiologically convincing manner.

Composite bone is lamellar bone deposited on a woven bone matrix. During rapid growth and wound healing, a highly porous, woven bone lattice grows out and captures blood vessels along an endosteal or periosteal surface. The woven lattice then fills the paravascular space with high-quality lamellae, resulting in reactive bone with adequate strength for load bearing (Fig 16–10, A and B). Depending on the rate at which the lattice forms, the finished product is a variation of fine cancellous compaction (primary osteons) or coarse cancellous compaction (whorling bone).[34] Lamellar compaction of composite bone is an

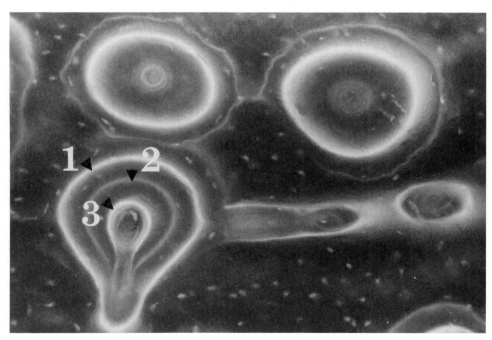

FIG 16–5.
Multiple fluorescent bone markers (1, 2, and 3) administered at 1-week intervals are a chronological record of cortical bone remodeling activity in a dog. (From Roberts WE, et al: *Calif Dent Assoc J* 15:54, 1987. Used by permission.)

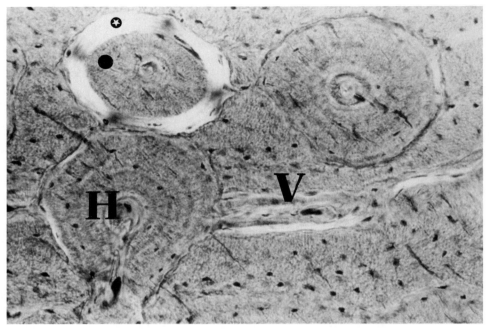

FIG 16–6.
Polarized-light illumination of the same 100-μm-thick mineralized section of bone in Figure 16–5 shows the variable orientation of collagen fibers;: circumferential fibers *(star)* within the recently remodeled cortical bone. Collagen orientation within bone matrix probably reflects the localized loading at the time the bone was formed. Haversian *(H)* and Volkmann's *(V)* canals are the vascular channels within cortical bone. (From Roberts WE, et al: *Calif Dent Assoc J* 15:54, 1987. Used by permission.)

important step in achieving stabilization of an implant during the rigid integration process.[35]

PHYSIOLOGIC ADAPTATION

To fulfill its dual functional role of support and metabolism, bone responds to a complex array of mechanical, bioelectrical, metabolic, and local mediators (cytokines and growth factors). Under steady-state conditions, osteoblast differentiation is mechanically mediated: that is, stress and/or strain dependent.[36] Surgical placement of a dental implant elicits an osteogenic response that is largely driven by local cytokines and growth factors. The initial healing response is apparently independent of direct mechanical control because bones heal optimally in the absence of functional loading. In fact, a relatively unloaded healing phase is preferable for osseous discontinuities such as fractures and dental implant interfaces. The vascularly dependent osteogenic process is easily disrupted by micromotion at a healing bone/implant interface.

Modeling is a surface-specific activity (apposition or resorption) that produces a net change in the size and/or shape of a bone (Fig 16–11). It is an uncoupled process, meaning that cell activation *(A)* proceeds independently to formation *(F)* or resorption *(R)*. The definition considers compacta and trabecular bone as blocks of tissue. It refers to a generalized change in overall dimensions of a bone's cortex or spongiosa. Modeling is a fundamental mechanism of growth, atrophy, and reorientation.

Remodeling is defined as turnover or internal restructuring of previously existing bone. It is a coupled tissue level phenomenon. Activation *(A)* of osseous

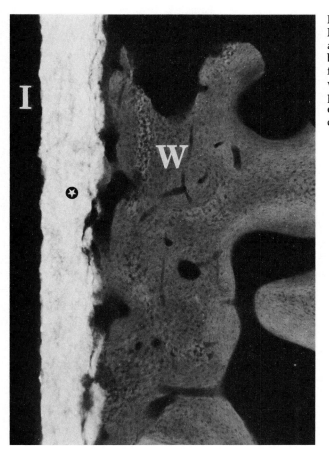

FIG 16–7.
Microradiograph of a mineralized section through woven bone *(W)* at the osseous interface of an implant *(I)* coated with high-density tricalcium phosphate. This is the peripheral portion of the periosteal callus in a rabbit.

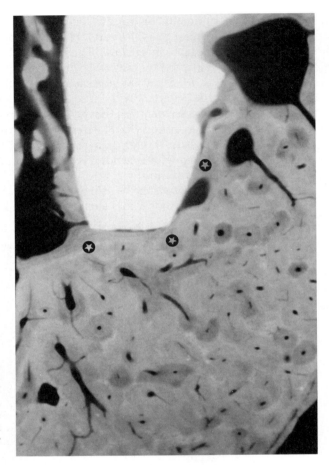

FIG 16–8.
Microradiographic image of a 100-μm-thick section shows that relatively mature lamellar bone *(stars)* is supporting a titanium implant in the mandible of a dog. (Adapted from Roberts WE, et al: *Angle Orthod* 59:247, 1989.)

precursor cells results in a sequence of active resorption *(R)*, quiescence or reversal *(Q)*, and formation *(F)*. The duration of the $A \rightarrow R(Q) \rightarrow F$ remodeling cycle (referred to as "sigma") is about 6 weeks in rabbits, 12 weeks in dogs, and 17 weeks in humans (Table 16–1). Remodeling includes all localized changes in individual osteons or trabeculae: turnover, hypertrophy, atrophy, or reorientation.

MICROSCOPIC EVALUATION

There is a direct relationship between the age of bone and its mineral density. Following a maturation phase of about 1 week, newly formed osteoid is mineralized by a large number of relatively small hydroxyapatite crystals. During this period of primary mineralization, osteoblasts deposit about 70% of the mineral found in mature vital bone. Secondary mineralization (the remaining 30%) is a noncellular crystal growth phenomenon that occurs over a period of months (Fig 16–12). The changes in mineralization can be followed by using high-resolution microradiography which is an overall physiological index of modeling and remodeling activity.

Precise quantitation of bone formation and turnover requires in vivo administration of multiple color, fluorescent markers (see Fig 16–5). Any bone mineralizing during the time that these calcium-binding agents are available will be permanently labeled. Utilizing the stereological principles of histomorphometry, the incidence of each label and the distance between labels reveals the three-dimensional time course of bone formation and turnover. This is a powerful tool for assessing interface development and bone adaptation to dental implants.

There is an important note of caution associated with assessing implant interfaces in mineralized sections. Neither brightfield nor polarized-light microscopy specifically resolves mineralized tissue. Brightfield is an index of tissue

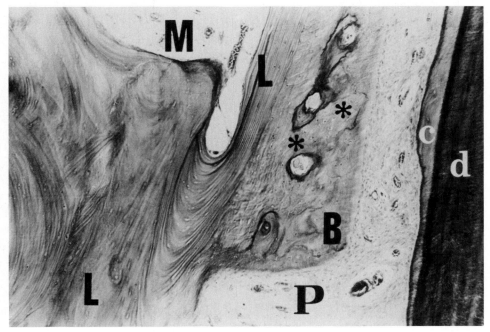

FIG 16–9.
Demineralized section of adult human periodontium shows cementum *(c)*, dentin *(d)*, periodontal ligament *(P)*, and marrow space *(M)*. Three types of osseous tissue are present: woven *(star)*; lamellar *(L)*; and bundle *(B)* bone. (From Roberts WE, et al: *Calif Dent Assoc J* 15:54, 1987. Used by permission.)

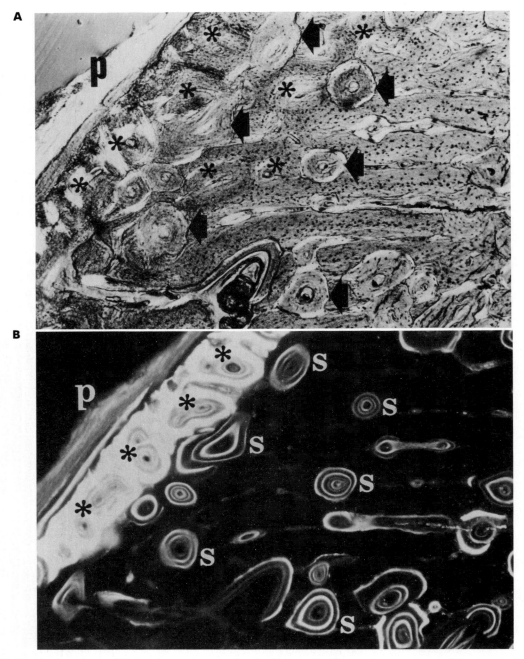

FIG 16–10. A, polarized light photomicrograph of rabbit cortical bone shows primary *(stars)* and secondary osteons near the periosteal surface *(p)*. A secondary osteon is distinguished by a scalloped, resorption arrest line *(arrows)* at its peripheral margin. **B,** viewing the same mineralized section with ultraviolet light reveals a series of intravital, multiple fluorochrome labels. The labels, administered at 1-week intervals, demonstrate growth (modeling) at the periosteal surface *(p)*. Primary osteons *(stars)* form irregular, whorling bone by the process of coarse cancellous compaction. Numerous secondary osteons *(s)* begin to remodel the primary compacta about 12 weeks after it is formed. (From Roberts WE, et al: *Calif Dent Assoc J* 15:54, 1987. Used by permission.)

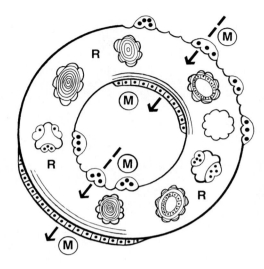

FIG 16–11.
This schematic drawing of a diaphyseal (midshaft) cross-section reveals differential sites of bone modeling *(M)* and remodeling *(R)*. Remodeling is turnover of previously existing bone. Modeling (change in shape or form) can be anabolic (formation) or catabolic (resorption). Bone modeling is the mechanism of differential growth and structural adaptation. (From Roberts WE, Garetto LP, DeCastro RA: *J Indiana Dent Assoc* 68:19, 1989. Used by permission.)

refraction. Both mineralized and nonmineralized tissues refract light. Tissue stains are helpful but still lack adequate specificity. With polarized light, parallel collagen fibers of fibrous connective tissue are similar in appearance to lamellar bone. Using either brightfield or polarized-light microscopy, it is not possible to rigorously determine if mineralized tissue (bone) is in contact with an implant (Fig 16–13).[37] High-resolution microradiography is the only proven method for assessing proximity of bone to the implant in histologic sections (Fig 16–14, A and B).

CORTICAL BONE

Cortical bone (compacta) is dense skeletal tissue that is composed of lamellar and composite bone. Similar to the midshaft of long bones, the mandible is

TABLE 16–1.

Cortical Bone Remodeling Cycle (in weeks)

	Rabbit	Dog	Humans
Activation (A)	< 0.5	0.5	< 1.0
Resorption (R)	1.0	1.5	2.0
Quiescent reversal (Q)	0.5	1.0	1.5
Formation (F)	4.5	10.0	13.0
$A \rightarrow R(Q) \rightarrow F$	6.0	12.0	17.0
Factor	×*	2×	3×

*Rabbit used as base value.

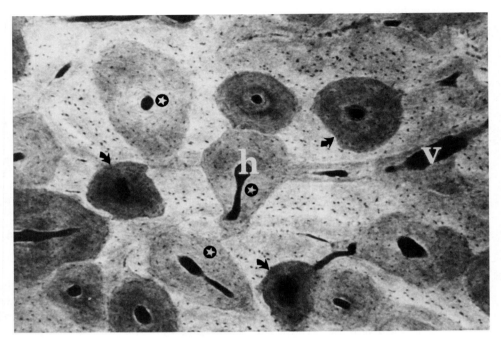

FIG 16–12.
Microradiography of a 100-μm-thick section demonstrates the vascular network of haversian *(h)* and Volkmann's *(v)* canals in the compact bone of a dog. Radiolucent (young) secondary osteons are in the primary stage of mineralization *(curved arrows)*. A progression of secondary mineralization *(stars)* is noted in older secondary osteons.

essentially a curved tube of compact bone. As an independent bone with no other osseous support, the mandible must be relatively rigid because mastication involves substantial bending and torsion.[38] Overall cortex diameter and thickness are dictated by the loading history (see Fig 16–4). Mass of the compacta is more related to peak strain than to repetitive loading. Overload hypertrophy (really "hyperplasia" with respect to bone) results in increased bulk and strength. This is the reason weightlifters have larger bones and muscles than marathon runners. From a dental perspective, chronic bruxers, habitual clenchers and others with high biting strength have relatively large jaws and thick compacta. Conversely, low biting strength corresponds to less dense jaw structure.

Slow growth of periosteal surfaces (anabolic modeling of the structural fraction) results in layers of circumferential lamellae that partially or completely encircle the bone (Fig 16–15). More rapid growth (5 to 10 μm/day) results in the capture of periosteal blood vessels by a lattice of woven bone. Subsequent lamellar bone formation concentric to the captured vessels produces an array of regular primary osteons (see Fig 16–10). Production of this type of composite bone is referred to as *fine cancellous compaction.*[34]

Very rapid periosteal apposition (>10 μm/day) results in increasingly irregular primary compacta. Blood vessels are pulled away from the periosteal surface by the rapid appositional rate, resulting in primary osteons with a streaming or whorling pattern. This type of primary compacta is an example of *coarse cancellous compaction.*[34] Irregular primary osteons are characteristic of the initial healing stage following implantation into bone.

Remodeling (turnover) of compact bone results in formation of secondary osteons, which are concentric lamellar structures with a peripheral scalloped margin (see Fig 16–10). The latter is a resorption arrest line, indicating the limit of bone resorption prior to being filled with new lamellar bone. Scalloped margins of secondary osteons are called cement lines because a fine layer of

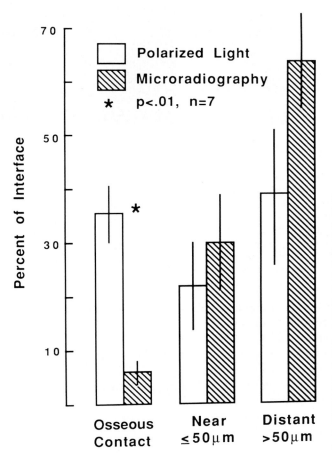

FIG 16–13.
Histomorphometric analysis of the mineralized sections in Figures 16–8 and 16–14 (100 μm thick) by polarized-light microscopy and microradiography reveals a substantial discrepancy between what appears to be osseous interface in transmitted light and what is mineralized interface (attenuated x-rays). Clinically successful implants, such as those shown in Figures 16–8 and 16–14 may have as little as 10% direct bone contact at the interface; about 30% of the interface has bone within 50 μm. (From Roberts WE, et al: *Angle Orthod* 59:247, 1989.)

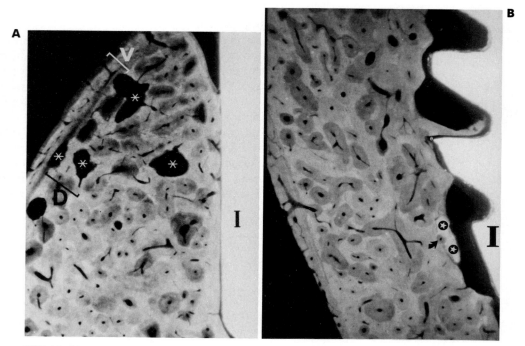

FIG 16–14.
A, Microradiograph of the cervical region of titanium implant *(I)* with a cylindrical emersion profile. This is the early loading phase (20 weeks after implantation, 13 weeks loaded) in a dog (same subject as Fig 16–8). The porosity *(stars)* is remodeling space related to postoperative RAP, which last about three sigma (36 weeks) in dogs. At least a portion of the subperiosteal bone may have been devitalized *(D)* by periosteal stripping at implantation. New vital bone *(V)* was deposited during the healing process (From Roberts WE, et al: *J Indiana Dent Assoc* 68:19, 1989). **B,** apical region of same implant shown in **A** reveals minimal direct bone contact. A hypermineralized sequestrum *(stars)* is probably residual to the original implantation procedure. Over time this "natural bone graft" will be remodeled away. Note the new secondary osteon *(arrow)* cutting into the sequestrum. *I* = implant.

polysaccharide-rich cementing substance is evident between old and new bone. When bone remodels adjacent to an implant, cementing substance may provide mechanical adhesion at the interface.

Bone can form or resorb at any endosteal or periosteal surface. Osseous tissue is incapable of interstitial growth because it is a rigid mineralized structure. Neither can it grow against a pressure gradient because compression compromises the periosteal blood supply. Turnover of compact bone requires internal access by way of tunneling osteoclasts. The cutting and filling cones of evolving secondary osteons are the mechanism of cortical bone remodeling (Fig 16–16). Continuous remodeling of the metabolic fraction (see Fig 16–15) provides a constant source of elemental calcium.

The coupled $A \rightarrow R(Q) \rightarrow F$ sequence of remodeling begins with an activation phase *(A)* of hours to days when osteoclasts form a cutting head. Circulating preosteoclasts (derivatives of marrow promonocytes) cross the blood vessel wall, enter the connective tissue, and form osteoclasts. Although osteoclasts are recruited to bone surfaces by way of marrow and the circulation, osteoblasts are formed within the tissue from paravascular connective tissue cells. A more complete discussion of the cell kinetics of osteoblast and osteoclast formation has been published.[39]

The cutting cone progresses through compacta at a velocity of about 30 μm/day. During the resorption phase *(R)*, the cutting cone opens a cavity of approximately 120 to 180 μm in diameter. Once the resorption cavity is complete, there is a variable quiescent *(Q)* phase: a few days in rabbits, 1 week in dogs and 1 to 2 weeks in man. The quiescent phase occurs between the cessation of

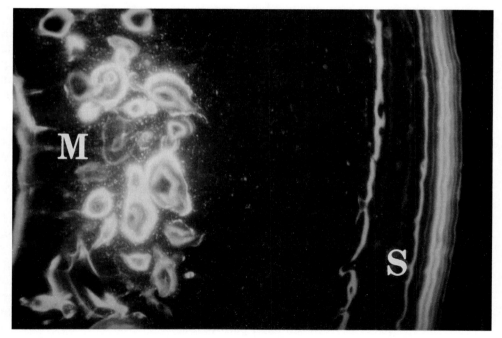

FIG 16–15.
Multiple fluorochrome labeling (2-week intervals) shows anabolic modeling of the structural fraction *(S)* to increase strength of the femur of a late adolescent female rabbit. Remodeling of the metabolic fraction *(M)* provides a continual source of elemental calcium. (From Roberts WE, Garetto LP, Katona TR: Principles of orthodontic biomechanics: metabolic and mechanical control mechanisms. In Carlson DS, Goldstein SA, editors: *Bone biodynamics in orthodontic and orthopedic treatments,* Ann Arbor, 1992, University of Michigan Press, pp 189–256. Used by permission.)

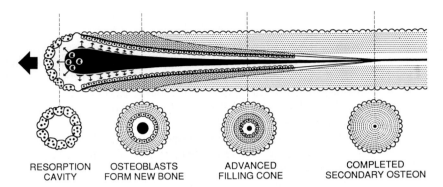

RESORPTION CAVITY   OSTEOBLASTS FORM NEW BONE   ADVANCED FILLING CONE   COMPLETED SECONDARY OSTEON

FIG 16–16.
Schematic drawing of a cutting/filling cone (evolving secondary osteon) demonstrates the mechanism of cortical bone remodeling. (Adapted from Roberts WE, et al: *Am J Orthod* 86:95, 1984.)

osteoclastic resorption and the beginning of osteoblastic bone formation. During this period occasional mononuclear cells (possibly macrophages) are noted along the resorbing surface. They may be finishing the resorptive process and/or preparing the surface for subsequent bone formation. Covering previously resorbing surfaces with cementing substance allows new bone to adhere to old bone.

The bone formation phase *(F)* of remodeling is the major variable between species. The cavity is filled in 4.5, 10, or 13 weeks in rabbits, dogs, and humans, respectively. Thus, the average duration of the $A \rightarrow R(Q) \rightarrow F$ remodeling cycle increases in proportion to the size of the animal. Using the rabbit ($\times$) as a base, the factors for similar physiological events in dogs and humans are 2 and 3 times, respectively (see Table 16–1).

The *vascularity* of cortical bone has important physiological ramifications. Diffusion through bone is effective only up to about 0.1 mm. To maintain internal vitality of osteocytes, the vascular supply of compact bone is organized into haversian canals (aligned along the long axis of the bone) and Volkmann's canals (aligned perpendicular to the bone's long axis) (see Fig 16–12). Concentric bone lamellae form around neurovascular bundles, resulting in a repetitive osteonal structure. Canaliculi radiate from the center of the osteon, providing cellular processes and diffusion pathways for logistical support of osteocytes.

Nutrient vessels (arteries and veins) provide blood circulation for the marrow cavity, trabecular bone, and specialized structures such as the base of the growth plate (primary spongiosa). The inferior alveolar artery and vein are the nutrient vessels of the body of the mandible. The mandibular condyle has separate nutrient vessels penetrating primarily at muscle attachments. Although the haversian/Volkmann network provides a collateral circulation within the compacta, it is highly tortuous and easily compromised by surgical trauma and postoperative inflammation. A portion of the arterial supply and all the venous return are by way of the periosteum. Stripping periosteum creates vascular stasis and compromises the vitality of the cortex.

Periosteum is the vital reactive layer of connective tissue covering cortical bone. Retraction of attached mucosa usually involves a full thickness mucoperiosteal flap. When periosteum is stripped, the osteogenic layer immediately adjacent to the bone surface is destroyed and the blood supply of underlying compacta is compromised. Minimal stripping, consistent with sound surgical principles of access and soft tissue management, is an important consideration in implant dentistry.[23]

Split-thickness flaps are utilized in the palate to avoid undue compromise of the osteogenic layer. Also, loose alveolar mucosa can be retracted, leaving the periosteum intact. In the latter case, excision and removal of periosteum over the operated bone is usually the most conservative approach. This procedure preserves the osteogenic capacity of adjacent periosteum.[35] Specific studies of surgical procedures are needed to define the osteogenic compromise of each approach.

TRABECULAR BONE

Spongy, cancellous, and trabecular bone are synonymous terms for low-density osseous tissue. Mature trabeculae are composed of lamellar bone. Vascular support of trabecular bone is derived from adjacent marrow because trabeculae are avascular. Trabecular bone is a relatively low-mass, selectively oriented skeletal tissue that is particularly efficient in resisting compression. Vertebral bodies and the maxilla are good examples of compressively loaded bones (Fig 16–17). There is a function-related tendency for trabeculae to align along lines of stress. Strength of trabecular bone depends on trabecular thickness (mass), orientation, and connectivity.[30]

Trabeculae within the marrow cavity of expanding compacta, such as the body of the mandible, are created by selective resorption of the endosteal surface (see Fig 16–4). Finger-like projections remodel into typical trabeculae. Intramembranous bones such as the maxilla form trabeculae in a similar manner. The osseous margin of growing sutures is composed of compact bone. The endosteal side of the cortical margin is converted into primary cancellous structures by selective resorption.

Trabecular bone remodels according to a coupled $A \rightarrow R(Q) \rightarrow F$ sequence that is essentially identical to cortical bone (Fig 16–18, A and B). Probably because of predominant metabolic control, the appositional rate for trabecular bone remodeling is remarkably constant, about 0.6 μm/day.[40] In contrast, the formation

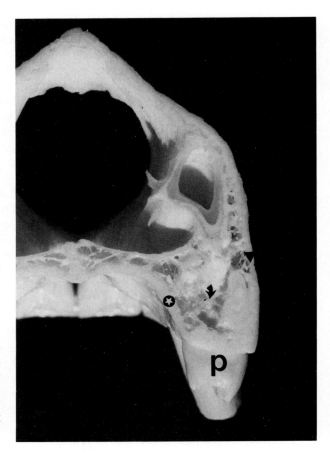

FIG 16–17.
Cross-section through the premolar *(p)* region of an adult monkey maxilla shows the thin buccal plate *(triangle)*, thicker palatal plate *(star)*, and relatively sparce trabeculae in the interradicular area *(curved arrow)*.

rate for subperiosteal lamellar bone is variable, up to 1.0 μm/day. The latter is a modeling process that responds to the peak strains of functional loading. The high rates of bone turnover in human alveolar processes and maxillae noted in bone scans[27] apparently reflect the remodeling of trabecular bone.

According to changing functional demands, trabeculae reorient along lines of stress (Wolff's Law) to provide maximal strength with minimal mass.[30] Remodeling of trabecular bone continues at a rapid rate throughout life (20% to 33%/yr). Trabecular bone remodeling provides a constant flux of calcium for metabolic purposes.[41]

With age there is a tendency to resorb more bone than is replaced. This results in an absolute decrease in spongiosa volume (catabolic modeling) as well as a decrease in the size and number of trabeculae (remodeling). When trabeculae of the secondary spongiosa are lost because of disease or aging, they are not readily

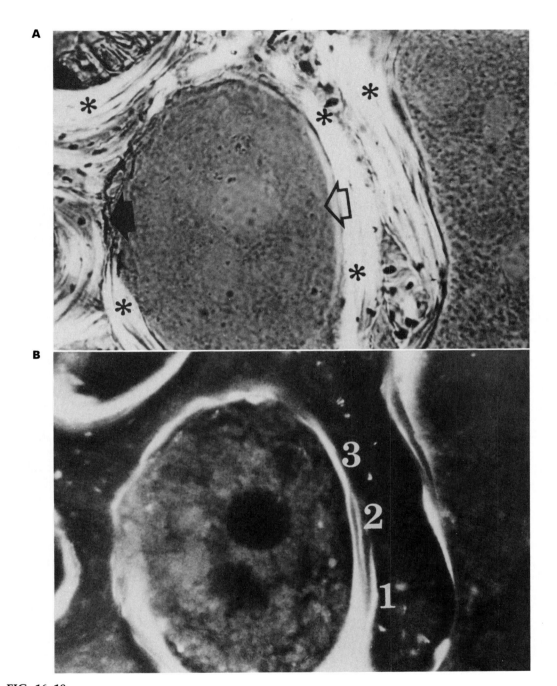

FIG 16–18.
A, Polarized light photomicrograph of trabecular bone shows recently remodeled foci *(stars)* of new bone deposited on a scalloped, resorption arrest line. The *solid arrow* to the left shows an active resorbing surface. The *open arrow* on the right shows an active bone forming site. The A → R(Q) → F sequence is similar to half of an evolving secondary osteon (Figure 16–16). **B,** ultraviolet fluoresence microscopy of the same specimen reveals four labels administered at weekly intervals. Numerous sites have one or two labels indicating some bone formation during the labeling period. The trabeculum to the right has three distinct labels (1, 2, and 3), indicating active bone formation.

replaced.[31] A relative osteopenia is classified as osteoporosis if symptoms of skeletal failure occur. Wrist, spine, and hip fractures are the most common problems. Conserving skeletal mass with proper diet, exercise, and hormonal supplements is currently the most effective means of maintaining adequate skeletal support.[22]

Low-density trabecular bone is common in edentulous areas of the atrophic maxilla where it is important to minimize surgical preparation. Once the cortical plate is penetrated, implants can often be installed without further preparation. Press-fit cylinders, plasma sprayed with hydroxylapatite or titanium, and self-tapping threaded implants are the most popular designs for poor quality trabecular bone. To maximize stability during the healing phase, it is often desirable to engage the opposite cortex with the apical threads of the implant.

BONE-IMPLANT INTERFACE

Anabolic modeling on bone surfaces is the first osseous healing reaction following implantation of a biocompatible device into cortical bone. Similar to fracture healing, a bridging callus forms at the periosteal and endosteal surfaces (Fig 16–19). Under optimal conditions (minimal trauma and vascular compromise) the callus originates within a few millimeters from the margin of the implantation site. In rabbits the lattice of woven bone reaches the implant surface in about 2 weeks and is sufficiently compacted and remodeled by 6 weeks to provide adequate resistance to loading. There is no definitive data for the early healing process in humans. Extrapolating from relative durations of the remodeling cycles (6 weeks vs. 4 months), timing for the primary callus (woven bone) may be similar to rabbits but the remodeling-dependent maturation process probably requires three times longer (up to 18 weeks).

If periosteum is stripped, the callus must originate in the nearest untraumatized osteogenic tissue.[42] Because healing reactions are self limiting, extensive loss of the osteogenic (inner) layer may preclude periosteal bridging.[35] Reapproximating retracted periosteum when the wound is closed positions the nonosteogenic fibrous (outer) layer near the implant. A compromised osteogenic reaction, associated with a defect in the periosteal margin of bone, favors invasion of fibrous connective tissue. Extensive stripping of periosteum substantially inhibits the initial healing response. Even though stimulating cytokines and growth factors are released from the blood clot at the surgical site, essentially no competent osteoprogenitor cells survive periosteal stripping. These cells must be reintroduced by ingrowth of new vascular tissue. Therefore, the surgeon should minimize periosteal trauma consistent with adequate access and appropriate soft tissue management.

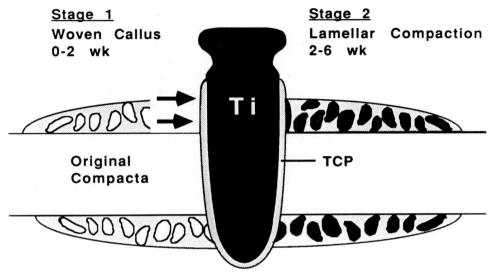

Stage 1
Woven Callus
0-2 wk

Ti

Stage 2
Lamellar Compaction
2-6 wk

Original Compacta

—— **TCP**

FIG 16–19.
Initial stages of implant healing and interface development are shown in a schematic drawing of a tricalcium phosphate *(TCP)* = coated titanium (Ti) implant in rabbit compacta. Woven callus is being formed during stage 1 (0 to 2 weeks). Stage 2 (2 to 6 weeks) is the period of lamellar compaction when the callus matures and achieves sufficient strength for loading. In humans, stages 1 and 2 are complete in 6 and 18 weeks, respectively. (From Roberts WE: *J Dent Educ* 52:804, 1988.)

Efficient reduction of an osseous defect by a bridging callus requires relative stability of the approximating segments. An unloaded healing phase (two-stage implantation procedure) is widely used to prevent extensive functional movement during healing. However, there are other important biomechanical considerations: (1) mechanical retention of the implant within the wound; (2) approximation of the periosteal margin of the cortex to the implant surface; and (3) functional flexure of the implanted bone. Healing implants in functioning bones are never really "unloaded."

The initial callus reaction near the implant is primarily driven by local cytokines and growth factors; however, the overall size and extent of the periosteal callus is mechanically dependent. A surgical defect weakens the bone and, as a result, may increase peak strains at a distance from the surgical site. Bursts of new bone formation (extensions of the callus) are often noted around the bone.[35] Remodeling of the callus begins early in the healing period. According to the principle of adequate strength with minimal mass, the callus reduces in size and reorients as internal maturation and strength are attained.[35]

Interface remodeling is essential in establishing a viable interface between the implant and original bone. As shown in Figure 16–20, about 1 mm of compacta adjacent to the osseous wound dies postoperatively despite optimal surgical technique. This is probably the result of inflammation and the relatively poor collateral circulation within cortical bone. Dead bone is not useless tissue; it provides important structural support during the initial healing phase. However, it must be replaced with vital bone to strengthen the interface and provide adaptable tissue for long term maintenance.

Remodeling of the nonvital interface is achieved by cutting/filling cones emanating from the endosteal surface. The mechanism is similar to typical cortical remodeling except that the cutting/filling cones are oriented perpendicular to the usual pathway (long axis of the bone). In longitudinal sections, cutting/filling cones occasionally deviate from the plane of the interface, turn 90 degrees, and form a secondary osteon perpendicular to the interface.[43] At the same time the interface is remodeled, the adjacent nonvital cortex (viewed in cross-section) is penetrated by typical cutting/filling cones (see Fig 16–20).

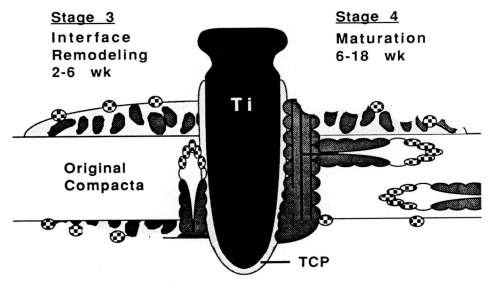

FIG 16–20.
Stage 3 (2 to 6 weeks) of healing and interface development begins at the same time the callus is completing lamellar compaction (Stage 2), but it is a morphologically distinct series of events. The callus starts to resorb, and remodeling of the devitalized interface begins. In all studies to date, the cutting heads penetrate from the endosteal surface. During stage 4 (6 to 18 weeks) the compacta matures by a series of modeling and remodeling processes: (1) interface remodels; (2) adjacent bone remodels; and (3) callus completes resorption (modeling). In man, stages 3 and 4 are complete in 18 and 54 weeks, respectively. (From Roberts WE: *J Dent Educ* 52:804, 1988.)

TABLE 16–2.

Time Course of Interface Development for Endosseous Implant in Cortical Bone

Stage	Rabbit (wk)	Human (3×) (wk)
Surface modeling		
Stage 1: woven callus	2	6
Stage 2: lamellar compaction	6	18
Remodeling; maturation		
Stage 3: interface remodeling	6	18
Stage 4: compacta maturation	18	54

*Initial healing (surface modeling) occurs at about the same rate as in rabbits.

Maturation of the interface and supporting bone requires an elapsed time after implant placement of about 3 sigma (12 months). The first 4 months (1 sigma) is the initial relatively unloaded healing process. The bone maturation phase requires an additional 2 sigma (8 months). Maturation to achieve maximal strength of interfacial and supporting bone involves completion of two physiological transients: the regional acceleratory phenomenon (RAP), and secondary mineralization of the newly formed bone. Extensive remodeling (RAP) in cortical bone is a well-known healing reaction to surgical wounding.[44] In general, remodeling sites decrease with increasing distance from the wound.[25] Stiffness and strength of lamellar bone are directly related to mineral content.[30] Full strength of bone supporting an implant is not achieved until the secondary mineralization process is complete, about 12 months (54 weeks) after the bone is formed (Table 16–2). Because of the RAP and the time restraints of secondary mineralization, maturation of a cortical bone implantation site requires approximately 1 year (4 months of healing plus 8 months of progressive loading).

Long-term maintenance of the rigid osseous fixation involves continuous remodeling of the interface and supporting bone. Bone, like other relatively rigid materials, is subject to fatigue.[25, 30] Repetitive loading results in microscopic cracks (microfractures). If allowed to accumulate, these small defects can lead to structural failure. Because osteoclasts preferentially resorb more highly mineralized tissue, cutting cones tend to remodel the oldest and presumably most weakened bone. This physiologic mechanism helps to maintain structural integrity indefinitely. Human cortical bone normally remodels at a rate of about 2% to 10% per year depending on site.[41] The interaction of mechanical and metabolic factors in controlling adult bone remodeling is not well understood. As shown in Figures 16–21 A and B, cortical bone around a loaded endosseous implant progressively remodels, but the long-term kinetics are unknown.

The histologic events for the four stages of interface development are summarized in Figures 16–19 and 16–20. The timing of each stage was established in the femoral cortex of young adult rabbits (6 to 18 month of age). Human equivalents are extrapolated according to the duration of the remodeling cycle.[35]

A   B

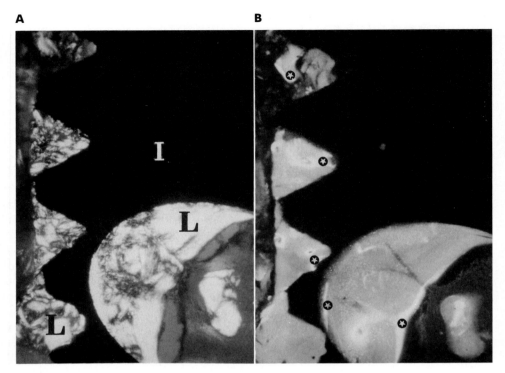

FIG 16–21.
A, polarized-light microscopy of a titanium implant recovered after about 4 years in a human mandible shows the mature lamellar nature of bone *(L)* at and near the interface of the implant *(I).* **B,** ultraviolet fluorescense microscopy reveals multiple sites of new bone formation *(stars)* labeled by demeclocycline administered shortly before biopsy. (From Roberts WE, Marshall KJ, Mosary PG: *Angle Orthod* 60:135, 1990.)

SUMMARY

Physiologic principles govern all aspects of implant healing and long-term function. An understanding of the fundamental physiology, metabolism, and biomechanics of bone is essential for clinicians placing and restoring these devices. A thorough physiologic assessment of the patient and the implantation site is an important part of the diagnostic process. Basic scientific information regarding the healing mechanism of bone in response to implantation is well known. However, definitive studies documenting the differential response are lacking for even the most fundamental design differences: threaded vs. cylindrical and hydroxylapatite-coated vs. uncoated titanium. A carefully controlled study is needed in which biomechanical properties can be compared with the histologic response resulting from basic differences in implant design.

Acknowledgments

This work was supported by National Institute of Dental Research Grant DE09237, National NASA Grant NCC 2-594, the International College of Oral Implantologists, and the Indiana University Foundation.

Special thanks to Drs. David Brown and Thomas Katona for their help with the manuscript.

REFERENCES

1. Sharawy M: *Companion of applied anatomy,* ed 2, 1990, Augusta, Ga, Medical College of Georgia Printing Service, pp 1–103.
2. Hickey JC, Zarb GA, Bolender CL: *Boucher's prosthetic treatment for edentulous patients,* ed 9, St Louis, 1982, CV Mosby.
3. Atwood DA, Coy WA: Clinical cephalometric and densitometric study of reduction of residual ridges, *J Prosthet Dent* 26:280–299, 1977.
4. DuBrul EL: *Sicher's oral anatomy,* St Louis, 1982, CV Mosby.
5. Atwood DA: Some clinical factors related to rate of resorption of residual ridges, *J Prosthet Dent* 12:441–450, 1962.
6. Atwood DA: Reduction of residual ridges: a major oral disease entity, *J Prosthet Dent* 29:266–279, 1971.
7. Bays RA: The pathophysiology and anatomy of edentulous bone loss. In Fonseca RJ, Davis WH: *Reconstructive preprosthetic oral and maxillofacial surgery,* Philadelphia, 1986, WB Saunders, pp 1–17.
8. Brookes M: *The blood supply of bone,* London, 1971, Butterworths.
9. Rhinelander FW: Circulation of bone. In Bourne GH, editor: *The biochemistry and physiology of bone,* New York, 1972, Academic Press, pp 1–77.
10. Hellem S, Ostrup LT: Normal and retrograde blood supply to the body of the mandible in the dog. II: the role played by periosteo-medullary and symphyseal anastomoses, *Int J Oral Surg* 10:31–42, 1981.
11. Bell WH, Levy BM: Revascularization and bone healing after anterior mandibular osteotomy, *J Oral Surg* 28:196–203, 1970.
12. Bell WH: Biologic basis for maxillary osteotomies, *Am J Phys Anthropol* 38:279–290, 1973.
13. Bell WH: Revascularization and bone healing after anterior maxillary osteotomy: a study using adult rhesus monkeys, *J Oral Surg* 27:249–255, 1969.
14. Castelli WA, Nasjleti CE, Diaz-Perez R: Interruption of the arterial inferior alveolar flow and its effects on mandibular collateral circulation and dental tissues, *J Dent Res* 54:708–715, 1975.

15. Perint J: Surgical anatomy and physiology: detailed roentgenologic examination of the blood supply in the jaws and teeth by applying radiopaque solutions, *J Oral Surg* 2:2–20, 1949.
16. Williams PL, Warwick R: *Gray's anatomy,* Br ed 36, Philadelphia, 1980, Saunders.
17. Bell WH: Biologic basis for modification of the sagittal ramus split operation, *J Oral Surg* 35:362–369, 1977.
18. Castelli W: Vascular architecture of the human adult mandible, *J Dent Res* 42:786–792, 1963.
19. Bradley JC: Age changes in the vascular supply of the mandible, *Br Dent J* 132:142–144, 1972.
20. Bradley JC: A radiological investigation into the age changes of the inferior dental artery, *Br J Oral Surg* 13:82–90, 1975.
21. Roberts WE et al: Bone physiology: evaluation of bone metabolism, *J Am Dent Assoc* 122:59–61, 1991.
22. Roberts WE et al: Bone physiology and metabolism in dental implantology: risk factors for osteoporosis and other metabolic bone diseases, *Implant Dent* 1:11–21, 1992.
23. Roberts WE et al: Bone physiology and metabolism, *J Calif Dent Assoc* 15:54–61, 1987.
24. Midgett RJ, Shaye R, Fruge JF: The effect of altered bone metabolism on orthodontic tooth movement, *Am J Orthod* 80:256–262, 1981.
25. Martin RB, Burr DB: *Structure, function, and adaptation of compact bone,* New York, 1989, Raven Press.
26. Baron R, Vignery A, Horowitz M: Lymphocytes, macrophages and the regulation of bone remodeling. In Peck WA, editor: *Bone and mineral research: annual 2,* Amsterdam, 1984, Elsevier, pp 175–243.
27. Reddy MS et al: Detection of periodontal disease activity with a scintillation camera, *J Dent Res* 70:50–54, 1991.
28. Weiner S, Traub W: Bone structure: from angstoms to microns, *FASEB J* 6:879–885, 1992.
29. Gowen M: *Cytokines and bone metabolism,* Boca Raton, Fla, 1992, CRC Press.
30. Currey JD: The mechanical adaptations of bones, Princeton, NJ, 1984, Princeton University Press.
31. Roberts WE, Gonsalves M: Aging of bone tissue. In Holm-Pedersen P, Loe H, editors: *Geriatric dentistry,* Copenhagen, 1986, Munksgaard International, pp 83–93.
32. Linkow LI, Dorfman JD: Implantology in dentistry: a brief historical perspective, *NY State Dent J* 57:31–35, 1991.
33. Weiss CM: Tissue integration of dental endosseous implants: description of comparative analysis of the fibro-osseous integration and osseous integration systems, *J Oral Implant* 12:169–214, 1986.
34. Enlow DH: *Principles of bone remodeling,* Springfield, Il, 1963, Charles C Thomas.
35. Roberts WE et al: Osseous adaptation to continuous loading of rigid endosseous implants, *Am J Orthod* 86:95–111, 1984.
36. Roberts WE, Morey ER: Proliferation and differentiation sequence of osteoblast histogenesis under physiological conditions in rat periodontal ligament, *Am J Anat* 174:105–118, 1985.
37. Roberts WE et al: Rigid endosseous implants for orthodontic and orthopedic anchorage, *Angle Orthod* 59:247–256, 1989.

38. Bouvier M, Hylander WL: Effect of bone strain on cortical bone structure in macaques *(Macaca mulatta),* *J Morphol* 167:1–12, 1981.
39. Roberts WE, Garetto LP, Katona TR: Principles of orthodontic biomechanics: metabolic and mechanical control mechanisms. In Carlson DS, Goldstein SA, editors: *Bone biodynamics in orthodontic and orthopedic treatment,* Ann Arbor, 1992, University of Michigan Press, pp 189–256.
40. Melsen F, Mosekilde L: The role of bone biopsy in the diagnosis of metabolic bone disease, *Orthop Clin North Am* 12:571–602, 1981.
41. Parfitt AM: The physiological and clinical significance of bone histomorphometric data. In Recker RR, editor: *Bone histomorphometry: techniques and interpretation,* Boca Raton, Fla, 1983, CRC Press, pp 143–223.
42. Melcher AH, Accursi GE: Osteogenic capacity of periosteal and osteoperiosteal flaps elevated from the parietal bone of the rat, *Arch Oral Biol* 16:573–580, 1971.
43. Roberts WE: Bone tissue interface, *J Dent Educ* 52:804–809, 1988.
44. Frost HM: The regional acceleratory phenomenon: a review, *Henry Ford Hosp Med J* 31:3–9, 1983.

Chapter 17

Spread of Dental Infection in the Head and Neck

Mohamed Sharawy
Carl E. Misch

SIGNIFICANT COMPLICATIONS AND IMPLANT DENTISTRY

Few significant complications are associated with implant dentistry. However, identification of potential problems that can be life threatening are in the best interest of all concerned. Death has been reported in dental practice and has been related to air emboli and spread of infection. These complications have a similar foundation: the vascular-lymphatic network and fascial planes. Routes associated with these potential situations are reviewed in this chapter.

There are three stages in the development of infection in the head and neck region: the development, extension, and complication stages. The *development stage* permits the infection to spread through the bone and form an abscess under the periosteum (subperiosteal abscess). A subperiosteal implant may be associated with this complication without the infection coming from within the bone. Most often, exudate has been present around the permucosal of the implant. On rare occasion, a fibrous tissue surrounded implant becomes infected and the infection may spread through the bone from a retrograde direction. For the most part, implant infection begins from the permucosal region and spreads in an apical direction. Also, an implant placed in an infected immediate extraction site may become involved in retrograde infection.

The *extension stage* of the development of infection occurs when the subperiosteal abscess penetrates the periosteum and extends to the fascial spaces, producing a cellulitis or fascial abscess. Mandibular subperiosteal implants most often produce this entity in the posterior region, along the posterior body of the mandible. In maxillary subperiosteal or sinus augmentation surgeries this stage of infection may develop along the lateral aspect of the maxilla, just below the zygomatic arch. On rare occasion, this extension stage has been observed under the anterior mental region from endosteal implants placed through the inferior border of the mandible.

The *complication stage* results when the infection spreads and causes cavernous sinus thrombosis, brain abscess, neck and mediastinal involvement, pleurisy, or pericarditis.

The principle routes for the spread of dental infection are through four mechanisms:

1. Bacteremia permits the infectious process to spread by way of the blood vessels.
2. Infection may spread to the walls of the veins, which may also thrombose and create a condition referred to as thrombophlebitis. Lack of valves in the head venous system allows retrograde flow of blood and may involve the cavernous sinus, and the pterygoid and/or pharyngeal plexus with infected thrombi.
3. The lymph vessels are very prevalent in the head and neck, and invasion into these structures may lead to metastatic inflammation of both regional and more remote lymph nodes.
4. Once the infection is outside the bone, the loose areolar connective tissue produces a path of least resistance into the various surgical spaces of the head and neck and mediastinum. The muscle connections and fascial compartments limit or direct the path of infection.

Subperiosteal implants often extend beyond muscle attachments and/or fascial planes. Infections associated with primary struts should be closely supervised and aggressively treated, because the infection may spread by continuing beyond these structures. Endosteal implants are most often positioned beyond the apices of natural teeth. As a result, infections beyond their apices may perforate bone beyond the usual limiting borders associated with the roots of teeth.

PATHOLOGIC ENTITIES

The definition of specific terms that describe infections of the head and neck provide keys to methodology of treatment and improved communications. An *acute cellulitis* involves inflammation of the areolar connective tissue and loose subcutaneous tissues. *Lymphadenitis* describes the condition when the regional lymph nodes become inflamed, enlarged, and tender. The node may become suppurated, break through the capsule, and involve the surrounding tissues.

Abscess formation results when tissues break down and leukocytes die, thus forming pus. Staphylococci and streptococci are the usual bacteria involved in this process; however, a more varied population is prevalent in sinus infections. *Phlegmon* describes any cellulitis that does not go on to suppuration. In this condition, the inflammatory infiltration of the subcutaneous tissue leads to accumulation of foul-smelling, brownish exudate. Hemolytic streptococci are usually present. A *chronic cellulitis* follows an acute cellulitis and may be the result of inadequate treatment or a subvirulent organism with no suppuration. A *chronic abscess* is a well-encapsulated entity caused by a subvirulent organism. In this case, a bone sequestrum or retained root tip are the more common sources of the infection. A *chronic skin fistula* is a sign of retained focus of infection. This has been observed by the authors in the mandible, associated with infection of both endosteal and subperiosteal implants, with patients who have poor dental awareness and lack of implant maintenance. A *noma* starts as a gangrenous stomatitis and spreads to adjacent bone and muscles, causing lysis and necrosis of tissue. This rare condition perforates the cheek, floor of the mouth, or both, and is usually seen in debilitated individuals.

MAXILLARY INFECTIONS (FIGS 17–1 AND 17–2)

Acute suppurative periapical abscesses in the maxilla may penetrate the alveolar bone and form a *subperiosteal abscess* under the periosteum. If the abscess penetrates the periosteum above the attachment of the buccinator muscle, it

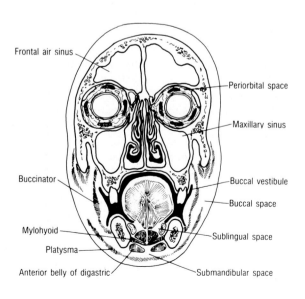

Frontal air sinus

Buccinator

Mylohyoid

Platysma

Anterior belly of digastric

Periorbital space

Maxillary sinus

Buccal vestibule

Buccal space

Sublingual space

Submandibular space

FIG 17–1.
Diagram of coronal section of the head at the molar region anterior to the mandibular rami. Head surgical spaces are labeled.

FIG 17–2.
Diagram of horizontal section of
the head shows the close relation
of the pterygomandibular space
to the parapharyngeal space.
Note that infection of the buccal
space can spread posterolaterally
into the masseteric space and
posteromedially into the pterygomandibular space. The visceral
space, perivertebral space, and
carotid sheath fascia are shown.

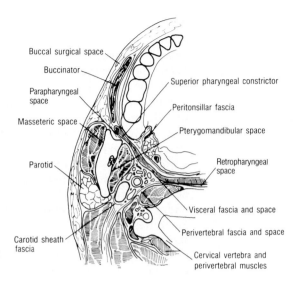

causes a buccal abscess. If the abscess continues to spread, it may involve the skin,
forming a cutaneous abscess. The infection may progress superiorly and involve
the temporal region. Downward extension may involve the submandibular space.
If the abscess perforates the buccal alveolar bone and periosteum below the
attachment of the buccinator muscle, the abscess wall appears intraorally in the
buccal vestibule and forms a gingival or alveolar abscess.

Palatal extension of the infection is rare. Usually it is from lingual roots of the
upper molars, forming a palatal abscess. On occasion, an implant may perforate
the palatal bone and cause an infection that may be evident at a later date.

The maxillary sinus may become invaded by an infection of the maxillary
teeth, resulting in an acute sinusitis. Radiographs reveal a clouded sinus resulting
from formation of pus. More frequently, sinus subantral graft surgeries may
penetrate an infected antrum, with subsequent extension of the infection into the
whole implanted region.

The loose, fat-containing connective tissue of the lips and cheeks is
continuous and is traversed by the muscles of facial expression, which arise from
the bones of the face, traverse the subcutaneous tissue, and end in the skin. These
muscles, with their thin perimysium, play a role in directing the spread of
infection. Dental or implant abscesses that erode and perforate the outer compact
lamella of bone sometimes find their way through the subcutaneous tissue to the
skin.

Most often, maxillary dental infections involve four regions of the maxilla:
upper lip, canine fossa, buccal space, and infratemporal space.

Lip

The lip contains weak and small muscles, but this does not limit the spread of infection. Infection of the base of the upper lip is most often caused by infection of the maxillary central region, which produces first a collateral edema, then a cellulitis of the upper lip. The abscess usually forms on the oral side of the orbicularis oris muscle in the buccal sulcus, and may extend upward between the levator anguli oris and levator labii superioris. The side of the nose and lower lid of the eye may then swell. In these cases, a potential exists for the development of a cavernous sinus thrombosis by spread of infection by way of the angular vein to the superior ophthalmic vein, to the cavernous sinus.

Treatment is usually by incision and drainage. A horizontal incision is made down to the bone in the apex area of the involved tooth or implant. The tooth or implant is then extracted, or the tooth is treated endodontically and a rubber drain is inserted within the incision. An implant is evaluated for mobility and, if present, is usually extracted. A stable implant may remain and be evaluated after the infection is controlled.

Infection of Canine Fossa

This condition is frequently caused by the spread of infection from the maxillary canine and premolars. The nasolabial fold is obliterated, and edema of the eyelids results. The infection forms between the levator labii superioris and orbicularis oris anteriorly and the buccinator posteriorly. This same space can be drained intraorally by making an incision at the fluctuant swelling in the buccal sulcus and the insertion of a clamp to drain the canine space superiorly.

Infection of Buccal Space

The buccal space lies between the skin of the cheek and buccinator, and contains a fat pad that extends upward and inward between the muscles of mastication, filling the retrozygomatic fossa and infratemporal space.

Abscesses of the second and third maxillary molars above the attachment of the buccinator frequently involve the buccal space. The infection may extend superiorly to the temporal space, or inferiorly to the submandibular space, or posteriorly to the masticatory spaces (see Fig 17–2).

Skin incision at the highest point of fluctuance, with blunt dissection to obtain adequate drainage of the space, is recommended.

Infratemporal Space

The infratemporal space lies below a horizontal plane drawn through the zygomatic arch and is bounded laterally by the ramus of the mandible and medially by the medial pterygoid muscle. The infratemporal space includes the pterygomandibular space between the ramus and medial pterygoid muscle, postzygomatic space, and pterygomaxillary fossa.

Infections of the maxillary teeth or endosteal implants extending above the attachment of the buccinator muscle can spread into the postzygomatic or infratemporal space. Infections of the mandibular second and third molars are more likely to infect the pterygomandibular part. Infection of this space, fortunately, is not common. It is serious because of the complications that can follow.

Infratemporal space infection may involve the pterygoid plexus of veins and subsequently the cavernus sinus. The infection may also spread through the infraorbital fissure and cause periorbital infection.

The temporal fossa, which is almost completely filled by the temporalis muscle and covered by the temporal fascia, may become involved from extension of an infection of the infratemporal space. Such involvement causes a painful swelling of the region, elevating the temporalis fascia and preventing opening of the jaw.

Incision and drainage constitute the treatment of choice. Whether an intraoral or extraoral incision is made will depend on the presence or absence of trismus, the decision whether the intraoral approach is adequate for drainage of deep pockets of pus, and whether or not the maintenance of drainage from the intraoral site would constitute a health hazard from aspiration.

Incision and drainage by an intraoral approach is usually made by incising the mucosa medial and parallel to the ascending ramus along the anterior border of the medial pterygoid muscle. The surgical spaces are then approached by blunt dissection in a posteromedial direction for the pterygomandibular and parapharyngeal spaces, in an upward direction for the temporalis space, and posterolaterally into the masseteric space. Extraoral incision at the angle of the mandible is recommended for more adequate drainage of these spaces. The temporalis space may also be drained by a skin incision parallel and superior to the zygomatic arch in order to avoid injury to the zygomatic branches of the facial nerve.

A decision has to be made in individual cases as to whether the maxillary implants should be removed or conservatively treated by curretage of the infected granulation tissue and close monitoring of the progress of healing.

MANDIBULAR INFECTIONS (SEE FIGS 17–1 AND 17–2)

In the mandibular dental or implant infections, the mylohyoid muscle attachment on the medial surface of the mandible and the buccinator attachment on the outer surface of the mandible play an important part in limiting or directing the spread of infection.

The line of origin of the mylohyoid muscle begins close to the lower border of the mandible and ascends posteriorly and diagonally across the inner surface of the mandible to the socket of the last molar. The apical level of the roots of the incisors, canines, and premolars is always above the mylohyoid line. The third molar reaches below, the second sometimes, and the first rarely. If a periapical abscess of the incisors, canines, and premolars perforates the lingual plate of the mandible, it will involve the floor of the mouth above the mylohyoid muscle and cause sublingual abscess or cellulitis. If the infection originates from the third molar (and sometimes the first and second molars), the subcutaneous connective tissue of the submandibular space is invaded, with the potential of spreading the infection backward to the parapharyngeal space, causing a descending cervical cellulitis. A lingual perforation of the periapical abscess of the mandibular molars is an exception because of the lingual inclination of these teeth; position the root tips closer to the buccal plate. Endosteal implants in the anterior and posterior regions may extend beyond the mylohyoid muscle attachment and often are positioned more lingually than the roots of teeth. Infections may therefore penetrate the bone and appear in the submandibular space.

Mandibular infections spread to the submandibular space, the parapharyngeal space, the parotid space, the carotid space, and the sublingual spaces—all of which communicate.

Circumscribed Mandibular Abscess

This abscess is generally from a mandibular premolar and is seen at the side of the mandible, anterior to the facial artery. It is not usually palpable under the skin and at times closely adherent to the mandible. The abscess is usually drained by a skin incision made parallel with the lower border of the affected area of the mandible, followed by a blunt dissection with a hemostat and placement of a rubber drain. This region may also be involved with a mandibular subperiosteal implant.

Subperiosteal implants may cause swelling in the region, unassociated with infection. Instead, a traumatic inflammation caused by the implant casting rubbing against the buccinator muscle may cause local swelling. Incision and drainage is not indicated. The condition is usually caused by hyperfunction due to overly aggressive eating episodes. Heat application coupled with brief avoidance to masticate on the affected side usually reduces the swelling and returns the region to normal within 1 to 3 days.

Infection of Submandibular Space

The submandibular space is frequently involved as a result of spread of dental infections, osteomyelitis, and fracture of the angle of the mandible. The submandibular space is found between the mylohyoid muscle and the skin and is bound by the posterior part of the mandible laterally.

The involvement of this space is usually from infection related to deciduous or permanent molars extending through the bone below the mylohyoid muscle or descending beneath the periosteum, from a periodontal abscess or pericoronitis, or from around the outer aspect of the mandible. Subperiosteal or endosteal implants may be placed into or close to the sublingual space. The lingual strut of the first molar post should be placed above the mylohyoid attachment when possible, to limit any potential infection from spreading directly into the submandibular space. Sublingual infection may also migrate on the surface of mylohyoid muscle and descend beyond its posterior border to the submandibular space. Conversely, infection from the submandibular space may spread around the posterior part of the mylohyoid into the sublingual space, to the adjacent parotid space and parapharyngeal space. When both the submandibular and sublingual spaces are involved, the floor of the mouth and tongue are elevated. In these cases, the tongue may retrude and cause difficulty in breathing.

Submandibular infection usually is drained by a skin incision 1 cm below the inferior border of the mandible, posterior to the facial artery. The areas anterior and posterior to the submandibular gland are explored by a hemostat. A rubber drain is placed.

Infection of Masticatory Spaces (see Fig 17–2)

The masseteric space is found between the fascia and the masseter muscle. The lateral wings of the subperiosteal implant extend along the lateral portion of the ramus. Infection of the ramus permucosal posts may extend in this region. The pterygomandibular space is found between the ramus of the mandible and the medial pterygoid muscle. The temporalis space is found between the thick temporalis fascia and the temporalis muscle.

Infection in the buccal space may spread in a posterolateral direction to involve the masseteric space or in a posteromedial direction to involve the pterygomandibular space, or may migrate superiorly along the temporalis tendons to involve the temporalis space. Infection of the muscles will lead to myositis. The patient usually complains of trismus and pain on opening of the jaw. Infection from the pterygomandibular space commonly spreads to the parapharyngeal space.

Infection of Sublingual Space (see Fig 17–1)

There are two sublingual spaces lying above the mylohyoid on each side of the median raphe. There is no natural barrier to the spread of infection from one sublingual space to the other. The sublingual abscesses are generally derived from an infected tooth in the anterior part of the jaw. The infection emerges on the lingual side of the mandible above the mylohyoid. This will lead to swelling of the floor of the mouth, elevation of the tongue, and difficulty and pain on swallowing.

The sublingual space is drained by an incision made at the base of the alveolar process of the mandible in the lingual sulcus so that the sublingual gland, lingual nerve, and submandibular duct will not be injured. A hemostat is passed down between the sublingual gland and the geniohyoid muscle. If no pus is found, a subperiosteal abscess on the inner surface of the mandible should be investigated; if found, incision of the periosteum is made. The drain should be sutured; as it may become displaced by the tongue.

Infection of Submental Space

This space lies within the boundaries of the submental triangle, which is bound by the anterior bellies of digastric muscles laterally and the hyoid bone inferiorly. Pus accumulates between the skin and platysma inferiorly and the mylohyoid muscle covered by suprahyoid fascia superiorly. Posteriorly, the space extends to the submandibular space. The infection forms an abscess or cellulitis emerging below the chin.

This space is drained by transverse incision below the mandible along skin folds, and a hemostat inserted forward and backward to open the entire area.

Ludwig's Angina

This distinct clinical entity is characterized by a deep, tender swelling of both the submandibular and sublingual spaces, swelling of the floor of the mouth, and elevation of the tongue.

This condition is usually a nonsuppurative cellulitis that originates in the submandibular space and spreads rapidly toward the floor of the mouth. It is caused almost exclusively from mandibular molar teeth because they reach below the mylohyoid ridge. An apical infection may spread directly to the submandibular space and from there extend to adjacent regions by continuity. The subperiosteal implant does not extend below this structure beyond the first molar, so the risk of infection below the muscle is reduced. The main danger from this infection is asphyxiation as a result of rapidly increasing respiratory embarrassment caused by swelling and displacement of the tongue backward and edema of the glottis. Early in the disease there is no pus, thus no fluctuation. If pus does form, it will be found between the mylohyoid and geniohyoid or between the geniohyoid and genioglossus. This will make swallowing and speech more difficult.

Bilateral incisions of the submandibular spaces with a blunt dissection into the submental region are needed. An incision into the submental space through the mylohyoid muscle should also be made. A clamp is inserted toward the base of the tongue to explore the sublingual space. A through-and-through drain should be placed between the submandibular spaces.

Infection of Parotid Space

This space contains the parotid gland and lies between two layers of deep fascia. It is in direct communication with the parapharyngeal and submandibular spaces. The infection may start within the parotid as in septic parotitis or result from spread of dental infection. The condition causes pain on eating and swallowing, and there is purulent discharge from the parotid duct.

To establish drainage of the parotid space, an incision is made around and below the angle of the mandible. The space is entered with a clamp, and a drain is placed.

Infection of Parapharyngeal Space

This space extends upward between the lateral wall of the pharynx and the medial surface of the medial pterygoid muscle. Behind the medial pterygoid muscle the parapharyngeal space widens considerably and reaches laterally to the styloid process with its muscles, and to the deep surface of the parapharyngeal space around the anterior and posterior borders of the medial pterygoid muscle. The patient usually experiences difficulty and pain during swallowing. The swelling of the tonsillar area can usually be seen intraorally. The infections may easily disseminate either upward through various foramina at the base of the skull, producing brain abscesses, meningitis, or sinus thrombosis, or downward along the carotid sheath or the visceral space toward the mediastinum.

This space is more commonly involved from acute infection around the mandibular third molar or from extension of pterygomandibular abscess, pharyngitis, tonsillitis, and parotitis.

The lateral or parapharyngeal abscess can be drained by intraoral incision of the lateral pharyngeal wall if there is no trismus, or by skin incision at the anterior border of the sternomastoid muscle at the level of the hyoid bone, followed by dissection along the posterior border of the posterior belly of the digastric muscle to the parapharyngeal space.

Infection of Perivisceral and Perivertebral Surgical Spaces of Neck

Deep cervical fascia surround the pharynx, larynx, trachea, esophagus, and thyroid gland and extend through the thoracic inlet into the mediastinum. There is a potential space between the fascia and the viscera, called the perivisceral space. The peripharyngeal, peritracheal, and periesophageal areas are all parts of the perivisceral space. Cervical vertebrae and perivertebral muscles are similarly surrounded by a deep cervical fascia known as the perivertebral fascia. There is a potential space between the perivertebral fascia and the perivertebral muscles known as the perivertebral space or "dangerous space." The space continues into the mediastinum. Infection in the perivisceral and/or perivertebral spaces commonly spreads into the thoracic mediastinum and may cause pleurisy, pericarditis, and lung abscesses. Urgent incision and drainage are therefore recommended. The spaces can be accessed through an incision of the skin along the anterior border of sternomastoid muscle below the hyoid bone, followed by retraction of the muscle and carotid sheath and blunt dissection of the spaces and placement of a drain. A tracheostomy or cricothyroidotomy is also performed if there is respiratory obstruction caused by the spread of infection to the peritracheal space.

Infection of Carotid Sheath

The carotid sheath is a fascial condensation around the internal jugular vein, the vagus nerve, and the common and internal carotid arteries. It lies deep to the sternomastoid.

The infection could spread to the carotid sheath from the submandibular space, infratemporal space, parotid space, and parapharyngeal space. Involvement is frequently associated with thrombosis of the internal jugular vein. This condition is serious as there is no anatomic barrier to downward spread of infection to the mediastinum. An incision is made over, and extending below, the region involved along the anterior border of the sternomastoid muscle, generally above the omohyoid muscle. If the internal jugular vein is thrombosed, it is ligated below its lowest limit of involvement to prevent further descent of the infection.

COMPLICATIONS OF TREATED AND UNTREATED INFECTIONS OF FACE AND NECK

Cavernous Sinus Thrombosis

Cavernous sinus thrombosis is one of the major complications of infection of the head and neck. It may occur from infection of the upper or lower jaw. The prognosis was poor prior to penicillin; 90% to 100% of patients died of advanced toxemia or meningitis in 5 days. The dentist should be able to recognize the early signs of cavernous sinus thrombosis and refer the patient immediately for hospital care by a specialist.

Cavernous sinus thrombosis may be caused by direct extension from the infratemporal space through the foramina or through the bone by osteomyelitis caused by staphylococcal infection or by venous thrombi originating in the venous system. One of three pathways is usually involved: the facial vein, angular vein, and/or superior ophthalmic vein to cavernous sinuses; the deep facial vein, pterygoid plexus of veins, emissary veins to cavernous sinuses; or the maxillary veins, inferior dental veins, pterygoid plexus of veins to cavernous sinuses.

The clinical signs and symptoms usually include all or a combination of some of the following: edema of the eyelids; hemorrhagic skin of nose and eyelids; ophthalmoplegia due to involvement of cranial nerves III, IV, and VI; burning and tingling sensation of the forehead due to involvement of nerve V_1; proptosis due to periorbital edema; chills, fever, restlessness, and severe headache.

Brain Abscess

A brain abscess may result from bacteremia or by direct spread of infection, and may occur as single or multiple abscesses, not always on the same side as the involved tooth or implant. Clinical signs consist of convulsive seizure, headache, stupor, slurred speech, and hemiparesis. Meningitis may develop, and death may occur in 2 to 6 weeks.

LYMPHATIC SPREAD OF INFECTION

The lymphatic circulation begins with blind-ended capillaries that drain the tissue fluid and carry it to larger vessels and eventually to two main lymphatic ducts (left thoracic and right common lymphatic ducts), which drain finally into the venous blood at the root of the neck. The lymphatic vessels are interrupted by lymph nodes. Each region of the body has a primary lymph node group that drains it. The knowledge of the regional nodes permits the diagnosis of the hitherto hidden site of infection. Although the sites of regional lymph nodes are fairly constant, there is great variability in their number and size.

Submental Lymph Nodes

The unpaired group of submental nodes lies between the hyoid bone and the anterior bellies of the digastric muscles in the submental triangle. They drain the middle part of the lower lip, the skin of the chin, and the tip of the tongue. Lymph from the lower incisors and the gingiva in this region flows at least partly into the submental nodes.

Submandibular Lymph Nodes

The submandibular lymph nodes are located in the submandibular triangle between the two bellies of the digastric muscle and the lower border of the mandible. They can be subdivided into an anterior, a middle, and a posterior group, each represented by one large or two or more smaller lymph nodes. Some of these nodes located in the submandibular niche (the space between the mylohyoid muscle and the medial surface of the mandible) are hidden by the body of the mandible and can be palpated only by pressing the finger upward on the inner surface of the lower jaw. This manipulation is facilitated with the patient's head tilted forward and toward the side being examined.

The anterior submandibular node or nodes are found along the submental vein close to the chin. The middle group is always represented by two or three small nodes situated around the anterior facial vein and facial artery, above the submandibular salivary gland. The posterior group of submandibular lymph nodes is located behind the anterior facial vein.

The submandibular lymph nodes collect the lymph of the upper and lower teeth with the exception of the incisors of the lower jaw, the lymph from the upper and lower lips with the exception of the middle part of the lower lip, the lymph from the anterior parts of the nasal cavity and palate, and finally, the lymph from the body of the tongue. Because of their relation to the teeth, the submental and submandibular lymph nodes are sometimes described as dental lymph nodes. The submandibular lymph nodes drain into the superficial and deep cervical lymph nodes.

Accessory lymph nodes are frequently associated with the submandibular lymph nodes and are closely related to the submandibular salivary gland. They are situated inside the capsule of the gland or even in its interlobular connective tissue (paramandibular lymph nodes).

Cervical Lymph Nodes

Cervical lymph nodes are found along the external and internal jugular veins. A subdivision into superficial and deep groups is made according to the relation of the nodes to the deep fasciae of the neck. The superficial cervical lymph nodes are, as a rule, restricted to the upper region of the neck, and are found in the angle between the mandibular ramus and the sternocleidomastoid muscle. These superficial nodes receive the lymph directly from the ear lobe and the adjacent part of the skin, and are secondary to the preauricular and postauricular lymph nodes.

The deep cervical lymph nodes may be subdivided into an upper and lower group, the latter sometimes are termed "supraclavicular lymph nodes." If a continuous chain of nodes accompanies the internal jugular vein, the omohyoid muscle is taken as the arbitrary boundary between the upper and lower deep cervical lymph nodes. In addition, each of these two groups again is subdivided into an anterior (or medial) and a posterior (or lateral) group. Superior and inferior deep cervical lymph nodes, situated in front of or covered by the sternocleidomastoid muscle, are classified as anterior or medial deep cervical lymph nodes; those situated in the posterior triangle of the neck behind the sternocleidomastoid are posterior or lateral deep cervical lymph nodes.

The deep cervical lymph nodes are primary sites for the drainage of the base of the tongue, the sublingual region, and the posterior part of the palate. They are secondary and tertiary nodes into which the lymph of the auricular, submental, and submandibular and accessory nodes of the face empty, also the lymph from the viscera of the neck. The two lymph nodes that are normally palpable are the jugulodigastric (tonsil) lymph node and the jugulo-omohyoid (tongue) lymph nodes.

The superior deep cervical lymph nodes send their lymph into the inferior deep cervical or supraclavicular lymph nodes. The lymph on the right side is then collected by the right common lymphatic duct, and the left side by the thoracic duct. The two main lymphatic vessels empty on either side into the "venous angle," where the internal jugular and subclavian veins unite; thus the lymph enters the venous system by way of brachiocephalic veins.

Conclusion

The complications from spread of dental infection are described in detail in this chapter, to make the implantologist aware of the potential danger of involving the surgical spaces of the head with infection from dental origin. The early signs of infection need to be recognized and considered urgently, especially when swallowing and/or breathing of the affected patient are compromised. Also, early signs of cavernous sinus thrombosis need to be recognized and the patient referred immediately to a specialist.

SUMMARY

Endosteal implants are usually inserted beyond the apex position of natural teeth. Subperiosteal implants traverse natural barriers of infection when extended beyond muscle attachments. Intraoral infections may extend to the base of implants, which may cause more concern than infections of natural teeth.

The implant dentist must be aware of the changes in the patient's symptoms as infection progresses and, when indicated, refer the patient immediately to a specialist for treatment. As discussed in this chapter, the infection may start as a painful swelling in the face region with little or no change in the ability of the patient to open the mouth, swallow, or breath, and with only mild signs of toxemia. The dentist has to be extremely alert to the possibility of a progression of the infection to involve the masticatory spaces, parapharyngeal spaces, perivertebral, perivisceral spaces, and similar areas, with accompanying signs and symptoms such as the inability to open the mouth, and the compromise of vital signs such as breathing. When this occurs, the patient should be hospitalized without hesitation.

Chapter 18

Tissues Surrounding Dental Implants

Robert A. James
Ralph V. McKinney, Jr.

TISSUE-IMPLANT BIOLOGIC SEAL

History and Function

Dental implants provide a unique treatment modality for the replacement of lost dentition. This is accomplished by the insertion of a relatively inert material (a biomaterial) into the soft and hard tissue of the jaws, thereby providing support and retention for dental prostheses.

Evidence of successful dental implantation can be seen in early civilizations, [1] and innovative dental practitioners who attempted the design and insertion of such devices published in modern literature as early as the late 19th and early 20th centuries.[2–7] However, these practitioners stood alone in their valiant attempts to investigate this line of treatment and their ideas were not well accepted by the practicing and investigative dental communities.

During the developmental years, implant dentists began to recognize that for implants to be successful and survive for extended periods of time in the hostile environment of the stomatognathic system, there had to be an effective biological adaptability between the implant material and the tissues of the jaws. Particularly, it became obvious that the role of the gingival epithelium and its interface with the implant posts was of considerable importance because initial breakdown of tissue usually was first seen around posts, with the onset of inflammatory reactions followed by destructive necrotic processes. Thus Weinmann theorized the concept of a seal around dental implants.[8] More recently, Lavelle[9] and others have emphasized the necessity for the attached gingiva to appropriately adapt to the implant, providing a barrier to the movement of bacteria and oral toxins into the space between implant posts and biological tissues. Although implant dentists began to recognize this was an important area, they were sometimes frustrated in their attempts to prevent the development of inflammation and bacterial ingress in this critical attached gingival zone. Much of this frustration developed because of the lack of scientific data and the failure to appreciate the joint roles of biomaterial surfaces and physiologic tissue response.

James and Kelln[10] were the first to begin a systematic scientific study to investigate this seal phenomena. Using a combination of light microscopy and electron microscopy, they were able to show that the gingival epithelium regenerated a series of epithelial cells following surgery that were consistently similar to those seen in the natural tooth crevicular epithelium and junctional epithelial zones. Other reports showed the presence of hemidesmosomes associated with the regenerated epithelial cells and the presence of an Oricin-positive deposition on the implant surface that suggested the presence of a dental cuticle-like or basal lamina-like structure that would assist in creating a positive attachment between gingival epithelium and the implant surface and that this mechanism developed very rapidly following implantation.[11, 12] In addition, they showed the presence of connective tissue fibers apical to this epithelial interface and discussed the role of these fibers in supporting the surface epithelium.[10] These types of studies were carried out in further detail by McKinney and co-workers, who positively identified the regeneration of the attached gingiva and its ability to form a gingival sulcus lined by crevicular (sulcular) epithelium.[13–17] These findings have been substantiated by numerous others using various biomaterials; thus the presence of a gingival attachment apparatus with epithelial components similar to that seen around natural teeth has been firmly established.[16–22]

The concept of the role of the gingival epithelium in forming a biologic seal is one of great importance in implant dentistry. All dental implants, whether endosteal, transosteal, or subperiosteal, must have a superstructure or coronal portion supported by a post that must pass through the submucosa (lamina propria) and the covering stratified squamous epithelium into the oral cavity. This permucosal passage creates a "weak link" between the prosthetic attachment and the predicted bony support of the implant. This permucosal zone is the area where initial tissue breakdown begins that can result in eventual tissue necrosis and destruction around the implant.

Subperiosteal implants, although not inserted into the bone of the jaw, do rest on the surface of the jaw bone and share in common a post that penetrates the fibrous connective tissue stroma (lamina propria and periostium) and covering epithelium. While the relation to the soft tissue is identical in most respects and therefore subject to the same insults as posts from endosteal implants, the load transmission to the bone is different, and the effect on the underlying bone is probably modified. The significance of the relationship between the pergingival disease process and that of the osseous tissues will be addressed later in this chapter, but it is clear that all types of pergingival implant modalities in use today are faced with the need for an effective biological seal.

The biological seal thus becomes an important and pivotal factor in dental implant longevity. The seal as a physiological barrier, must be effective enough to prevent the ingress of bacterial plaque, toxins, oral debris, and other deleterious substances taken into the oral cavity. All these agents are known initiators of tissue and cell injury and must be prevented from gaining access into the internal environment that provides support for the implant device.

If the seal is violated, it is probable that the adjacent soft tissues will become inflamed. This will be followed by osteoclastic activity of the underlying hard tissue and chronic resorption of the supporting bone. With continued loss of the supporting bone, the discrepancy will fill with granulation tissue and the implant will become increasingly mobile, resulting in percolation or pumping action of the bacterial toxins and degenerative agents further into the internal environment surrounding the implant.[23] Finally, sufficient destruction will occur to give rise to an acute suppurative inflammation or acute inflammation with pain, particularly upon mastication, or extensive mobility that renders support of the dental prosthesis impractical. If degenerative processes are allowed to progress to this extent, the only effective treatment is removal of the implant and debridement of the lesion. Furthermore, if sufficient bone is lost to this destructive procedure, subsequent support of additional implants or other restorative devices may be severely compromised.

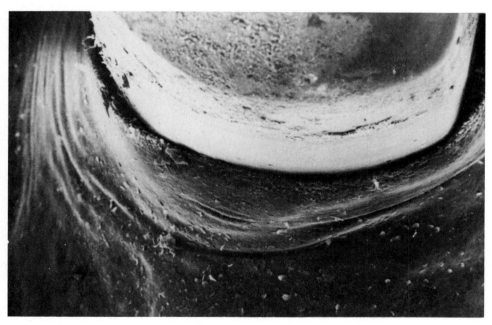

FIG 18–1.
Scanning electron micrograph of an endosteal dental implant in a healed alveolar ridge, demonstrating the healed gingiva and formation of the free gingival margin and gingival sulcus.

Seal Formation

Current concepts of the biological formation of this transmucosal seal indicate that a series of events occur following implant surgery. The attached gingiva regenerates around the implant forming an epithelial "cuff," more appropriately termed the free gingival margin (Fig 18–1). Even though this area has been edentulous, in some cases for long periods of time, the regenerating epithelium forms the free gingival margin complete with free gingival groove and a gingival sulcus.[15] The epithelium regenerates into this sulcus and forms nonkeratinized sulcular (crevicular) epithelium and a zone of epithelial cells at the base of the sulcus that interface the implant surface (Fig 18–2). These regenerated cells have the same morphology as the junctional epithelial cells seen around natural teeth.[15, 16] These epithelial cells at the base of the sulcus produce a series of biological attachment structures that are recognized as part of normal cell biology and physiology. This latter attachment mechanism involves the formation of a basal lamina collagenous structure composed predominately of type IV col-

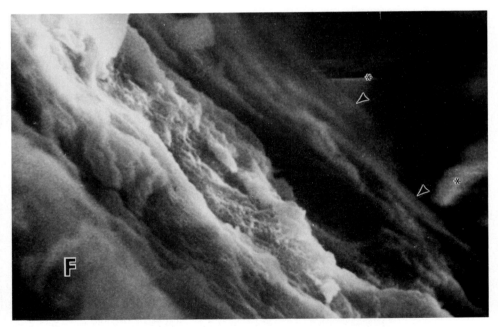

FIG 18–2.
Scanning electron micrograph of the most apical portion of a regenerated gingival sulcus around an endosteal implant. The free gingival margin exhibiting keratinized surface cells is indicated at *F*, and the apical aspect of the sulcus against the implant is indicated by the *arrows*. (White marks indicated by the *asterisks* on the implant face are electron discharge artifacts.)

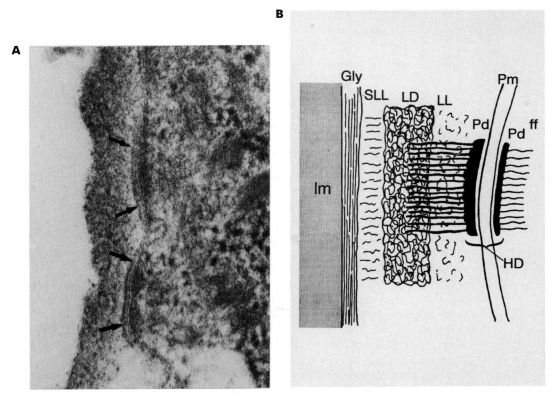

FIG 18–3.
A, transmission electron micrograph shows hemidesmosomes located next to a dental implant post made of surgical-grade vitallium. Implant had functioned in a monkey for 3 months. (Original magnification × 130,000.) (From James RA, Schultz RL: *J Oral Implantol* 1974; IV(3):294. Used by permission.) **B,** attachment component of the gingival epithelium to the implant face as determined from interpretation of transmission electron microscopic studies of the biological seal zone. *Pm* = plasma membrane; *HD* = hemidesmosome; *Pd* = peripheral density; *ff* = fine filaments, *LL* = lamina lucida; *LD* = lamina densa; *SLL* = sublaminal lucida; *Gly* = glycocalyx; *Im* = implant.

lagen.[17] Also developed are hemidesmosomes, which are the attachment plaques to hold epithelial cells to the basal lamina (Fig 18–3,A). In addition, the epithelial cells produce an enzyme called laminin, which serves as an additional molecular bonding agent between the epithelial cells and the various component layers of the basal lamina.[24, 25] The basal lamina component layers are the lamina lucida next to the epithelial cell plasma membrane, next is the lamina densa, followed by the sublamina lucida and a glycosaminoglycan structure on the implant called the linear body (see Fig 18–3). The structures forming the biologic seal are listed in Table 18–1.

TABLE 18–1.

Biological Structures Creating Biological Seal Following
Surgical Placement of an Implant

Epithelial cell with cell membrane
Basal lamina outside cell membrane
    Lamina lucida
    Lamina densa
    Sublamina lucida
Hemidesmosomes on cell membrane
    Peripheral densities
    Pyramidal particles
    Fine filaments
Linear body on implant face

Although collagenous components of the linear body cannot physiologically adhere to or become embedded into the implant biomaterial as they do in the living cementum of the tooth, the high content of glycosaminoglycans (mucopolysaccharides) in the linear body that coats the dental implant has sufficient "stickiness" or gluelike properties to form a biologically active and trauma-resistant attachment at the base of the regenerated gingival sulcus. The longevity of this regenerated structure can be demonstrated by measuring and probing the peri-implant gingival sulcus in long-term implant trials and the successful longevity of many different types of implants that have been placed and followed by critical clinical analysis for many years.[26–29]

Thus the biological seal around dental implants is a definitive entity that must be present to prevent external toxins and agents of the oral cavity from moving into the internal environment of the jaw. The seal serves as an effective barrier to maintain these two distinct environments separate in the peri-implant environment.[30] The dentist must use good dental prophylaxis procedures and instruct the patient in adequate home care to maintain the gingival tissues and preserve the biological seal in a viable and healthy state.

SUPPORT AND LOAD-TRANSFER MECHANISMS

Bone is the biological component within which endosteal and transosteal implants function and on which subperiosteal implants function. Composed of 75% inorganic calcified matrixes, bone is the principal load-bearing organ of vertebrate animals. Consequently, knowledge about bone and its role in implant support must be understood. It not only provides stabilization of the teeth but also cushioning of mastication forces.

Bone must respond in several ways to successfully support an implant. Because most endosteal implants are placed in edentulous areas, the bone must initially be trephined, or drilled, in order to provide a receptor site for the implant. It must respond to osteotomy in a positive manner in order to allow appropriate bone healing to occur. Recent studies have indicated that use of slow-speed rotary cutting instrumentation with internal irrigation provides the least amount of cell damage to bone during the cutting procedure.[31] However, this finding is disputed by others who claim that standard dental rotary cutting procedures with copious externally applied irrigation are just as successful in the healing of bone.[32] There is agreement, however, that there must be minimum elevation of bone temperature during cutting. Following the osteotomy, the bone then must heal around the endosteal implant surface.

With the attachment of a prosthetic device, the bone next experiences the effects from loading the implant. In the case of a one-stage endosteal implant these forces may be applied at any time. Some protocols delay this event until approximately 8 to 12 weeks after insertion of the implant, while others follow a schedule similar to two-stage devices.

With the two-stage devices, the prosthetic loading procedures are usually instituted 4 to 6 months after initial insertion of the implant. When the prosthetic load is placed on the implant, the load is transferred to the bone. Some studies have shown that this load transfer may initiate bone resorption.[33] When threaded implants are used, stress is concentrated around the thread tips, and there is growing evidence that bone in this area may show evidence of active resorption with the development of a highly cellular fibrous stroma that contains no calcified tissue[33, 34] (Fig 18–4). This may indicate that all the recently healed bone has been reabsorbed under the pressure of the prosthetic device and has been replaced with an active fibrocellular connective tissue. Beginning ossification in this fibrocellular stroma has even been observed, which further indicates that activity in this fibrocellular tissue can restore new calcified tissue in approximately 5 to 6 months.[33–35]

Following healing, and restoration of a bone interface, the bone must now be maintained in a healthy state to provide continued long-term support for the implant and prosthesis. Maintenance of healthy bone is predicated on maintenance of good oral health and retention of the established biological seal. The stages of critical bone turnover and healing parameters are summarized as follows:

1. Initial surgery, preparation of osteotomy
2. Bone healing; cellular response and reestablishment of bone-implant interface following surgery
3. Mature bone interface following completion of healing and remodeling of repair bone
4. Prosthetic loading; bone subjected to occlusal forces
5. Bone reabsorption around implant in response to loading; bone replaced with fibrocellular stroma

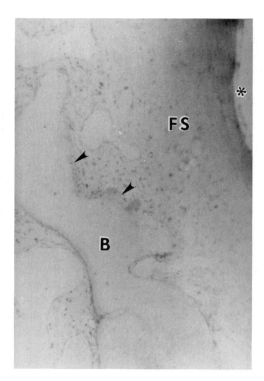

FIG 18–4.
Immediate endosteal peri-implant bone response to prosthetic loading. The bone (**B**) has undergone resorption (*arrows*) and is replaced with a fibrocellular stroma (**FS**) next to the implant (*asterisk*).

6. Ossification begins in fibrocellular stroma
7. Ossification complete; commencement of remodeling in repair bone
8. Mature bone once again interfaces the implant
9. Maintenance of bone in a healthy state by oral hygiene, disease control, and avoidance of occlusal disharmonies

Bone response to the subperiosteal implant is slightly different. In this procedure, the bone is not subjected to an osteotomy that may produce heat and damage the bone cells. However, the elevation of an extensive full thickness flap results in the stripping off of the attached gingiva with lamina propria and underlying periosteal covering from the bone. This temporarily separates the tissues that provide the nutrient supply to the osteoblastic cells and the outer surface of the cortical bone. This surgical technique may disrupt enough nutrient blood supply to allow necrosis of bone osteocytes to occur. With the death of these cells, focal areas of the bone could become nonvital and be eventually reabsorbed by phagocytic cellular activity that is constantly occurring. Thus, in the absence of functional stress stimulation, discrepancies in the adaptation of the subperiosteal substructure to bone could occur and with the passage of time could be attributed to this bone reaction phenomena. The osteoblasts lining the endosteal surfaces of the jaw bone usually become quite active in response to the surgical manipulation of the periostium and respond by initial osteoclastic activity followed by deposition of new bone on the interior surface of the lamellar and cortical bone. Thus the thickness and quantity of the alveolar process may remain approximately stable. From this one may speculate that the repositioning of bone from outer cortical plate to inner bone endosteal surfaces could leave a subperiosteal framework ill fitting. However, superimposition of functional stress on the bone as a result of the placement of the implant could counteract bone loss subjacent to the periosteum. As with any implant, the goal is to restore function to the supporting bone and thus ensure its preservation through the normal remodeling process. The well-established, long-term favorable history of the complete mandibular subperiosteal implant would indicate its frequent meeting of that goal. Current speculation regarding the reaction of the jaw bone to subperiosteal implant placement is summarized as follows:

1. The dissection of the subperiosteum from the bone during implant surgery disrupts the blood supply to the outer cortical bone.
2. The two-stage surgical impression procedure for standard subperiosteal implants disrupts this blood supply twice.
3. The surgical disruption of the outer periosteum stimulates osteoblastic activity of the bone cells lining the internal endosteal layers.
4. The disruption of the periosteum and the stimulation of osteoblastic and osteoclastic activity following implant surgery results in remodeling of the outer cortical alveolar bone under the subperiosteal implant.
5. This remodeling phenomena may give rise to some of the irregularities in terms of framework fit that occur later in the subperiosteal implant function.
6. The alveolar bone will respond to adverse occlusal forces with potential resorption or remodeling of bone during the service period of the implant.

There can be no question as to the reality that any dental implant of any design or material that has supported a prosthesis for several or more years has been load bearing and that some form, method, or mechanism of load transfer has indeed been developed by the host to transmit the occlusal forces to the bone. Two mechanisms have been discussed whereby this phenomenon occurs: (1) the development of an ankylotic-like relationship between the implant and the bone, and (2) the development of an intermediate ligamental system. There has been much discussion as to which is preferable, with most authors preferring the ankylotic state (frequently referred to as osseointegration or a derivative thereof); however, there should be no doubt as to their existence, even though some authors still question the ability of an organism to develop a ligamentous support in the absence of a preexisting periodontal ligament.[36]

The direct bone-implant interface without intervening connective tissue was described as early as 1939 by Strock[37] and more recently by Branemark et al.[38]

A connective tissue structure interposed between dental implants and bone has been a long-recognized entity,[39, 40] but its role in load transfer was considered to be only as some form of cushion or pad. Jahn was the first to describe it as a hammoch-like suspensory ligament.[41] Since then its load transfer mechanism for blade-form and subperiosteal implants has been well described.[23, 42]

It is recognized that bone is ideally suited to withstand compressive loading, whereas ligaments and tendons are best suited to transfer tensile loads. This significant difference must be kept in mind, and in the ensuing years, as we attempt to determine which mechanism may be most desirable, we cannot deny that both are viable.

In recent years the actual distribution of stress in the bone surrounding dental implants has received considerable interest. Studies in this area have relied on photoelastic stress analysis and finite element analysis and seem to be consistent in showing the locations of stress concentrations.[43-49] Such concentrations are shown to be subjacent to the posts of subperiosteal implants regardless of the direction of the force. However, with endosteal implants, the stress concentrations are greatest in the crestal bone when subjected to lateral or transverse forces, and greatest in the apical area under normal or axial loads. Additionally, it has been demonstrated by these methods that implants supported by a ligament do not show the same stress concentrations. It is difficult to model a true ligament or tendon with either of these methods; therefore, most work is being done with ankylosed, root form implants.

One of the weaknesses of conclusions drawn from these types of studies lie in the assumption that stress concentrations lead to breakdown of the hard tissue. To date, no study has been able to define at what point overloading occurs (the so-called physiologic limit); however, some estimates may be made.[50] It is accepted that bone development is stimulated by stress (Wolff's Law), and it is thus possible that stress concentrations in the bone surrounding dental implants result in increased density of bone in these areas. Indeed, it must be assumed that if the stress concentrations do not exceed the physiologic limit of the bone, increased density of the bone in these areas is likely to occur,[52] and there is considerable anecdotal evidence to support this assumption. However, in the case of ankylosed implants, if the physiologic limit of the bone in the emergence zone is exceeded, then vertical bone loss can be expected to occur. This would be followed by an apical extension of the junctional epithelium, which would result in deepening of the sulcus and the establishment of more pathogenic flora.[50]

The rapidity at which the sulcus deepens may also be dependent on the post diameter as well as the surface texture. These factors will be discussed under the topic of the interrelationship between the support and the biologic seal.

As stated earlier, plate form and subperiosteal implants can function either in an ankylosed state or by way of a suspensory ligament or tendon. The inability of a root form implant to function in a ligament may possibly be explained on the basis of biomechanics. The deflection of a viscoelastic material such as a tendon or ligament increases exponentially with its length (Fig 18–5). Therefore, based on the size alone, a ligament that must extend around the smallest possible root form implant will be at least three times as long as one around the strut of a plate-form or subperiosteal implant. This would result in stretch and deflection of the ligament of 27 to 36 times that of the shorter one and would most likely be beyond the scope of physiologic load bearing for the device. Additionally, the ligament supporting a plate form or subperiosteal implant strut is captured and cannot slip, whereas a ligament around a root form implant would be uncaptured and thus would slip over the surface under normal loading and thus fail to be load bearing.

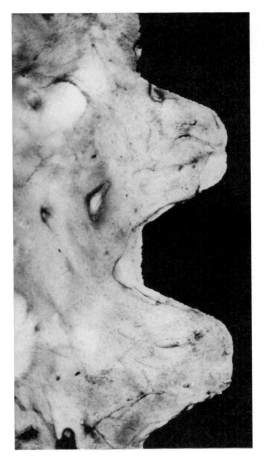

FIG 18–5.
Light photomicrograph showing direct bone interface and adaptation to a titanium endosteal implant following implantation and healing.

As to which is most desirable, it seems intuitive to these authors that load bearing by way of a direct bone-implant interface is the preferable means in that greater loads and more favorable load distribution to the bone should be able to occur. However, there are those who argue that the ligament is preferred because of its damping effect during dynamic loading.

To a certain extent, it appears to be within the hands of the clinician to control which method of load bearing will be established by the host. Relative movement during healing has been shown to be the determining factor.[51] If the implant is loaded so that the implant moves relative to its surrounding bone during the healing phase, then a tendon or ligament will occur around a plate or subperiosteal implant. If the implant is allowed to heal without relative movement, then ankylosis can be expected to occur.

The recognition that a direct bone interface is required for root form endosteal implants has led to the development of two-stage dental implants in which the infrastructure of the device is implanted in the bone in a submerged manner in order to minimize the opportunity for relative movement to occur and thus allow undisturbed interface healing to take place. Following a healing period of 4 to 6

FIG 18–6.
Light photomicrograph revealing healed struts of trabecular (cancellous) bone in direct interface with a ceramic implant following surgical placement, healing, and prosthetic loading.

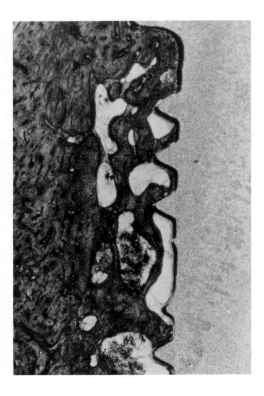

months, the coronal end of the implant is uncovered and the superstructure or second stage of the implant is placed. A one-stage endosteal implant left in a free-standing mode is subject to some degree of pressure from the patient's tongue, cheek, lips, or from mastication of a bolus of food. Pressure against the implant can result in relative movement between the implant and the bone that will disturb the cells involved in bone healing. Unsplinted one-stage root form implants are most prone to such movement, which leads to unsatisfactory adaptation of bone to the implant (Figs 18–5 and 18–6).

INTERRELATIONSHIP BETWEEN SEAL AND SUPPORT

The transmucosal passage of dental implants make them unique from other orthopedic devices. Their survival in a load-bearing capacity while remaining partially exposed to the oral environment is dependent upon the establishment and maintenance of both a biological seal and a load-bearing mechanism. It is convenient to study these two phenomena (seal and support) separately, and this separation can probably be carried out without significant loss of understanding as long as one deals only with their development and structure. However, one cannot examine the pathologic processes within the bony crest without immediately recognizing their interdependence.

Crestal bone loss has been a consistent finding associated with all types of dental implants. The cause of this bone loss has been the subject of considerable discussion and has been attributed to many factors, most of which are still poorly understood. Most theories that attempt to explain this phenomenon fall into two types, one based on principles of mechanical engineering and the other on the autoimmune response of the host. The former looks at the physical properties of the implant material and tissue mechanics, and is led to certain conclusions consistent with the principles of static and dynamic loading. The latter looks at cellular and tissue behavior when subjected to bacterial insult. It seems probable that both approaches have merit and that causality involves an intimate interaction between both aspects of the problem. It is in this area where both seal and support come together that recognition of their interrelation is critical, and it is the belief of these authors that the confusion stems from our attempts to separate them in our thinking.

If one looks at the areas of load concentrations, discussed earlier, one may be led to believe that crestal bone loss is a result of stress concentrations in the emergence zone. However, if one looks at the bacterial flora surrounding dental implants as compared to the natural dentition, one may be led to believe the cause of crestal bone loss is tantamount to periodontal disease.[53–56]

In all probability these two approaches are interrelated and either may on occasion be the primary etiologic factor and the other the secondary. It is probably very dangerous to base clinical therapy on the belief that it is only one or the other.

It can be speculated that an ankylosed implant is less prone to crestal bone loss from bacteria than one functioning in a ligament in that there is greater restriction to a deepening sulcus. Likewise, it can be speculated that an ankylosed implant is more prone to crestal bone loss from crestal stress concentrations than one functioning in a ligament.

Even if the cause of crestal bone loss is similar to that of periodontal disease, conditions may be more favorable around an implant than a tooth, in that nonporous metal surfaces are less likely to accumulate concentrations of endotoxin than are their porous cementum counterparts. A porous surface will permit the rapid establishment of a septic condition when it communicates with the oral cavity,[57] and it is generally agreed that a smooth or polished surface is desirable for an implant post in the pergingival area. Less apparent is the significance of the post diameter in this area, especially if the post diameter is greater than 3.0 mm.

The hemidesmosomal attachment discussed earlier provides a seal against the outside environment. This seal around teeth is protected by Sharpey's fibers extending from the gingival fibers into the tooth, and both implants and teeth are further protected by alternating bands of epithelium and connective tissue in the surrounding gingival cuff. These alternating bands form a viscoelastic system that provides mechanical protection of the hemidesmosomal seal against tearing, which could result from displacement of the cuff by mechanical forces applied within the sulcus (e.g., those exerted by toothbrush bristles or popcorn husks, or hydraulic pressure from a dental hygiene irrigating device [Prophy-Jet]). This tissue effect must follow basic mechanical laws.

As discussed previously relative to the supportive ligaments of implants, the total amount of physical deformation of such a system increases exponentially with the length of the ligament, and because the hemidesmosomal seal only has this circumferential band of tissue to provide mechanical protection against tearing, with no fibers extending into the implant, it can be argued that an implant with a large diameter post will be more prone to violation of this seal from tissue pull than will an implant having a smaller diameter.[58] Clinically, tissue pull around the small-diameter posts associated with some root form, blade form, and most subperiosteal implants is seldom seen, whereas it is a common finding around the larger diameter posts of other implants.

The argument that bone loss in the emergence zone of ankylosed implants (sometimes called saucerization) is due to mechanical overload may be thought to be compromised by the fact that while stress concentrations occur at both the apex and the crestal area, bone loss occurring in the apex is rarely observed clinically, whereas it is a common finding in the crestal area. However, the recognition that loss in the crestal area may be secondarily infected by bacteria—whereas this is unlikely to occur at the apex and, as noted earlier, is reversible—still leaves us uncertain of the primary cause.

One therefore must conclude that neither the biomechanical factors nor the bacterial factors can be ignored, and to do so can lead to serious errors. Ignoring the bacterial role in the pandemic condition of peri-implant disease leads clinicians to the indiscriminate use of overhanging margins and a cavalier approach to poor oral hygiene. Ignoring the possibility of a biomechanical cause can lead a clinician to inappropriate loading. Still, it seems to these authors, that the bacterial factors are more frequently ignored clinically.

SUMMARY AND CONCLUSIONS

A biological seal is a unique phenomena that occurs in the jaws and peri-implant tissues of patients as a result of implant treatment. This biological phenomena is the regeneration and adaptation of biologic cells and tissues to the surfaces of a relatively inert implanted biomaterial. The formation of this biological seal is paramount to the longevity and successful service of the implant and prosthesis system. The biological seal is the tissue barrier created by the body to prevent the ingress of foreign material and bacterial toxins from the oral cavity into the internal environment of the gingival tissues and jaw bone. The biological seal must be maintained by sound oral hygiene and prophylactic procedures. Initial evidence of potential trouble leading to infection and loss of implant will first occur in the zone of the biological seal. The dentist must be cognizant of the signs of inflammation and excess crevicular fluid production and take appropriate measures to correct the occlusal disharmonies or hygiene maintenance problems that are contributing to the breakdown of this seal. Once the biological seal is restored to a healthy state, the long-term prognosis for the implant system is excellent.

Bone is the basic foundation for all dental implant systems. It provides stability for implant devices and the prostheses that they support. The endosteal implant must be placed with careful attention to surgical procedures so as not to damage the delicate cell viability and nutrient blood supply to the bone, which is composed of 75% inorganic calcified matricies. Attention must be paid to maintaining bone in a healthy state during surgical manipulations, impression procedures for subperiosteal implants, initial phases of prosthetic loading, and long-term maintenance. The dentist must understand that bone is an active biological tissue that undergoes periodic resorption and remodeling periods in response to various factors, including occlusal and other forces. If the dentist keeps this biologic activity of bone in mind during surgical and prosthetic procedures, and establishes sound maintenance and recall programs in patients with uncompromised autoimmune responses, the bone can be expected to be maintained in a healthy state, thus assuring long-term serviceability for such dental implants.

REFERENCES

1. Anjard R: Mayan dental wonders, *Oral Implant* 9:423, 1981.
2. Gramm CT: Implantation of foreign objects in the maxilla, *Dent Dig* 4:832, 1898.
3. Lewis TG: Implantation, *Dent Cosmos* 31:385, 1889.
4. Payne C: Gold capsule implantation, *Pacific Dent Gaz* 8:653, 1900.
5. Greenfield EJ: Implantation of artificial roots for crown and bridge work, *Dent Rev* 28:1–7, 1914.
6. Strock AE: Experimental work on a method for the replacement of missing teeth by direct implantation of a metal support into the alveolus, *Am J Orthod* 25:467–472, 1939.
7. Dahl G: Dental implants and superplants, *Rassegna Trimestrale Odont* 37:1952.
8. Weinmann JP: Biological factors influencing implant denture success, *J Implant Dent* 2:12–15, 1956.
9. Lavelle CLB: Mucosal seal around endosseous dental implants, *J Oral Implant* 9:357–371, 1981.
10. James RA, Kelln E: A histopathological report on the nature of the epithelium and underlining connective tissue which surrounds implant posts, *J Biomed Mat Res* 5:373, 1974.
11. James RA, Schultz RL: Hemidesmosomes and the adhesion of junctional epithelial cells to metal implants: a preliminary report, *J Oral Implant* 4:294–302, 1974.
12. Swope EM, James RA: A longitudinal study on hemidesmosome formation at the dental implant-tissue interface, *J Oral Implant* 9:412–422, 1981.
13. Koth DL, McKinney RV Jr: The single crystal sapphire endosteal dental implant. In Hardin JF, editor: *Clark's clinical dentistry,* Philadelphia, 1981, JB Lippincott, chapter 53.
14. McKinney RV Jr, Koth DL: The single crystal endosteal dental implant: material characteristics and 18-month experimental animal trials, *J Prosthet Dent* 47:69–84, 1982.
15. McKinney RV Jr, Steflick DE, Koth DL: The biological response to the single crystal sapphire endosteal dental implant: scanning electron microscopic observations, *J Prosthet Dent* 51:372–379, 1984.
16. McKinney RV Jr, Steflik DE, Koth DL: Ultrastructural surface topography of the single crystal sapphire endosseous dental implant, *J Prosthet Dent* 51:372–379, 1984.
17. McKinney RV Jr, Steflik DE, Koth DL: Evidence for a junctional epithelial attachment to ceramic dental implants:a transmission electron microscopic study, *J Periodontol* 56:579–591, 1985.
18. Listgarten MA, Lai CH: Ultrastructure of the intact interface between an endosseous epoxy resin dental implant and host tissue, *J Biol Buccale* 3:13, 1975.
19. Ogiso, M et al: Investigation of hydroxyapatite ceramic implant under occlusal function, *J Dent Res* 60A:419, 1981.
20. Hausson HA, Albrektssan T, Branemark PI: Structural aspects of the interface between tissue and titanium implants, *J Prosthet Dent* 50:108, 1983.
21. Gould T, Westbury L, Burnette D: Ultrastructural study of the attachment of human gingiva to titanium in vivo, *J Prosthet Dent* 52:418, 1984.
22. Hashimoto M et al: Ultrastructure of the peri-implant junctional epithelium on

single-crystal sapphire endosseous dental implant loaded with functional stress, *J Oral Rehabil* 16:261–270, 1989.

23. James RA: Tissue response to dental implant devices. In Hardin JF (editor): *Clark's clinical dentistry,* Philadelphia, 1986, JB Lippincott, chapter 48.

24. Campbell JH, Terrarova VP: Laminin: molecular organization and biological function, *J Oral Pathol* 17:309–323, 1988.

25. McKinney RV Jr, Steflik DE, Koth DL: The epithelium dental implant interface, *J Oral Implant* 13:622–641, 1988.

26. Smithlof J, Fritz ME: The use of blade implants in a selected population of partially edentulous adults: a 15-year report, *J Periodontol* 58:589–593, 1987.

27. Albrektsson T et al: Osseointegrated oral implants: a Swedish multicenter study of 8,139 consecutively inserted Nobelpharma implants, *J Periodontol* 59:287–296, 1988.

28. Koth DL et al: Clinical and statistical analyses of human clinical trials with the single crystal alumina oxide endosteal dental implant: five-year results, *J Prosthet Dent* 60:226–234, 1988.

29. James RA et al: Subperiosteal implants, *Calif Dent Assoc J* 16:10–14, 1988.

30. McKinney RV, Jr, Steflik DE, Koth DL: Per, peri, or trans? *J Prosthet Dent* 52:267–269, 1984.

31. Lavelle C, Wedgwood D: Effect of internal irrigation on frictional heat generated from bone drilling, *J Oral Surg* 38:499–503, 1980.

32. Matthews LS, Hirsch C: Temperature measured in human cortical bone when drilling, *J Bone Joint Surg* 54:297–308, 1972.

33. McKinney RV Jr, et al: Histological results from a comparative endosteal dental implant study, *J Dent Res* 66(spec issue):186, 1987.

34. Steflik DE, McKinney RV Jr, Koth DL: Ultrastructural comparisons of ceramic and titanium dental implants in vivo: a scanning electron microscopic study, *J Biomed Mater Res* 23:895–909, 1989.

35. Steflik DE, McKinney RV Jr, Koth DL: Light and scanning electron microscopic characterizations of the apical support system to endosteal dental implants, Transactions of the 15th Annual Meeting, International Manufacturing Society for Biomaterials, Lake Buena Vista, Fla, 1989, vol 12, p 62.

36. Ten Cate AR: Biological determinants in implant design, *Int Dent J* 39:108–112, 1989.

37. Strock AE: Experimental work on a method for the replacement of missing teeth by direct implantation of a metal support into the alveolus, *Am J Orthod* 25:1465, 1939.

38. Branemark P-I et al: Osseointegrated implants in the treatment of the edentulous jaw: experience from a 10-year period, *Scand J Plast Reconstr Surg* 11(suppl 16), 1977.

39. Herschfus L: Histopathologic studies of five year implants in dogs, *J Implant Dent* 4:12–21, 1957.

40. Bodine R, Melrose R, Grenoble D: Long-term implant denture histology and comparison with previous reports, *J Prosthet Dent* 35:665–673, 1976.

41. Jahn E: Bindegewebige aufhangung bei lattimplantaten: Vorlaufige Mitteilung. *Schweiz Monatsschr Zahnheilkd* 85:1143, 1975.

42. Weiss CM: A comparative analysis of fibro-osteal and osteal integration and other variables that affect long-term bone maintenance around dental implants, *J Oral Implant* 13:467–487, 1987.

43. Jones SD, Travis C: Load-transfer characteristics of mandibular subperiosteal implants, *J Prosthet Dent* 42:211, 1979.
44. Bidez MW, Staphens BJ, Lemons JE: An investigation into the effect of blade dental implant length on interfacial tissue stress profiles. In Spilker RL, Simon MR, editors: *Computational methods in bioengineering,* Proceedings of the American Society of Mechanical Engineers Winter Annual Meeting, Chicago, Nov 17–Dec 2, 1988.
45. Siegele D, Soltasz U: Numerical investigations of the influence of implant shape on stress distribution in the jaw bone, *Int J Oral Maxillofac Implants* 4:333–340, 1989.
46. French AA et al: Comparison of peri-implant stresses transmitted by four commercially available osseointegrated implants, *Int J Periodontol Rest Dent* 9:221–230, 1989.
47. Rieger MR et al: Alternative materials for three endosseous implants, *J Prosthet Dent* 61:717–722, 1989.
48. Rieger MR, Mayberry J, Brose MO: Finite element analysis of six endosseous implants, *J Prosthet Dent* 63:671–676, 1990.
49. van Rossen IP et al: Stress-absorbing elements in dental implants, *J Prosthet Dent* 64:198–205, 1990.
50. Roberts WE et al: Rigid endosseous implants for orthodontic and orthopedic anchorage, *Angle Orthodont* 59:247–256, 1989.
51. Brunski J: The influence of functional use of endosseous dental implants on the tissue-implant interface. I: histological aspects, *J Dent Res* 58:1953, 1979.
52. Roberts WE, Garetto LP, DeCastro RA: Remodeling of devitalized bone threatens periosteal margin integrity of endosseous titanium implants with threaded or smooth surfaces: indications for provisional loading and axially directed occlusion, *J Indiana Dent Assoc* 68:19–24, 1989.
53. James RA: The support system and the pergingival defense mechanism of oral implants, *J Oral Implant* 6:270, 1976.
54. Lekholm U et al: The condition of the soft tissues of tooth and fixture abutments supporting fixed bridges, a microbiological and histological study, *J Clin Periodontol* 13:558–562, 1986.
55. Apse P et al: Microbiota and crevicular fluid collagenase activity in the osseointegrated dental implant sulcus: a comparison of sites in edentulous and partially edentulous patients, *J Periodontol Res* 24:96–105, 1989.
56. Becker W et al: Clinical and microbiologic findings that may contribute to dental implant failure, *Int J Oral Maxillofac Implants* 5:31–38, 1990.
57. Kent JN, Homsy CA: Pilot studies of a porous implant in dentistry and oral surgery, *J Oral Surg* 30:608, 1972.
58. James RA: Basic principles of endosteal dental implant design. In Hardin JF, editor: *Clark's clinical dentistry,* Philadelphia, 1981, JB Lippincott.

Chapter 19

Pharmacologic Considerations in Implant Dentistry

Daniel E. Becker
Paul A. Moore

GENERAL PRINCIPLES

The introduction of dental implant therapy into a dental practice requires not only the use of rigorous prosthetic and surgical techniques but also a clear understanding of dental therapeutics. Patients requiring implants have frequently had unfavorable dental experiences, have avoided routine dental care, and may be quite apprehensive of the implant procedures and outcomes. A large number of these patients are older adults who are concurrently taking medications for chronic diseases and who may have compromised healing and immune responses. A clear understanding of the indications and contraindications of dental therapeutic agents is essential to maximize patient comfort and surgical success. This chapter provides a guide of the dental pharmacotherapeutics that may be specifically useful to practitioners who are incorporating dental implants into their practice. It cannot replace more extensive references on specific agents and therapies.

Pharmacokinetics

Pharmacokinetics is a division of pharmacology that deals with drug absorption, distribution, biotransformation, and elimination. In essence, these processes reflect the body's effects on the drug. Pharmacodynamics pertains to the actions and effects a drug exerts on the body. An overview of these principles is followed by a synopsis of drug classes having particular importance for the implant dentist.

Drug Absorption

The term "bioavailability" refers to the portion of an administered drug that reaches the systemic circulation in active form and is thereby available for distribution to the intended tissue. The bioavailability of a drug is influenced mostly by its absorption and the properties of the pharmaceutical preparation.

Absorption is the process by which drug molecules leave the site of administration and enter the systemic circulation. Oral and topical administrations require that the drug diffuse across the cell membranes of epithelium; therefore, the drug must exhibit some degree of lipid solubility. Ionized (charged) molecules are water soluble and are therefore absorbed poorly. However, water solubility is not as detrimental following intramuscular (IM) and subcutaneous injection because the drug molecules can dissolve in extracellular fluid and diffuse between the loosely joined endothelial cells. Connective and adipose tissue at the injection site may delay the rate of absorption by impeding access to the capillary endothelium. Absorption is not required when drugs are administered intravenously.

To achieve effective serum concentrations, doses for a drug administered orally (PO) are generally greater than those for any parenteral route. Following absorption through gastric or intestinal mucosa, the drug enters the portal system and must pass through the liver before it gains access to the systemic circulation. In such cases, drugs are subjected to "first-pass metabolism," and this may reduce its subsequent bioavailability. Additional reasons for differences in oral and parenteral administration include slow dissolution, poor lipid solubility, binding to foods, and degradation in gastric juices. Drugs absorbed through, or injected into, oral mucous membranes bypass the portal circulation and avoid significant first-pass metabolism. This provides the rationale for sublingual administration of nitroglycerin tablets.

Distribution

Following absorption, drugs are distributed to most body tissues in proportion to the tissue's perfusion and the drug's solubility or affinity for the particular tissue. For example, both diazepam and tetracycline are distributed to skeletal muscle because of the high perfusion of this tissue. However, diazepam also distributes to fatty tissues, whereas tetracycline has great affinity for calcium ions in bone and cartilage. The intended target organ may receive only a modicum of the total amount absorbed. For convenience, nontarget tissues are viewed as reservoirs for drug storage.

Distribution to brain tissue is impeded by tighter capillary endothelial junctions and the presence of pericapillary glial cells.[1] Therefore, drugs must be lipid soluble if they are to produce effects on the central nervous system (CNS). The capillary network of the placenta is analogous to that found in the brain, favoring the diffusion of lipid-soluble drugs. Still, one should suspect that a fetus is potentially exposed to all medications taken by the mother. For this reason, most drugs should be avoided, if possible, during pregnancy.

Most drugs bind to plasma proteins, and this influences their availability for distribution to the target site. Acidic drugs are primarily bound to albumin, whereas basic drugs bind to alpha-1-acid glycoprotein. When bound to these proteins, drugs are "trapped" or stored within the plasma and cannot undergo distribution or elimination.[2] During the research and development of a drug, scientists calculate the percentage of protein binding in order to establish dosage recommendations. Significant reductions in plasma proteins may allow increased intensity of drug effect unless dosage is reduced, but this consideration is often overstated. This is particularly true regarding geriatric patients, who comprise a significant portion of an implant-related dental practice. Although geriatric patients are generally more sensitive to drug effects, diminished plasma protein is not a factor provided the patient is healthy otherwise.[3] Age-related reductions in hepatic blood flow and renal function and decrease in lean body mass are more significant explanations for heightened sensitivity and residual drug effects in geriatric patients.[4]

Drug Metabolism

Metabolism, or biotransformation, refers to chemical changes of the drug molecule. In general, biotransformation converts lipid-soluble molecules into water-soluble metabolites that are more suitable for renal elimination. The principal site for drug biotransformation is the microsomal enzyme system of the gut wall and liver. However, we must appreciate that enzymes are ubiquitous and therefore provide countless additional sites at which reactions can occur. For example, the plasma esterases are responsible for hydrolysis of many esters, including succinylcholine and procaine.

The pharmacologic activity of drug molecules vary, as do the ability of the drugs to produce beneficial and harmful effects. The activity and toxicity of the parent drug (molecular structure at the time of administration) must be distinguished from that of its metabolites: "metabolism" and "detoxification" are not synonymous. For example, prednisone is a very useful anti-inflammatory agent that is inactive as a parent drug and must undergo hepatic biotransformation to prednisolone, its active metabolite. So-called "prodrugs" must be administered orally to assure adequate hepatic biotransformation. In contrast, diazepam (Valium) is active as a parent drug and is also biotransformed to several active metabolites. These include desmethyldiazepam, which is eliminated more slowly than diazepam, the parent drug. In certain cases, metabolites produce effects different from those of the parent compound. Normeperidine is an active metabolite of meperidine that acts as a CNS stimulant. Because it is eliminated more slowly than its parent compound, prolonged use of meperidine may result in CNS toxicity.

Microsomal enzymes are critical for drug biotransformation, and certain consequences may follow inhibition or induction of their activity. The decreased microsomal activity associated with aging and liver disease certainly warrants a dose reduction for most medications. Also, patients may receive several prescriptions, often from different practitioners. Thus a comprehensive knowledge of each drug's influence on microsomal enzyme activity is required.

Drug Excretion

The principal route for drug elimination is renal excretion, but molecules that remain lipid soluble are excreted in feces. Other routes are generally regarded as insignificant. Because human milk may account for 1% or 2% of maternal drug elimination,[5] consideration should be given to any medication prescribed for patients who are nursing.

Elimination half-life ($t_{1/2}$) is the time necessary for the plasma concentration of a drug to decrease by 50%. The value of this parameter is often overestimated. One must not assume that $t_{1/2}$ and duration of clinical effect necessarily correlate. For example, the half-life for diazepam (Valium), along with its active metabolite desmethyldiazepam, may vary from 24 to 90 hours, yet its sedative and anxiolytic effects are shorter than that for another benzodiazepine, lorazepam (Ativan), whose half-life ranges only 8 to 25 hours.[6, 7] The fact that drug remains in the body does not assure that it is present in adequate concentration at the target tissue. Therefore, $t_{1/2}$ does not predict the duration of clinical effects.

Impressive ranges in $t_{1/2}$ also illustrate the fact that it alone is not a precise indicator for the overall clearance of a drug. It varies according to each patient's renal and hepatic function, and also by his or her body composition, which influences the drug's volume of distribution. A patient having a large percentage of body fat will retain lipid-soluble drugs longer because of drug storage.[8] For example, diazepam is a lipid-soluble drug having an extremely variable $t_{1/2}$. One should anticipate prolonged elimination in a geriatric patient for two reasons. With aging, body composition contains a greater proportion of fat, and both renal and hepatic clearance are reduced.

Two generalizations can be made regarding elimination half-life. A reasonably consistent plasma concentration will follow four or five doses, provided each is administered after one half-life. Conversely, following discontinuation, five half-lives must pass before the drug can be regarded as essentially eliminated.[1]

Pharmacodynamics

The term "effect" is simply the physiologic changes a drug produces. Two examples of drug effects would be "decreased heart rate" and "sedation." Drug "indications" reflect the conditions suffered by the patient and essentially represent the opposite of drug effects. In the examples given, drug indications could include tachycardia and insomnia.

Drugs are incapable of producing a single effect. All produce a variety of effects, some that are desirable and others that are not. Desired effects are generally described as "primary," and others are arbitrarily designated as "side effects" or "adverse effects." Furthermore, a particular effect may be regarded as primary in one patient, but adverse in another. The constipating effect of opioids (narcotics) is a bothersome side effect when these drugs are being used to manage pain. However, this same effect is desired when using opioids to manage diarrhea.

Dose-Response Considerations

The intensity of a drug's primary effect is referred to as "efficacy." When choosing between drugs of comparable cost and safety, preference must be given to the one demonstrating greatest efficacy. "Potency" refers to the quantity of drug required to produce an effect. Potency does not reliably correlate with efficacy or toxicity.[1] Unfortunately, the term is frequently misused as a synonym for efficacy. Drugs belonging to the same class generally produce comparable efficacy, provided one administers equivalent doses. Such doses are designated as "equipotent." Meperidine (Demerol) is more potent than codeine. When administered by the same route, using equipotent doses (i.e., 75 and 120 mg, respectively), they exhibit comparable analgesic efficacy and side effect profile.[1] The potency and efficacy of similar drugs can be compared using a dose-response curve (Fig. 19–1).

Drug Action

The mechanism by which a drug produces an effect is described as its "action." In many cases, drug action involves an interaction with specific macromolecular components of cells. These components are operationally defined as "receptors." Most receptors are protein in structure and represent the cellular component with which endogenous molecules interact to produce normal physiologic responses.

Drugs have been synthesized to interact with receptors in two manners. Those that bind to the receptor and initiate a response are called "agonists." Others able to bind to receptors but unable to initiate a response are called "antagonists" and function clinically as blockers, denying agonists or endogenous ligands access to the receptor.

In addition to receptor mechanisms, drugs may also produce effects by interacting with enzymes that regulate specific metabolic pathways. Drugs that increase a particular enzyme's activity are called "enzyme inducers"; while those that diminish enzyme activity are called "enzyme inhibitors." Although this concept may resemble that described for receptor mechanisms, it must be distinguished, because enzymes are not regarded as structural components of cells.

Aspirin provides an excellent example of enzyme inhibition. Most of its effects have been explained by an inhibitory effect on cyclooxygenases that convert

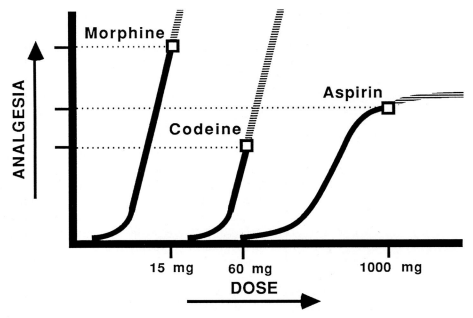

FIG 19–1.
Summary of dose-response relationships for three analgesics: morphine, codeine, and aspirin. Recommended dosages are limited by respiratory depression with morphine, nausea with codeine, and maximum analgesic response with aspirin. At therapeutic doses morphine 15 mg IM is more effective than aspirin 1,000 mg PO, and aspirin 1,000 mg PO is more effective than codeine 60 mg PO.

arachidonic acid to prostaglandins. Prostaglandins are involved in the production of pain, fever, and inflammation. By inhibiting the enzymes responsible for prostaglandin synthesis, aspirin produces analgesic, antipyretic, and anti-inflammatory effects.

MANAGEMENT OF POSTOPERATIVE PAIN

Dentists have traditionally relied on the aspirin-like and morphine-like drugs to minimize postsurgical pain. After surgery, pain and inflammation frequently occur, and multiple strategies, both pharmacologic and behavioral, are essential to optimize patient comfort. Because surgical procedures for the placement of dental implants are often extensive and involve manipulation of bone and periosteum, significant postoperative pain is likely to occur. Additionally, because implant surgery is not a common oral surgical procedure (e.g., dental extractions), most patients have some anxiety regarding the overall surgical outcome that may amplify their discomfort. A thorough explanation of the procedure and expected postoperative sequelae is an essential part of postoperative pain management.

As more is understood about the mechanism of action for analgesics and as newer analgesics are marketed, the traditional classifications for analgesic drugs become less acceptable. The terms "peripheral" and "central" have traditionally been used for describing the aspirin-like and morphine-like agents. However, both classes exert their analgesic action through complex mechanisms that involve both the central and peripheral nervous systems. The term "opioids" has been used to describe agents that have actions similar to that of opium and interact with morphine receptors. Although this may be an accurate term, its counterpart, "nonopioid," is confusing and not very specific.

The term "nonsteroidal anti-inflammatory drugs (NSAIDs)" has gained acceptance in recent years, in part due to the many analgesics and antiarthritics that have been marketed to compete with aspirin. Yet the term NSAID does not accurately describe the mechanisms of all peripheral analgesics (notably acetaminophen). With an appreciation for the problems associated with analgesic terminology and a lack of any clear consensus, this section will use the term "opioid" to describe agents that produce analgesia similar to morphine, and the term "nonopioid" to describe acetaminophen and the aspirin-like analgesics.

Nonopioid Analgesics

Bradykinin, histamine, and oxidation products of arachidonic acid released in response to tissue injury are implicated in the development of inflammation and pain. Cell damage that occurs during surgery releases a fatty acid (arachidonic acid) from disrupted membrane phospholipids by an enzyme called phospholipase. This arachidonic acid reacts with molecular oxygen in the presence of cyclooxygenase to produce a variety of biologically active factors, including prostaglandins, prostacyclins, thromboxanes, leukotrienes, and HPETEs (hydroperoxyeicosatetraenoic acids).

The prostaglandins have many inflammatory functions depending on their specific chemical structure and the targeted organ system.[9] Prostaglandin E_2 appears to play a major role in the initiation of pain and swelling. This prostaglandin can sensitize pain receptors, thereby contributing to the development of hyperalgesia at the site of tissue injury. Hyperalgesia following surgery is characterized by spontaneous pain, decreased pain threshold, and increased sensitivity to suprathreshold stimuli. Tenderness is the most obvious sign of hyperalgesia.

Prostaglandins also enhance the edema and pain initiated by bradykinin and histamine.[10, 11] The edematous response that occurs following surgery is a result of vasodilatation and increased vascular permeability, allowing blood elements to flow from the vascular compartment into the interstitial space. Edema is the result of fluid transferred from vascular spaces to the extracellular tissue. The prolonged duration of postsurgical pain results in part from this plasma extravasation, which replenishes inflammatory mediators such as bradykinin. While prostaglandins potentiate the actions of bradykinin, bradykinin in turn stimulates the synthesis of prostaglandins. This feedback relationship contributes to the duration of the clinical signs of inflammation, which persist far beyond the time course associated with the tissue damage of the dental procedure.

The mechanism of action of NSAIDs is believed to result primarily from inhibition of the synthesis of prostaglandins from arachidonic acid.[12] By inhibiting the enzyme cyclooxygenase, conversion of arachidonic acid to prostaglandins is interrupted. It is proposed that by limiting the synthesis of prostaglandins in traumatized tissue, the hyperalgesia and edema associated with acute inflammation can be minimized.

The nonopioid agents most useful and most frequently prescribed for analgesia are listed in Table 19–1. Although other agents such as naproxen, ketoprofen, and flurbiprofen are available, a clear therapeutic advantage to these has yet to be demonstrated. All of these agents, with the possible exception of acetaminophen, have anti-inflammatory properties. It is interesting to note that the dose of a NSAID that provides maximum analgesia may not be adequate in preventing swelling. Generally the dose to manage swelling in arthritis is two to three times the dose that provides maximum analgesia.

Acetaminophen has gained popularity in the past 20 years as an over-the-counter analgesic and as a component of many prescription compounds. Its pharmacologic spectrum differs distinctly from those of the classic NSAIDs such as aspirin, ibuprofen, and diflunisal. Although it provides analgesic and antipyretic effects comparable to aspirin, at equivalent doses acetaminophen has little anti-inflammatory activity.

Unlike aspirin, acetaminophen does not erode the gastrointestinal mucosa and has little effect on platelet aggregation and bleeding. Clearly this latter distinction is important when considering extensive implant surgery. An increase

TABLE 19–1.

Nonopioid Analgesics

Agent	Dose (mg)	Regimen	Comment
Ibuprofen	200–400	q4h	Limited effect on hemostasis; low incidence of gastrointestinal (GI) upset; excellent analgesia for moderate pain
Acetaminophen	650–1,000	q4–6 h	Alternative when allergy to aspirin; little anti-inflammatory effect
Diflunisal	500	1,000 mg stat; then q8–12 h	Long-acting; slow onset; excellent analgesia for moderate pain
Aspirin	650–1,000	q4–6h	Increased bleeding; GI upset common

in oozing under full thickness flaps caused by the use of aspirin can only compromise healing and the overall success of surgery.

Because prostaglandin E_2 is a stimulus for bone resorption, NSAIDs may play a role in periodontics and implant dentistry. Investigations are under way of newer NSAIDs (such as flurbiprofen) for use as adjunctive therapy to slow bone loss associated with rapidly progressing periodontitis and to improve osteointegration of dental implants. The use of NSAIDs to improve surgical outcomes may become the accepted standard of care in the near future.

Preoperative NSAIDS

Use of nonopioid analgesics prior to or immediately following surgery to diminish postoperative sequelae has become more common in recent years. The agents most frequently studied have been acetaminophen and ibuprofen.[13, 14] Because aspirin can significantly alter normal hemostasis, it is obviously not recommended for prophylactic therapy. The justification for using a prophylactic regimen relies on three possible mechanisms. The first is that cyclooxygenase inhibition might be more effective prior to surgical trauma and the initial production of prostaglandins. Second, when administered prior to surgery, the agent has time to be absorbed and for adequate levels to be established in the blood by the time local anesthesia dissipates. Last, because the newer NSAIDs have anti-inflammatory properties, the amount of swelling and trismus that occur postoperatively may be reduced.

Although the anti-inflammatory efficacy of NSAIDs after surgery is modest, overall patient comfort has been shown to improve. A recent review of prophylactic NSAID therapy in dentistry concluded that, when moderate pain and swelling is expected, ibuprofen 400 mg is the drug of choice.[15] Although 1,000 mg of acetaminophen has been shown to significantly decrease postoperative pain following third molar extractions, the anti-inflammatory effects of ibuprofen may provide added benefit.[14] Other agents such as flurbiprofen and diflunisal have also been shown to be effective. If swelling is expected to be severe enough to possibly compromise the surgical outcome, a more aggressive anti-inflammatory therapy using steroids is recommended (description below).[16]

Opioid Analgesics

Few drugs have had greater acceptance in medicine and dentistry than the opioid analgesics. Morphine, the primary derivative of opium, is the standard for all other analgesics. Its predominance in therapeutics, dating back to the third century BC, is particularly impressive when compared with the numerous alternative analgesics that have been introduced into practice in recent years. There are no analgesic agents more effective than the opioids in relieving severe acute pain. The NSAIDs provide valuable alternatives, particularly for mild to moderate postoperative pain. However, the relative safety and efficacy of these recently marketed analgesics will ultimately be judged by their comparability to opioid analgesics.

Although a specific site of action for opiates had been postulated for many decades, morphine-binding sites within the nervous system were demonstrated only recently.[17] The distribution of these receptors is not ubiquitous in the CNS but is limited to specific regions implicated in the perception of pain. The search for endogenous ligands with opiate receptor–binding properties culminated in the isolation of a group of polypeptides, termed endorphins.

The properties of the endorphins are remarkably similar to those of morphine. Endorphins produce not only analgesia but also the undesirable properties of the opioids such as respiratory depression, physical dependence, and tolerance. Endorphins, as well as the exogenous opioid analgesics, appear to inhibit neurotransmission along central pain pathways, probably by inhibiting the release of an excitatory pain transmitter. Additionally, peripheral actions of opioids in blocking pain and inflammation have been recently described.[18]

At equianalgesic doses, the spectrum of CNS effects produced by the opioid analgesics are remarkably similar. These include analgesia, drowsiness, respiratory depression, euphoria, pupillary constriction, stimulation of the chemoreceptor trigger zone for emesis, and suppression of the cough reflex. Peripheral responses to morphine and its congeners include increased intestinal smooth muscle tone, increased uterine tone, and bronchial constriction. Release of histamine, causing peripheral vasodilation and hypotension, is common, particularly following intravenous administration of opioid analgesics.

The analgesic property of all opioid analgesics is dose-related. The dose-analgesia relationships for morphine, codeine, and aspirin are shown in Figure 19–1. The curve for aspirin, as well as the other NSAIDs, displays a plateau. Increasing the dose of aspirin beyond the plateau provides little additional relief of pain. Analgesic doses of 650 to 1,000 mg represent the maximal response that can be achieved. On the other hand, morphine and codeine do not have a plateau in their analgesic response curves. The customary doses for morphine (10 mg IM) and codeine (60 mg PO) do not represent the maximally effective dose, but the point above which a significant incidence of side effects is first noted. An IM dose of 20 mg of morphine will provide greater pain relief as well as a significant degree of respiratory depression. An oral dose of 120 mg codeine will also provide more relief of pain. However, an unacceptable number of patients may report nausea and vomiting at this dose.

Patient Instructions

The pharmacologic effectiveness of any analgesic is maximized by providing accurate and thorough postoperative instructions. If clear written and oral instructions are not provided, patient compliance will probably be unsatisfactory. Noncompliance associated with antibiotic therapy may effect healing and surgical success. Noncompliance associated with analgesics results in added discomfort during the postoperative period.

A recent study of pain following oral surgery found the regimen for administration to be important.[14] Instructions to take analgesics as needed (prn) provided better pain relief than fixed interval (e.g., every 4 hours) instructions, even though identical doses of analgesics were consumed. A probable explanation for the enhanced analgesia is based on patient expectations. Fixed interval instructions imply a need for the medication. A patient assumes that, if strong analgesics are required, severe pain must be an expected outcome of surgery. On the other hand, instructions that the analgesic should be taken "when and if they are needed" may not establish painful expectations.

An effective strategy for prescribing analgesics postoperatively is illustrated in the following instructions:

> Before the local anesthetic wears off, I recommend taking two 200-mg ibuprofen tablets [name an over-the-counter product if you like]. Continue with this when and if you need relief. For many of my patients this provides adequate pain relief.
>
> In addition, I'm providing you with a prescription for a stronger analgesic in case you are not getting adequate relief from the ibuprofen. You can have it filled immediately if you want. If you are having any problems, feel free to call me.

These instructions provide analgesic instructions adequate for the relief of either moderate or severe pain without establishing unfavorable expectations. The need for a stronger opioid combination prescription can thereby be minimized.

Drug Interactions

Concomitant drug therapy is likely to augment a patient's response to opioids, possibly producing severe adverse effects (Table 19–2). The phenothiazines, monoamine oxidase inhibitors, and tricyclics are most commonly implicated in unexpected increases in sedation and narcotic respiratory depression. This known supra-additive interaction necessitates that a practitioner avoid prescribing opiates to patients taking these agents. The depressant effects of narcotics can also be increased by concomitant administration of alcohol, barbiturates, benzodiazepines, and antihistamines.

Protocol for Selection of Analgesic

Because there are numerous opioid analgesics available, the process of selection can appear somewhat perplexing. In implant dentistry, one can place these agents into three discrete categories, according to recipient, thereby

TABLE 19–2.

Adverse Drug Interactions Involving Opioids

Interacting Agent	Resulting Effect
Barbiturates Alcohol Benzodiazepines Anesthetics Chloral hydrate	Enhanced sedation and CNS depression
α-Adrenergic blockers	Exaggerated hypotension
Phenothiazines Tricyclic antidepressants	Supra-additive enhancement of CNS and respiratory depression
Monoamine oxidase inhibitors	Following meperidine, unexpected excitation, delirium, hyperpyrexia and convulsions

simplifying the process of selection: hospitalized patients with severe pain; dental outpatients with severe pain; and dental outpatients with moderate pain. The drug of choice for each of the following circumstances is listed first. Alternative analgesics and agents with special indications are also provided.

RELIEF OF SEVERE PAIN IN HOSPITAL PATIENTS

Hospitalized patients with severe or moderately severe pain can be best managed using the parenteral opioid agents (Table 19–3). In this controlled setting, patients can be administered larger doses of narcotics because possible adverse reactions can be recognized and managed. Nausea and vomiting (problems seen more frequently in ambulatory patients) are minimized because patients remain recumbent. Also, because these patients can be monitored throughout the day, agents with longer durations can be used.

RELIEF OF SEVERE PAIN IN DENTAL OUTPATIENTS

The available agents for managing severe acute pain in dental outpatients are shown in Table 19–4. The agents can be administered orally and have slightly lower potential for intravenous drug abuse. The doses are generally well tolerated, although nausea is sometimes reported. These agents are almost always

TABLE 19–3.

Analgesics for Hospitalized Patients With Severe Pain

Agent	Route	Adult Dose (mg)	Duration (hr)
Morphine sulfate	IM	10–15	4–5
Meperidine (Demerol)	IM	80–100	2–4

marketed in combination with peripheral analgesics, such as aspirin or acetaminophen, to achieve the most favorable response. The newer NSAIDs, such as ibuprofen and diflunisal, are not presently formulated in combination with codeine or its derivatives.

Oral meperidine is sometimes considered to be a possible alternative to the codeine analogues. The usual dose of 50 to 100 mg administered orally is significantly less effective than the same dose given parenterally. The routine use of oral meperidine is not recommended because it provides no advantage over a codeine preparation in terms of analgesia and because increased abuse potential may attract drug-abusing patients to the dental office.

RELIEF OF MODERATE PAIN IN DENTAL OUTPATIENTS

The agents most commonly prescribed for moderate pain are combinations of codeine (at lower doses) and nonopioid analgesics. It should be noted however, that most of the patients having mild-to-moderate pain can be managed with NSAIDs alone (Table 19–4).

Propoxyphene (Darvon) is a popular analgesic marketed in a variety of preparations that include different doses and combinations. The analgesic

TABLE 19–4.

Analgesics for Dental Patients

Agent	Route	Adult Narcotic Dose (mg)	Duration (hr)
Patients with severe pain			
Acetaminophen 650 mg with codeine 60 mg (Tylenol 3), 2 tablets	PO	60	4
Acetaminophen 500 mg with oxycodone 5 mg (Tylox)	PO	5	6
Patients with moderate pain			
Acetaminophen 650 mg with codeine 30 mg (Tylenol 2), 2 tablets	PO	30	4–5
Ibuprofen 400 mg (Advil), 2 tablets	PO	200	4

properties of propoxyphene are minimal and are frequently difficult to demonstrate in controlled drug trials. It appears to have no advantage over peripheral analgesics with or without lower doses of codeine.

Pentazocine (Talwin) is a benzomorphan analgesic with agonist and mild antagonist activity. Although doses of 50 mg are reportedly equivalent to 60 mg of codeine, routine use in moderate pain is limited by its unique and unpleasant side effects, which include mental disturbances, anorexia, disorientation, and possible hallucinations.

MANAGEMENT OF POSTOPERATIVE SWELLING

The basis for pain management following dental implant surgery has been provided in the previous section of this chapter. Swelling may be particularly significant when implant surgery is prolonged and when large areas of gingiva and oral mucous are manipulated. Although edema normally occurs postoperatively and is a functional part of the healing process, when swelling is severe, healing may be compromised. Trismus associated with swelling may inhibit adequate oral hygiene and may limit food intake. When excessive, oral and pharyngeal swelling may inhibit normal respiratory function.

Many of the management strategies used to limit swelling after implant surgery are nonpharmacologic. A careful history prior to surgery may reveal recent use of aspirin or aspirin-containing medications. The use of aspirin is known to significantly affect hemostasis for up to 7 to 10 days after ingestion. Poor hemostasis can aggravate healing and induce submucosal bleeding. Although the effect is usually not severe, swelling and higher incidences of ecchymosis have been reported when aspirin is administered prior to surgery.[19] It is highly recommended that patients receiving dental implants be instructed to avoid aspirin for 5 to 7 days prior to implant surgery.

Additionally, careful surgical technique is effective in limiting tissue damage and subsequent swelling. Care should be taken to avoid prolonged periods of tissue elevation and retraction. Ice packs applied immediately following surgery may have additional benefit.

Nonsteroidal anti-inflammatory agents may limit the edema associated with bony impaction removal.[20] Swelling following implant procedures should similarly be reduced by a preoperative NSAID such as ibuprofen. However, the anti-inflammatory effect of preoperative ibuprofen is modest at best. If the surgery is expected to produce significant swelling, a short-term therapeutic regimen of an anti-inflammatory steroid is recommended.

Glucocorticosteroids appear to inhibit all phases of inflammation. They block the increased capillary permeability produced by histamine and kinins, and therefore decrease edema. Capillary dilatation, migration of leukocytes, and phagocytosis are decreased. Kinin generation is also inhibited. Furthermore,

TABLE 19–5.

Corticosteroid Regimen for Managing Postoperative Dental Swelling

Agent	Route	Dose (mg)	Timing
Dexamethasone; (Decadron)	PO	9	Morning of surgery
	PO	6	1 day after surgery
	PO	3	2 days after surgery

steroids activate the synthesis of a protein inhibitor of phospholipase, thereby blocking the formation of arachidonic acid. Therefore, the pathways for the formation of prostaglandins, thromboxanes, prostacyclins, leukotrienes, and HPETEs are inhibited.

Several authors have evaluated the efficacy of glucocorticoids for oral surgical procedures.[21, 22] Hooley and Francis[23] performed a clinical study of swelling following mandibular third molar extraction. This double-blind, randomized, patient-controlled study observed six times less edema with steroid treatment. In addition, patients treated with glucocorticoids had half the pain and half the trismus experienced by the control group. Skjelbred and Lokken[24] reported that even when the corticosteroid was injected 3 hours after oral surgery, swelling was reduced 47% compared to a placebo. Trismus was less significant when steroids were administered. In addition, an average of 11 codeine tablets were taken for pain in the steroid treatment group compared to 26 tablets with the placebo treatment.

Several factors should be considered when using steroids for surgery. The chosen steroid should have minimal mineralocorticoid effects. The drug should be administered before surgery, allowing ample time for drug distribution to provide an optimal reduction of arachidonic acid at the time of wounding. It is preferably given in the morning, when cortisol is naturally released by the body. This schedule interferes least with the normal adrenocortical system. The postoperative regimen should not exceed 3 days. Because edema peaks in 48 to 72 hours, prolonged therapy has little benefit. A 5-day steroid intake diminishes the normal release of cortisol up to 5 additional days after steroid therapy.[25]

The dose should probably not exceed 300 mg of cortisol equivalence the morning of surgery, which corresponds to the maximum reported amount of natural glucocorticoid released during trauma, surgery, or infection. The dose should be reduced the 2nd day, and further reduced the 3rd day, because the intended effect on days 2 and 3 is directed to the edema feedback loop, which decreases with time. An acceptable regimen that fulfills these criteria is shown in Table 19–5. Utilizing this approach to short-term steroid use, the practitioner will optimize the benefits and minimize any risks. Those preferring parenteral administration can use an 8-mg intravenous preoperative dose of dexamethasone phosphate followed postoperatively by 8 mg of a long-acting repository acetate formulation for intramuscular or submucosal injection. Glucocorticosteroids are contraindicated if the patient has a history of tuberculosis, ocular herpetic simplex, acute glaucoma, peptic ulcer or diabetes, or if active infection exists.

As the science of implantology evolves, techniques will inevitably become more invasive. This is particularly true for maxillary surgery, where entry into nasal and maxillary sinuses introduces concern regarding inflammation and infection of mucous membranes. The judicious use of anti-inflammatory agents and antibiotics should be considered the first-line agents for prophylaxis when surgery involves the sinus cavities. If discomfort from sinus congestion occurs despite these preventive measures, one might consider a decongestant to reduce mucosal swelling. In this case, a nonprescription, 1% phenylephrine nasal spray should provide satisfactory relief.

Currently there is no published evidence supporting the preoperative use of antihistamines and/or decongestants to reduce postoperative discomfort or to improve healing associated with sinus membrane congestion. Furthermore, it is doubtful that antihistamines would be beneficial because histamine is not as significant a mediator in trauma-induced congestion as it is in allergic forms of rhinitis. However, the anticholinergic action of most antihistamines may be useful if the patient experiences serous or mucous drainage.

LOCAL ANESTHESIA

The availability of effective amide local anesthetics (Table 19–6) has dramatically improved the public's image of the dental profession and has

TABLE 19–6.

Amide Local Anesthetics Used in Dentistry

Local Anesthetic	Concentration (%)	Vasoconstrictor
Lidocaine (Xylocaine)*	2	None (plain)
	2	Epinephrine 1:50,000
	2	Epinephrine 1:100,000
Mepivacaine (Carbocaine)†	2	Levonordefrin 1:20,000
	3	None (plain)
Prilocaine (Citanest)*	4	Epinephrine 1:200,000
	4	None (plain)
Bupivacaine (Marcaine)†	0.5	Epinephrine 1:200,000
Etidocaine (Duranest)*	1.5	Epinephrine 1:200,000
Articaine (Ultracaine)‡§	4	Epinephrine 1:200,000
	4	Epinephrine 1:100,000

*Astra Pharmaceutical Products, Westboro, Mass.
†Cook-Waite Laboratories, New York.
‡Hoeschst Canada Inc, Montreal.
§Available in Canada and Europe.

permitted the development of many of the sophisticated surgical outpatient procedures now available to dental patients. The ester local anesthetics, such as procaine and tetracaine, have little utility in clinical practice because they are less reliable and have greater allergenicity.

In the United States, profound surgical anesthesia is most commonly induced using a 2% lidocaine–1:100,000 epinephrine formulation. This preparation is the "gold" standard for all other agents. It has a rapid onset of 2 to 3 minutes and a duration of surgical anesthesia approximating 60 to 90 minutes. Preparations of lidocaine with 1:50,000 epinephrine do not provide a significantly longer duration. Mepivacaine is considered an excellent second choice to lidocaine with epinephrine. The 3% preparation without vasoconstrictor has a rapid onset and provides satisfactory surgical anesthesia in most cases. When a vasoconstrictor is to be avoided, mepivacaine is an excellent alternative. The primary disadvantage of 3% mepivacaine plain is its somewhat shorter duration when compared to lidocaine with epinephrine.

Long-acting Anesthetics

During the past 20 years, two long-acting amide local anesthetics, bupivacaine and etidocaine, have found a place in the dentist's armamentarium. These agents, with their unique anesthetic characteristics, play a valuable role in the overall management of surgical and postoperative pain.[26]

Although many variables exist that prevent comparing results among investigators, the abundance of published information regarding long-acting local anesthetics as used in dentistry permits one to assess their advantages and disadvantages. The agents currently available in the United States in 1.8-cc dental cartridges are 0.5% bupivacaine 1/200,000 epinephrine (Marcaine) and 1.5% etidocaine 1/200,000 epinephrine (Duranest). Both agents have been used extensively and have been shown to be safe and effective. Soft tissue anesthesia and the period of painlessness following the long-acting local anesthetics is 2 to 3 times that of standard agents. Soft tissue anesthesia following mandibular blocks lasts 6 to 8 hours and following maxillary infiltration lasts 4 to 6 hours.[27–31] Although, the onset times for mandibular block anesthesia may be somewhat longer for bupivacaine,[28, 31] onset times are clinically acceptable for both agents. The durations of pulpal anesthesia following maxillary infiltrations using bupivacaine and etidocaine do not appear to be longer than lidocaine.[32, 33] Because the epinephrine concentrations are lower for bupivacaine and etidocaine, increased bleeding during surgery has been demonstrated.[30] When moderate to severe pain is expected, the long-acting agents can delay the onset of pain, reduce its severity, and decrease the need for strong oral analgesics.

The rationale for using a long-acting local anesthetic should be clearly explained to the patient. Overall patient satisfaction with this pain management strategy requires careful patient selection and preparation.

Safety

Many comprehensive evaluations of local anesthetic toxicity have been reported. The earliest and most common response to local anesthetic overdose is CNS excitation. Initially a feeling of lightheadedness or dizziness occurs. Auditory and visual disturbance may also be noted. The patient may become disoriented and develop slurred speech, tremors, muscle twitching, and generalized convulsions. Generalized central nervous system depression follows, with loss of consciousness and respiratory arrest. The cardiovascular-depressant effects of local anesthetics, such as decreased myocardial contractility, decreased peripheral resistance, hypotension, and circulatory collapse, may also be seen.[34]

Although true allergic reactions to amide local anesthetics are rare, life-threatening toxic reactions due in part to local anesthetic overdose have been reported in dentistry.[35, 36] Toxic reactions to local anesthetics in dentistry occur most frequently in children, in whom the relative anesthetic doses are generally higher.

Over the past 20 years, there have been an exceedingly small number of reported toxic reactions to the use of local anesthetics in dentistry. Considering the number of injections that are given each year, the incidence of local anesthetic toxicity in dentistry is remarkably low, and should be kept in that perspective. When used within recommended dosage guidelines (Table 19–7) life-threatening reactions to local anesthetics are essentially nonexistent.

Vasopressors

With the exception of mepivacaine and prilocaine, most local anesthetics induce some degree of vasodilation.[37] To limit their systemic uptake and improve the overall clinical characteristics, vasoconstrictors are added (see Table 19–7).

The most common vasoconstrictor added to local anesthetics is epinephrine. This naturally occurring sympathomimetic stimulates both alpha and beta adrenergic receptors of the sympathetic nervous system. The alpha stimulation provides the profound vasoconstriction, which is required to prevent absorption of the local anesthetic from its site of injection. The vasoconstrictor used in mepivacaine formulations is levonordefrin. Although almost identical in structure

TABLE 19–7.

Maximum Safe Dosage Recommendations for Local Anesthetics in Implant Dentistry

Agent	Maximum Safe Adult Dose (mg)	mg/1.8 mL Cartridge	Maximum Safe Cartridges
2% lidocaine (1:100,000 epinephrine)	300–500	36	8–14
3% mepivacaine (no vasoconstrictor)	300–500	54	6–9
0.5% bupivacaine (1:200,000 epinephrine)	90	9	10

and activity to epinephrine, levonordefrin is less potent and therefore must be administered at a higher dose (1:20,000) to be equally vasopressive to epinephrine.

A vasoconstrictor is an essential addition for local anesthetics that produce vasodilation. The presence of a vasoconstrictor improves the profoundity and increases the duration of anesthesia. In addition, the vasoconstrictor decreases the rate of system absorption of the local anesthetic, thereby decreasing systemic toxicity.

Epinephrine and levonordefrin have both alpha and beta adrenergic activity. The beta stimulation of these agents can produce cardiac stimulation and some smooth muscle relaxation. Both agents can increase heart rate, myocardial oxygen consumption, and cardiac irritability and should be limited or avoided in patients with cardiovascular disease, significant hypertension, and unmanaged hyperthyroid disease.

Blood loss during oral surgery, although rarely life-threatening, may effect visualization of the surgical field. In some surgical procedures, such as periodontal surgery and implant surgery, a clear operating field is essential. Nonpharmacologic strategies are recommended to aid in clearing blood from the operating site and facilitating visualization. The use of the vasoconstrictor in local anesthetics to provide hemostasis must be done conservatively because healing may be effected by the ischemia and subsequent oozing that may occur.[38]

ANTIMICROBIAL AGENTS

Antibiotics have undeniable importance in managing implant-related infection. Furthermore, their preoperative use has gained wide acceptance as preventing infection during implant surgery. Adverse effects attributed to antibiotics are surprisingly infrequent, but most agents are associated with varying degrees of nausea and dyspepsia. Broader spectrum agents may allow overgrowth of nonsusceptible organisms, which can lead to various superinfections. Vaginal infection due to overgrowth of *Candida albicans* is a common example.

Beta Lactam Derivatives

The penicillins and cephalosporins have many similarities. Each molecule consists of a beta lactam ring that confers its bacteriocidal action on cell wall synthesis. Unfortunately, an increasing number of microbial species are resistant because they secrete enzymes that cleave this beta lactam ring, rendering the molecule inactive. Beta lactamases are secreted by a variety of microorganisms, including *Haemophilus influenzae, Staphylococcus aureus,* and several *Pseudomonas* species. Many of these enzymes have been isolated and are subclassified as either penicillinases, cephalosporinases, or both.[39]

Allergy is the most common side effect attributed to beta lactam antibiotics. In rare cases, patients allergic to penicillin may also experience allergic reactions to the cephalosporins. For those having documented allergy to penicillins (positive skin tests), the incidence of cross-allergenicity to first-generation cephalosporins is approximately 2% to 5%.[40] Results of skin testing are seldom available, and the following guidelines have been suggested.[41] If the patient relates an episode that was merely pruritic, or any rash was maculopapular, an immunologic mechanism is unlikely. In such cases, it is reasonably safe for the patient to receive cephalosporins. However, all beta lactam derivatives should be avoided if the rash was urticarial or an anaphylactoid reaction is described.[41, 42]

Penicillin G is highly degradable in gastric acid and for this reason it is generally administered by parenteral routes. It is very active against the gram positive cocci implicated in most oral infections. The phenoxymethyl derivative of penicillin, designated penicillin V, is more acid-stable and has become the standard penicillin for oral use. Its spectrum is similar to that for penicillin G, but it is less active against *Nisseria* species and several anaerobes.

Many microbial species otherwise sensitive to penicillin are resistant because they synthesize penicillinase. This is particularly true for strains of *S. aureus*, over 90% of which are resistant to penicillin G and V. Penicillin derivatives have been synthesized that are not inactivated by beta lactamases. These "penicillinase-stable" agents include oxacillin and dicloxacillin. Their selection should be guided by culture and sensitivity data because their activity against *Streptococcus viridans* species is less than that of the conventional penicillins.[1]

Ampicillin was the first penicillin derivative to exhibit an extended spectrum of activity. This includes several gram negative organisms, such as *H. influenza* and *Escherichia coli,* respectively implicated in sinus and urinary tract infections. Amoxicillin is a derivative that demonstrates greater oral bioavailability than ampicillin or penicillin V.[43] For this reason, amoxicillin may rival penicillin V as a first-line agent for oral infections.

All extended-spectrum penicillins are susceptible to the action of penicillinases. Clavulanic acid is a beta lactam molecule with weak antimicrobial action, but strong affinity for beta lactamases. It can be combined with these agents to act as a "suicide molecule," protecting the penicillin from beta lactamases. Augmentin is one such product and consists of clauvulanic acid compounded with amoxicillin. It is a very expensive product and should be used only when culture and sensitivity data reveal penicillinase-producing species.

The first generation of cephalosporins have a spectrum of activity resembling that of ampicillin. A significant exception is that they resist the destructive action of beta lactamases produced by most strains of *S. aureus*. However, this species is rarely implicated in oral infections; therefore, the cephalosporins are wisely relegated as substitutes for patients having a history of minor allergic reactions to penicillins.

Erythromycins

Erythromycin is active against most penicillin-sensitive microbes, and therefore is the standard antibiotic for patients allergic to penicillin. Erythromycin base is the active molecule but is also prepared as several salts and esters to improve gastrointestinal tolerance and absorption. For example, the absorption of erythromycin ethylsuccinate (EES) is minimally reduced when food is present and this is its principal advantage.

There is considerable confusion regarding equivalent doses for the various formulations.[43] Erythromycin salts are biotransformed to free base in the gut wall, while esters are biotransformed in plasma. In recommending the ester EES, the recent American Heart Association's guidelines for endocarditis prophylaxis failed to account for this difference. Former guidelines suggested 1,000 mg of erythromycin base. The current recommendation is 800 mg EES, which is only equivalent to 500 mg erythromycin base.[44]

Regardless of the preparation selected, erythromycins produce a high incidence of nausea and are bacteriostatic at conventional doses. These characteristics may be unattractive when high doses are required for severe infections or when a patient is severely immunocompromised and requires bacteriocidal activity.

Clindamycin

Clindamycin has reliable activity against both aerobic and anaerobic cocci, as well as most bacteroides species including *Bacteroides fragilis*. These pathogens are frequently isolated from severe orofacial infections. Its cost and propensity to induce antibiotic-associated, pseudomembranous colitis (PMC) limit its routine use.

Antibiotic-associated diarrhea and PMC represent superinfections generally caused by *Clostridium difficile*. If diarrhea and/or abdominal cramping occur during clindamycin therapy, the drug should be discontinued. Antidiarrheal medications should be avoided because they hinder fecal elimination of the pathogen. If the condition persists after 3 days, the patient should be assessed medically for fluid and electrolyte status. The patient will likely be treated with oral vancomycin which is active against *Clostridium* and has limited absorption, confining its action to the intestinal lumen. PMC has occurred as late as 6 weeks following clindamycin use and has also occurred following the use of erythromycins, tetracyclines, and beta lactam antibiotics.[45]

Tetracyclines

Tetracyclines have a wide spectrum of activity, but microbial resistance has increased to the extent that they are first-line agents in but a few incidences. Sinus and respiratory infections caused by *H. influenzae* and *pneumonocci* are notable exceptions because most of these strains remain sensitive. Notably, there is less antimicrobial resistance to doxcycline and minocycline than other more conventional tetracyclines.

Tetracyclines are active against most of the microorganisms implicated in gingival and periodontal disease. Also, following systemic administration, tetracyclines exhibit high bioavailability in the gingival sulcus.[46] For these reasons they are primary agents for treating periodontal disease and infections around implant posts. Their efficacy for managing intrabony infections is questionable, considering their inactivity while chelated with calcium complexes.[47, 48]

Tetracyclines are known well for their propensity to discolor developing teeth and promote opportunistic *Candida* infections. They also increase skin sensitivity to sunlight, leading to intense sunburn and generalized erythema. Doxycline shares these side effects but offers several advantages. It is well absorbed in the presence of food and has an extended elimination half-life which reduces dosing intervals. It is eliminated primarily in feces, which is particularly attractive for patients having hepatic or renal compromise.

Metronidazole

Metronidazole is bacteriocidal against most anaerobic organisms. It is ineffective as a sole agent for mixed oral infections because it is inactive against aerobic and facultative streptococci. However, it may be combined with penicillin when managing severe infections.[49] Patients should be cautioned to avoid alcoholic beverages while taking this medication, as disulfiram-like reactions have been reported. These consist of severe nausea and abdominal cramping due to the formation of a toxic compound resembling formaldehyde.

THERAPEUTIC CONSIDERATIONS

The most common pathogens implicated in oral infections have been isolated, and the most appropriate antibiotics are established.[50–52] For these reasons, the initial selection of an antibiotic is largely empirical rather than guided by culture and sensitivity data. A summary of useful agents is provided in Table 19–8. When possible, surgical drainage should accompany antibiotic therapy. A two-step approach to antibiotic selection is illustrated in Figure 19–2. If there is a poor response to empiric agents, further selection of antibiotics should be guided by culture and sensitivity data.

TABLE 19–8.

Suggested Agents for Empiric Therapy of Implant-Related Infections

Antibiotic	Dosage	Comments
Penicillin V	500 mg qid	Agent of choice for mild to moderate intraoral infections (amoxicillin may be preferred because of superior bioavailability)
Erythromycin	500 mg qid	Standard alternative for patient allergic to penicillin
Cefadroxil	500 mg bid	Alternative to erythromycin for penicillin-allergic patient negative
or cephalexin	500 mg qid	for anaphylaxis or if patient is significantly immunocompromised
Metronidazole	250–500 mg tid	Added to penicillin V if infection does not respond to monotherapy
Clindamycin	300 mg tid	Alternative to penicillin plus metronidazole for refractory infections; may be agent of choice for severe orofacial infections
Doxycycline	100 mg bid/qid	Agent for low-grade chronic infection around posts, that is, infections mimicking periodontal infections; bid dosing on day 1 followed by once daily is the most common regimen

PROPHYLAXIS CONSIDERATIONS

Antibiotics are used not only to treat existing infection but also to prevent infection following surgical or invasive diagnostic procedures. This practice is justified if patients are immunocompromised or are at risk for developing bacterial endocarditis. The routine use of antibiotics for surgical prophylaxis is more controversial.

Surgical and invasive diagnostic procedures always carry a risk for introducing bacteria into the bloodstream (bacteremia). This is of little consequence unless

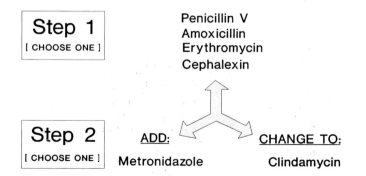

FIG 19–2.
Two-step approach to empiric selection of antibiotics for oral infections, including those related to dental implants. Doxycycline may be used as an alternative step 1 agent for chronic infections around implant posts. If the patient does not respond or the condition deteriorates with empiric therapy further selection must be guided by culture and sensitivity data.

a patient has some deformity of the endocardial surface. Valvular lesions, prosthetic valves, and ventricular septal defects are examples of such deformities. In any of these cases, it is possible for microorganisms to colonize on the defect and culminate in a bacterial endocarditis. The American Heart Association recommends that patients at risk receive prophylactic antibiotics prior to dental and other surgical procedures.[44] The antibiotics recommended are those that are most active against microbes likely to be introduced during the particular procedure. The most recent guidelines for prevention of bacterial endocarditis are found in Table 19–9. Although penicillins are generally preferred, erythromycin and clindamycin are acceptable alternatives for patients having penicillin allergy.

Many surgeons administer antibiotics routinely to prevent wound infections. Routine surgical prophylaxis is effective in some cases but, if used improperly, constitutes a flagrant misuse of antimicrobial drugs.[1] During lengthy oral surgical procedures it is often difficult to strictly maintain aseptic conditions; for this reason, it may be appropriate to administer an antibiotic preoperatively to decrease the likelihood of postoperative infection. Antibiotic prophylaxis for implant surgery has been reviewed recently.[53, 54] An adequate blood titer should be present at the time of surgical incision and should be initiated no more than 2 hours preoperatively. Coverage need only be sustained for 24 to 48 hours.[55–57] Prolonged coverage may encourage growth of resistant organisms that compromise long-term success of the implant.[58] Logical regimens can be derived from those suggested for prevention of bacterial endocarditis. Several options for oral regimens are summarized in Table 19–10. For those preferring an intravenous regimen, 1 g of cephazolin is attractive because of its 8-hour duration. This can be followed with an oral cephalosporin or amoxacillin to complete the regimen.

TABLE 19–9.

Antibiotic Prophylaxis of Bacterial Endocarditis*

Drug	Adult Dosing Regimen
Amoxicillin	3.0 g orally 1 hr before surgery and 1.5 g 6 hr after initial dose
Erythromycin (EES)	800 mg orally 2 hr before surgery and 400 mg 6 hr after initial dose
Clindamycin	300 mg orally 1 hr before surgery and 150 mg 6 hr after initial dose

Child Weight (lb)	Dose Adjustment for Child
> 60	Use adult dose
30–60	Use one half adult dose
< 30	Use one fourth adult dose

*Recently revised guidelines for prevention of bacterial endocarditis. Amoxicillin is preferred over penicillin V because of its superior bioavailability. Parenteral regimens are no longer required for patients having prosthetic valve replacements. (Adapted from Dajani et al: *JAMA* 1990; 264:2919–2922.)

TABLE 19–10.

Suggested Oral Antibiotic Regimens for Surgical Prophylaxis

Preparation	Dosing Schedule
Penicillin V	2 g, 1 hr before surgery; 1 g q 6 hr × 3
Amoxicillin	2–3 g, 1 hr before surgery; 1 g, q 6 hr × 3
Cephalexin	2 g, 1 hr before surgery; 1 g q 6 hr × 3
Clindamycin	450 mg, 1 hr before surgery; 150 mg q 6 hr × 3

Oral Contraceptive Controversy

Most of the antibiotics used for oral infections have been implicated in scattered reports of oral contraceptive failure. The proposed mechanism for this interaction is interference with the enterohepatic activation of estrogen, thereby reducing its bioavailability. However, studies have failed to demonstrate reduced serum levels of estrogen in patients receiving any antibiotic other than rifampin, an anti-tuberculosis agent.[59–61] Szoka and Edgren[62] found no association between penicillin use and oral contraceptive failure in reports published through 1987. The current edition of *Drug Interaction Facts,* published by Facts and Comparisons (1991), considers the interaction to be only "possible." There is no documentation to classify the interaction as "established," "probable," or even "suspected." To date, there is no legal evidence to mandate a discussion of "informed consent" when prescribing antibiotics for oral infections. However, until the issue is convincingly resolved, it may be wise to advise a patient of the controversy.

The dentist should resist temptations to prescribe expensive "designer" preparations, based on anecdotal suggestions by colleagues or sales representatives. Inappropriate use of such agents significantly impacts the $2.4 billion spent annually on oral antibiotics.[63]

SEDATIVE ANXIOLYTICS

Stress reduction is critical if the dentist is to properly perform the meticulous surgery involved with implant placement. Sedatives and anxiolytics are underused despite the fact that fear and apprehension are principal reasons for patients acquiring their edentulous status. A variety of agents are currently available for oral preoperative sedation. When used properly they have an impressive margin of safety and calm the patient during the surgical procedure.

Benzodiazepines

For oral sedation, there is little reason to consider drug classes other than the benzodiazepines. Their efficacy is comparable to the barbiturates, and their therapeutic index (safety) is greater. They act at specific receptor sites to potentiate the generalized depressant effect of gamma aminobutyric acid (GABA).[64] There is little scientific evidence to substantiate any claims for superior sedative or anxiolytic efficacy among the benzodiazepines currently available. Therefore, the basis for selection is based on pharmacokinetic, rather than pharmacodynamic, reasons.

One distinguishing feature of the benzodiazepines is their conversion to active metabolites. This difference is probably insignificant during short-term use[6, 7]; however, it may be prudent to avoid products having active metabolites when sedating the elderly or those patients with renal and hepatic compromise. Given the number of agents currently marketed, this recommendation is easily followed.

There is considerable variability in elimination half-lives among the benzodiazepines (Table 19–11). However, the clinician is cautioned not to equate this with duration of clinical effect. Their degree of lipid solubility varies and this correlates with distribution half-life (alpha $T_{1/2}$) rather than elimination half-life (beta $t_{1/2}$). Distribution more accurately predicts duration of clinical effect.[6-8] Simply stated, the more lipid-soluble agents have the fastest clinical onset and the shortest duration of clinical effect.

Unfortunately, there are few well designed studies that establish equipotent oral doses of benzodiazepines for preoperative sedation. A recent study compared triazolam at 0.125, 0.25, and 0.5 mg with diazepam at 5, 10, and 15 mg, but only the highest triazolam dose was consistently effective.[65] The sedation and anterograde amnesia associated with most benzodiazepines is beneficial for preoperative use, but should emphasize the importance of a responsible adult escort for the patient during the postoperative period.

Miscellaneous Agents

Antihistamines (H_1 blockers) such as hydroxyzine 100–200 mg or promethazine 25–50 mg may also be used for preoperative sedation. Although their

TABLE 19–11.

Benzodiazepines for Oral Sedation

Factor*	Triazolam (Halcion)	Diazepam (Valium)	Lorazepam (Ativan)
Active metabolites	No	Yes	No
Elimination T½ (hr)	2–3	20–100†	8–24
Onset (initial) (min)	20–30	30–45	45–60
Onset (peak) (min)	75	90	120
Duration (hr)	1–3	2–4	4–6
Sedative dose (PO) (mg)	0.25–0.5	10–20	2–4

*Initial onset times and durations are estimates of the author regarding clinically useful sedative effects. Peak onset reflects published data regarding peak plasma concentration following oral administration. Doses should be halved for the elderly or significantly compromised.
†Including active metabolite, desmethyldiazepam.

TABLE 19–12.

Suggested Protocol for Oral Preoperative Sedation

1. To assure a restful night's sleep before the appointment, one may prescribe a dose approximately half that planned for preoperative use.
2. Full dose is taken 30 to 60 minutes before time of scheduled appointment and patient escorted to office. It may be wiser to administer triazolam (Halcion) in the office because of its rapid onset.
3. If sedation is inadequate, titrate nitrous oxide to end point.
4. Patient must have adult escort at discharge.

sedative efficacy is inferior to the benzodiazepines, their anticholinergic and antiemetic actions may have prophylactic as well as therapeutic use.[66] Their sedative action is due to central blockade of the excitatory transmitters, acetylcholine, and histamine. For this reason, their combination with GABA potentiators, such as the benzodiazepines, will likely produce an enhanced effect. However, combination regimens are better reserved for intravenous titration techniques because precise oral dosing is virtually impossible. An oral sedation protocol that can be combined with nitrous oxide-oxygen titration is summarized in Table 19–12. This technique is preferable to sequential oral doses because the precise amount of additional increments cannot be estimated. If an oral dose must be repeated, it certainly should be delayed until the peak onset of the initial dose has passed. There is little evidence that IM administration has a significant advantage over oral preoperative regimens.[67]

It is difficult to avoid a biased word against the use of opioids for oral sedation. Given the fact that opioids are greater respiratory depressants than the benzodiazepines or antihistamines,[68] and given the difficulty of accurately selecting an appropriate dose for combined oral regimens, opioids are best reserved for carefully titrated intravenous techniques.

REFERENCES

1. Gilman AG et al, editors: *Goodman and Gilman's the pharmacological basis of therapeutics,* New York, 1990, Pergamon Press, pp 11, 26, 67, 497, 1077, 1041.
2. Wood M: Plasma binding and limitation of drug access to site of action, *Anesthesiology* 75:721–723, 1991.
3. Montamat SC, Cusack BJ, Vestal RE: Management of drug therapy in the elderly, *N Engl J Med* 321:303–309, 1989.
4. Rousseau P: Pharmacologic alterations in the elderly: special considerations, *Hosp Formul* 22:543–545, 1987.
5. American Academy of Pediatrics, Committee on Drugs: Transfer of drugs and other chemicals into human milk, *Pediatrics* 84:924–936, 1989.
6. Greenblatt DJ, Shader RI, Abernathy DR: Current status of benzodiazepines (part 1), *N Engl J Med* 309:354–358, 1983.

7. Greenblatt DJ, Shader RI, Abernathy DR: Current status of benzodiazepines (part 2), *N Engl J Med* 309:410–416, 1983.

8. Greenblatt DJ: Elimination half-life of drugs: value and limitations, *Annu Rev Med* 36:421–427, 1985.

9. Hargreaves KM, Troullos ES, Dionne RA: Pharmacologic rationale for the treatment of acute pain, *Dent Clin North Am* 31:675–694, 1987.

10. Basran GS et al: Evidence in man of synergistic interaction between putative mediators of acute inflammation and asthma, *Lancet* 24:935–937, 1982.

11. Mense S: Sensitization of group IV muscle receptors to bradykinin by 5-hydroxytryptamine and prostaglandinE$_2$, *Brain Res* 225:95–105, 1981.

12. Vane JR: Inhibition of prostaglandin synthesis as a mechanism of action for aspirin-like drugs, *Nature* 231:232–235, 1971.

13. Dionne RA, Cooper SA: Evaluation of preoperative ibuprofen for postoperative pain after removal of third molars, *Oral Surg* 45:851–856, 1978.

14. Moore PA et al: Analgesic regimens for third molar surgery: pharmacologic and behavioral considerations, *J Am Dent Assoc* 113:739–744, 1986.

15. Jackson DL, Moore PA, Hargreaves KM: Preoperative nonsteroidal anti-inflammatory medication for the prevention of postoperative dental pain, *J Am Dent Assoc* 119:641–647, 1989.

16. Misch CE, Moore PA: Steroids and the reduction of pain, edema and dysfunction in implant dentistry, *J Oral Implant* 6:27–31, 1989.

17. Pert CB, Snyder SH: Opiate receptor: demonstration in nervous tissue, *Science* 179:1011–1014, 1973.

18. Hargreaves KM, Dubner R, Joris J: Peripheral actions of opiates in the blockade of carrageen-induced inflammation. In *Pair research and clinical management*, vol. 3, Amsterdam, 1988, Elsevier Science Publishers, pp 55–60.

19. Hepso HU et al: Double-blind crossover study of the effect of acetylsalicylic acid on bleeding and postoperative course after bilateral oral surgery, *Eur J Clin Pharmacol* 10:217–225, 1976.

20. Lokken P, Olsen I, Norman-Pedersen K: Bilateral surgical removal of impacted lower third molar teeth as a model for drug evaluation: a test with ibuprofen, *Eur J Clin Pharmacol* 8:209–216, 1975.

21. Huffman CG: Use of methylprednisolone sodium succinate to reduce postoperative edema after removal of impacted third molars, *J Oral Surg* 35:198–199, 1977.

22. Pedersen A: Decadron phosphate in the relief of complaints after third molar surgery, *Int J Oral Surg* 14:235–240, 1985.

23. Hooley JR, Francis FH: Bethamethasone in traumatic oral surgery, *J Oral Surg* 27:398–403, 1969.

24. Skjelbred P, Lokken P: Post-operative pain and inflammatory reactions reduced by injection of corticosteroid, *Eur J Clin Pharmacol* 21:391–396, 1982.

25. Bahn SL: Glucocorticoids in dentistry, *J Am Dent Assoc* 105:476–481, 1982.

26. Moore PA: Long-acting local anesthetics: a review of clinical efficacy in dentistry, *Compendium Continuing Educ Dent* 11:22–30, 1990.

27. Chapnick P, Baker G, Munroe CO: Bupivacaine anesthesia in oral surgery, *Can Dent Assoc J* 7:441–443, 1980.

28. Nespaca JA: Clinical trials with bupivacaine in oral surgery, *Oral Surg* 42:301–307, 1976.

29. Trieger N, Gillen GH: Bupivacaine anesthesia and postoperative analgesia in oral surgery, *Anesth Prog* 20:23–27, 1979.
30. Linden ET et al: A comparison of postoperative pain experience following periodontal surgery using two local anesthetic agents, *J Periodontol* 10:637–642, 1986.
31. Moore PA, Dunsky JL: Bupivacaine anesthesia: a clinical trial for endodontic therapy, *Oral Surg* 55:176–179, 1983.
32. Danielsson K, Evers H, Nordenram A: Long-acting local anesthetics in oral surgery: an experimental evaluation of bupivacaine and etidocaine for oral infiltration anesthesia, *Anesth Prog* 32:65–68, 1985.
33. Teplitsky DE, Hablichek CA, Kushneriuk JS: A comparison of bupivacaine to lidocaine with respect to duration in the maxilla and mandible, *Can Dent Assoc J* 6:475–478, 1987.
34. Liu PL et al: Comparative CNS toxicity of lidocaine, etidocaine, bupivacaine and tetracaine in awake dogs following rapid intravenous administration, *Anesth Analg* 62:375–379, 1983.
35. Goodson JM, Moore PA: Life-threatening reactions after pedodontic sedation: an assessment of narcotic, local anesthetic and antiemetic drug interaction, *J Am Dent Assoc* 107:239–245, 1983.
36. Reynolds F: Adverse effects of local anesthetics, *Br J Anaesth* 59:78–95, 1987.
37. Lindorf HH: Investigation of the vascular effect of newer local anesthetics and vasoconstrictors, *Oral Surg* 48:292–297, 1979.
38. Sveen K: Effect of the addition of a vasoconstrictor to local anesthesia solution on operative and postoperative bleeding, analgesia and wound healing, *Int J Oral Surg* 8:301–306, 1979.
39. Sykes RB: The classification and terminology of enzymes that hydrolyze beta-lactam antibiotics, *J Infect Dis* 145:762–765, 1982.
40. Guill MF: Allergic drug reactions: identification and management, *Hosp Formul* 26:582–589, 1991.
41. Shepherd GM: Allergy to beta-lactam antibiotics, *Immunol Allergy Clin North Am* 11:611–633, 1991.
42. Donowitz GR, Mandell GL: Beta-lactam antibiotics (2 parts), *N Engl J Med* 318:419–426, 490–500, 1988; also letters, *N Engl J Med* 319:520–521, 1988.
43. AMA Department of Drugs: *Drug evaluations annual 1992.* Chicago, 1992, American Medical Association, pp 1260, 1354.
44. Dajani AS et al: Prevention of bacterial endocarditis: recommendations by the American Heart Association, *JAMA* 264:2919–2922, 1990; also letters, *JAMA* 265:1686–1688, 1991.
45. Bartlett JG: Antimicrobial agents implicated in *Clostridium difficile* toxin-associated diarrhea or colitis, *Johns Hopkins Med J* 149:6–9, 1981.
46. Genco RJ: Using antimicrobial agents to manage periodontal diseases, *J Am Dent Assoc* 122:31–38, 1991.
47. Montgomery EH: Antibacterial antibiotics. In Neidle EA, Kroeger DC, Yagiela JA (editors): *Pharmacology and therapeutics for dentistry,* St Louis, 1985, CV Mosby, p 565.
48. Pallasch TJ: The healing pattern of an experimentally-induced defect in the rat femur studied with tetracycline labeling, *Calcif Tissue Res* 2:334–342, 1986.
49. Peterson LJ: Principles of antibiotic therapy. In Topazian RG, Goldberg MH (editors): *Oral and maxillofacial infections,* Philadelphia, 1987, WB Saunders, p 153.

50. Hunt DE, Meyer RA: Continued evolution of the microbiology of oral infections, *J Am Dent Assoc* 107:52–54, 1983.
51. Labriola JD, Mascaro J, Alpert B: The microbiologic flora of orofacial abscesses, *J Oral Maxillofac Surg* 41:711–714, 1983.
52. Moenning JE, Nelson CL, Kohler RB: The microbiology and chemotherapy of odontogenic infections, *J Oral Maxillofac Surg* 47:976–985, 1989.
53. Becker DE: Principles of antimicrobial prophylaxis during surgical placement of implant prostheses, *J Oral Implantol* 14:467–471, 1988.
54. Peterson LJ: Antibiotic prophylaxis against wound infections in oral and maxillofacial surgery, *J Oral Maxillofac Surg* 48:617–620, 1990.
55. Classen DC et al: The timing of prophylactic administration of antibiotics and the risk of surgical-wound infection, *N Engl J Med* 326:281–286, 1992; also Wenzel RP: Preoperative antibiotic prophylaxis, editorial, *N Engl J Med* 326:337–339, 1992.
56. Kaiser AB: Antimicrobial prophylaxis in surgery, *N Engl J Med* 315:1129–1138, 1986.
57. Scher KS et al: Duration of antibiotic prophylaxis—an experimental study, *Am J Surg* 151:209–212, 1986.
58. Leviner E et al: Development of resistant oral viridans streptococci after administration of prophylactic antibiotics: time management in the dental treatment of patients susceptible to infective endocarditis, *Oral Surg Oral Med Oral Pathol* 64:417–420, 1987.
59. Back DJ, Orme ML: Pharmacokinetic drug interactions with oral contraceptives, *Clin Pharmacokinet* 18:472–484, 1990.
60. Murphy AA et al: The effect of tetracycline on levels of oral contraceptives, *Am J Obstet Gynecol* 164:28–33, 1991.
61. Neely JL et al: The effect of doxycycline on serum levels of ethinyl estradiol, norethindrone, and endogenous progesterone, *Obstet Gynecol* 77:416–420, 1991.
62. Szoka PR, Edgren RA: Drug interactions with oral contraceptives: compilation and analysis of an adverse experience report database, *Fertil Steril* 49(5 suppl 2):31S–38S, 1988.
63. Frieden TR, Mangi RJ: Inappropriate use of oral ciprofloxacin, *JAMA* 264:1438–1440, 1990.
64. Snyder SH: Drug and neurotransmitter receptors: new perspectives with clinical relevance, *JAMA* 261:3126–3129, 1989.
65. Baughman VL et al: Effectiveness of triazolam, diazepam, and placebo as preanesthetic medications, *Anesthesiology* 71:196–200, 1989.
66. Becker DE: Management of nausea and vomiting: physiological, pharmacological, and therapeutic considerations, *J Am Dent Assoc* 115:292–294, 1987.
67. Nicolson SC et al: Comparison of oral and intramuscular preanesthetic medication for pediatric inpatient surgery, *Anesthesiology* 71:8–10, 1989.
68. Becker DE: The respiratory effects of drugs used for conscious sedation and general anesthesia, *J Am Dent Assoc* 119:153–156, 1989.

Part III

Implant Treatment

Chapter 20

Edentulous Alveolar Ridge Augmentation and Restorative Grafting

PREPROSTHETIC SURGERY INVOLVING BONE GRAFTING

Philip J. Boyne

Maintenance of edentulous alveolar ridges after loss of teeth and/or after bone graft augmentation of deficient edentulous areas has been a consistent clinical problem for many years. The persistence of this problem, together with the demographic shifts in population groups, has increased the number of patients requiring rehabilitation of the jaw and enhanced the need for the delivery of this type of qualitative health care to an aging population.

In this section of the chapter the nature of the problem is described, discussing what is known concerning alveolar bone repair and regeneration. A brief review of past clinical failures in dealing with the problem is given. Such failures have largely resulted from a lack of attention to known patterns of healing and to anatomic and physiologic factors operating in the alveolar bone of the mandible and maxilla. Inadequacies of past surgical techniques have also resulted from lack of appropriate research in areas of important osseous healing phenomena.

PREPROSTHETIC SURGERY INVOLVING BONE GRAFTING

Preprosthetic surgery is an important aspect of the surgical rehabilitation of the edentulous and the partially edentulous patient presenting with severe alveolar atrophy, and of the postresection oncologic patient presenting with the totally or partially resected mandible and/or maxilla. Classic methods of preprosthetic rehabilitation have involved bone grafting with particulate and other forms of autogenous osseous material, followed by vestibuloplasty to provide vestibular depth for later construction of conventional prosthesis.[1] In the fully resected mandible and the hemi-resected mandible, the use of these procedures has been facilitated in the past by the use of titanium mesh implants to control the regenerating bone and to contain the bone graft material.[2]

Bone grafting techniques of the alveolar portion of the jaws should be based on a clear understanding of the anatomic and physiologic nature of alveolar ridge bone itself.

Use of Bone Grafts to Restore Ridges

In the past, patients presenting with excessively resorbed alveolar ridges underwent grafting procedures with autogenous bone using either one-piece iliac crest grafts or rib grafts. These grafts, although maintaining the ridge for a short period of time—up to 1 to 3 years—were almost uniformly subjected to a similar resorptive process as in the case of the original bony ridge. The grafted areas were not maintained over an acceptable postoperative course.

Use of Particulate Ceramic Implants in Restoring Alveolar Ridges

Another approach to this bone resorption problem was to graft with a nonliving bone substitute such as hydroxylapatite (HA). Hydroxylapatite particles when used alone do *not* produce bone regeneration of the ridge; rather, fibrous tissue routinely surrounds such HA particles. An artificial ridge therefore is produced that is composed of a *mass of hydroxylapatite and connective tissue* lying above the previous bony ridge. In excessively resorbed ridges, these implants of HA have not been successful, and the substitution of HA particles for living bone grafts has not been met with uniform success. The mass of HA particles is subject to micro and macro movements, which are inconsistent with good prosthodontic base support and which lead to discomfort, dysesthesia, and paraesthesia.[3, 4]

Use of Particulate Ceramic Implants Together With Autogenous Cancellous Bone

A third approach was to utilize HA particles with particulate autogenous marrow and cancellous bone grafts in an attempt to produce a more lamellated structure of the alveolar ridge to slow the resorptive process. This procedure, particularly when porous HA is used, has been clinically more successful than the complete substitution of autogenous bone grafts by synthetic HA materials.

It appears that particles of porous HA, when appropriately combined with autogenous iliac crest grafts in a composite transplant, will result in a more lamellated bone product at the recipient site. Such a lamellated or cortical bone structure tends to resist resorption when subjected to the function of either a removable or a nonremovable prosthesis.

Use of Xenografts in Restoring Alveolar Ridges

A porous xenogenic bone material that has been shown to be successful in slowing the resorption of ridges has been produced from a bovine source. This bone material, obtained from animals, is subjected to a process that removes all organic material, leaving only the inorganic portion which is largely HA but may contain other inorganic material as well depending on the manufacturing process. Because this inorganic product has the porosity of normal bone and has some carbonate and tricalcium phosphate in addition to the HA component, there tends to be some osteoclastic resorption of the material. This slow resorptive process, together with a favorable remodeling and bone rebuilding response, continues over a long period of time. During the time that the particles of biologic xenogeneic mineral are slowly resorbing and remodeling, the alveolar ridge is being maintained.[5] Thus we have a graft material which by itself has no osteoinductive effect but when combined with autogenous bone may produce an optimal type of xenograft-autograft composite material bringing about alveolar ridge maintenance.

Use of Endosteal Implants in Maintaining Alveolar Bone

A more recent development in preprosthetic surgery has evolved with the application of endosteal implants to posttraumatic bone lost, postoncologic surgery, postatrophic bone loss, and more minor types of reconstruction. The use of endosteal implants has led to new investigations of osseous repair and the response of host bone to the insertion of metal implants within the bony mass of the mandible and maxilla. This application of metallic endosteal implants has led to considerable discussion of the histologic process of integration of bone-to-metal surfaces, the nature of the interface phenomena between metal and surrounding host bone, and the possible effect of such bony response on the maintenance of alveolar bone.

SUMMARY

The clinic problems of lost alveolar bone are best addressed by preventive measures of retaining teeth in place. If tooth extraction is necessary, placement of slowly resorbable porous HA in the particulate form (1- to 2-mm particles) in the surgical extraction socket can be effective in maintaining bone.

The restoration of lost alveolar bone can best be addressed by restoration of the ridges with autogenous particulate cancellous bone mixed with xenografts of biologic slowly resorbable porous bone mineral.

The use of titanium endosteal implants to preserve existing alveolar bone and to maintain grafted areas is also advocated.

The anatomic and physiologic basis for these surgical techniques is that change in the histologic structure of bone is necessary to return the osseous tissue to the maximally supportive structure existing prior to teeth extraction and if possible to actually increase the relative amount of cortical bone in the ridge bone structure.

Further improvements in the anatomic position of the ridge crest in relationship to the opposing ridge is also helpful in reducing further bone loss and in aiding in the construction of a functional "bone sparing" prosthesis.

RESIDUAL RIDGE AUGMENTATION

Carl E. Misch

The facial plate of bone is remodeled or lost after tooth extraction, disease, or trauma to a greater extent than the lingual cortical bone. The labial bone over the natural teeth is much thinner than its lingual counterpart. Periodontal diseases create intrabony pockets on the lingual supporting bone, but are responsible for the complete loss of the overlying labial process. Dehiscence of the labial plate may naturally occur as a consequence of tooth eruption, movement from orthodontic therapy, or parafunction. Tooth trauma, vertical fractures, apicoectomy, poorly fitted margins, subgingival tooth preparation, and extractions also affect the labial plate more often than the thicker palatal bone.

The placement of the maxillary anterior teeth is more critical for ideal esthetics, phonetics, and function. The alveolar bone of the premaxilla is rapidly recontoured after the loss of the natural teeth. There is a 40% to 60% decrease in the crest width within the first 3 years after tooth loss.[6] As a result, the 8 mm wide anterior crest of the maxilla is reduced to approximately 4 mm, and this width decrease continues until it is common to find less than 3 mm within 5 years after extraction.[7] The labial plate of bone is then located lingual of its original location. Available bone width and height are major factors for implant selection, placement, and longevity. Any modality capable to improve the available bone dimension in the premaxilla should be considered.

The labial periosteal covering should remain intact during tooth extraction. The cells of the inner layer of the periosteum are responsible for the bone remodeling. Whenever the periosteum is reflected, the cells are injured and require regeneration before the remodeling process.[8] The cortical bone receives over 80% of its arterial blood supply from the periosteum, and 100% of its venous return.[9] Careful tooth elevation and extraction are indicated to minimize trauma and bone loss. Surgical extractions should segment the teeth, rather than remove bone. If bone removal is obligatory, it should be at the expense of the portion of the lingual wall, not the fragile labial process. All fibrous tissue from periodontal disease or endodontic origin should be completely removed from the socket by curettage after tooth extraction. These soft tissues impair bone formation and delay bone healing for extended periods.

The sequence of events that replaces bone in the alveolar process after tooth loss is not completely understood. There are critical steps, however, that influence the clinical end result. The ability to control or influence bone growth in this region has become more predictable in recent years. The addition of bone and bone substitutes after tooth extraction is a factor under the control of the dentist, and improves the topography and anatomic condition of the residual ridge for implant placement. In this section of the chapter, pertinent bone graft terminology is reviewed and the clinical use of different alloplasts, allografts, and autogenous bone for alveolar ridge maintenance and augmentations is clarified.

BONE AUGMENTATION

Osteoconduction

Bone is capable of repair through physiologic remodeling or healing processes after an injury, which include tooth extraction or implant placement. Bone augmentation materials can be incorporated into this process to assist or stimulate bone growth in areas where it disappears as a result of pathologic, traumatic, or physiologic processes. These bone substitutes can act on the host bone through three different mechanisms: osteoconduction, osteoinduction, and/or osteogenesis. Osteoconduction characterizes bone growth by apposition, from and on existing bone. Therefore, this process must occur in the presence of bone or differentiated mesenchymal cells. The healing of bone around an osteointegrated implant is an osteoconductive process and follows typical phases of remodeling at the bone-implant interface.[10]

Osteoconductive materials are biocompatible. Bone or soft tissue can develop by apposition to these materials without evidence of toxic reaction.

The most common osteoconductive materials in implant dentistry are alloplastic products. Alloplastic materials are exclusively synthetic, biocompatible products developed to cover a broad range of indications. They come in a great variety of textures, particle sizes, and shapes that are readily available. They may be separated into ceramics, polymers, and composites. The most frequently used are the ceramics, which may be bioinert (aluminum oxide and titanium oxide) or bioactive (calcium phosphate materials). Bioinert ceramics do not exhibit direct bonding with the host bone and are mechanically held in contact to the bone. Bioactive ceramics are the largest family of alloplasts used for bone augmentation and include hydroxylapatite (HA) and beta tricalcium phosphate. A chemical contact between the host bone and the grafted material has been demonstrated.[11–15] There are two categories of osteoconductive materials for tissue maintenance or augmentation, nonresorbable and resorbable. If these materials are placed under the skin, or surrounded by fibrous tissue, they do not grow bone. The material will remain relatively unchanged, or resorb. The sequence is summarized as follows:

1. Bone Augmentation by Osteoconduction:
   a. Differentiated cells (osteoblasts) grow next to the surface by apposition.
   b. Alloplasts (most common):
      (1) Synthetic (ceramic, polymer, composite).
      (2) Biocompatible:
         (a) Bioinert:
            i Mechanical bone contact.
            ii "Osteointegration."
            iii Aluminum oxide, titanium oxide.
         (b) Bioactive:
            i Ceramics.
            ii Hydroxylapatite and tricalcium phosphate (most common).
            iii Chemical contact.
   c. Allografts:
      (1) Same species, different genotype.
      (a) Frozen bone (irradiated).

Dense HA has become a popular bone substitute. This material has been described as nonresorbable and osteophilic when in a highly dense crystalline structure.[11] In the presence of bone, a direct bone-HA interface may be observed.[12] This finding is more common when fibrous tissue is impeded by bone or small pore size membranes from first contacting the HA surface. It appears the source of the growing blood vessels determine the contacting tissue. Fibrous tissue can grow 0.5 mm daily, compared with bone, at 50 μm per day; thus, the result favors soft tissue. When HA is placed on top of cortical bone, the bottom layer may have bone at the interface, but the majority of material is encapsulated by fibrous tissue.

When the HA is placed into a bone preparation or tooth socket, or covered with a small pore membrane, the tissue interface is more likely bone.

Dense HA is an inorganic material and cannot grow or rigidly fixate itself to an implant surface. It is also a very hard, ceramic-like material that is difficult to cut with a knife or bur. Therefore, when dense, particulate HA is placed into bone, its purpose is usually to obtund the space, maintain the bone volume and shape, or support a soft tissue–borne removable prosthesis. If an endosteal implant is desired in the bone-HA region, a diamond drill and high-speed handpiece may be required to modify the HA. A common placement of dense particulate HA with endosteal implants is on the facial plate to improve the soft tissue contour. This material is also used for ridge augmentation for denture support.[16, 17]

The second type of osteoconductive materials are resorbable when placed into bone or soft tissue. Their primary indication is when bone can first grow next to the material and then replace it, similar to the creeping substitution found in natural bone remodeling.[14] These materials are usually very porous and amorphous HA products, or calcium phosphate combinations. It should be noted that all HA products resorb in the presence of low pH (infection) at a similar rapid rate, similar to that of any calcium phosphate combination. HA and resorption rates are as follows:

1. Structure:
   a. Dense, crystalline:
      (1) Least resorption.
   b. Amorphous:
      (2) Faster resorption.
2. Porosity:
   a. Dense:
      (1) Least resorption.
   b. Macroporous:
      (1) Fifteen percent pore spaces.
      (2) Large holes.
   c. Microporous:
      (1) Thirty percent pore spaces.
      (2) Small holes.
      (3) Faster resorption.
3. pH:
   a. Low pH (infection).
      (1) All $CaPO_4$ compounds (including hydroxylapatite) resorb rapidly.

Osteoconductive materials also include organic sources such as highly irradiated or frozen bone. The resorbable and nonresorbable manufactured inorganic products are easily obtained; do not risk contamination or allergic reaction, disease transmission, or the need of an additional surgical site; and are the most common osteoconductive materials used in dentistry.

Osteoinduction

An osteoinductive material is capable of inducing the transformation of undifferentiated cells into osteoblasts or chondroblasts, in an area where this is not expected behavior. Osteoinductive materials are more contributory to bone formation during the remodeling process.[18] The most common osteoinductive materials in implant dentistry are bone allografts. A bone allograft is a hard tissue from an individual of the same species as the recipient but of different genotype. The advantage of such materials is the elimination of the donor site in the patient and availability, which permits its use in large quantities. It is obtained from cadavers, processed and stored in various shapes and sizes in bone banks for future uses. There are three types of allografts: frozen, freeze-dried, and demineralized freeze-dried.

Frozen bone is obtained from cadavers and directly frozen and stored. It may also be irradiated to decrease the immune reaction within the recipient.[10, 19] It primarily is osteoconductive and is rarely used in implant dentistry.

Freeze-dried bone includes an additional desiccating step. The inorganic matrix has been maintained, but osteoclasts are required to release the bone growing factors, because of the remaining calcium and phosphate salts. The osteoclasts may induce bone resorption in the region and makes the product more unpredictable.[20] Freeze-dried bone also works primarily through an osteoconductive process.

Demineralized freeze-dried bone (DFDB) is also obtained from a cadaver. The process to form DFDB is specific, and wide variation may alter the result. Cortical and/or trabecular bone is harvested from a disease-free person. The bone is washed in distilled water and ground to a particle size of 75 to 500 μm. The powder is demineralized in 0.6N hydrochloric or nitric acid for 6 to 16 hours. After dehydration, it is often sterilized in ethylene oxide and freeze-dried to further decrease the antigenicity. Several tests are performed to evaluate the safety of the process, and the acid demineralization process destroys any known viruses and pathogens. The calcium and phosphate salts are removed from the bone in the acid-reducing process. The bone remaining from this treatment still possesses the organic osteogenic growth factors in the matrix necessary for bone formation, including bone morphogenetic protein (BMP), platelet derived growth factor, and transforming growth factor.[21] The cortical bone contains most of the BMP in bone.[22] Because the salts are removed from the bone, the nonsoluble proteins may be released to the environment without osteoclastic activity. As a result, more undifferentiated cells may transform into osteoblasts, and the bone forming process is osteoinductive.

If an osteoinductive material is placed under the skin, the material will be replaced by small quantities of bone. Therefore, it is used when the environment is less prone to form bone. It may also be used with autogenous or osteoconductive materials, which results with more bone formation than without DFDB.

Osteogenesis

Osteogenesis refers to a material capable to form bone, even in the absence of local undifferentiated mesenchymal cells. Osteogenic graft materials are composed of living bone cells, which produce large amounts of growth factors for bone. At present, autogenous bone is the only osteogenetic material available. Autogenous iliac bone grafts, or local bone grafts from the maxillary tuberosity, ascending ramus, or mental symphysis, are the most common donor sites. The medullary or trabecular bone contains the bone cells in greatest concentration. The cells should be stored in sterile saline, lactated Ringer's solution, or sterile 5% dextrose and water to maintain cell vitality. Distilled water is contraindicated for this purpose, and venous blood is not as effective as saline or dextrose and water.[22] Because the graft material requires an additional operative site, it is used when conditions for growth of bone are poor and/or in conjunction with the other materials if more volume is required.

Autogenous bone has an inorganic matrix, primarily of HA, which contains osteocytes, osteoblasts, osteoclasts, and osteogenic proteins.[17] The membranous bone harvested from the mandibular symphysis represents an excellent source of autogenous bone, with excellent properties as to early revascularization, high BMP potential, and numbers of living cells. Small graft regions of one to four teeth may be augmented by this procedure (see Chapter 26).

The mechanism of bone growth with autogenous bone includes all three methods. The living cells, primarily from the trabecular region, may actually live and form an osteoid product. However, a source of blood supply and cell numbers greatly influence the result. This osteogenic effects process diminishes within 4 weeks. As the bone resorbs, it may release BMP and other proteins to form bone with the osteoinductive process. This begins approximately after 6 weeks and lasts as long as 6 months.[23] The cortical bone is the primary source of these proteins. A thick cortical plate on the graft may prevent fibrous tissue from invading the area and acts like a small pore membrane in guided regeneration. The scaffold of the autogenous bone graft may also form bone with the osteoconductive effect as new bone forms with creeping substitution.

Application

The graft material selected for maintenance of ridge form after tooth extraction is related to availability and to the needs of the patient. An extraction socket with five healthy walls of bone will heal with vital bone in approximately

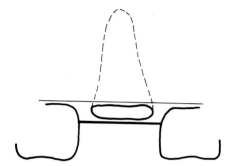

FIG 20–1.
Extraction site (or cyst on lateral aspect of
bone) may form a five-wall defect. Resorbable
alloplast is used to maintain bone volume.

4 to 6 months, depending on the root size and patient's health (Fig 20–1). The
blood clot that forms will constrict, and the surrounding bone will permit
reestablishment of the blood supply, followed by bone formation but of decreased
width. However, the labial bone loss in width will be less dramatic when the
socket is filled with a graft material. The socket should be filled with a resorbable
material if an implant may be placed in the region after healing. Calcium
phosphates and/or porous HA are often used for this purpose. Collagen may be
placed over the extraction site to limit the loss of bone graft material. Expensive
membranes are not required because five walls of bone are present. The
interdental papillae on each side are separated, and sutures are placed over the
extraction socket to contain the blood clot and graft material. If a removable
prosthesis is used to replace the missing tooth, it is not removed for 3 days to
further protect the loss of the graft.

An alternative is to remove the tooth at one appointment, but place the graft
2 months later. This option allows primary closure, makes sure no infection is
present, and allows the doctor to evaluate the number of existing walls before the
graft procedure. As a result the fee and appropriate time period for the patient
may be discussed before the treatment. The disadvantages include an additional
surgery and a delay of 2 months.

Four to six months are usually required before reentry and implant
placement, depending on the extraction socket size. The socket may not be
completely healed in the center, but the 4 mm implant osteotomy will be against
living bone cells on the periphery. Bone cells may be harvested from the drill
during the osteotomy and packed over and around the implant site. Primary
closure is possible after implant placement because the extraction socket is
covered with attached gingiva within 2 months after tooth extraction.

The loss of one wall of healthy bone (usually the labial or the apex) requires
additional grafting elements for osseous reformation without dramatic decrease
in bone width (Fig 20–2). Fifty percent of an osteoinductive material (DFDB),
should be added to the resorbable osteoconductive calcium phosphates. If all

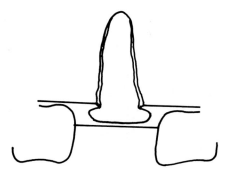

FIG 20–2
Loss of a labial plate from the extraction socket results in a four-wall defect. DFDB is added to the bone and covered with DFDB and resorbable alloplast. A membrane also may be used to cover this layered graft.

DFDB is used, it is often lost through the incision line or resorbed too rapidly to permit bone formation to replace the missing wall of bone. A layer of DFDB is placed on the bone. This is covered with DFDB mixed with the alloplasts. It is more important to place a sheet of laminar bone, or small pore membrane, over the labial aspect of the graft if primary closure cannot be achieved after the extraction. If the tooth was removed 2 months previously, the graft primary closure and the decreased risk of infection are benefits. A 5- to 6-month healing period is suggested before reentry and implant placement.

The loss of two or more bony walls of vital bone requires incorporation of an autogenous component to the graft for a more rapid, predictable graft site (Fig 20–3). The greater the defect, the more autogenous bone is added to the graft material. When autogenous bone is added to the graft, it is placed directly on the underlying bone. A blood supply from bone must be established to maintain vitality of the living cells and obtain their osteogenic effect. The osteoinductive effect of living bone does not begin for several weeks (when osteoclasts remove the salts around the organic matrix). Therefore, DFDB is placed over the autogenous bone to start the osteoinductive process more rapidly. On top of the DFDB a microporous HA or tricalcium phosphate mixed with DFDB may be used.

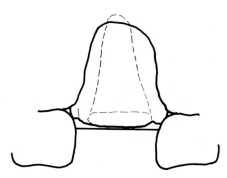

FIG 20–3.
Loss of bone on the lateral aspects of the extraction site may result in a two- or three-wall defect. Autogenous bone, then DFDB, then DFDB and resorbable alloplast and a membrane may restore the volume of bone.

If significant volume is important for the graft site, a small pore membrane may be placed over this layered graft technique. This prevents the blood vessels from the overlying fibrous tissue from invading the graft and forming fibrous tissue instead of bone.

Four or five walls of missing bone are treated as an onlay graft and often require autogenous cortical and trabecular bone on top of the residual ridge. Demineralized freeze-dried bone may be used around the autogenous graft along with DFDB and alloplast and a small pore membrane to complete the layer graft approach (see Chapter 27). If a block of bone graft is used, the thick cortical plate may act as a membrane. Four to six months elapse before reentry and implant placement when most all the graft is autogenous bone used in the grafted site.

Grafting of future implant sites is summarized as follows:

1. Five-wall defect:
   a. Examples:
      (1) healthy tooth extraction.
      (2) cyst on lateral aspect of bone.
   b. Use inexpensive resorbable alloplasts.
   c. Wait 4 to 6 months before reentry for implant.
2. Four-wall defect:
   a. Example: loss of labial wall on extraction site.
   b. Use demineralized freeze-dried bone (DFDB) on bone.
   c. Use DFDB and calcium phosphate (CaPO$_4$) on top of DFDB.
   d. Wait 5 to 6 months for reentry
3. Two-wall to three-wall defect:
   a. Example: periodontal infected tooth extraction.
   b. Autogenous bone chips on bone.
   c. DFDB on top of autogenous graft.
   d. DFDB and CaPO$_4$ on top layer.
   e. Small pore membrane when larger volumes are desired.
4. One-wall defect:
   a. Example: onlay graft.
   b. Autogenous bone block on bone (both cortical and trabecular).
   c. DFDB on autogenous graft.
   d. DFDB and CaPO$_4$ on top layer and sides of bone block.
   e. Small pore membrane if cortical bone thin or not present on bone block.

The same rationale for ridge augmentation is used without extraction sockets. Osteoconductive and osteoinductive materials will form bone when placed *into* bone. An onlay graft of HA and DFDB or DFDB alone is not as predictable and therefore not suggested for augmentation prior to endosteal implants. Onlay grafts with autogenous bone as the major component of the graft material improves the amount of bone formed. Intraoral sources of bone are usually preferred when small regions require augmentation. If adequate amounts of autogenous bone are not available, the edentulous ridge may be split with an osteotomy, bone wedges used to increase the width (keeping the periosteum intact on the lateral sides), and then autogenous bone, DFDB and porous HA or calcium phosphate placed within the bone. Reentry is similar to that for an extraction socket with a missing wall (5 to 6 months) and is related to the size of the graft (see Chapter 26).

Results to increase residual bone width and/or height with only small pore membranes are variable. A study in animals indicated that height augmentation was less predictable than width augmentation, and augmentations ranged from 0.5 mm to 4 mm.[24] Short-term clinical trials are expressing similar findings. Therefore, it is suggested the membrane be used with as much autogenous bone as practical for an onlay graft to increase width and/or height. In addition, the augmentation should usually be performed before implant placement, especially in the premaxilla. Although more time and additional surgery are required, the results are more predictable. The osteotomy of the implant may still be performed at the augmentation surgery. But the purpose of the osteotomy is to harvest additional autogenous bone to mix with DFDB, not to place an implant. When several millimeters of bone width and height are desired, the reentry implant surgery after 5 to 6 months may require additional ridge augmentation when the implant is placed. Again, the bone is harvested during the osteotomy and used in the augmentation/implant insertion procedure.

HYDROXYAPATITE FOR MAXILLARY ANTERIOR ALVEOLAR RIDGE AUGMENTATION

A maxillary complete denture is a satisfactory replacement for missing teeth for many completely edentulous patients. However, once a mandibular implant support restoration is fabricated, the patient becomes more aware of the lack of stability, support, and/or retention of the removable maxillary prosthesis. The successful restoration with a soft tissue–supported removable prosthesis depends on several conditions. The anatomy of the edentulous arch foundation is the primary criterion for prosthesis support and stability. Several modalities are available to improve the prognosis of the restoration on a compromised support area. However, varied soft tissue impression techniques, altered occlusal schemes, and a broad range of removable prosthetic concepts show limited improvement of the final restoration.

Surgical techniques can help improve the soft tissue–supported prosthesis in the maxilla. These include vestibuloplasty, free soft tissue grafts, and alveolar ridge augmentation. Autogenous bone grafts for ridge augmentation are a viable alternative in the atrophic maxilla, if implants are placed at the time or shortly after the graft surgery. If the autogenous graft is used only for improved soft tissue support, resorption is a major problem. As much as 90% of the grafted bone resorbs sporadically within 3 to 5 years following augmentation surgery.[16, 19] The soft tissue–supported denture needs repeated relining and rebasing procedures to maintain ridge contact. The resultant soft tissues become highly mobile and unsupported by the resorbing ridge. The patient often complains of recurrent soft tissue abrasions, and of mobile, unstable, and poorly retentive prostheses.

Dense nonresorbable HA is classified as a nonresorbable ridge augmentation material. It is a relatively common commercial cleaning product, used also in toothpaste. Hydroxyapatite comprises many components of the stomatognathic system. Enamel is 96% HA; dentine, 70% to 80%; and cementum, 50% to 60%. The inorganic portion of bone is also made of this material. Dense hydroxyapatite is inert, biocompatible, and does not induce any inflammatory or foreign body reactions when implanted in the tissues. There is no evidence of immune response or local or systemic toxicity.[16]

Bone can grow to the surface of HA without any interposing connective tissue, and an ionic bond may actually form between the host bone and the implanted material.[16, 17] However, when HA is placed on top of cortical bone, fibrous tissue, not bone, surrounds most of the particles not in contact with the host bone. Sharawy found that a mixture of DFDB and HA improved the relationship between bone and that material around the particles.[21] Dense, block HA has surgical advantages, but has not given routine predictable results.

Hydroxyapatite has been overused for ridge augmentation, especially in the mandible, with the result of poorer soft tissue anatomy and prosthesis support than before augmentation.[25] Thus, improved surgical procedures specific for the maxillary anterior edentulous patient using HA and DFDB ridge augmentation are discussed.

Indications

Ridge augmentation is rarely indicated for the mandibular arch. The mandibular denture moves 10 mm during function, compared with approximately 2 mm movement for the complete maxillary denture.[26] Ridge augmentation alone does not provide enough improvement for successful mandibular denture support. In addition, sore spots are more common on the thinner, nonmobile tissues; migration of the augmentation is of great occurrence; and paresthesia of the mental nerve is a concern.[25] Permucosal implants achieve much greater support, retention, and stability for the mandibular denture. On the other hand, the maxillary edentulous arch and complete denture can often benefit from ridge augmentation. The maxilla can be divided into three regions: left and right posterior segments, and the anterior segment. The posterior maxilla rarely requires ridge augmentation for improved ridge shape or contour. The tuberosity region usually maintains ridge form. The posterior palatal seal area of the denture is not primarily dependent on the posterior ridge form. The posterior buccal space is usually present to give lateral stability in the posterior region, regardless of posterior ridge contour.

The anatomy of the premaxilla is primarily responsible for varying degrees of stability found in maxillary dentures. The loss of teeth causes bone to first resorb in width. In this region, the incisive papilla eventually becomes the most anterior part of the edentulous ridge. This landmark is 5 to 7 mm behind the labial crest of bone when central incisors are present. After the initial 40% to 60% of the ridge width is lost, the height and width of the anterior edentulous ridge becomes considerably diminished. Because the maxillary anterior teeth are placed anterior and inferior to the landmark, instability occurs as a result of moment loads against the teeth.

Once the ridge width is decreased, the anterior vertical height of bone is the primary dimension that prevents anterior rotation of a removable prosthesis and loss of posterior seal. Anterior forces against the maxillary prostheses are common. They occur in all mandibular excursions, especially in anterior incision of food. When food is between the teeth, the occlusion can not stabilize a denture; the bolus of food acts as a pivot region for denture rotation. Hence, the chewing cycle, or incision of food, may cause maxillary anterior denture instability. As a result, the premaxilla is the most common region of the maxilla that resists denture movement during function and improves stability of the removable prosthesis.

Denture Criteria

The width of the ridge is the primary region that contributes to denture stability and support under vertical pressures.[27] The crest of the ridge is best suited for vertical forces. Selective pressure impression techniques take advantage of this primary area of support.[28] Broader ridges encourage greater distribution of occlusal forces and cause less tissue changes on the alveolar ridge.

A secondary area of denture support and stability is the premaxilla.[29] The anterior third of the palate is able to resist the anterior movement of the denture, and presents adequate attached tissue (e.g., without glands) to be loaded by the prosthesis. The vertical walls of the anterior premaxilla are beneficial for retention of the maxillary denture (Fig 20–4).

Many factors are involved with denture retention, including saliva, valve seal, muscle attachments and tonus, and denture adaptation. Edentulous maxillae vary widely in these factors, but the ability to maintain a border seal during function is much greater than with a mandibular denture and compensates for other limiting retention factors.[30]

Ridge Shape

The portion of the edentulous anatomy most likely to change after augmentation is the ridge form. In many instances the incorrect assumption has

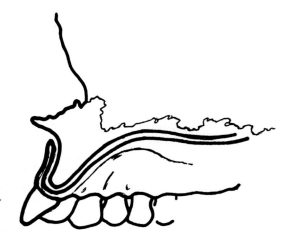

FIG 20–4.
The premaxilla is a secondary area of denture support, and improves stability by resisting anterior movement during mandibular excursions.

been made that the larger the alveolar ridge the better the retention and stability of the denture. As a result, many alveolar ridge augmentations have resulted in greatly increased ridge size, but a decrease in retention and stability. Therefore, it is most important to appreciate the shape of the ridge in developing the relation between stability and support criteria for a maxillary removable prosthesis.

Alveolar ridge shape may be classified related to retention. The V-shaped ridge is poorest for retention or support. This is a common ridge form resulting from ridge augmentation surgery which oversizes the ridge with particulate HA. The ideal ridge form for retention has parallel lateral and medial walls. The greater the ridge wall is parallel in height, the greater the retention. This shape and dimension also improves lateral stability. Lateral movement of the prosthesis is limited by the parallel walls, even if vertical displacement occurs. Therefore, both retention and stability are affected by the lateral aspect of the ridge contour (Fig 20–5).

FIG 20–5.
A, a square ridge form is best for retention and stability. The parallel walls resist lateral movement, and height is related to retention. **B,** a V-shaped ridge (often resulting from bone loss in width before the height is significantly affected) is poorest in retention and stability. It should be converted to a square arch form *(dashed line)* on the lingual aspect of the ridge with HA ridge augmentation.

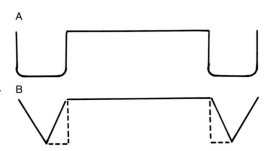

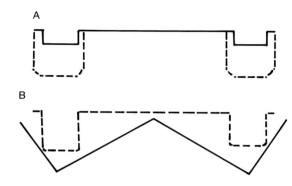

FIG 20–6.
A, an atrophic ridge with a flat palate has excellent properties for support of a denture. **B,** conversion to a V-shaped ridge with HA augmentation is incorrect because it provides poorer support, retention, and stability. Instead, the flat ridge should be augmented to a greater height, but maintaining a broad flat crest *(dashed line)*.

The best ridge form to oppose vertical denture movement is a flat, broad ridge crest, parallel to the opposing force at the ideal vertical dimension. The least stable is the V-shaped ridge at an angle to the opposing force. Hence, support and stability are affected by ridge shape and ridge augmentation should be designed to provide a square-shaped ridge form (Fig 20–6).

Tissue Type

The type of supporting tissue is also an important parameter in considering HA ridge correction. The amount of tissue movement over the bone can directly affect denture stability and formation of tissue abrasions.

The oral mucosa has classically been described as a movable, unattached, nonkeratinized mucosa or as a nonmobile, attached keratinized mucosa. These categories are oversimplified for denture support. It has been recognized that attached keratinized mucosa may increase in thickness as a consequence of bone resorption, primarily in the anterior maxilla. This tissue thickness often exceeds several millimeters and becomes highly mobile. Although classified as attached gingiva, it serves as a poor denture base. Likewise, unattached, nonkeratinized tissue may become thick and nonmobile tissue by placing HA between the bone and periosteum. This tissue then can serve as a good quality denture supporting base. Therefore, important qualities of tissue for denture support relate to thickness and mobility, not necessarily to its histologic surface condition.

Ridge augmentation with HA can decrease the amount of ridge resorption. The dense material can bond to the cortical bone and increase the amount of support. Because HA does not resorb as easily as bone, the surrounding bone resorbs less. Clinical experience demonstrates longer periods between necessary relines of the maxillary prosthesis. The primary long-term goal of premaxillary augmentation is to achieve a square ridge shape, which can oppose the forces of the opposing arch. Other benefits are a reduction of soft tissue movement, a decrease in the rate of resorption, and the maintenance of the vertical component of the anterior ridge.

PROCEDURE

Various techniques have been proposed for subperiosteal placement of HA for ridge augmentation. The most common procedure is to primarily introduce it on the labial aspect of the resorbed ridge.[16] This technique in theory is appropriate, because the ridge width is lost almost completely from the labial, and the maxilla narrows as the mandible widens during resorption.

However, this approach is usually incorrect, except for labial undercuts of a Division A ridge form. The anterior valve seal region of the denture is often compromised, and when a vestibuloplasty may be necessary, it requires a second surgery. Diffusion of HA into adjacent areas needed for valve seal retention, or into areas outside the extension area of the denture is not uncommon. Excessive ridge width and/or height with a labial approach may compromise placement of artificial teeth with impact on esthetics, phonetics, or function.

The maxillary Division A ridge with high muscle attachment usually has both height and width of bone to support the prosthesis. On occasion, labial undercuts may compromise retention and increase soft tissue abrasions. As a result, the labial undercut areas may be filled in with HA to improve the ridge contour. The Division B and C-w anterior ridge is ideally indicated for HA/DFDB ridge augmentation. The Division B augmentation is to the lingual side and squares the ridge form. The Division C-w is also on the lingual, but increases the ridge height and width. A vestibuloplasty may be performed as indicated. The Division D and C-h ridges are least suited for HA augmentation. Although these ridges are in greater need, the poor ridge form does not resist future migration of the HA in the labial fold. Hence, long-term success is compromised.

Lingual-Crest Technique

A technique designed primarily to enhance ridge form was developed by Misch in 1983.[31] The lingual crest technique offers the primary advantages of unaffected anterior valve seal, labial flange contour, and a combined vestibuloplasty option. Migration of HA is limited, as is height and width over extension. The technique may also be used on partially edentulous Kennedy-Applegate Class IV patients.

The arch shape is first determined. An incision is made from the nasal spine to the incisive papilla in the tapered or ovoid shape, whereas incisions in the canine eminence to the lingual incline of the ridge are made in a square arch shape (Fig 20–7).

A full-thickness subperiosteal opening is accomplished first on the labial of the incision area for approximately 5 mm, then over the crest of the ridge and into the papilla and/or palatal region. A 2 Molt elevator is introduced into the initial opening, and is used to elevate the periosteum along the lingual alveolar ridge.

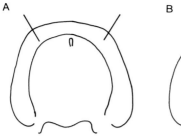

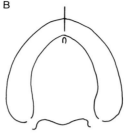

FIG 20–7.
Access incision for augmentation is made in the canine region for the square arch **(A)** and in the midline for the tapered or ovoid arch **(B).**

This is performed bilaterally to the region of the first premolar. The 2 Molt elevator then may proceed toward the crest of the ridge. A constant effort is made to square the ridge form, rather than over zealous reflection. A 4 Molt elevator then reflects the same surgical site, slightly expanding the tunnel or envelope of reflection. The reflection is only large enough to introduce a small HA syringe and square the ridge form (Fig 20–8).

Particulate dense HA mixed with one-third volume DFDB and the patient's blood is then loaded in a HA syringe. The DFDB is an osteoinductive material, and the HA is an osteoconductive material. The patient's whole blood mixed with these materials will form a coagulum, and help prevent initial migration.

The syringe and graft material are introduced into the subperiosteal tunnel. The slight labial reflection improves entry of the syringe into the surgical site. The syringe is positioned as far distal in the tunnel as reflected. The graft material is

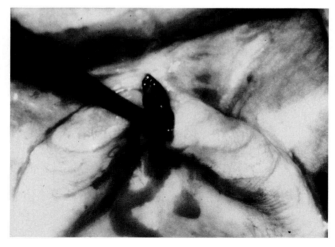

FIG 20–8.
An elevator is introduced into a subperiosteal tunnel on the lingual aspect of the premaxilla. An attempt is made to square the ridge form.

then injected into the subperiosteal tunnel while the syringe is slightly withdrawn. An attempt is made to densely pack the augmentation material into the surgical tunnel while the fingers shape the ridge form. Only one and one-half to three syringes are needed per side for a typical augmentation. The amount is far less important than the square ridge form that is developed. The ridge form should remain square and the tissue firm even with positive pressure. If not, additional HA should be introduced into the tunnel. Three-0 vicryl sutures are used to approximate the initial incision(s), with interrupted sutures on the labial and interrupted horizontal mattress sutures on the crest and lingual incision (Fig 20–9).

Vestibuloplasty

If a vestibuloplasty is needed to improve the height of the labial ridge form, it may be accomplished during the same surgery. The graft material is not introduced on the labial, so any vestibuloplasty technique may be performed without compromise or HA migration. The most common technique incises the tissue just above the junction of the mucoperiosteum. The muscle attachments and tissue are reflected to the level of the periosteum and above the height of the desired vestibule. Some relapse of vestibular height is common so the height is usually extended several millimeters above the final desired amount. A free tissue graft may be applied to the split tissue technique, or the area can heal by secondary epithelialization. If an autogenous tissue or allograft freeze-dried graft

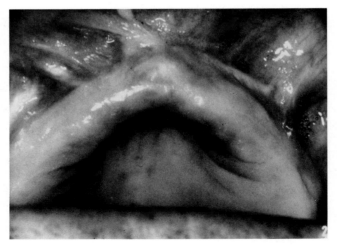

FIG 20–9.
Anterior ridge forms several months after HA and DFDB augmentation. The ridge form is broader and firmer than before surgery.

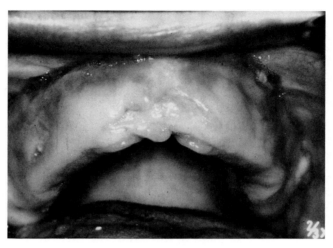

FIG 20–10.
Vestibuloplasty may be performed at the same time as lingual augmentation. Freeze-dried skin or autogenous tissue graft will improve vestibule height over the long term.

is placed over the surgical site, less vertical relapse of the vestibuloplasty occurs (Fig 20–10).

Surgical Stent

Several techniques allow the patient to wear a prosthesis immediately following surgery. The first option is to use the patient's existing denture. Acrylic is first added to the external surface of the anterior palatal portion of the prosthesis. The crest and lingual areas of the denture are then generously relieved prior to surgery. The posterior palate and ridge areas are not modified. At the end of the surgical augmentation, the denture is inserted into the patient's mouth. The denture should seat in the posterior region as before, and the maxillary teeth and lips are compared to the presurgical evaluation. If it is not similar, more acrylic in the anterior region must be removed. Once adequate relief is obtained, a chairside rigid acrylic reline material is used, especially on the labial flange, if a vestibuloplasty was performed. This material will help support the HA graft and prevent crestal migration of the vestibuloplasty. The borders of the reline are then slightly shortened, smoothed, and polished, and the surgical areas are slightly relieved 1 to 2 mm. A tissue conditioner then may be placed into all relieved regions and muscle molded for proper extension. Sterile petroleum jelly may be applied to the sutures to prevent entrapment during acrylic reline or soft tissue conditioning procedures.

The second alternative uses a transitional prosthesis fabricated from an altered presurgical impression. Clay or other medium is added to the crest and lingual arch to simulate the final surgical result. The cast is duplicated, and a transitional prosthesis fabricated. The palatal region is made of clear acrylic, so direct vision may be used to determine excess pressure in any region. This restoration is also evaluated after surgery, and modified as needed, similar to the previous technique.

Postoperative Instructions

The patient is instructed to leave the maxillary prosthesis in place for the next 10 to 14 days. Antibiotics are prescribed as routine, along with analgesics, ibuprofen, and steroids. The patient may brush the denture while in place. Use of oral rinses is not encouraged during the first 48 hours, since incision line closure is delayed because of the HA at the surgical site. Swelling or ecchymosis is not unusual, especially if a vestibuloplasty is simultaneously performed.

The patient is usually in good spirits and the vestibuloplasty is generally healed at 2 weeks. The sutures may remain in place on the lingual portion of the area for an additional 1 to 2 weeks. The tissue conditioner is removed and replaced by a soft liner. The esthetics, phonetics, and occlusion are evaluated and compared with those characteristics in the presurgical state.

A full liquid diet is generally indicated for the first 2 weeks following surgery; this is modified to a masticatory soft diet for the following 2 to 4 weeks. The prosthesis is worn as little as possible after the initial 2 weeks, and the tongue and other structures that may place pressure on the augmentation are carefully evaluated. The final impression may generally be made 2 months after surgery. A reline is often needed 6 to 9 months after surgery. A metal base prosthesis should not be fabricated before 9 months after surgery.

Complications

The most common complication is the separation of tissue at the lingual crestal region during the surgical tunnel preparation. This is usually of no long-term consequence, and will not significantly alter the end result. The procedure should continue if this occurs, as initially directed. Once the area is reflected, direct vision can ensure that the periosteum is elevated. The tissue is sutured along the crestal separation using horizontal mattress sutures. This restores the tunnel and enables the graft material to be packed into position.

The migration of HA particles through the incision line occurs with enough frequency to be considered a side effect or consequence of dense packing of the material. The patient should be notified before surgery that sandlike particles can be found under the denture for as long as several weeks. This condition may lead to a soft tissue depression along the incision line.

A mobile augmented ridge after healing may result from several causes. The most common is prosthesis mobility during healing. The HA augmentation should be treated like other implants. A rigid, nonmobile material during healing results in a stable ridge for support, stability, and retention. If the prosthesis is not stable, especially in occlusion with a bruxism patient, other methods must be employed to limit movement. For example, a surgical stent without teeth may be wired or screwed into place for the initial 2 weeks of healing. This rigid stent should not compress the tissue, causing necrosis, but should be sufficiently stable to protect the bone-implant interface. Once the stent is removed, a transitional prosthesis is worn primarily for esthetics.

Another factor that causes mobility of the augmented ridge is placement of the graft material above the periosteum. Because the tunnel approach is a blind surgical technique, repeated evaluation at the time of surgery is necessary to ensure subperiosteal augmentation placement.

The augmented ridge should be firm to palpation before the sutures are placed. If the ridge is mobile, further condensing of the graft into the tunnel will improve the situation. Occasionally the hyperplastic tissue in the anterior maxilla is so thick, even dense compaction of the graft will not limit tissue mobility. This tissue may be surgically recontoured to a thinner amount at the time of surgery or shortly thereafter. Delaying the tissue recontouring may cause prosthesis mobility and resultant ridge mobility.

An augmented ridge that is mobile at 2 to 4 weeks is much easier to correct at that time rather than waiting additional months hoping for improvement. The original surgical procedure may be repeated, and the ridge firmness improved.

Overzealous subperiosteal tunneling, or on occasion too aggressive packing of the DFDB and HA, may result in placement of the material beyond the square ridge form. The placement of a horizontal mattress suture through the base of the ridge form may constrict the material from migration during initial healing. A similar suturing approach may help to form the square ridge form for C-w ridges, where some height and form are developed with the augmentation. In this case, however, the sutures are placed primarily to improve the ridge form, rather than to limit migration.

Premaxillary HA augmentation is not predictable for Division C-h or D arches. The complete lack of vertical premaxilla does not provide resistance to anterior denture displacement or movement. As a consequence, anterior HA migration or entire ridge movement may occur even months after the augmentation process appeared successful. These patients often require endosteal implants for additional stability of the removable prosthesis. However, more extensive procedures, which include subantral augmentation and/or nasal elevation and augmentation, are often required prior to endosteal implant placement.

CONCLUSION

A maxillary denture is satisfactory for the majority of completely edentulous patients. However, once a mandibular implant–supported restoration is fabricated, many patients become more aware of the lack of stability, support, and retention of the maxillary denture. Techniques to improve these conditions are therefore warranted. The premaxilla is a secondary area of support involved with retention and stability. Ridge augmentation with HA and DFDB can improve this critical region and improve the conditions required for denture satisfaction.

REFERENCES

1. Boyne PJ: Preprosthetic surgery for the older patient. *J Am Dent Assoc* 1987 (spec issue): Jan-Feb, p 17.
2. Boyne PJ: The use of marrow particulate grafts and titanium implants in the reconstruction of resected mandibles, in Jacobs JR (ed): *Maxillofacial Trauma: An International Perspective,* vol 19. Praeger, 1983, pp 212–218.
3. Boyne PJ: Current clinical experience with Durapatite. Proceedings of Symposium on Alveolar Ridge Augmentation in Edentulous Patients. Princeton, NJ, Communications Media for Education, 1985, pp 3–11.
4. Kent JN, Quinn JH, Zide MF, et al: Alveolar ridge augmentation using nonresorbable hydroxylapatite with or without autogenous cancellous bone. *J Oral Maxillofac Surg* 1983; 41:629–642.
5. Boyne PJ: Comparison of porous and nonporous hydroxylapatite and xenografts in the restoration of alveolar ridges. Proceedings of ASTM Symposium on Implants, Nashville, 1987, pp 359–369.
6. Pietrowkowski J, Massler M: Alveolar ridge resorption following tooth extraction, *J Prosthet Dent* 17:21–27, 1967.
7. Tatum OH: The Omni implant system, abstract, Alabama Implant Congress, May 7, 1987.
8. Roberts EW: Bone physiology and metabolism, *Can Dent Assoc J* 75:54–61, 1987.
9. Chanavez M: Blood supply to the cortical bone, abstract, Alabama Implant Study Group, Birmingham, Alabama, May 1991.
10. Fonseca RJ, Davis W: *Reconstructive preprosthetic oral and maxillofacial surgery,* Philadelphia, 1986, WB Saunders.
11. Jarcho M: Calcium phosphate ceramics as hard tissue prosthetics, *Clin Orthop* 157:259, 1981.
12. LeGeros RZ: Calcium phosphate materials in restorative dentistry, a review, *Adv Dent Res* 2:164–182, 1988.
13. LeGeros RZ: Properties of commercial bone grafts compared to human bone and new synthetic bone biomaterials, abstract, Annual Meeting of the Society for Biomaterials, 1983, p 86.

14. Rejda BV, Peelen JCJ, Grot K: Tri-calcium phosphate as a bone substitute, *Bioengineering* 1:93, 1977.
15. Judy WK: Multiple uses of resorbable tri-calcium phosphate, *New York Dent J* 53:1983.
16. Kent JN et al: Correction of alveolar ridge deficiencies with non-resorbable HA, *J Am Dent Assoc* 105:993–1001, 1982.
17. Boyne P: Impact of durapatite as a bone grafting material in oral and maxillofacial surgery, *Compendium Continuing Educ Dent* 2(suppl):583–586, 1982.
18. Cook SD et al: Interface mechanics and histology of titanium hydroxyapatite-coated titanium for dental implant application, *Int J Oral Maxillofac Implants* 2:15–22, 1987.
19. Converse JM, editor: *Reconstructive plastic surgery, principles and procedures in correction, reconstruction and transplantation,* ed 2, Philadelphia, 1977, WB Saunders.
20. Hurt WC: Freeze-dried bone homografts in periodontal lesions in dogs, *J Periodont Dent* 39:89, 1968.
21. Sharawy M: Allografts and bone formation, International Congress of Oral Implant, World Meeting, London, May 1991.
22. Marx RE: Principles of hard and soft tissue reconstruction of jaws, abstract ML 315, American Association of Oral and Maxillofacial Surgery, New Orleans, 1990.
23. Fonseca RJ, Frost D, Zeitler D, et al: Reconstruction of edentulous bone loss. In Fonseca RJ, Davis WH, editors: *Reconstructive preprosthetic oral and maxillofacial surgery,* Philadelphia, 1986, WB Saunders, pp 117–165.
24. Misch CE, Sarnachiaro O, Sharawy M: Monkey pilot study: Ridge augmentation using small pore membranes and bone substitute, in press.
25. Desjardins RP: Hydroxyapatite for alveolar ridge augmentation: indications and problems, *J Prosthet Dent* 54:374–383, 1985.
26. Smith D et al: The mobility of artificial dentures during communication, *J Prosthet Dent* 13:839–856, 1963.
27. Luthra SP: Measurement of the area of the maxillary basal seat for denture, *J Prosthet Dent* 30:25–27, 1973.
28. Boucher CO: Complete denture impression based upon the anatomy of the mouth, *J Am Dent Assoc* 31:1174–1181, 1944.
29. Hickey J, Zarb G, Bolender C: *Boucher's prosthodontic treatment for edentulous patients,* ed 9, St Louis, 1985, CV Mosby, p 123.
30. Tyson KW: Physical factors in retention of complete dentures, *J Prosthet Dent* 18:90–97, 1967.
31. Misch C: Alveolar ridge augmentations, American Academy of Implant Dentistry, Western District, Las Vegas, Nevada, March 29, 1985.

Chapter 21

Root Form Implants

Carl E. Misch

Root form implants are the design most often used in restoration of the partial or complete edentulous patient. Root form implant history dates back thousands of years and includes civilizations such as the ancient Egyptians and Incas. Maggiolo introduced the more recent history in 1809 using gold in the shape of a tooth root.[1] In 1887 Harris reported the use of teeth made of porcelain into which lead-coated platinum posts were fitted.[2] Many materials were tested, and in the early 1900s Lambotte fabricated appliances of aluminum, silver, brass, red copper, magnesium, gold, and soft steel plated with gold and nickel. He identified the corrosion of several of these metals in body tissues related to electrolytic action.[3]

The first root form design that differed significantly from the shape of a tooth root was the Greenfield latticed cage design in 1909, made of iridoplatinum.[4] The surgery was designed to use a calibrated trephine bur to maintain an inner core of bone, and the implant crown was not added to the implant root for several weeks. Reports indicate this implant had a modicum of survival.

Surgical cobalt chrome alloy was introduced to oral implantology in 1938 by Strock, when he replaced a maxillary left incisor single tooth, an implant that lasted over 15 years.[5] In 1946 Strock designed a two-stage screw implant that was inserted without a permucosal post. The abutment post and individual crown were added after complete healing.[6] The desired implant interface at this time was described as "ankylosis," which may be equated to the term rigid osseous fixation. The first submerged implant placed by Strock was still in function 40 years later.

Bone "fusing" to titanium was first reported in 1940 by Bothe and co-workers.[7] Branemark began extensive experimental studies in 1952 on the microscopic circulation of bone marrow in situ. These studies lead to the dental implant application in the early 1960s, and 10-year implant integration was established in dogs without significant adverse reactions to hard or soft tissues.[8] Studies in humans began in 1965, followed for 10 years, and reported on in 1977.[9] No other person in recent history has influenced root form implant concepts more than Branemark. The documentation of past clinical case studies, research of material, design, surface characteristics, surgery and bone physiology, healing of soft and hard tissues, and restorative applications from Branemark's laboratory were all unprecedented. Adell et al.[10] published their 15-year clinical case series report in 1981 on the use of implants in the completely edentulous jaws. Approximately 90% of the reported mandibular implants were still in function at this time.

There are currently over fifty types of root form implant designs. Consistent in their philosophy is the desire for clinical rigid fixation corresponding microscopically to a direct bone-to-implant interface, without intervening fibrous tissue over a portion of the implant body.

IMPLANT DESIGN

The selection of the implant design is first determined by the prosthesis. The patient presents to the dentist for teeth, not implants. Once the prosthetic options are explored and selected (FP-1 to RP-5; see Chapter 4), and the available bone permits root form use in the ideal or optional abutment sites, the retention mechanism is designed (screw or cement) from the implant to the prosthesis, and the angulation expected between the implant and the abutment post is calculated.

The implant system should have a separate implant body and prosthodontic abutment to permit a two-stage surgical approach, separated by the hard tissue healing process (see Chapter 2). This criterion is present in the vast majority of implant systems. It is also suggested implant systems in clinical use have undergone evaluation for more than 5 years. This permits observation by the profession, and slight design or instrument modifications as needed. In addition prosthodontic protocol and laboratory training would have been well established by this time.

A solid screw design with a blunt apex offers significant advantages to the practitioner with limited experience or limited availability of different implant systems. A number of manufacturers provide this design. The solid screw has a long history of success. The load capabilities are tried and tested in the most common diameter of 3.75 mm. Various lengths range from 7 mm to 20 mm, but lengths from 10 mm to 16 mm are the most widely used to provide adequate initial and long-term fixation. A solid screw permits the preparation and placement of the implant in dense cortical bone as well as fine trabecular bone. The surgery may be easily modified to accommodate to both extremes. The solid screw permits the implant to be removed at the time of surgery if placement is not ideal. A solid implant may perforate the inferior border of the mandible, nares, or maxillary sinus without inherent complication if the apex is smooth or blunted. The solid screw may be spray coated with titanium or hydroxyapatite to increase surface area, microlocking of bone, or biochemical properties related to the surface

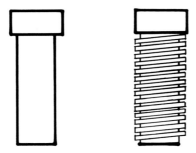

FIG 21–1.
Screw-type implant with a blunt apex *(right)* has twice the surface area as a smooth, press-fit implant of equal diameter and height *(left)*. Either design may be coated with hydroxylapatite or plasma spray.

coating. Some manufacturers also provide slightly smaller and larger implant diameters for use in anatomic or surgical complications. A solid screw also permits the implant to be easily removed at the second stage surgery if angulation or crestal bony contours are not adequate for long-term prosthesis success.

A "press-fit" or "tap-in" implant design system offers the advantage of ease of placement, even in difficult access locations. For example, in the posterior of the maxilla in very soft D-4 bone, a 70:1 handpiece is needed to insert a threaded implant design rather than a hand wrench. Otherwise the very soft bone will displace during the handratchet procedure and the implant will not be rigid. A "press-fit" implant may be placed by hand even in the softest bone. Another location the press-fit system has benefits is the single tooth implant, especially if the crown height of the adjacent teeth is large. Extenders are needed for the bone preparation in these situations, as well as additional armamentarium to insert a threaded implant. Press-fit systems are also easier and faster to place, because bone tapping, the speed of rotation, and the direction of force in implant insertion are less relevant. However, most press-fit implants require a "bioactive" or increased surface area coating for retention in the bone. If these same materials were placed on a threaded design, the surface area of bone contact would be more than twice the smooth press-fit design. The greater the surface area of the bone-implant contact, the better the support system for the prosthesis (Fig 21–1).

MANDIBULAR SURGICAL TECHNIQUE

Once the implant is selected, the achievement of rigid fixation is primarily the responsibility of the implant surgeon. To maintain this interface the restoring dentist must work closely with the patient, the laboratory, and the maintenance professionals.

The most common location for root form implants in the edentulous patient is in the anterior mandibular region between the mental foramina. This chapter will describe the surgery for a Type I Division A or B; Type II Division A, C or B, C patient; or Type III Division A, B, C or B, B, C bone category. The surgery descriptions are for ideal bone density. The modifications of surgical approach related to bone density are specifically addressed in the following chapter. The type and amount of support for the prosthesis is determined first. If a FP-3 or RP-4 prosthesis is planned (see Chapter 4), five root form implants are indicated (see Chapter 12) in the A, B, C, D, and E positions.[11] A panographic radiograph is evaluated for disease, bone height, and foramina location. A lateral radiographic view is evaluated for bone height and angulation. A surgical template is fabricated to indicate incisal edge position of the final restoration. This template helps determine the implant location and angulation.

The patient is prepared for surgery with medications typical for implant surgery. Bilateral inferior alveolar block anesthesia is administered with a long-acting anesthetic. Intraoral and extraoral scrubbing with betadine or chlorhexidine are performed by the scrubbed assistant. A surgical scrub and gowning is performed by the doctor during the patient preparation. Upon return to the operatory, the patient's final drapes are positioned and the surgical site evaluated for depth of local anesthesia. The surgical gloves are rinsed and wiped with sterile saline to remove any powder or contaminant that may inadvertently have been placed in the surgical and/or on the implant surface. Infiltration anesthesia with 2% lidocaine with 1:100,000 epinephrine is deposited into the labial and lingual mucoperiosteum, and controls the depth of anesthesia, provides vasoconstriction of peripheral arteries, and anesthetizes the inferior aspect of the mandible, which is innervated by cervical nerves.

Soft Tissue Reflection

After anesthesia is achieved, the soft tissues and ridge height are evaluated. The lingual aspect of the mandible is palpated for severe undercuts, and compared with the patient's lateral cephalogram. Identification of the approximate position of the mental foramen permits anterior incision line design in moderate to severe atrophy mandibles and allows more rapid reflection in regions around this landmark. The mandibular foramen region may be located by several methods. Palpation for the depressed foramen is the most variable. The overlaying tissues usually prevent adequate feeling to identify the foramen with certainty. Before the patient is surgically draped for the procedure, an imaginary line may be drawn between the pupils of the eyes. A perpendicular line may be then mentally drawn through each pupil (Fig 21–2). This vertical line will pass through the infraorbital foramen and mental foramen. A surgical pen marks the soft tissue over the mental foramen region. If the patient is draped and the eyes cannot be used as a landmark, a forefinger is placed next to the ala of the nose. The foramen region corresponds to a vertical line drawn one finger width distal to the ala.

Opening of the incision line is the most common immediate postoperative complication. The surgical incision is designed to limit this problem. If the crest

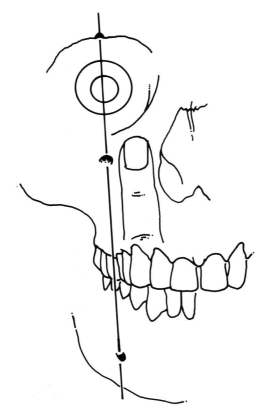

FIG 21–2.
Locating mandibular foramen region.
Vertical line through the pupils of the
patient's eyes passes through the infraorbital and mental foramen. Fingerwidth
lateral to the nasal colar also is on this
vertical landmark.

of the ridge is above the floor of the mouth and there is greater than 3 mm of
attached gingiva on the crest of the ridge, a full-thickness incision is made
bisecting the attached tissue and scoring the bone from the first molar to the first
molar region. If less than 3 mm of attached gingiva exist on the ridge the
full-thickness incision is placed posterior to the foramen to the lingual of the
attached tissue. This places a zone of attached tissue to the lateral aspect of the
posterior incision line and provides greater resistance of the sutures to the
buccinator muscle in the molar-premolar region. In the advanced resorbed
mandible (Division D), the mental foramina and mandibular canal are dehiscent.
The lingual approach to the crest of the ridge usually avoids these structures.
However, care is taken to prevent inadvertent incision and postoperative
paresthesia in the region.

The anterior portion of the incision in patients with close anatomic position
of the floor of the mouth is a split-thickness incision that crosses the ridge 5 mm
anterior to the mental foramina and proceeds in arc form at least 10 mm from the
crest at the midline. The lip is stretched taut, to stretch the muscle fibers in the

region and permit sharp dissection in a horizontal fashion (Fig 21–3). Tissue pick-ups elevate the split mucosa and permit a full-thickness incision through the periosteum approximately 5 mm below the crest of the ridge. A sharp periosteal elevator reflects the periosteum several millimeters over the crest of the ridge. All fibrous tissue is removed from the crest of the edentulous ridge. A moist surgical sponge rubbed across the crestal surface eliminates most fibrous adhesions.

The surgical flap is reflected to the lingual, and retraction sutures with 2-0 silk hold it in position. The right canine region is tied to the left molar area, and vice versa. This improves visibility, negates surgical assistant retraction efforts, and reduces trauma to the thin periosteal lingual tissue.

The exact locations of the mental foramina and associated nerve, artery, and vein are then identified. This is an important surgical landmark. Because the primary incision was extended to the first molar region, the approach to the foramen can be from both anterior and posterior, which facilitates its identification. Once the periosteum is reflected off the residual crest, a moist surgical sponge can be used to separate the periosteum from the dense labial cortical plate. This permits rapid exposure of the nerve complex without trauma from instruments or periosteal elevation.

The panoramic radiograph is observed to visualize an anterior loop of the mandibular canal past the mental foramen. This occurs approximately 12% of the time for an average anterior distance of 5 mm.[12] A probe may be inserted inside

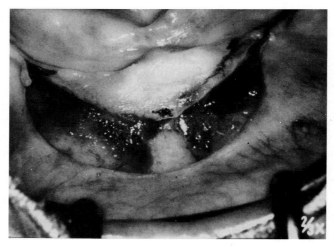

FIG 21–3.
Crest anatomy level with the floor of the mouth. A split thickness incision anterior to the mental foramen is used. The tissue is elevated approximately 10 mm before an incision through the periosteum permits a full thickness reflection.

and along the distal half of the foramen to determine if the nerve enters from the posterior within this structure. If no nerve entry is felt along the distal one-half, the nerve must loop anteriorly and enter from the anterior aspect of the foramen. Probing the anterior half of the foramen is not diagnostic because the mental vascular complex continues anterior from the foramen to innervate teeth and bone. A score mark is made on the crest of the ridge to delineate the most anterior position of the mandibular nerve. This may correspond to the foramen or the anterior loop of the canal, whichever is more anterior. These lines mark the boundaries of the posterior surgical implant placement. The most distal portion of the implant will be placed 2 mm anterior to this border. Once the periosteum is reflected, the cells must regenerate from the unreflected portion before crestal bone healing can occur.[13] Therefore, adequate reflection to identify all landmarks is necessary, but overzealous reflection increases soft tissue trauma and delays callous formation over the implant and crestal bone healing.

An osteoplasty of the crest of the ridge is often indicated, especially in Division B bone. This may be accomplished with a bone rongeur or a slow-speed (2,000 rpm), high-torque handpiece under copious amounts of sterile saline until 5 mm width in the implant sites is obtained. The osteoplasty eliminates any fibrous tissue on the crest and ensures adequate width for implant placement. If several millimeters of bone must be removed to obtain the necessary width, additional resorption is probable during healing. Consider countersinking the implant below the remaining bone crest in these instances to prevent loading of the implant with the soft tissue–borne prosthesis during healing. Remember, the prosthesis must replace the vertical bone height removed during the osteoplasty. Whenever an osteoplasty is performed, the bone is harvested and stored in sterile saline in case an autogenous graft is required during the surgical procedure.

Implant Site Preparation

Rotary instruments are used to prepare the implant site. Regardless of implant design or manufacturer, several surgical concepts are important to obtain initial rigid fixation. Much care and effort are taken to limit trauma to the surrounding hard tissues. Bone is very susceptible to heat[14]; therefore, a conscious effort is made to control temperature elevation every time a rotary bur is placed in contact with bone. A coolant, such as sterile saline, is used as a profuse irrigant. This acts as a lubricant, removes bone particles from the implant site, and most importantly reduces the temperature at the cutting surface. Distilled water should not be used, as rapid cell death may occur in this medium.[15] It is not critical if internal or external irrigation is used. Each has advantages. The portal of the internal cooled burs that exits at the apex often becomes clogged once the bur is in the bone greater than a 5 mm depth. Cleaning is most difficult, and the bur may retain organic contaminants in the trephine from a previous surgery. Excessive pressure during drilling may prevent saline from flowing. The external irrigant may not be applied at the cutting surface, but instead on the shank of the bur. Either technique may be used satisfactorily, with patience and care.

The rotation speed of the bur and the torque of the handpiece must permit bone preparation without too much force or time. Eriksson and Albrektsson[14] determined 2,000 rpm as the maximum speed at which the bur should rotate. They reported bone death when a temperature of 40° C is applied for 7 minutes or when a temperature of 47° C is applied for 1 minute.[14] Time and temperature are interrelated critical factors in implant site preparation. The very soft (D-4) bone can be prepared with speeds of below 800 rpm, whereas the hardest bone (D-1) usually requires at least 1,500 rpm to proceed in timely fashion.

To err on the side of safety, the surgeon should allow the cutting surface of the bur to contact the bone only 5 out of every 8 seconds. The following procedure can be used. The surgical assistant quietly counts for five seconds while the bur is progressing in the bone. The surgeon uses a pumping action to prepare the osteotomy. Every time the surgeon stops or lifts the handpiece longer than a few seconds, the counting may begin again. If the assistant reaches 5 seconds, a gentle touch by the assistant on the back of the surgeon's hand reminds the surgeon to pause a few moments before continuing again.

The pressure used against the bone should neither be so hard as to stall the bur, nor so light that the bur only creates heat and does not prepare the bone. Different amounts of pressure are used in response to the density of the bone. Enough pressure should be used to proceed at least 0.5 to 1 mm every 5 seconds. If this is not achieved, smaller diameter drills are indicated for initial preparation. In addition, new drills and higher speeds (up to 2,000 rpm) may also be of secondary help. Bone chips should be removed frequently in dense bone to maintain optimal cutting action.

Five implant sites are planned for mandibular overdentures, regardless of the two to five being placed. This permits insertion of additional implants in the future if needed. A guide drill marks the initial implant site location in the midline. If the intended prosthesis is a FP-1, the center implant is placed off the midline toward the most distal foramen.

The boundary score lines on the crest of the ridge that correspond to the anterior position of the mandibular canal are identified. A pilot hole on the crest of the ridge is placed 4 to 5 mm medial to each distal score line (if the implants are 4 mm or less in diameter), which determines the center of the distal implant. This provides 2 mm of surgical error away from the mandibular nerve during bone preparation and implant placement. The distance between the center pilot hole and distal pilot holes are then divided equally. This should leave at least 6 to 7 mm between each center of the implant sites. The surgical guide template is placed in position, and the location and ideal angulation for the implant are determined. The ideal angulation is perpendicular to the plane of occlusion, and corresponding to the cingulum position of the teeth for a screw-retained superstructure.

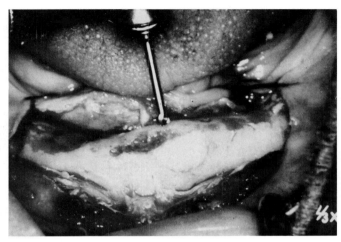

FIG 21–4.
Pilot drill is used to map out all the implant sites before starting the implant osteotomies. Adequate distance from the nerves and each implant is 2 mm. Therefore, 4-mm-diameter implants require center pilot holes that are at least 6 mm from each other and 4 mm from the mandibular nerve.

The pilot drill is usually a number 2 round bur used to evaluate the density and thickness of cortical bone on the crest of the ridge, if any remains after the osteoplasty. The pilot drill can also be used for initial bone preparation in the narrow ridge. This bur can prevent lateral perforations because it will roll away from the harder inner cortical plate and stay within the softer trabecular bone, if a light touch is used (Fig 21–4).

A small diameter drill is then used to continue the bone preparation. The center implant site is prepared first. Angulation is checked in a labiolingual direction with a template and also in the mesiodistal dimension with guidance from an assistant at the foot of the chair. Do not prepare the osteotomy while the template is in place. The implant site must have adequate bone on the labial and lingual. This requires direct vision and careful observation. A pumping motion is used to prepare the site to the radiographically determined depth. However, this dimension is reevaluated and may be changed at this time. The bone preparation should proceed into the opposing landmark, in this case the inferior cortical plate or the lingual plate of the mandible, dependant on the angulation of the anterior mandible and the incisor edge position of the teeth. Therefore, if the preselected length does not reach the opposing landmark, the operator should attempt to drill to the next height of the implant body in the system. If the opposing landmark is perforated, the osteotomy length prior to perforation is noted (Fig 21–5).

Root form implants are provided in preestablished heights, dependant on the specific system. The implant should be at least 10 mm long. The implant should

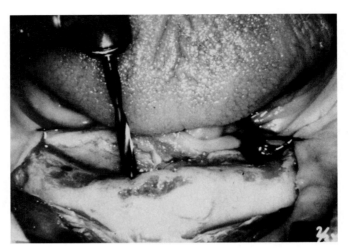

FIG 21–5.
Small-diameter bone drill used to begin the implant osteotomy. Direction, bone density, and implant height are determined with the use of this initial drill.

not perforate the mandible more than 2 mm, to avoid irritating the soft tissue. If the implant has a sharp apex, even slight perforation may irritate the tissues.

Gauge lines inscribed on the shank of the drills correspond to the height of the implant. Some systems make the drill depth 1 mm longer than the implant (a 13-mm implant has a corresponding line 14 mm on the drill). Other systems make the implant 1 mm shorter than the corresponding drill gauge (a 13-mm implant is really 12 mm; the drill line is 13 mm). Some manufacturers make the depth line of the drill the same as the implant. This variance in corresponding depths becomes critical when preparing bone sites over the mandibular canal or when exact measurements are required.

A small diameter direction indicator is used in the initial implant site and evaluated for any minor needed adjustments. The surgical guide template is placed, and the implant angulation and position are evaluated for the final prosthesis (Fig 21–6). If the angulation is beyond 30 degrees or the osteotomy is too lingual or may impinge on the incisal edge, correction of the angulation should precede any further bone preparation. The most distal implant sites are prepared next, using the direction indicator for parallelism in all planes. Direction indicators are placed in the distal sites, and the implant surgeon proceeds to the intermediary locations. Direction indicators may also be used to tamponade profuse bleeding from an implant bone drilling site until the implant is placed. This technique is useful to the surgeon in maintaining adequate vision and decreasing surgical blood loss.

If a bone drill becomes locked in the bone during preparation, the handpiece should not be wiggled back and forth to disengage the bur. This may increase the size of the bone preparation, injure bone cells and cause necrosis, or separate the drill above or below the bone. Instead, the rotation of the drill in the handpiece is reversed, or the drill is disengaged from the engine and rotated counterclockwise with a forceps.

A drill of intermediate diameter is used next for the implant bone preparation, especially if the superior cortical bone is dense and thick. Gradual increases in drill diameter reduce the amount of pressure and heat transmitted to the bone. Direction indicators are placed in bone sites medial and/or lateral to implant sites being prepared. Minor corrections in angulation should be accomplished during this drilling step. The final drill diameter is used to prepare the implant receptor site. This step is the most critical for initial insertion and healing. The bone surrounding this drill will be in direct contact with the implant. Copious amounts of saline, very light pressure, reduced handpiece speed compared with the speed used in the previous steps, and use of direction indicators in adjacent sites to maintain correct angulation all improve the final result. Because bur remnants may remain in the bone during the osteotomy, the final drill should be coated with titanium nitride or a similar material. If one marginal crest of bone is higher than the other (usually the lingual), the drill preparation is measured from the most inferior edge when the implant body is desired to be below the crest of the ridge.

The implant surgeon must select at this time the height of the final implant placement. If the cortical bone is thick, the overlying tissue is thick, and the patient

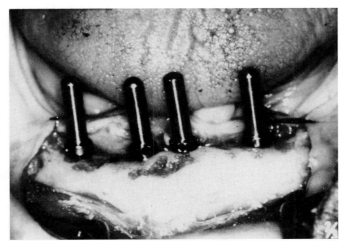

FIG 21–6.
Direction indicators are placed in the osteotomies to evaluate angulation when the surgical guide template is inserted to evaluate angulation and placement.

has no parafunctional habits to transmit stress to the implant during healing, the implant and healing cover height are less important. If the overlying tissue is thin, the superior cortical plate was removed during the osteoplasty, and the remaining bone is soft and fine trabecular, the implant and healing cover must be placed below the bone crest. As a result, the final osteotomy height must be increased. A critical step in obtaining clinical rigid osseous fixation after initial placement is to maintain a rigid bone-implant interface without micromovement from original placement to the second stage surgery. The implant does not have to be submerged below the bone to achieve this result. The implant does not even need to be below the soft tissue to obtain this type of interface. However, it is more at risk, and the chances that trauma may result in movement at the interface increase in proportion to the elevation of the implant and healing cover above the bone.

The crestal collar of any system, regardless of dimension, should be placed in contact with crestal cortical bone. Many implant systems present a wider crestal collar design. For these systems one may need an additional step in the bone preparation, with a crestal countersink drill in areas of crestal cortical plates.

If there is no marginal cortical bone, and especially if the trabecular bone is soft, the implant is inserted without a marginal countersink operation. This compresses the marginal rim and adds rigidity to the implant during initial healing (Fig 21–7).

If a threaded implant system has been selected to support the prosthesis, the implant surgeon next decides whether a bone tap is indicated before implant

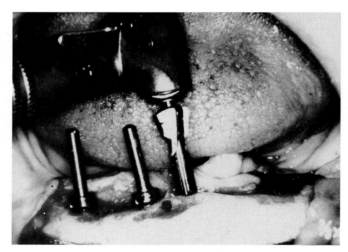

FIG 21–7.
Crestal counter sink drill is used when the crestal collar of the implant is greater than the body and cortical bone is present on the crest or if cortical bone will interfere with final implant placement.

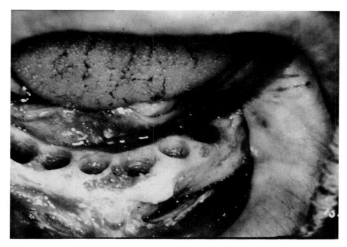

FIG 21–8.
A bone tap has threaded the bone for a more passive implant body placement. Slow drill speeds and use of irrigation decrease the heat and pressure generated against the bone, which will initially contact the threaded implant body.

insertion. The very dense (D-1) bone requires a bone tap for the entire implant height. With thick superior and inferior cortical plates and trabecular bone in between, a bone tap is also required for the entire height, unless the inferior cortical plate is not used for the implant bone site. If only the superior cortical plate is used to provide initial rigidity of the implant, the bone tap is used only in this section. A thin cortical plate or absence of this structure means that the bone tap is contraindicated because it decreases the initial stability of the implant.

Whenever the bone tap is required, it should prepare the bone at very slow speed (under 25 rpm) under copious amounts of irrigant. This may be accomplished with a hand ratchet, or a slow-speed, high-torque contra-angle handpiece (70:1 or 200:1 reduction). It is imperative that the angulation and light vertical pressure used on the ratchet or handpiece follow the same path as the final drill preparation for the entire depth; otherwise, the tap may inadvertently stray in the trabecular bone and compromise the final implant placement. The direction indicators are very beneficial in helping one maintain correct angulation (Fig 21–8).

The hand position of the surgeon is important to maintaining constant force and direction during the threading process. One hand holds the handpiece or ratchet, while the thumb of the other hand is directly over the tap; the index finger retracts the lip so vision is not obscured; and the middle finger is placed under the mandible in direct path of the osteotomy. The bone tap is cleaned with saline before each new site is prepared. If a ratchet is used, care must be taken to let the handle rotate around the insertion pin, not pull or lever the pin and connected tap as it rotates.

Implant Placement

The implant sites are irrigated with saline and suctioned, and the implants are now ready to be inserted. Excess saline or blood is removed from the implant crypt so it is not hydraulically pushed into the bone during implant insertion. The direction indicator pins may still be needed in adjacent sites to guide the implants in the correct angulation in soft trabecular bone. The implant surface has been prepared by the manufacturer to be clean and uncontaminated with any foreign debris. Handling the implant is poor protocol and may alter the surface chemistry. Instead, the implant is placed directly into the implant site by means of a preattached insertion mount. Some manufacturers require the surgical team to attach the implant mounts before placement.

Once the first threads of the implant body engage the bone, the same drill speed used to tap the bone is used to insert the implant. The surgeon's hand position is identical to that maintained during the bone tapping procedure. Sterile saline may be used after the implant has begun its descent into the implant osteotomy. The hand ratchet is used at the end of implant insertion to check the final stability of the implant body. The marginal cortical bone should seal the implant without voids or cracks. The surgeon should not overtighten the implant in place. Too much force used to tighten the implant in its final position may destroy the entire implant thread-to-bone profile.

The first stage cover (screw) is then inserted into the implant body. If this cover is threaded into position, care is taken not to overtighten it. The stress transmitted may rotate the implant body and also make the cover removal complicated at the second stage surgery (Fig 21–9).

Soft Tissue Adaptation

The crest of the bone is evaluated for any sharp edges, and a rongeur or file is used as indicated. The surrounding bone is also evaluated, because final soft tissue contour is very relevant to its position. The surgical site is thoroughly irrigated with saline, including the depths of the tissue reflection, to remove any debris or bone fragments. The lingual retraction sutures are cut and removed. The tissues are approximated without tension and a 3-0 Vicryl interrupted suture is placed at the midline. An interrupted modified vertical mattress, interrupted horizontal mattress, or a continuous suture begins at the distal of the primary incision. It is important that the labial periosteum be joined to the lingual periosteum. Surface epithelium should not contact the periosteum along the suture line, as this may result in delayed healing and incision line opening. The

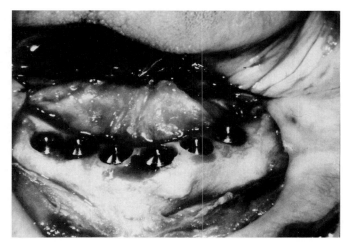

FIG 21–9.
Implant body is threaded into position, and a first stage cover (screw) is inserted. The level of the implant body with the crest is related to parafunction, bone density, and the final prosthesis.

sutures should be placed approximately 3 to 5 mm from the incision line, and 3 to 5 mm apart.

Postoperative Procedures

Following surgery, the patient's mouth is rinsed with saline, and moist gauge sponges are rolled and inserted over the surgical site. Several other 4 × 4-inch gauze sponges are rolled together and placed intraorally between the arches. Pressure is placed on the gauze packs for approximately 1 hour. A panoramic radiograph is taken at the conclusion of surgery and developed while the transitional prosthesis is modified. The radiograph is closely evaluated to ensure proper implant placement and the relationship of the implant to opposing landmarks or surrounding structures. On rare occasions it has been necessary to remove the suture and reposition an implant after analysis of the panoramic radiograph. It is far better to perform this surgery while the patient is still anesthetized and the soft tissue is not healed than to wait for a future appointment. Because the implants and primary healing covers are often placed after an osteoplasty, the labial flange of the denture is overextended and therefore shortened 5 mm, and the intaglio surface of the denture is aggressively relieved 3 to 5 mm. A tissue conditioner replaces the acrylic. The tissue conditioner is also relieved over the implant sites. The patient may wear his or her denture during the healing process. Incision line opening is a possible consequence of wearing the denture during the first two postoperative weeks; however, this is rarely a problem if the denture is properly modified, and the patient wears it primarily for social encounters. The patient must, however, not use denture adhesives or other products which may enter the incision line.

The denture is not worn at night, and the conditioner is coated with vaseline or soaked in water to maintain its pliable nature. The usual course of events after the procedure is uneventful. There is occasional edema in the floor of the mouth, accompanied by minor hematoma formation. However, the edema may extend extraorally, and include the chin, especially if the inferior cortical plates were perforated. An occasional short-term paresthesia of the lip is possible. Analgesics are recommended the first few days following the procedure.

The patient returns in 14 days for suture removal and observation. Although vicryl sutures resorb, this requires 6 to 8 weeks, and on rare occasion small fistulas form in this time frame. Any fistula, regardless of cause, affects the pH in the area and can cause bone loss. Therefore, the sutures are removed at this 14 day postoperative visit.

If a minor opening in the incision line is observed, do not reapproximate and suture the area. Instead, the cause of the incision opening should be determined. If the design of the removable prosthesis is involved in the cause, this condition is corrected. The patient rinses two to three times daily with chlorhexidine and within a few days to weeks the tissue will granulate in without compromise to the implants.

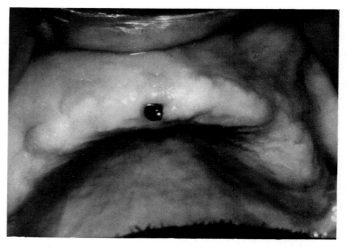

FIG 21–10.
Exposed first stage cover screw during healing does not require surgical correction. The most common reason for exposure is pressure from the soft tissue–borne prosthesis. The denture should be recontoured so no contact is present on the implant body.

Tissue conditioners are selected for the 2 weeks following surgery because they are able to change dimensions the first 24 to 36 hours under pressure. As a result, excess tissue force in any region will cause modification of the material. However, these products become more rigid faster, and harbor more bacteria, than tissue liners. Therefore, the conditioners are removed at the suture removal appointment, and a soft tissue liner is placed.

If the implants become exposed during the healing period, no attempt should be made to cover them. Implant exposure alone does not alter the success of rigid fixation. The soft tissue over the top of the implant has little to do with the bone forming on the surface of the implant (Fig 21–10). However, if the cause of the exposure was pressure on the implant from the prosthesis, this is a problem that may cause micromovement of the implant. Therefore, whenever an implant becomes exposed through the tissue, external forces over the implant should be eliminated. The denture is relieved and a soft tissue liner is placed which is also relieved in this region. A chlorhexidine rinse is also indicated to reduce bacteria growth in the sulcus and surrounding implant soft tissue region.

SECOND STAGE SURGERY: UNCOVERY

The initial surgery and healing process ideally result in a rigidly fixated implant, proper abutment position, no crestal bone loss around the implant, adequate zones of attached gingiva, soft tissue thickness less than 3 mm, and no tenderness or discomfort under vertical or lateral forces. The second stage implant (uncovery) surgery permits the direct evaluation or attainment of these goals.

The second phase surgery should not be underestimated for the total success of treatment. An opportunity exists to correct poor implant placement, inadequate crestal bone healing and soft tissue defects, or poor soft tissue relationships. The final restoration should not be placed in short-term or long-term jeopardy at the expense of compromised initial conditions. When full arch implants are uncovered the patient is prepared for surgery in a manner similar to the original surgery. In general, discomfort, swelling, and risk of infection occur at a lesser degree than at the original surgery. However, if corrective procedures are indicated during surgery, they should not be compromised by poor preparation.

The initial incision is designed to place attached gingiva on each side of the permucosal abutment. The full-thickness incision therefore bisects the remaining attached tissue on the crest of the ridge. The attached tissue and incision are usually more lingual than the actual implant site. The incision continues at least 5 to 10 mm bilaterally distal to the last implant placed (Fig 21–11). A full-thickness envelope flap design permits reflection of the periosteum for direct implant observation. The elevators are not positioned against the

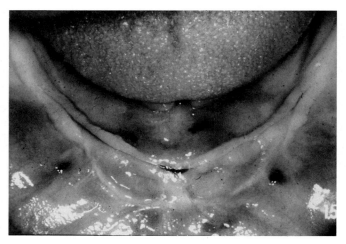

FIG 21–11.
A full-thickness incision is made which bisects the attached gingiva and extends beyond the location of the implant.

endosteal implant body or first stage cover (screws) during this procedure. Instead, the lingual or palatal bone is used for leverage, and the facial tissues are pulled off the healed implant sites. The reflection is adequate to completely visualize the crestal implant site and reposition the attached tissue at the conclusion of the procedure (Fig 21–12).

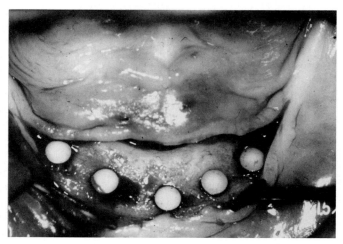

FIG 21–12.
A full-thickness reflection reveals the first stage implant covers and all surrounding bone.

The first stage covers are identified and the surrounding area closely evaluated. Any bone growth on the covers is removed with curettes or slow-speed rotary burs under sterile saline irrigation. All soft tissue is removed from around the implant body. If a vertical soft tissue defect is identified anywhere around the implant, a curette is used to remove the soft tissue from the defect. The bone, rather than the implant body, should be subject to the curette to remove the soft tissue. This loosely bound and unorganized tissue is relatively easy to remove at this time. The implant surface should not be scratched or contaminated during this procedure.

The first stage covers (screws) are removed, and the top of the implant body closely evaluated to make sure it is free of any bone or soft tissue over the edges. A 3- to 5-mm-high metal second stage permucosal extension is threaded completely flush into the body. The rigid fixation of the implant body is tested for resistance to torque with only 10 N/cm force (half to two thirds the final force for the abutment) against the threaded extension. Be careful! The torque force to remove the permucosal extension is usually greater than the force to tighten. There is primarily weak, unorganized woven bone at the surface of the implant at this time. Bone is weakest against torsion or shear. Too great an initial rotation force may loosen the implant, even if direct bone contact is present. When a lateral force of 5 lb is applied to the permucosal extension, no clinical movement should be noted (Fig 21–13).

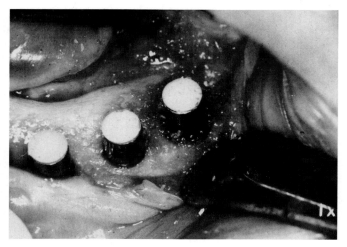

FIG 21–13.
Permucosal extensions are threaded into the implant bodies at one half to two thirds the final torque and tested for mobility with a lateral force of 5 lb. The most distal implant had a vertical defect of 3 mm and is filled with autogenous bone harvested from the surrounding region.

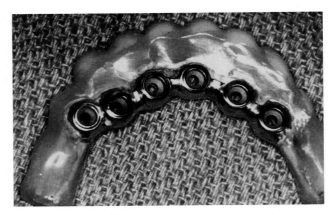

FIG 21–14.
Implants were placed too lingual in relationship to the incisal edge of the teeth. As a result the implants are offset loaded, the hygiene conditions are poor, the acrylic may fracture, the tongue space is encroached upon, and the distance between the most anterior and most posterior implants is reduced.

Once the implant is uncovered, and a permucosal extension is placed into the implant body, the prosthetic template is inserted and the implant position evaluated. An implant body in a position that completely compromises the prosthesis should not be maintained (Figs 21–14 and 21–15).

The surrounding bone is evaluated. In the case of a vertical bone defect there are two surgical options, depending on size. An osteoplasty may eliminate the vertical defect if it is minimal, and the reduced bone-implant interface does not compromise the prosthetic support or esthetics. This is the most predictable method by which to eliminate a vertical defect, but converts it into a horizontal deficiency.

FIG 21–15.
Implants placed in correct relationship to the teeth permit improved conditions compared with the restoration shown in Figure 21–14.

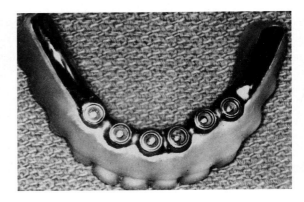

A vertical pocket greater than 3 mm is usually grafted or, if it represents one-third or more of the total implant height, the implant is removed. At this time, the implant body is not contaminated by microorganisms if it has been under soft tissue until the uncovery procedure. If no soft tissue dehiscence is present, the full-thickness reflection has exposed areas of vital bone not involved in the implant body support. This bone may be harvested and packed into the vertical pocket (after the soft tissue has been removed). The defect and surrounding area are overpacked. Another alternative is to place a wedge into the bone several millimeters from the implant body. Tapping the wedge into place will spread the bone up against the implant body. The wedge region is surrounded by bone and will heal without consequence. This technique can place living bone adjacent to the implant body. If the amount of defect is moderate in depth or area, a small pore membrane is placed over the defect and the soft tissue is reapproximated. This prevents soft tissue ingrowth into the defect, and provides greater bone graft healing time in the absence of fibrous tissue against the implant surface.

A horizontal defect of bone around the implant body is also handled one of two different ways. The soft tissue may be apically repositioned so the implant body is more permucosal. If threads or a rough surface are present above the bone, a white stone and abrasives are used to smooth the region and reduce future plaque accumulation. A cement-retained prosthesis may extend to and be placed on the implant body in esthetic regions. Horizontal bone loss for more than one-third of the implant body indicates the removal of the implant.

The second option to address horizontal bone loss grows bone above the crest and is used when the final prosthesis is FP-1 and/or additional bone-implant interface is required to withstand the forces exerted on the prosthesis. To improve the amount of bone formation several steps may be taken. The first is to add autogenous bone to the graft. In most cases, bone is harvested and placed on the crest, then demineralized freeze-dried bone (DFDB) is placed over the graft, and also mixed with 30% to 50% porous hydroxylapatite (HA). The HA will help maintain the graft above the bone crest and next to the implant body during bone formation. A small pore membrane is also placed over the site to increase the amount of bone height formation in the area. The tissue is approximated with primary closure. The second stage uncovery is delayed for approximately 4 months, depending on the size of the graft.

Dense HA and DFDB may also be added to the labial bone surface for fixed prostheses when the maxillary lip or pontic position requires greater support or contour for esthetics. The prosthetic template is placed over the implant site and should represent the desired lip support region to determine the amount of HA labial graft required.

Several options exist for implant removal. The implant may be removed, and if enough implants remain, the prosthesis is still fabricated. The prosthesis may be converted to a removable RP-4 or RP-5 restoration to decrease force transfer to the superstructure in amount and duration. An additional implant may be placed in an optional implant location at the same time as the implant removal. The implant may be removed and a larger diameter implant simultaneously inserted with a different angulation or deeper within the osteotomy. The implant may be removed, the site augmented, and an additional implant placed months later. The treatment of choice attempts to best satisfy the conditions for the prosthesis, without compromise.

The thickness of the overlying tissue is then evaluated. Soft tissue greater than 3 mm thick will result with a less than ideal pocket depth around the implant. The tissue is relieved from the periosteal surface, until it is approximately 2 mm thick.

The width of the attached tissue is addressed last. If less than 3 mm of attached gingiva is present and the crestal bone is in excellent condition around the implant, the incision bisects the thin zone of attached tissue and the labial portion is approximated to the sole facial aspect of each implant. The lingual flap approximates the lingual aspect of each permucosal extension. Loose, interrupted sutures are placed between the implants. The section in between is allowed to heal by secondary intention. In this manner attached gingiva forms between the implants, and the original attached tissue width is now divided between the facial and the lingual implants (Fig 21–16).

A second option to increase the zone of attached gingiva at the second stage surgery is to use a split-thickness incision at the time of uncovery. Once the implant body is evaluated as previously addressed, a free tissue graft from the palate, or freeze-dried skin is placed and sutured around the second stage permucosal extensions.

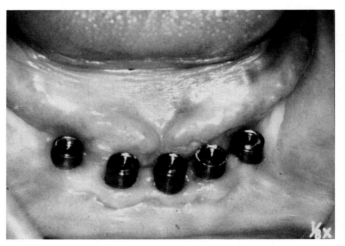

FIG 21–16.
Lack of attached tissue in Figure 21–11 was improved by allowing the tissue to granulate in between the unapproximated tissue after the permucosal extensions were placed.

A third option to increase the zone of attached tissue is to harvest an open gingival sleeve from the palate. The open region is 3.5 mm in diameter and is slid over the top of the permucosal extension and on top of the underlying bone or split thickness incision.

A fourth option is to place dense HA around the permucosal extension before approximating the tissue. This does not increase the zone of attached gingiva, but makes the nonkeratinized tissue less mobile. However, this technique may also increase the gingival sulcus around the implant.

A non-eugenol periodontal dressing may be added over the top of the permucosal extensions, but is not required. The transitional prosthesis is aggressively recontoured to avoid premature loading of the permucosal extensions. A tissue conditioner is placed in the prosthesis and is checked to make sure it is several millimeters thick over the implant sites. The tissue conditioner is then relieved over the permucosal extensions and in any region of secondary intention soft tissue healing.

The sutures are removed in 2 weeks. The soft tissue is not completely keratinized and healed at this time, and is still slightly inflamed. The second stage permucosal extensions are removed and replaced by the final abutment for screw or abutment for cement. An indirect impression transfer coping is placed into the abutment for screw. Vertical pressure is placed on the implants to make sure no tenderness is present. The surrounding gingiva may have a gingiplasty with a diamond bur to shape an interdental papilla around the implant abutments for FP-1 prostheses or to reduce the depth of an implant sulcus.

A preliminary irreversible hydrocolloid or elastic impression is made of the implants. The indirect impression transfer coping or abutment for cement is removed, and the second stage permucosal extension replaced.

The patient is scheduled to be seen again in 1 to 4 weeks, depending on the original density of bone determined during surgery. Density category D-1 separates all future prosthetic steps by 1 or more weeks, D-2 by 2 or more weeks, D-3 by 3 or more weeks, and D-4 by 4 or more weeks (see Chapter 22) for a cement-retained fixed prosthesis.

The indirect impression transfer coping and/or implant abutment analog (for screw or for cement) are placed into the preliminary impression, which is poured with dental stone. The purpose of this step is to fabricate the final impression tray and begin the fabrication of a transitional prostheses if a fixed restoration is indicated (see Chapters 28 to 30).

SUMMARY

Root form implants placed in an anterior mandible are the most often observed in the completely edentulous patient. It is an excellent region to begin a learning curve in implant surgery because the landmarks are clear, access is good, and bone density often permits more flexibility in technique. The step-by-step approach described in this chapter allows excellent results for implant-supported prostheses.

The second phase surgery permits the direct evaluation of the hard and soft tissues condition. The fabrication of the final prosthesis should begin with ideal abutment support. This includes an absence of crestal bone loss or defects, rigid fixation, no discomfort upon loading, adequate zone of attached gingiva, pocket depths less than 3 mm, and acceptable implant body position for the intended prosthesis. The second stage surgery is an opportunity to evaluate these conditions and, if they are not present, create them before prosthesis fabrication starts. The final restoration should not be compromised at the onset. On occasion, this requires additional time and surgeries. However, the alternative is a higher risk of future complication, which will require even more time, cost, and effort to correct or improve.

REFERENCES

1. Maggiolo *Manuel de l'art dentaire, (Manual of dental art)*, Nancy, France, 1809, C. Lefevre.
2. Harris LM: An artificial crown on a leaden root, *Dent Cosmos* 55:433, 1887.
3. Lambotte A: New instruction for the banding of bones: "banding with a screw," *J Chir Ann Soc Belge Chir* 9:113, 1909.
4. Greenfield EJ: Implantation of artificial crown and bridge abutments, *Dent Cosmos* 55:364–430, 1913.
5. Strock AE: Experimental work on direct implantation in the alveolus, *Am J Orthod Oral Surg* 25:5, 1939.
6. Strock AE, Strock MS: Further studies on inert metal implantation for replacement, *Alpha Omega,* Sept 1949.
7. Bothe RT, Beaton LE, Davenport HA: Reaction of bone to multiple metallic implants, *Surg Gynecol Obstet* 71:598–602, 1940.
8. Branemark PI: Osseointegration and its experimental background, *J Prosthet Dent* 50:399–410, 1983.
9. Branemark PI: Osseointegrated implant in the treatment of the edentulous jaw, experience from a 10-year period, *Scand J Plast Reconstr Surg* 16(suppl): 1977.
10. Adell R et al: A 15-year study of osseointegrated implants in the treatment of the edentulous jaw, *Int J Oral Surg* 6:387, 1981.
11. Misch CE: Implant overdenture relieves discomfort for the edentulous, *Dentist,* Jan/Feb, 1989, pp 37, 39.
12. Misch C, Crawford E: Predictable mandibular nerve location—a clinical zone of safety, *Int J Oral Implant* 7:37–40, 1990.
13. Robert EW: Bone physiology and metabolism, *J Calif Dent Assoc* 15:54–61, 1987.
14. Eriksson RA, Albrektsson T: Temperature threshold levels for heat-induced bone tissue injury, *J Prosthet Dent* 50:101, 1983.
15. Marx RE: Principles of hard and soft tissue reconstruction of the jaws, Abstract ML 315, American Association of Oral and Maxillofacial Surgeons, New Orleans, 1990.

Chapter 22

Density of Bone: Effect on Treatment Planning, Surgical Approach, and Healing

Carl E. Misch

The density of available bone in an edentulous site has a primary influence on treatment planning, implant design, surgical approach, healing time, and initial progressive bone loading during prosthetic reconstruction.[1, 2] Endosteal implants achieve predictable success with rigid fixation. A direct bone-implant interface has been demonstrated with a variety of endosteal implant designs and materials. Three requirements are necessary for rigid fixation: atraumatic bone preparation,[3] close approximation of living bone to the biocompatible implant surface,[4] and absence of movement at the interface during healing.[5] Bone density is a most important parameter at the implant site for initial fixation and lack of movement, and is least in control of the surgeon.[6]

The bone density may be grossly estimated by radiographic evaluation with tomograms; conventional dental radiographs, using periapical, panoramic, or lateral cephalometric studies, are less diagnostic.[7] However, the easiest and most accurate method by which to evaluate bone clinically is at the time of surgery. The presence and thickness of a crestal cortical plate and the density of trabecular bone are easily determined during implant osteotomy preparation. The density of the bone is determined by the initial bone drill, and evaluation continues until final implant placement.

HISTORY

The term "available bone" is particularly important in implant dentistry, and describes the width, height, length, and angulation of the edentulous area considered for implants. Sufficient quantity of bone is the primary condition for the use of endosteal implants. In addition, available bone is also described in density, which reflects the hardness of the bone.

When a tooth is lost, the alveolar bone starts to lose dimension and density.[8] The spacing of trabeculae in relation to variable forces of mastication was discussed by MacMillan in 1926.[9] Levels of bone density are directly related to stress: the greater the physiological stress, the denser the bone. When the tooth is lost, and hence does not transmit any stress, the local alveolar process begins to remodel, and more bone is resorbed than formed because the requirements of the bone to handle stress are reduced. In general, bone loss occurs with immobilization or decreased stress in the body.[10, 11] The longer time span the alveolar bone is edentulous, the less trabeculae are present. This decrease begins within a few months, continues long term, and affects both cortical and trabecular bones.[12, 13]

Branemark and Zarb[14] listed four bone qualities found in the jawbone. Quality 1 was comprised of homogeneous compact bone. Quality 2 had a thick layer of compact bone surrounding a core of dense trabecular bone. Quality 3 had a thin layer of cortical bone surrounding dense trabecular bone of favorable strength. Quality 4 had a thin layer of cortical bone surrounding a core of low-density trabecular bone. Irrespective of the different bone qualities, all bone was treated according to the same standard procedures.[14] Using this protocol causes as much as 50% implant failure, especially in softer bones.[15]

Misch defined four bone density groups, which vary in both macroscopic cortical and trabecular bone types. The regions of the jaws with different densities are often consistent. The surgical protocol, healing, treatment plans, and progressive loading time spans are unique for each bone density type.[1, 2, 16]

BONE DENSITY CLASSIFICATIONS

Bone may be classified into four macroscopic decreasing density groups[17]:

1. Dense compact
2. Porous compact
3. Coarse trabecular
4. Fine trabecular

The dense and porous compact components are found on the outer surface of bone and include the crest of an edentulous bone segment. Coarse and fine trabecular bone are found within the outer shell of compact bone, and occasionally on the surface of an edentulous ridge (see Chapter 16).

The four decreasing macroscopic densities describe and establish four categories of bone located in the edentulous areas of the maxilla and mandible. The regional locations of the different densities of cortical bone are more consistent than the highly variable trabecular bone. In this chapter the usual anatomic site, treatment plan, surgical considerations, and optimal healing time, are discussed relative to each bone group, based on extensive clinical experience.

Dense Compact (D-1) Bone

The very dense (oak or maple-like) bone is composed of almost all dense compact, and labeled D-1. The resorbed anterior mandible (Division C or D) often consists of this bone type, which represents the basal bone of the symphysis. Dense compact bone is also found on the thick lateral aspects of anterior mandibles with adequate to abundant bone volume. Implants placed on the lingual aspect of the anterior mandible often are placed within D-1 bone (Fig 22–1).

This bone maintains its shape and density because of the stress from muscle attachments and torsion of the mandibular skeletal system. This bone has a reduced nutrient system compared with the other bone categories, because it contains little trabecular bone.

This dense bone type presents several advantages for implant dentistry. Composed of histologic lamellar bone, it is highly mineralized and able to withstand greater loads. The lamellar bone may heal with little interim woven bone formation, ensuring excellent bone stability even after trauma. As a result, implants may be removed and reinserted if necessary at the surgical procedure. A threaded, titanium implant in the anterior mandible has proved to be very predictable long term, with success above 94%.[4, 18]

A threaded implant provides immediate fixation and ensures the dissipation of stresses to resist functional forces long term when in cortical bone. The percentage of bone at the implant interface is greatest in this bone type and approximates 80%. As a result, shorter implants can bear greater loads than in any other bone density.

Dense compact bone also presents several disadvantages which should be considered. The implant height is often limited to less than 12 mm in the atrophic mandible, and the crown-implant ratio is greater than 1. As a result, force factors applied to the implant-prosthetic system should be evaluated to determine if stress reducing factors should be incorporated in the prosthesis.

Dense compact bone is more difficult to prepare for endosteal implants than any other bone density (Table 22–1). The bone is easily overheated during implant osteotomy procedures, because rotary drills are less performant and progress with more difficulty. This bone density may require greater bur revolutions (up to 2,000 rpm) to obtain adequate depth penetration. If too light a force is applied on the bone, the drill will rotate without penetrating, and only generate heat. The

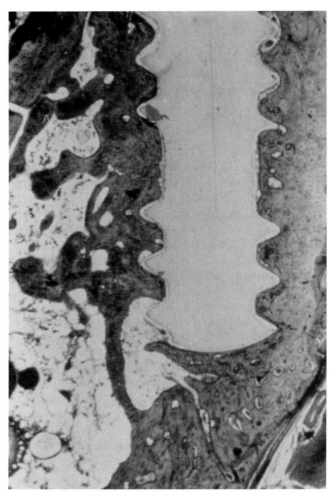

FIG 22–1.
Single crystal implant placed in the lingual cortical plate on the right side and apex represents D-1 bone with the greatest average bone implant contact, compared with other bone densities. (Courtesy of Dr. Ralph McKinney.)

surgeon should apply enough force to permit the drill to proceed at least 0.5 to 1 mm every 5 to 10 seconds.

Both the higher rpm and greater pressure result in higher bone temperature during implant osteotomy preparation. As a result, several methods are employed to counter this effect. External and internal irrigation with cool sterile saline solution is suggested in order to reduce heat, help rinse bone particles away from the cutting surface, and act as a lubricant. Internal coolant is effective in this bone type only when the drill portal exit remains open and intermittent pressure is applied. Intermittent force is applied to the handpiece during bone preparation to reduce the amount of heat generation, which also depends upon the speed of drill rotation, drill sharpness, design, amount of force, and time. The use of new drills with improved design is even more critical for surgery in this bone than with other categories. The surgeon should pause approximately every 5 seconds to allow the limited blood supply access to the bone surgical site, to permit dissipation of heat, and to irrigate the area to reduce bone temperatures.

A gradual increase in bone drill diameter permits progressive removal of bone and limits heat, while decreasing the risk of bur entrapment in the bone, hence trauma and bur separation. Therefore, intermediate drill widths between the initial and final diameter are indicated. The drill width increase should be less than 0.75 mm at each step. This decreases the time required to prepare the osteotomy and decreases the heat generated.

TABLE 22–1.

Implant Osteotomy Preparation in Dense Compact (D-1) Bone

Overheating during osteotomy
    External and internal irrigation
    Cool saline irrigation
    Intermittent force on drill
    Pause every 3 to 5 seconds
    New drills
    Smaller drill sequences in width
Blood supply
    Periosteum provides most
    Limit reflection
Final osteotomy drill
    Width greater
    Height greater
    Slower rpm used
Titanium bone tap
    Short of full osteotomy depth
    Allows passive implant fit
    Prevents internal implant-body damage
    Removes drill remnants
Final implant placement
    Division C or D
        Total bone height with implant design for force transfer
        May require the smooth neck portion above bone
Slower healing rate
    Lamellar bone slower
    Fewer blood vessels
    5 months suggested

Because D-1 bone has fewer blood vessels than the other three types, it is more dependent on the periosteum for nutrition. The cortical bone receives the outer third of its arterial supply, and nearly all of its venous supply from the periosteum.[17] This bone density is almost all cortical. Therefore, delicate and limited periosteal reflection is indicated. Fortunately, there are few occurrences when facial undercuts are observed associated with D-1 bone densities. The bone width in the anterior mandible is abundant. The minimum area of reflection is of little surgical risk.

The final bone preparation size should be made slightly larger in both width and height, especially for the threaded implant. This reduces the risk of microfracture or trauma between the implant threads during insertion, which may lead to fibrous tissue formation at the bone-implant interface. If a drill of slightly greater diameter is not available with the implant system for either intermediate or final preparations, the implant surgeon may remove, then guide the rotating bone drill into final position several times. The final drill should be used at reduced speed (revolutions per minute) to further decrease heat generation.

A titanium bone tap should be used in D-1 bone prior to insertion of the threaded implant. The implant should not be threaded to the full depth of the osteotomy; this causes it to "bottom out" and set up many microfractures along the implant interface. The bone tap permits a more passive implant placement and prevents the internal aspect of the implant body from being damaged with the insertion wrench or implant body mount prior to abutment insertion. Drill remnants are more likely to be left in the implant osteotomy during preparation in dense bone and/or with a new drill and cutting edge. The titanium bone tap removes these remnants and decreases the risk of long-term corrosion from dissimilar metal contacting within the bone. Once the threaded implant is introduced into the osteotomy and in final position, it is unthreaded one-half turn to ensure that there is no residual stress along the bone interface. This step is only used in D-1 bone, because too much initial stress may form at the interface with even one extra rotation.

The final placement of the implant in relation to the crest of the ridge is related to its design. The neck of the implant is often smooth and designed to provide minimum stress and/or support to the implant system. The D-1 dense compact bone is stable during healing, but often of decreased height. Therefore, the actual support system of the implant may be increased in Division C or D limited height bone type by not countersinking the implant below the crest of the ridge. The smooth portion of the implant body may even be placed above the ridge if no load is applied to the implant to cause micromovement during healing. A countersink drill is used corresponding to the final implant placement, often short of the final depth, to permit placement of the implant above the crestal bone, and obtain bone proximal to the smooth neck. This approach is beneficial only when the implant body extends the entire height of available bone and only the smooth implant

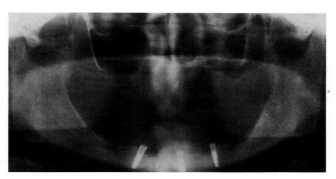

FIG 22–2.
Fourteen-mm implants are placed into a 12-mm D-1 anterior mandible with 2 mm of the smooth implant body neck above the bone. This permits 12 mm of thread design for support, rather than 10 mm (17% more surface area in this example).

neck is above the bone. For example, for 11 mm bone height, a 13-mm threaded implant may be used, leaving the 2 mm smooth neck above the bone. There is an increase of over 35% surface area for load resistance, since this increases the implant design load to all 11 mm of bone, rather than using a 10-mm implant with 8 mm of thread (Fig 22–2).

Many of the cutting cones which develop from monocytes and are responsible for bone remodeling at the implant interface come from the blood vessels found in trabecular bone. Therefore, dense compact bone requires greater healing time. In addition, this bone density may establish lamellar bone after the initial trauma. Lamellar bone forms at the rate of 0.6 μm/day. Most other types of bone densities first form woven bone at the rate of 30 to 50 μm/day. Roberts reports that a 17-week period is required for bone to remodel and become 70% mineralized after an endosteal implant is inserted in a combined cortical and trabecular bone density.[17] Therefore, for complete regeneration of vital bone and rigid fixation to be maintained in this dense oaklike structure, 5 months healing time may be required before prosthodontic loading.

Once established, the interface in this bone density is load bearing and demonstrates lamellar bone. As a result, progressive bone loading is not as necessary in order to develop a stable condition. The restoring dentist may proceed as rapidly as desired to the final prosthesis after 5 months bone healing and uncovering of the implants.

Dense to Thick Porous Compact and Coarse Trabecular (D-2) Bone

The second density of bone found in the edentulous jaws (D-2) is a combination of dense to porous compact bone on the outside and coarse trabecular bone on the inside (Fig 22–3). The tactile feeling when preparing this

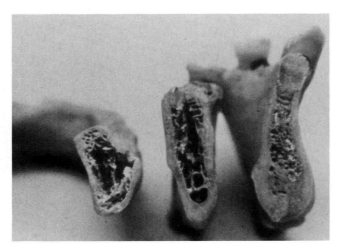

FIG 22–3.
Cross section of three different posterior mandibles: *right to left,* D-2 bone density, D-3 bone density, and after osteoplasty, D-4 density.

bone density is similar to preparations in spruce or white pine wood. This bone type occurs most frequently in the anterior mandible, followed by the posterior mandible. On occasion, it has been observed in the anterior maxilla, although the dense to porous compact bone is then found primarily on the lingual surface of the implant site.

D-2 bone provides excellent rigid healing, and osteointegration is very predictable. Most implant systems refer to this density of bone for their usual protocol. The dense to porous compact bone on the surface and lateral portions of the implant provide an initial rigid interface. Osteoplasty to gain additional width of bone prior to implant placement or countersinking does not compromise support, because the lateral cortical bone and coarse trabecular bone provide adequate support and blood supply. The implant may be placed slightly below the crest of the ridge without compromise or risk of movement at the interface during healing. The intrabony bleeding helps control overheating during preparation, and is most beneficial for bone-implant interface healing.

A threaded implant placed in the anterior mandible often engages the thick cortical bone at the edentulous crest, apex, and most of the lateral sides. This provides immediate stability, and proved long-term survival. The D-2 density of bone in the posterior mandible, does not provide apical cortical bone, as the inferior alveolar nerve limits implant height. A threaded titanium implant should attempt to engage lateral cortical bone during placement. Implant angulation may permit the use of the mandibular lingual plate to this effect. A hollow basket design has also proved effective at 95.3% for up to 10 years, when placed into coarse trabecular alveolar bone.[19] The titanium plasma-coated press-fit cylinder has also proved effective in this bone density. The primary advantage of a press-fit implant in this region is simplification of the surgical approach, especially if limited access is available.[20]

The anterior maxilla sometimes presents this bone density and is then treated very similar to the mandible with D-2 consistency. A threaded implant should engage the palatal cortical plate, where the labial cortical bone is thinner and porous. In addition, the apex of the implant should engage the thin cortical plate in the floor of the nose when a solid screw type system is employed. This is not indicated if a hollow cylinder implant is selected, as perforation of the bone and periosteum will compromise the ability to form bone in the internal basket.

The excellent blood supply and rigid initial fixation permit adequate bone healing within 4 months. Abutment placement and prosthodontic therapy may then commence. It should be noted that the time frame for initial bone healing is based on the density of bone, not on the location in the jaws. Therefore, a 4-month rigid healing phase is adequate for porous compact and coarse trabecular (D-2) bone, even when found in the maxilla.

The implant interface is well established at the 4-month healing interval. Bone-implant percentage is approximately 70%, especially when cortical bone engages the facial, lingual, and apical portions of the implant.

Progressive bone loading (see Chapter 28) is more important when the only cortical bone in contact with the implant is at the crest of the ridge. The amount of coarse trabecular bone around and in contact with the implant may be increased during a gradual loading intermediate prosthodontic process.

Porous Compact and Fine Trabecular (D-3) Bone

The third density of bone (D-3) is composed of the thinner porous compact bone and fine trabecular bone (see Fig 22–3). This bone density provides the surgeon with a tactile sense similar to drilling in balsa wood. It is usually found in the anterior or posterior maxilla, or in the posterior mandible. It may also be found in the Division B edentulous ridge with crestal D-2 thick cortical bone, which is removed when modified by osteoplasty to provide adequate width for root form implant placement.

The porous compact layer is thinner on the labial aspect of the maxilla and the fine trabecular pattern is more discrete in wider edentulous sites. The D-3 anterior maxilla is usually of less width than its mandibular counterpart. Implants of smaller diameter are often necessary.

The advantage of D-3 porous compact and fine trabecular bone is the implant osteotomy may be finished within 10 seconds for each drill size. The intermediate size drill and countersink drill and bone tap may be eliminated in the protocol. Blood supply is excellent and helps with cooling the osteotomy and during bone healing.

D-3 bone also has many disadvantages (Table 22–2). It is more delicate to manage than the previous two bone density types. Its preparation is almost too easy. The surgeon must be extremely careful to avoid undesired lateral perforations of the cortical bone during osteotomy procedures, especially on the thin labial porous compact of the maxilla. The sequence of implant drills may eliminate the intermediate or the final drill size required for D-1 bone. If the final size drill is used, it should not be inserted more than one time to avoid oversizing the preparation. If the system has a slightly narrower intermediate drill, it may be used as the final osteotomy width. The rotations of the drill may be reduced to less than 1000 rpm to improve the tactile sense of bone preparation. In addition, bone preparation must be made with care of constant direction, to avoid enlargement or elliptical preparation of the site. A common mistake which causes

TABLE 22–2.

Disadvantages of Porous Compact Fine Trabecular (D-3) Bone

Bone anatomy
   Anterior maxilla often is narrow
Osteotomy
   Lateral perforation
   Oversize by mistake
   Ovoid osteotomy
   Apical perforation
Bone-implant contact
   Approximately 50%
   Additional implant
Implant placement
   One time
   Level with thin crestal cortical bone
      More fixation
      More risk of load during healing
   Use high-torque handpiece to insert self-tapping threaded
      implant
Implant design
   Hydroxyapatite (HA) coated
      Increase bone contact
      Increased cost
   HA threaded
      Greater surface area
      More difficult to place
   Press-fit
      Easier to insert
      May expand bone
      If bullet shaped, has less surface area
Healing period
   Six months
      Increase bone contact
      Progressive loading more important than for D-2 or D-1

an enlarged site is the use of a finger rest during the osteotomy. Because the drill is often longer than 20 mm, a finger rest results in an arched pathway of the drill. In dense bone this arc will engage the side of the drill and stop the rotation before the crestal osteotomy is enlarged. In D-3 bone the arc pathway is not stopped and the osteotomy at the level of the crestal bone is of greater diameter than the final drill. If the implant design does not increase at the crestal region, a space results around the top of the implant. This surgical defect may heal with fibrous tissue rather than bone and cause an initial bony pocket.

To improve rigid fixation during healing, the opposing thin cortical bone of the nasal or antral floor is often used in the maxilla. If the original implant height determined before surgery does not engage the opposing cortical bone, the osteotomy is increased in depth until it is engaged, and even perforated. Slightly longer implants are placed in this approach, to further increase surface area of support. Sinus elevation and subantral augmentation with the Tatum technique are often indicated in the posterior maxilla to gain additional surface area of support.[21] The maximum use of vertical bone is more essential than in the previous categories. However, perforation into an infected sinus may cause retrograde infection and complications.

The implant should not be removed and reinserted, as initial rigid fixation may be compromised. The countersink drill and bone tap are not used, and the implant self-taps the soft, thin, trabecular bone to enhance initial stability. The amount of bone at the bone-implant interface is reduced, in comparison to bone types D-1 and D-2. If the lingual and apical cortical bone are not engaged at the time of implant placement, less than 50% of the implant surface may actually contact bone. An additional implant may be used to improve load distribution and prosthodontic support. If the only cortical bone is on the crest of the ridge, as in a posterior mandible, the implants are not countersunk below the crest in this density of bone. The thin porous compacta is more stable and provides more rigidity than the fine trabecular bone underneath. This is especially important in the mandible, where bone flexure toward the midline occurs during opening. The implant is placed up against the lingual cortical plate at the crest and through the opposing landmark in the maxilla, to take advantage of the denser cortical bone.

For a threaded implant, a high-torque (70:1 or greater) handpiece should be used rather than a hand wrench for implant self-tapping insertion. This decreases the risk of oversizing the osteotomy with an elliptical implant insertion, which usually accompanies hand wrench placement in softer bone. Do not tighten a threaded implant once inserted, because stripping the threads and decreased fixation is likely.

A hydroxyapatite (HA) coating on a threaded implant body is advantageous in soft bone conditions. The coating increases the amount of trabecular bone at the bone-implant interface, and may even accelerate the bone healing process.[22–24] The coated threaded implant provides more surface area than a bullet-shaped coated implant. A smaller size osteotomy also may be required for a press-fit implant, and also permit a slight expansion of the implant site during implant placement with the Tatum bone spreading approach.[25] The less dense bone may expand easier and permit larger diameter implants to be inserted.

The time frame for atraumatic healing is approximately 6 months. The implant interface develops prior to this time period. The extended time permits the implant to stimulate by its presence the formation of greater trabecular bone patterns. Additional time is allotted for their development, and an extended gradual loading period is recommended to improve this bone density.

Fine Trabecular (D-4) Bone

Fine trabecular (D-4) bone has very light density and little or no cortical crestal bone. It is the opposite spectrum of dense compact (D-1) bone. The most common location for this type of bone is the posterior maxilla of the long-term edentulous patient. These edentulous ridges are often very wide, but have reduced vertical height (Figs 22–3 and 22–4). This bone type is also present after osteoplasty for ridge width increase in D-3 bone, because the crestal cortical bone is removed during this procedure. The tactile sense of this bone is similar to styrofoam. It rarely is observed in the anterior mandible.

Fine trabecular bone presents the most arduous difficulty to obtaining rigid fixation, no matter which implant system is used. It is very porous and as a result, initial fixation of the implant presents only limited mechanical advantage. The implant surgeon should prepare D-4 bone with drills narrower than the dimension of the final implant body, without countersink drill. The initial drill to determine site depth and angulation is the only drill used in the bone. The bone

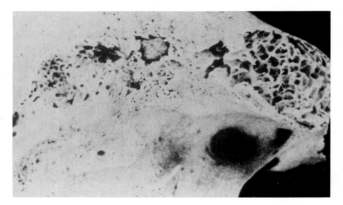

FIG 22–4.
Posterior maxilla often is wide, but has little to no cortical crestal bone and only fine trabecular bone (D-4 density).

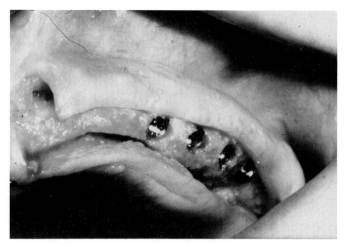

FIG 22–5.
D-4 bone has the implant body placed below the crest of the ridge. Lack of cortical bone and only fine trabecular bone gives little resistance to micromovement from even light loads during healing.

osteotomy is prepared with great care. The bone site is easily distorted, resulting in reduced initial stability of the implant.

The implant should self-tap the bone or shape the implant receptor site while being seated. Press-fit implants present an advantage, because it is difficult to thread an implant in soft bone with difficult access. If there is any cortical bone in the opposing landmark, it is engaged to enhance stability and simultaneously ensure the maximum length of implant. The requirement for maximum height of available bone is greater in D-4 bone than in other types. Sinus elevation and subantral augmentation are often indicated to significantly improve the surface area of support. In addition, subantral augmentation permits the implant to perforate the original sinus floor, composed of cortical bone. The implant should not be removed and reinserted: one-time placement is mandatory. The implant may be countersunk in this bone. No loss of initial stability occurs, as in D-3 bone, because there is an absence of any cortical lining on the surface. In addition, countersinking below the crest reduces the risk of micro-movement during healing in this very soft bone (Fig 22–5).

The amount of bone at the initial bone-implant interface is the lowest percentage of any of the bone types, and may range around 25% at the initial healing and uncovery of the implant (Fig 22–6). Additional implants are placed to improve implant bone loading distribution and permit prosthodontic rehabilitation, especially during the first critical year of loading.

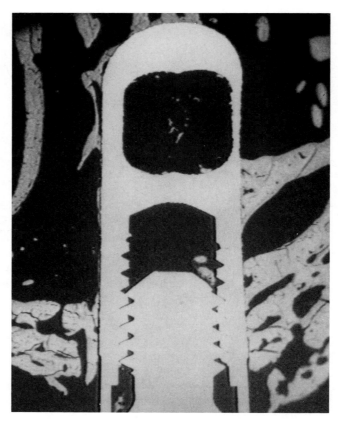

FIG 22–6.
D-4 bone has the lowest percentage of bone contacting the implant surface. As a result, greater stress is transferred to each region when the implant is loaded (Courtesy of Dr. R. Kraut, Montefiore Hospital).

The implant of choice in the wide posterior maxilla with D-4 bone is a greater diameter HA-coated implant. The inexperienced implant surgeon finds a press-fit implant advantageous, as the threaded implant does not self-tap with tactile feedback. However, the experienced surgeon may use a handpiece for implant placement, and the pressure for insertion corresponds to the speed of rotation. The HA-threaded implant can be more stable and provide twice the overall surface area than the bullet-shaped design. Ideally, the HA-coated implant should have an adequate substructure support system. The long-term maintenance of HA has not been determined. An underlying support design would protect the implant if the HA resorbed in the future. The larger diameter implant offers greater surface area for support, compresses the fine trabecular bone for greater initial rigidity, and has a greater chance to engage the lateral regions of cortical bone for support.

The healing and progressive bone loading sequence for D-4 bone require more time than the other three types of bone. Time is needed not only to allow bone to remodel at the surface but also to intensify its trabecular pattern. Hence, up to 8 months of undisturbed healing is suggested. For fixed restorations, one implant is used for each tooth replaced, and no cantilever prosthetic appliance is used with this bone density. An additional implant may be placed at the time of surgery in the molar region to further improve support the first critical year of loading.

SUMMARY

Bone remodels in relationship to the forces exerted upon it. Depending on the location of the edentulous ridge and the amount of time the area has been edentulous, the density of bone is variable. Clinically, the surgeon can correlate the hardness of the bone and the presence of a cortical plate with four different densities of bone. The typical locations of these different densities, the alteration in surgical technique with each type, and the advantages and disadvantages of each have been related to each density classification. Different bone densities correspond to unique treatment plans, healing requirements, and initial bone-implant interfaces. The dense compact bone of D-1 is similar to oak or maple wood. The thick porous compact and coarse trabecular D-2 bone is like drilling into white pine or spruce wood. The thin porous compact and fine trabecular bone D-3 is similar to preparations in balsa wood. The fine trabecular bone of D-4 is similar to osteotomies in styrofoam. The initial bone drilling is used to characterize implant site, depth, and angulation, the surgeon can distinguish between the four bone density types.

Type D-1 bone heals with a lamellar bone interface and has the greatest percentage of bone at the implant body contact regions: about 80%. Type D-2 bone heals with woven and lamellar bone, is adequately mineralized at 4 months, and often has approximately 70% bone touching the implant body. Type D-3 bone has about 50% of bone at the implant interface and benefits from HA on the implant body to increase this percentage. An additional 2 months (6 months total) is used for initial bone healing to permit a greater percentage of bone trabecular to form around the implant in D-3 bone. D-4 bone density has the least amount of trabecular at implant placement. However, an additional time period for bone healing and incremental loading of bone will improve the density and result in implant survival similar to that of other bone densities. Subantral augmentation is often required in addition to HA coating, and modified surgical approaches are used.

REFERENCES

1. Misch CE: Density of bone: effect on treatment plans, surgical approach, healing, and progressive bone loading, *Int J Oral Implant* 6:23–31, 1990.
2. Misch CE: Bone character: second vital implant criterion, *Dent Today* June/July 1988; 39–40.
3. Branemark PI, Albrektsson T: Microcirculation and healing of artificial implants in bone, Proceedings of the 2nd World Congress for Microcirculation, 1979, 2:59,60.
4. Adell R et al: A 15-year study of osseointegrated implants in the treatment of the edentulous jaw, *Int J Oral Surg* 10:387–416, 1981.
5. Brunski JB et al: The influence of functional use of endosseous implants on the tissue-implant interface: histological aspects, *J Dent Res* 58:1953, 1979.
6. Niznick G, Misch CE: The Core-Vent system of osseointegrated implants. In Clark JW, editor: *Clinical dentistry,* Philadelphia, 1987, Harper & Row.
7. McGivney GP et al: A comparison of computer-assisted tomography and data gathering modalities in prosthodontics, *Int J Oral Maxillofac Implants* 1:55–68, 1968.
8. Parfitt AM: Investigation of the normal variations in alveolar bone trabeculation, *Oral Surg Oral Med Oral Pathol* 15:1453–1463, 1962.
9. MacMillan HW: Structural characteristics of the alveolar process, *Int J Orthod Oral Surg* 12:722–730, 1926.
10. Allison N, Brooks B: An experimental study of the changes in bone which result from non-use, *Surg Gynecol Obstet* 33:250, 1921.
11. Geiser M, Treuta J: Muscle rarefication and bone formation, *J Bone Joint Surg [AM]* 40:282, 1958.
12. Kazarian LE, Von Gierke HE: Bone loss as a result of immobilization and chelation: preliminary results in *Maccacca mulatta, Clin Orthop* 65:67, 1969.
13. Minaire MC et al: Quantitative histological data on disuse osteoporosis: comparison with biological data, *Calcif Tissue Res* 17:57, 1974.
14. Branemark P-I, Zarb GA, Albrektsson T: *Tissue-integrated prostheses,* Chicago, 1985, Quintessence, p 201.
15. Jaffin RA, Berman CL: The excessive loss of Branemark fixtures in types IV bone: a 5-year analysis, *J Periodont* 1991.
16. Misch CE: Bone density and root form implants (manual), Dearborn, Mich, November 3–5, 1984, Quest Implant Inc.
17. Roberts EW et al: Bone physiology and metabolism, *J Calif Dent Assoc* 15:54–61, 1987.
18. Babbush C: Titanium plasma spray screw implant system for reconstruction of the edentulous mandible, *Dent Clin North Am* 30:117–131, 1986.
19. Babbush C: ITI endosteal hollow cylinder implant systems, *Dent Clin North Am* 30:133–149, 1986.
20. Kirsch A, Mentag P: The IMZ endosseous two phase implant system: a complete oral rehabilitation treatment concept, *J Oral Implant* 12:576–589, 1986.
21. Misch CE: Maxillary sinus augmentation for edentulous arches for implant dentistry—organized alternative treatment plans, *Int J Oral Implant* 4:7–12, 1987.
22. Block MS, Kent JK, Kay JK: Evaluation of hydroxylapatite-coated titanium dental implants in dogs, *J Oral Maxillofac Surg* 45:601, 1987.

23. Cook SD et al: Interface mechanics and histology of titanium and hydroxylapatite-coated titanium for dental implant application, *Int J Oral Maxillofac Implants* 2:1–15, 1987.

24. Block MS et al: Loaded HA-coated and grit-blasted titanium implants in dogs, Proceedings of the World Biomaterials Congress, April 1988.

25. Tatum H: Maxillary and sinus implant reconstructions, *Dent Clin North Am* 30:207–229, 1986.

Chapter 23

Plate Form Implants and Mandibular Posterior Surgery

Carl E. Misch

The elements necessary to achieve initial rigid fixation of a plate form implant include a biocompatible material, an acceptable implant design, atraumatic hard and soft tissue preparation and implant placement, and a healing period of 4 to 8 months without movement at the implant interface. The plate form implant is an endosteal implant designed for Division B edentulous ridges. The plate form or "blade-vent" implant is narrow in the buccolingual dimension, moderate in height, and has its greatest dimension and support in the horizontal dimension. It is one of the first implant designs that did not attempt to mimic the tooth root anatomy. The plate form implant has demonstrated the capability to develop a similar histologic interface to root forms in both animals and humans.[1, 2]

This chapter presents the history of the plate form design, indications for its use, tissue interface issues, and body and abutment design. Treatment plans and surgical placement are also discussed.

HISTORY

Roberts demonstrated the use of a custom plate form design in the mid 1960s, but did not publish any early reports.[3] Linkow first applied for a patent of a pre-made "blade-vent" implant with Edelmann in 1968.[4] He is almost solely responsible for its introduction and widespread use around the world. Many implant designs and approaches have been developed since then, including those of Cranin,[5] Weiss,[6] Viscido,[7] Hahn,[8] and Misch.[9]

INDICATIONS FOR PLATE FORM IMPLANT

The plate form implant presents several advantages. Because it uses a horizontal dimension for support, rather than ridge width and height, it may be utilized in long-term edentulous areas in spite of loss of bone width. A minimum amount of bone removal in the facial-lingual dimension is required prior to its placement. The horizontal dimension of the plate form is supported by bone on each side and provides a large surface area of support in spite of the Division B available bone. A typical plate form implant has 1.5 times the surface area of a Division A root form, and more than twice the area of a narrower Division B root form.

The narrow endosteal body of the plate form implant has holes, vents, or slots. Thus bone can grow through the implant within a few months to increase the surface area of support, rendering higher vertical load-bearing ability. The metal plate form implant may be bent to follow the curvature of the arch or the flare of the ascending ramus, allowing greater use of available bone. When engaging two different planes, the lateral stability of the plate form implant is enhanced.

The plate form implant may be indicated for Division B available bone, especially in the posterior edentulous mandible. This is not an uncommon condition, as approximately 20 million of partially edentulous Americans have mandibular posterior edentulism. The most common indication is an edentulous ridge between 2.5 and 5 mm wide, at least 10 mm high above the alveolar canal, greater than 15 mm length, with an angulation less than 20 degrees, and a crown-implant ratio less than 1. In general, the options for Division B are osteoplasty, small diameter root form or plate form implants, or augmentation. The posterior mandible often has decreased height because of the location of the inferior alveolar canal. As a result, inadequate height of bone for endosteal implants is present after osteoplasty and nerve repositioning has increased risk of paresthesia. Augmentation requires autogenous bone to be predictable in this region. Narrow diameter root forms require at least 3.5 mm of bone, and usually three or more Division B root form implants are required to replace even two molars.

Tissue Interface

In the past, plate form implantation used surgical techniques, design, and healing criteria which lead to a fibrous tissue interface, and some practitioners even encourage its presence.[10] High-speed bone preparation, poor stress transfer implant design, and immediate loading of the implant after placement all encouraged fibrous tissue formation between the bone and implant. In some plate form osteotomy procedures, high-speed dental handpieces are used, with rotations approximately 300,000 rpm. These speeds may overheat bone if preparation time in any region is not dramatically reduced and coolant is not abundant. However, bone prepared under these conditions can form next to an implant.[11]

The most important principle leading to a fibrous interface with the plate form implant is the concept of movement at the interface before bone formation and initial mineralization.[12] It takes approximately 18 weeks for bone with 70% mineralization to develop at the bone-implant interface.[13] Loading the implant with a prosthesis before this initial mineralization of bone increases possible implant micromovement and formation of a fibrous interface. Techniques to encourage development of fibrous tissue next to the implant included inserting and loading the implant and prosthesis at between 0 to 6 weeks. Consequently, movement at the interface occurred with high incidence. However, fibrous tissue formation around the plate form implant has proved to be predictable when used within specific conditions and guidelines. Kapur,[14] Schnitman,[15] and Smithloff et al.[16] report survival rates of approximately 85% for 3 to 15 years.

Brunski compared loaded vs. unloaded plate form implants in the same animal and reported that the plate form implant could heal with a direct bone interface when it was not loaded initially with a prosthesis.[12] Direct bone interfaces with plate forms have been reported to have been maintained in function for as long as 20 years in animals and in humans.[1, 2, 17] A bone cell of approximately 150-μm diameter only has a portion next to an endosteal implant. It cannot "tell" the gross geometric shape or trademark of the implant, or whether it is permucosal or submerged during the healing process. However, the osteoblast can "tell" if the implant is biocompatible, contaminated, or moving during initial healing. Hence, movement during healing is more influential on the amount and presence of fibrous tissue than the method of placement, design of an implant, or implant manufacturer. Higher success rates are reported with plate form implants with a rigid fixation. Hahn[8] and Misch[1, 9] report above 97% survival for 3 to 10 years (Fig 23–1).

There are many advantages to a direct bone-implant interface other than improved survival rate (Table 23–1). Long-term results are less dependent on peri-implant disease in the absence of fibrous tissue. This improves the quality of implant survival. Greater loads may be transferred to bone without increase in fibrous tissue and mobility to the implant, which further increases soft tissue complications. Clinical experience and reports demonstrate "saucerization" around fibrous tissue–supported plate forms as being typical.[16] Moderate bone loss is reported in almost half of instances at 5 years.[16, 18] This has not been observed with rigid fixation plate forms. In addition, clinical assessment of the implant is easier with rigid fixation, because the healthy implant is nonmobile. A

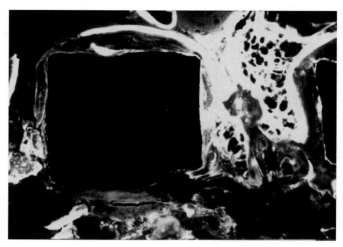

FIG 23–1.
Plate form implant in function for 1 year in a *Macaca fascicularis* monkey. Tetracycline label *(white regions)* demonstrates bone at the surface, with no evidence of fibrous tissue at the light microscopic magnification. (Histologic study courtesy of W.E. Roberts.)

healthy fibrous tissue implant may have a range of recordings from 0 to 2. As a result, the practitioner is able to assess conditions more clearly with rigid fixation before the several appointments and laboratory costs of the final prostheses are incurred. When mobility is permitted and encouraged, how much movement is acceptable? The amount of movement related to direction and force is variable, and additional assessment experience is required.

The primary causes of failure in traditional prostheses are dental caries and uncemented restorations. A plate form implant with a fibrous tissue interface often has greater mobility than the abutment teeth, especially when more than one tooth is splinted. As a result, the natural teeth have greater risk of cement failure and an unretained component of the prosthesis. This results with excess forces on the implant and increased risk of decay on the natural abutment tooth. The most common cause of failure with a rigid fixated plate form has been implant fracture. Past plate form designs have smaller diameter necks or permucosal extensions. Long-term fatigue fractures resulted. Later designs increased the post diameter and strength. As a result, material fracture has not been reported.

Implant Material

The initial support system of the plate form implant is related to the biomaterial, surgical placement, and healing conditions. A plate form implant design requires materials able to bend, yet have adequate strength. The plate form implant is usually fabricated from commercially pure titanium or its alloy, both capable of a direct bone-implant interface at the light microscopic level. Commercially pure titanium is easier to adjust or bend to follow the osteotomy, and may even bend to fit the implant site while being seated in final position. Hydroxylapatite (HA) may be placed on all or part of the body of the implant. Usually a HA-coated plate form will be shorter than a noncoated form because bending the implant body results in fracture of the coating.

Plate Form Implant Body Design

Biomechanical designs of the plate form implant vary greatly. Initial photoelastic studies indicated that the open vented apex or base design is more stressful to bone than the closed border design.[19] Most all current designs have a closed inferior border. The more holes or slots in the body of the implant, the more potential implant-bone interface area to distribute vertical forces. The horizontal slot design first introduced by Hahn[8] dramatically increased bone-implant surface area for force distribution. In addition, the horizontal slot allows bone to be loaded in compression, rather than shear. Because bone is strongest in compression and weakest with shear loads, the slot design offers significant advantage.

TABLE 23–1.

Characteristics of Interfaces

Fibrous tissue–implant interface
  High-speed bone preparation
  Load during healing
  Movement at healing interface
  Decrease surface area and/or load transfer designs
  85% implant survival
  Clinical mobility range 0 to 2
  "Saucerization" common
  Advantage: less treatment time
Bone-implant interface
  No movement during healing
  Delayed loading
  Increase surface area and/or load transfer design
  97% implant survival
  0 clinical mobility
  Advantages: cost and time of fabrication for the prosthesis performed after implant assessment
  Less peri-implant disease; higher quality of survival
  Less uncemented restoration or decay of natural abutment
  Higher implant survival
  Easier health assessment of implant

The crest of the edentulous ridge is more cortical and dense than the trabecular portion of the implant site. Lateral forces applied to the implant result in greater stress in the crestal region. The most superior strut of the grid implant design may be of greater height, to increase the surface area in contact with the denser crestal cortical bone.

The width of the implant is related to vertical support. An implant twice as wide gives twice the compressive support area of the implant if all other factors are equal, and if the implant has a direct bone-implant interface. Many plate form bodies are tapered, with the apical or base portion being narrower than the crestal portion. The wedge shape was required early in history, as the implant osteotomy was not prepared to full depth. Instead, the implant was driven into the bone as a nail is hammered into wood. The bone is widest at the base of Division B ridge. Hence, surface area may be increased by over 20% when the plate form width is equal on the crest and apex. Therefore, the plate form implant body of choice is an implant with holes or horizontal slots (with a greater height of the superior strut), a closed inferior border, that is as wide as possible, limited by the anatomic factors of a Division B ridge.

Design of Plate Form Implant Abutment Post

Plate form implants may have fixed or removable abutments for cement. The plate form implant with a removable abutment for cement presents the advantages of the one-piece fixed abutment blade-vent implant with a major additional factor. Low tissue profile healing decreases the threat of trauma from masticatory forces or the tongue during formation of the bone-implant interface. Atraumatic healing is paramount to the rigid osseous fixation process. Therefore, a low-profile permucosal extension during the first 4 to 8 months of bone healing (related to bone density) has advantage.

The number of permucosal sites on the plate form implant has undergone concept changes in the past few years. Because complications often originate at this location, past philosophy limited the number and size of permucosal sites.[5] Recent studies demonstrate that two abutment posts are more suited for force transfer.[20] Because the two abutment posts are splinted together in the prosthesis, the amount of occlusal force is being applied into more than one region of the implant, therefore reducing the amount of stress transferred at each site. Thus, two abutment posts are used whenever possible. Uncemented restorations are a common source of fixed prosthesis failure. The two abutment posts offer the additional advantage of increased retention of the final prosthesis.

The neck or permucosal extension from the implant body may be further redesigned to minimize stress at the crest. A thicker and more rigid post transmits more stress to the body of the implant.[21] Because plate form implants are used in narrow bone, the buccolingual dimension of the post cannot be dramatically increased without negating its use in Division B bone. However, increase in

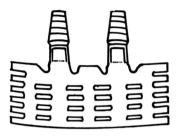

FIG 23–2.
Double-headed plate form implant with a horizontal slot design, with a permucosal post 4 to 5 mm in mesiodistal width and 2 to 3 mm above the most superior strut (which is wider than the remaining struts).

mesiodistal length of the permucosal neck can improve force transfer. The mesiodistal dimension of each abutment region of the permucosal neck may be greater than 4 mm. This not only reduces stress at the crest of bone, but also increases the long-term strength of the implant and reduces risk of fatigue fracture. The abutments may be designed with cement or screw retention of the final prosthesis. Use of FP1, FP2, and FP3 restorations have several advantages when abutments for cement are selected (see Chapter 29). Types RP-4 or RP-5 restorations often require an abutment for screws when implants are placed in a Division B ridge (see Chapter 29) (Fig 23–2).

Treatment Plan

The design of the plate form implant requires the span of two or more teeth in length. No clinical studies are reported with one endosteal implant of any shape or size (root form or plate form) as independent support for two or more teeth. Therefore, one endosteal implant, regardless of design or size, should not independently replace two or more teeth. Therefore, the plate form implant design should be splinted to other implants and/or teeth.

The most common region for plate form placement is the posterior mandible. Because this region receives greater forces than the anterior region and the missing molars had two roots to resist the natural forces, the endosteal treatment plans are altered, depending on the number of natural tooth roots missing. The third molar is never replaced and the second molar is rarely replaced, if these are the only posterior teeth missing (see Chapter 7). When the first and second molars are missing, the plate form is inserted so that the two abutment posts are positioned in the mesial half of the first and second molar crowns. The prosthesis is splinted to a healthy nonmobile second premolar, and replaces the first molar and only half of the second molar. The final restoration often appears as four premolars, to improve the embrasure spaces between the two abutments for cement, and does not replace the distal half of the second molar (Fig 23–3).

In a patient missing molars and second premolar, the plate form abutments are positioned in the distal half of the first molar and second premolar positions. The final prosthesis splints the natural nonmobile first premolar, to the second

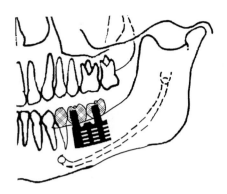

FIG 23–3.
Double-headed plate form replacing two molars has one post in the mesial half of the missing second molar and the other post in the mesial half of the first molar. The prosthesis splints a nonmobile second premolar to the mesial half of the second molar.

premolar and first molar implant abutments. The first molar crown may be designed to occlude with a mesial portion of the maxillary second molar to prevent exfoliation. The final prosthesis also appears as four premolars, but does not replace the crown of the second molar (Fig 23–4).

A patient missing molars and premolars has two treatment options. Ideally, a Division A or B root form implant is positioned in the first premolar region, anterior to the mental foramen. A plate form is then inserted so the two abutments project into the distal half of the first molar and second premolar region. The final prosthesis is completely implant supported, joining the root form and plate form implant. The prosthesis appears similar to that described in the previous scenario. The occlusal scheme is mutually protected or canine guided when opposing natural dentition. Because the canine tooth is not splinted in the restoration, lateral forces to the implant are eliminated during mandibular excursions (Fig 23–5).

The abutments of the plate form are positioned in the mesial half of the first molar and first premolar regions if an anterior endosteal implant cannot be inserted in the first premolar region. The final restoration should then join a

FIG 23–4.
Plate form implant replacing first molar and second premolar has one post in the distal of the first molar and other post in the second premolar region. The prosthesis splints a nonmobile first premolar to the distal of the first molar.

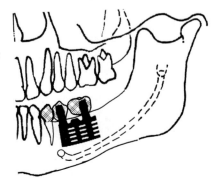

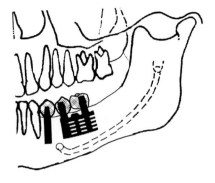

FIG 23–5.
Plate form implant replacing both premolars and molars uses a root form implant in the first premolar region and the plate form in the second premolar and distal of the first molar. The prosthesis is completely implant supported, from the root form to the first molar.

nonmobile canine tooth and extend only to the mesial half of the first molar. This restoration replaces only the first and second premolars and the anterior half of the first molar (Fig 23–6). If the natural abutment has clinical mobility, the treatment plan splints additional teeth (see Chapter 9).

Therefore, the treatment plan for plate form implants is modified in relationship to the remaining natural abutment and the number of teeth missing. The implant body replaces three roots of the missing natural dentition.

1. The mesial root of the second molar and two roots of the first molar when both molars are replaced.
2. The two roots of the first molar and one root of the second premolar when the first premolar remains.
3. The root form replacement of the first premolar and similar treatment plan when molars and premolar are replaced.
4. The least desirous treatment which replaces molars and premolars joins the canine tooth to the restoration, because lateral forces are introduced through the prosthesis to the implant body. The final prosthesis only ex-

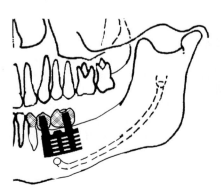

FIG 23–6.
Second (and poorer) option to replace molars and premolars places the plate form in the first premolar and mesial half of the first molar. The prosthesis splints a nonmobile canine tooth to the plate form implant and to the mesial half of the first molar.

TABLE 23–2.

Treatment Plans With Plate Form Implants

Replace two molars
    Abutments in mesial half of second molar and first molar
    Prosthesis splints nonmobile second premolar to mesial of second molar (four premolars)
Replace molars and second premolar
    Abutments in distal half of first molar and second premolar
    Prosthesis splints nonmobile first premolar to distal of first molar (four premolars)
Replace molars and premolars
    Place root form in the first premolar and plate form in the distal half of first molar and second
        premolar
    Prosthesis splints root form to distal half of first molar (four premolars)
        or
    Position abutments in mesial of first molar and first premolar position
    Splint a nonmobile canine tooth to the mesial half of the first molar (three premolars and
        canine)

tends to the mesial half of the first molar since three roots are being replaced by the implant (Table 23–2).

SURGERY IN POSTERIOR MANDIBLE

Because a primary indication for plate form implants is the edentulous Division B posterior mandible, the surgical procedure is described in this region. Many aspects of the surgical approach are also applied to root form surgery in wider bone.

The study models of the patient are duplicated and a diagnostic wax-up is made. This step is important in determining the position of the abutment posts for the prosthesis, the plane of occlusion, the height of the abutment for cement and whether they are adequate for long-term cement retention, the need for pontics, the angulation of the post in relation to the abutment teeth, and the length of the body of the implant. The study models, diagnostic wax-up, and panoramic radiograph are all available at the time of surgery.

The patient is premedicated as suggested for any implant surgery. The patient is anesthetized using a Gow-Gates or Akinosi block with long-acting anesthetic. This injection not only anesthetizes the inferior alveolar nerve, and usually the long buccal nerve, but equally as important, the mylohyoid nerve. This nerve is often responsible for the regional paresthesia occasionally observed even when adequate inferior alveolar blocks are accomplished. Postoperative discomfort is reduced with long-acting anesthetic agents.

The patient is prepared for surgery with a preoperative intra and extraoral betadine or chlorhexidine scrub. The surgical team also scrubs and gowns in the standard aseptic method. Care is taken to remove any powder or foreign bodies from the surgical gloves to limit contamination of the implant or surgical site.

Soft Tissue Reflection

The surgical region is checked for regional anesthesia with local infiltration of 2% lidocaine with 1:100,000 epinephrine. Local infiltration also decreases initial hemorrhage and offers better visibility during the soft tissue incision. This is important because the plate form implant has a permucosal extension at initial placement, so the initial incision will determine the amount of attached gingiva on the facial aspect of the implant abutments.

The primary incision is made on the crest of the ridge from the retromolar pad to the anterior tooth abutment. If there is 3 mm or more of attached gingiva on the crest of the edentulous ridge, the incision bisects this tissue. This places half of the attached gingiva on each side of the low-profile permucosal extensions, which will be just above the level of the tissue. If there is less than 3 mm of attached tissue on the crest, the incision is made lingually so at least 2 mm of the attached band of tissue will be bound to the facial aspect of the implant abutments. In this way the buccinator muscle does not impinge on the posts and does not cause opening of the incision line during the initial healing, or a muscle pull and gingival complications over the long term.

An accessory incision is made lateral to the retromolar pad and up the ascending ramus, inferior to the two attachments of the temporalis muscle. Another accessory incision is made in the sulcus around the abutment teeth to the area of the canine tooth, and occasionally a vertical release incision is made just distal to the mandibular canine. A full-thickness periosteal flap is reflected, exposing the underlying crest and lateral surface of the edentulous mandible in the region of the foramen (Fig 23–7). The lingual flap is reflected only a few millimeters, because reflection of the periosteum destroys the osteopotential cells of the periosteum which must be regenerated from the unreflected area before bone can be remodeled. However, the facial reflection should expose several millimeters of the lateral aspect of the edentulous ridge and the superior portion of the mental foramen. Almost all concavities in bone of the posterior mandible occur on the facial aspect, with the exception of the submandibular fossa. By exposing this area the implant surgeon is less likely to inadvertently perforate the bone, which would result in fibrous tissue formation next to the implant in the region. In addition, the mental foramen is always identified in mandibular posterior surgery to determine the zone of safety above the mandibular canal[22] (Fig 23–8).

The retromolar pad should be elevated to the lingual to expose the underlying bone when both premolars are present. The bone under the pad in this area is usually 4 to 5 mm wide and 5 to 7 mm in length. The region is palpated just inferior to the retromolar pad to distinguish anatomic landmarks. Severe undercuts

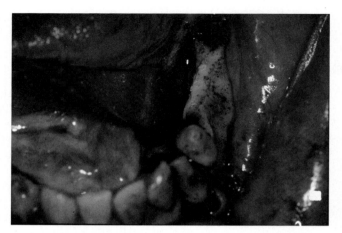

FIG 23–7.
Full-thickness reflection exposes a Division B edentulous posterior mandible.

inferior to this region are typical. If the anatomy permits, the extension of an additional 5 mm of implant length and 4 or more mm of implant height in this area improves the implant surface area. The retromolar pad reflection is not necessary when the implant also replaces premolars, since the more anterior implant position avoids the distal aspect of the implant from extending to this region.

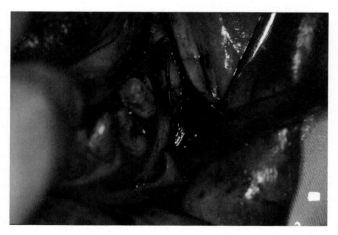

FIG 23–8.
Measuring rod is used to determine the "safe zone" height of bone from the top of the mental foramen to the crest of the ridge.

Predictable Mandibular Nerve Location: Clinical Zone of Safety

The risk of mandibular canal penetration during endosteal implant placement in the posterior mandible is a concern for both the implant surgeon and patient. At the time of surgery, intrusion into the mandibular canal results in an increase in hemorrhage, impairs visibility, and increases the potential of fibrous tissue formation at the surface of the implant. More important, the patient experiences altered nerve feeling in the form of anesthesia, paresthesia, or hyperesthesia. This may affect the patient's lifestyle during eating, kissing, and placing lipstick, and is a frequent cause for litigious action against the implant dentist. Consequently, the surgical landmark is often set 2 mm above the mandibular canal, in order to establish a surgical zone of error.

Literature Review

Several clinical approaches to the posterior mandible have been proposed using radiographic techniques. In the region of the first mandibular molar, the mandibular canal is often difficult to identify on a periapical or panoramic radiograph. A cortical lining of the canal is not always present in the molar region, and when present, it is in the region of the submandibular fossa, which approximates the facial and lingual cortical plates; the relative increase in density obscures the superior cortical lining of the mandibular canal. Fishel et al. found the mental foramen was only visible on approximately 50% of periapical radiographs.[23] On the other hand, Yosue and Brooks[24] showed that the mental foramen could always be identified on a panoramic radiograph. However, only 28% of the radiographs evaluated showed the accurate position of the foramen. The majority of panoramic radiographs illustrated the mental foramen as being significantly closer to the inferior border of the mandible than its actual position. In addition, the appearance of the foramen varied with the positioning of the mandible in relationship to the focal length used while obtaining the radiograph.[24]

A panoramic radiograph is often used to determine the height of the bone available over the mandibular canal. A 25% manufacturer-supplied magnified image of the implant is placed over the radiograph to select the desired size of implant to be inserted in the abutment positions. However, panoramic radiographs do not have a uniform magnification rate. Additional variables such as the patient's head position may significantly alter magnification, which may range over 55%.

At the time of surgery, the crest of the edentulous site is often modified by osteoplasty to increase the width of crestal bone. The premeasured height is reduced and its amount may be difficult to assess. The angulation of the bone in the posterior mandible progressively evolves from almost vertical in the premolar region, to 15 degrees in the first molar, and 25 degrees in the third molar region. A periapical radiograph cannot be parallel to all three of these planes, and foreshortening or elongation of the image is expected.

A surgical approach with no block anesthesia has been suggested.[25] Local anesthesia is achieved by infiltration into the surrounding soft tissues. The bone is then prepared without block anesthesia, as few sensory nerve fibers exist in this region, except those of the mandibular canal. The patient is instructed to notify the surgeon if sensation or discomfort is experienced, which theoretically correlates to the rotary instrument approaching the mandibular nerve. The infiltration surgical approach presents several disadvantages. The patient is not relaxed, and often apprehensive because the possible paresthesia complication is partly their responsibility. With this approach, sedation must be minimal to enable the patient to communicate intelligently during the procedure. The misinterpretation of a pressure phenomena or bur vibration raises the patient's and doctor's anxiety regarding nerve encroachment. Additional sensory mandibular nerve pathways are often present within the bone. These nerves innervate teeth, but little or no soft tissue of the face. Apprehension or misinterpretation by the doctor or patient with this technique can result in the selection of a short endosteal implant of lesser bone-implant surface area. This condition may lead to greater bone loss and failure, and is not recommended.

The placement of endosteal implants medial to the mandibular canal has been reported.[26] However, the position of the canal in a transverse plane is not reliable. The inferior alveolar nerve enters the medial aspect of the ramus above the lingula and exits on the lateral aspect of the mandibular body at the mental foramen. The crossover from medial to lateral aspects usually occurs in the third to second molar region. But this is highly variable. As a result, the general rule is to place the implant above the mandibular canal.

A computer generated tomogram (CT) series of films may represent an improved diagnostic tool for identifying bone width, height, and mandibular canal location. However, the cortical lining of the mandibular canal is often absent in the first molar region, and when present may be confused with a vascular region surrounded by trabecular bone. In addition, attempting to place an implant medial to the canal as a result of information from the CT image requires a precise control of the angulation of penetration at the crest of the edentulous ridge. Surgical error of a few degrees may result in perforation of the canal. Visualization of a few degrees is most difficult in the posterior regions of the mouth, when observing the mandible from the lateral aspect of the patient.

Materials and Methods

A zone of safety for the placement of posterior mandibular endosteal implants was established by Misch in 1980, by the evaluation of 530 consecutive panoramic radiographs of partially edentulous patients. In 1989, this evaluation was confirmed by Misch and Crawford with an additional 324 consecutive panoramic radiographs.[22] The zone of safety is defined as an area within the bone which can safely support implants without fear of impingement on the mandibular neurovascular bundle.

The zone of safety is measured as follows: line A is drawn parallel to the posterior plane of occlusion, at the level of the residual crestal ridge at its lowest point. Line B is drawn at the most superior aspect of the mental foramen parallel to line A. Lines A and B are joined with a perpendicular line C at the position of the foramen. All bone measured posterior to line C to the mesial half of the first molar is within the safe zone.

Results

The results of these studies indicated prevalence of the mandibular canal below the second line (B) on radiographs, using the landmark of the mental foramen. A zone of safety was observed 100% of the time mesial to the middle of the mandibular first molar. The most common position of the canal was 2 mm or more inferior to line B, drawn from the top of the foramen. The area below the zone of safety and above the mandibular canal allows an additional surgical safety zone that is usually greater than 2 mm. In the region of the distal half of the first molar, the mandibular canal was below line B in 97.5% of radiographs. In the region of the mesial half of the second molar, it was below line B in 43% of the radiographs and in the distal half of the second molar only 5.5% (Fig 23–9).

The position of the foramen is also an anatomic landmark for mandibular implant placement in the premolar region. An anterior loop of the mandibular canal occurs when the mandibular nerve proceeds inferior and anterior to the position of the foramen, then loops superior and distal to reach the foramen. An anterior loop was observed in 12% of the panoramic radiographs and averaged 5 mm in length anterior to the foramen (Table 23–3).

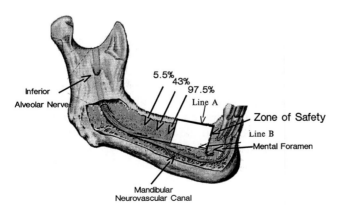

FIG 23–9.
The "safe zone" is determined by drawing *line A* parallel to the plane of occlusion at the crest of the residual ridge, and a parallel *line B* at the height of the mental foramen. A perpendicular line C determines the height of the safe zone up to the mid first molar region.

TABLE 23–3.

Mandibular Canal Location

Location*	Posterior Mandible†			
	Mesial 1st Molar	Distal 1st Molar	Mesial 2nd Molar	Distal 2nd Molar
+	324 (100)	316 (97.5)	140 (43)	18 (5.5)
0	0	6 (1.8)	166 (51)	134 (41)
−	0	2 (<1)	18 (5.5)	172 (53)
	Anterior Mandible			

Presence of anterior loop: 12% (5 mm average forward)
Absence of anterior loop: 88%

* + = within zone of safety; 0 = below zone of safety but not touching canal; − = touching or below top of canal.
† Data from 324 consecutive Panorex radiograph measurements. Numbers in parentheses are percentages.

Safe Zone Procedure

The zone-of-safety technique is used for endosteal implant placement in the posterior mandible. First, radiographic estimates of vertical bone height are made by measuring the distance between lines A and B in the safe zone and correcting this measurement due to magnification by using calibrated balls or wire ratios of magnification, or an arbitrary 25% magnification. This permits the evaluation of available bone height and a treatment plan to be developed and discussed with the patient prior to surgery. An implant height may be initially determined, with the understanding that the safe zone may be actually measured at the time of surgery and may be different because of osteoplasty or incorrect magnification allowance.

Bone Preparation

At the time of surgery, a mandibular block anesthesia is used, accompanied by oral or intravenous sedation, for patient and doctor comfort. The crest of the edentulous posterior ridge and the mental foramen are exposed. The edentulous ridge is evaluated, as is the position of the abutment posts. An abutment location point is made on the mid-crestal bone of the ridge with a rotary bur when root form implants are planned. If the ridge is Division B and a plate form is desired, the post locations are made on the facial of the ridge, since the osteoplasty for plate forms eliminates any crestal location point. If the edentulous ridge is narrower than 2.5 mm, an osteoplasty is performed with rotary burs under copious amounts of sterile saline. As a result, the crest width is increased, but at the same time the anatomic landmark of the mandibular canal is now closer to the remaining crest of bone.

The facial and lingual cortical plates of bone should be at the same level in the region of the abutment posts. The head of the implant is designed to rest on both cortical plates. If one side is higher than the other, only that plate will be in correct position when the implant is seated. Bone will form to the height of the lowest plate of bone. The height of the available bone is then determined, forward of the mesial half of the first molar. An imaginary line A is drawn parallel to the occlusal plane at the region of the mid first molar on the crest of the residual ridge after osteoplasty to a point over the mental foramen. Another parallel imaginary line B is established at the superior aspect of the mental foramen. The height of the available bone in the molar region corresponds to the height between these lines and the height of the endosteal implant in this region.

The radiograph is then evaluated to confirm and extend the zone of safety beyond the mid first molar region. If the canal appears to remain at the same distance as the zone of safety in the distal of the first molar region (97.5% of the time), the safe zone measurement is expanded to the distal root region. If the canal appears to rise 2 mm in the mesial of the second molar region (about 60%), the safe zone measurement is reduced accordingly in this region. The second molar region is almost always reduced from the safe zone measurement (94% of the time) and usually is 4 mm (or more) less than the safe zone height. The plate form osteotomy preparation may be started if adequate bone height is present. It is recommended to error on the side of safety, in the region past the mesial one-half of the first molar, using the panoramic X-ray as a guide. This clinical approach has been used successfully by the author and colleagues in over 5,000 surgical procedures without paresthesia.

The implant osteotomy may proceed in the region of the foramen to the same measurement as the top of the foramen without the implant osteotomy impinging on the nerve for three reasons. Although the crossover position of the mandibular canal from the medial aspect of the ramus to the lateral area of the body of the mandible is variable and may occur anterior to the second molar region, the mandibular nerve always exits the mandible facially at the foramen. Therefore, the implant osteotomy will be lingual to the canal and its contents in the foramen region. In addition, the mandibular foramen is cone shaped. The base of the cone is positioned to the facial, and its summit is toward the occlusal. Therefore, when the height measurement is made from the top of the external foramen, this represents the more superior portion of the cone shaped foramen. Thus the nerve is apical and lateral to the area of the implant osteotomy. In addition, the nerve exits from a path inferior to the foramen, so the nerve approaches below the height of the external measurement.

Once the measurement is made for vertical available bone, and correlated to the radiograph distal to the middle of the first molar region, the depth measurements of the implant osteotomy may be established every 5 mm, starting 2 mm distal from the last abutment tooth.

If the preselected implant size needs to be modified from that planned on the basis of the initial radiographic estimations, a different implant is selected at this time. A smaller implant is indicated over one too large, to eliminate the risk of paresthesia as a consequence of excess implant size. The available bone and implant should be at least 10 mm in height from the base of the abutment post to the inferior portion of the implant body from the mid first molar region forward.

A series of holes are prepared 5 mm apart and 5 mm deep. The pilot holes are positioned to form a straight line whenever possible. A surgical 557 bur has a cutting surface height of approximately 5 mm and is used as a depth gauge bur to prepare these pilot holes. Pilot holes should be angled to bisect the buccolingual cortical plates and parallel the lingual plate of bone, in order to avoid penetrating the submandibular fossa on the lingual aspect of the mandible. This is especially noted in the region of bone under the second to third molar, which often exhibits a severe lingual undercut. The pilot holes should be prepared with a moderate speed, high-torque handpiece under copious amounts of external sterile saline. The higher the revolutions per minute the less time the bur should be used on the bone and the more saline solution should be used, with longer intervals between bone preparation steps. An electric motor, with variable speed control and 1:3 ratio, and sterile saline pump can prepare the bone at a rotary speed between 40,000 and 60,000 rpm. The bur should not contact the same bone region for more than 3 seconds at any one time.

The next step is to connect the pilot holes in a plane parallel to the lingual plate of bone. A paint brush–like intermittent stroke, or continuous posterior to anterior movement, is suggested. The 557 surgical bur may be used to a depth of 8 mm in the osteotomy, before the shank of the bur prevents its further use. If any doubt exists regarding coolant in the osteotomy, additional sterile saline from the assistant is directed in the bone preparation (Fig 23–10).

A 700 XL bone drill, and if needed a 700 XXL bone drill, is used with copious amounts of saline to finish the depth of the osteotomy. Whenever possible the osteotomy should form a straight line not only on the crest but also within the entire body of the osteotomy. This may require the crestal bone preparation to be off center for part of the osteotomy. The bone osteotomy corresponds to the depth of the implant from its base to 2 to 3 mm above its shoulder, and to the abutment post for the restoration. This allows 2 to 3 mm of bone to form over the implant shoulder and around the permucosal posts of the implant after healing.

A bone disc may be used after the initial preparation to straighten and widen the osteotomy as needed. A channel guide is placed in the prepared osteotomy and slid in an anterior-posterior direction. Inaccurate planes within the osteotomy may be connected with the instrument. The depth is observed, to make sure steps or undercuts are not present.

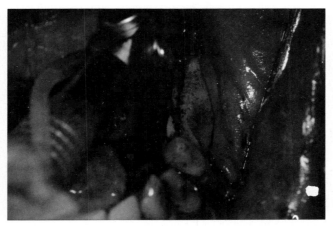

FIG 23–10.
Osteotomy is prepared with a series of burs using an intermittent paint brush stroke to the required depth, at a high-torque, moderate-rpm drill speed, and with copious sterile saline solution.

Plate Form Placement

The length and curvature of the implant are compared with the bone preparation, and accordingly bent or modified. The implant should fit passively for approximately one third of its final vertical position (Fig 23–11). While the plate form is partly in position, the abutment posts of the implant are checked to ensure that they are parallel in all planes to the most anterior fixed prosthesis abutment. Often the implant needs to be removed and the abutment posts bent facially approximately 10 to 15 degrees. Titanium-coated bending instruments are used whenever the implant is bent or modified, to limit metal contamination. Do not over bend an implant, or bend it in two different directions, to limit grain structure alteration and future fracture complications. The implant is then reinserted into the osteotomy.

Once in position the implant is lightly tapped vertically into position. If one end of the implant begins to seat deeper than the other, a shoulder set instrument is used to help seat it evenly. At the final placement, the implant shoulder should be 2 to 3 mm below the crest of the edentulous ridge. If the implant appears to be difficult to insert, the decision to remove it and reevaluate the osteotomy should be made before the implant body is level with the crest of bone. Otherwise more difficulty will result in removing the implant, and may damage the surrounding bone. The implant should be rotated in an anterior-posterior direction when it is necessary to remove, never buccolingual, as bone fracture is more likely in this direction.

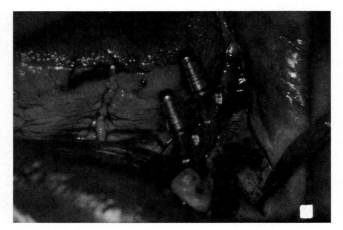

FIG 23–11.
Plate form implant is passively placed into the osteotomy to one third its depth. Angulation of posts to the most anterior abutment is evaluated and modified as required before final placement.

Care is taken to tap the implant in the same plane as the osteotomy. Because the seating instruments are placed on the implant from an anterior position to exit from the orifice, a common error is to drive the implant posterior as it is inserted. This not only results in the permucosal post too far distal, but may also position the implant body into the ascending portion of the alveolar canal, with resultant paresthesia. Tapping in a lingual direction may fracture the cortical plate during insertion.

The surgical assistant should brace the body of the mandible during the tapping procedure. The patient is also notified before this process. The tapping is firm, and similar in range to tapping a nail into white pine to balsa wood. Once the implant is seated, the shoulder of the implant body should be 2 mm or more below the lowest bone margin (Fig 23–12). The implant must be rigid when in final position, with no mobility clinically evident in any direction. The prosthetic abutment posts are then removed from the implant permucosal necks. Resorbable calcium phosphate mixed with saline and demineralized freeze-dried bone (DFDB) is packed into the osteotomy above and over the shoulder of the implant. These materials retard fibrous tissue from growing into the osteotomy over and around the implant from the overlying soft tissue, and bone is more likely to form over the shoulder and around the implant neck. The narrower the ridge, the greater risk of crestal bone loss and the more crucial is this step. If the ridge is particularly narrow, a putty mixture of DFDB is added to the lateral walls of bone before membrane placement. The DFDB may not augment the ridge width, but helps maintain its current dimension.

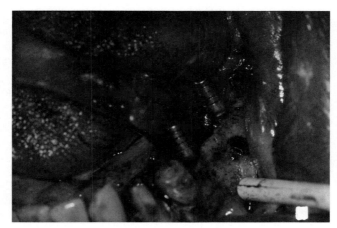

FIG 23–12.
Final position of the plate form implant places the abutment post on the crest of the ridge. The implant must be rigid when in this position.

A barrier or membrane is placed over the Division B ridge, and the permucosal abutment posts project through the barrier (Fig 23–13). Resorbable barriers such as collagen or laminar bone have an advantage, as surgical removal is not indicated after initial bone healing. The first stage cover screws are placed onto the necks of the implant body and help maintain the membrane.

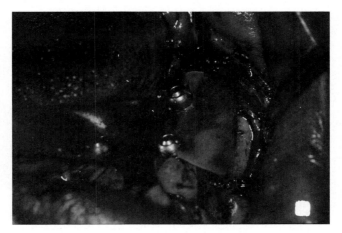

FIG 23–13.
Mixture of resorbable calcium phosphate and DFDB is placed above the plate form and within the osteotomy. A barrier or membrane (laminar bone strip) is placed over the edentulous ridge, and healing covers are placed on the abutment posts.

The tissues are approximated and sutured with 3-0 vicryl. A continuous locking suture, nonlocking suture, or interrupted sutures may be placed. The accessory incisions are often closed first to ensure proper tissue placement after reflection. Carefully ensure that opposing periosteal tissues are in contact, not epithelium or graft material.

A panoramic radiograph is taken at the conclusion of each endosteal implant surgery. If inadequate placement is observed or infringement on the mandibular canal is evident, the implant placement should be corrected at this time.

Immediate Postoperative Instructions

The patient's postoperative course is usually without consequence. Medications as previously discussed are administered. Rest, ice, pressure, elevation (RIPE) and protection of the area from any force (eating, tongue) are emphasized. The patient is asked to return in 14 days. The site is flushed and wiped with saline and the sutures are then removed.

Healing Period

The submerged or low-profile healing period of the plate form implant is similar to that of other endosteal implants designed to achieve a direct bone-implant interface. The mandibular plate form implant usually remains unloaded for approximately 4 to 6 months. During this time the patient is reminded to avoid any force on this healing implant. This is especially critical if the patient wears a removable prosthesis. Experience has shown that a hole

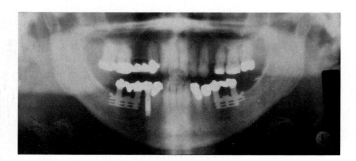

FIG 23–14.
Panoramic radiograph of bilateral plate form implants in place. The right side has a root form in the first premolar and plate form abutments in the second premolar and distal half of the first molar. An implant-supported restoration splints the plate form and root form. Canine crowns, independent from the implant restorations, modify the mandibular excursions to eliminate any posterior lateral forces on the implants. The plate form implant in the left posterior mandible places abutment posts in the second premolar and distal first molar region. A fixed prosthesis splints a nonmobile first premolar to the implant.

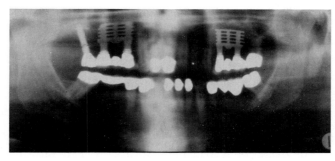

FIG 23–15.
Bilateral plate form implants in the maxilla after subantral augmentations. The implants are splinted to a nonmobile second molar on the left and a second molar root form implant on the right. This allows the canines to be independent and to disclude the posterior restorations in excursions while eliminating lateral forces on the implants.

should be placed all the way through a partial denture over the region of the implant post. The restoration can then proceed following progressive bone loading phases for cemented prostheses (Figs 23–14 and 23–15).

CONCLUSION

In the past, most techniques utilized with the plate form implant resulted in a fibrous tissue or a peri-implant ligament support system. This support system has proved to be effective for abutments of fixed prostheses. However, several studies indicate that a direct bone interface is more desirable whenever possible. To achieve this result, the techniques may be slightly modified. Advantages, indications, and support system of the plate form implant allow the practitioner to develop treatment plans for the narrow edentulous ridge. The incorporation of these principles has shown that the plate form implant can achieve a direct bone-implant interface in animal and human patients. As a result, long-term success may be obtained in the narrow edentulous alveolar ridge for implant-supported prostheses.

REFERENCES

1. Misch CE: Osseointegration and the submerged blade-vent implant, *J Houston Dist Dent* Jan:12–16, 1988.
2. Viscido A: The submerged blade implant—a dog histologic study, *J Oral Implant* 5(2):195–209, 1974.
3. Roberts R: History of the Ramus Frame implant, Alabama Implant Congress, Birmingham, Alabama, May 1985.

4. Linkow LI: U.S. Patent No. 3, 465, 441, 1969.
5. Cranin AN: The Anchor oral endosteal implant, *J Biomed Mater Res* 235(suppl 4): 1973.
6. Weiss C: The physiologic, anatomic, and physical basics of oral endosseous implant design, *J Oral Implant* 10(3):459–486, 1982.
7. Viscido A: Submerged function predictive endosteal blade implants, *J Oral Implant* 15:195–209, 1974.
8. Hahn J: Clinical experience with the Titanodent subcortical implant system, *J Oral Implant* 11(1):72–88, 1983.
9. Misch CE: Blade vent implant: still viable, *Dent Today* 8(9):34, 42, 1989.
10. Weiss CM: A comparative analysis of fibro-osteal and osteal integration and other variables that affect long-term bone maintenance around dental implants, *J Oral Implant* 13:467, 1987.
11. Scortecci G: The Disk-Implant, a histologic perspective, Alabama Implant Congress, Birmingham, Alabama, May 1986.
12. Brunski JB: The influence of functional use of endosseous dental implants on the tissue-implant interface: clinical aspects, *J Dent Res* 58:1953, 1979.
13. Roberts WE et al: Bone physiology and metabolism, *J Calif Dent Assoc* 15:54–61, 1987.
14. Kapur KK: Veterans Administration co-operative dental implant study—comparison between fixed partial dentures supported by Blade-Vent implants and partial dentures, *J Prosthet Dent* 59:499–512, 1987.
15. Schnitman P et al: Three-year survival rates, blade implants vs. cantilever clinical trials, abstract, *J Dent Res* 67(special issue):347, 1988.
16. Smithloff M, Fritz ME: The use of blade implants in a selected population of partially edentulous adults: a ten-year report, *J Periodontol* 53:413–415, 1981.
17. Linkow LJ, Donath K, Lemons JE: Retrieval analysis of a blade implant after 231 months of clinical function, *Implant Dent* 1:37–43, 1992.
18. Armitage JE: Risk of blade implants. In Schnitman PA, Shalman LB, editors: *Dental implants: benefit and risk,* National Institutes of Health Publ 81, 1531, Bethesda, Md, 1980, U.S. Public Health Service, pp 294–304.
19. Vajda TT, Fung JY: Comparative photoelastic stress analysis of four blade type endosteal implants, *J Oral Implant* 8(2):257–269, 1979.
20. Bidez MW: Stress distribution within endosseous blade implant systems as a function of interfacial bonding conditions (dissertation), University of Alabama at Birmingham, 1988.
21. Misch CE: A three-dimensional finite element analysis of two blade implant designs (thesis), University of Pittsburgh, November 1989.
22. Misch CE, Crawford E: Predictable mandibular nerve location: a clinical zone of safety, *Int J Oral Implant* 7(1):37–40, 1990.
23. Fishel D et al: Roentgenologic study of the mental foramen, *Oral Surg Med Oral Pathol* 41:682–686, 1976.
24. Yosue T, Brooks SL: The appearance of mental foramina on panoramic and periapical radiographs, *Oral Surg Oral Med Oral Pathol* 68:488–492, 1989.
25. Heller AL: Blade implants, *Can Dent Assoc J* 16:78–86, 1988.
26. Linkow L: Mandibular implants: a dynamic approach to oral implantology, New Haven, Conn, 1978, Glarus, pp 10–12.

Chapter 24

Mandibular Complete Subperiosteal Implants

Carl E. Misch

The mandibular complete denture is the most unstable, unretentive, conventional prosthesis fabricated in routine dental practice. During function, the typical mandibular denture moves five times more than the maxillary denture. The patient with advanced atrophy presents the additional problems of thin mucosa, high muscle attachments, increased vertical replacement of the prosthesis, poor muscle coordination, speech difficulties, denture adhesive solubility and general failure, and adverse psychological influences on normal lifestyle.

Oral implantology is often used to improve the support system for the mandibular complete edentulous patient. A common axiom used in implant dentistry is to use endosteal implants whenever the prosthetic and bone anatomic conditions permit. However, endosteal implants are not always the implant of choice for the completely edentulous patient.

The subperiosteal implant is designed to rest on top of the bone, under the periosteum. Rather than gaining endosteal support as teeth or most alloplastic implants used in the body, this implant distributes stresses from the prosthesis to large areas of bone surface, in comparison to a snowshoe. A customized casting, made of surgical metal, adheres to the bone with a combination of fibrous tissue and bone support, and has permucosal abutment posts and intraoral bars to attach a prosthesis.

INDICATIONS

In this chapter, the prosthodontic support for mandibular arches with Division C bone in the anterior region and C or D bone in the posterior sections is considered. A complete mandibular subperiosteal implant provides support for

511

a completely implant supported restoration (RP-4). If this prosthesis is required to satisfy the needs or desires of the patient, consideration of implant support should include this implant design. The complete implant supported restoration is very stable. Because the prosthesis is removable, the moderate to advanced atrophy may be replaced with the prosthesis, without compromise for hygiene or esthetics. RP-5 restorations rest on the soft tissue in the posterior mandible, and often have complications in Division C or D ridges. Therefore, many edentulous patients with poor posterior ridge anatomy should not be restored with an RP-5 restoration. Whether root forms or subperiosteal forms are used, an RP-4 prosthesis is indicated. An FP-2 or FP-3 fixed prosthesis for Division C patients often compromises hygiene or esthetics, does not permit removal in case of parafunction, and is usually not indicated in the mandible. The subperiosteal implant patient has Type I Division C, Type II Division C,D or Type III Division C,D,C bone anatomy. This volume of bone requirements may often be satisfied with endosteal or subperiosteal implants. A practitioner may select either support system in many of these patients. However, there are additional factors to evaluate other than available bone. These other factors include angulation, skeletal relationship of the jaws, bone width, anterior defects, time, cost, and arch form.

The available bone height is measured in relation to the trajectory or angulation of bone in reference to the prosthetic abutment and the direction of load from occlusion. The crest of the edentulous ridge to the inferior aspect of the anterior mandible may measure 15 mm, but if the angulation needed to attach a prosthesis or load the implant is improper, the bone is not adequate for endosteal implants. In addition, severe angulation places the endosteal implant under the anterior section of the tongue or within the vestibule. Compromises of offset loading, hygiene, speech, and prosthesis design are all a consequence. The subperiosteal implant has a superstructure bar attached to the underlying substructure. The bar may be designed to be ideally positioned for the prosthesis, which may not be over the crest of the residual ridge. Hence, the angulation of bone does not compromise the implant placement, or the superstructure design when subperiosteal implants are used as a prosthetic support system.

On rare occasions the width of the entire anterior Division C mandible is insufficient for endosteal root form implants. More often, for adequate width of bone for root forms to be obtained, an osteoplasty results in less than 8 to 10 mm of height. The subperiosteal implant does not have a width requirement, although modification of the abutment strut design is indicated when decreased width is present.

Anterior endosteal implants placed in an edentulous mandible may fail for a number of reasons. An anterior defect may remain in the bone after their removal, especially if this failure occurred from peri-implant disease after many years of service. Impacted teeth (usually canines) may also leave anterior defects when removed from the anterior mandible. The localized defect may compromise adequate numbers of future endosteal implant placement to obtain longevity of the prosthetic support. The subperiosteal implant may be designed around these defects because it is a custom device.

Occasionally, time is a factor in patient treatment. The patient may desire a more stable mandibular prosthesis for a particular social event. Rigid fixated endosteal implants and the associated prosthesis require 5 months or more to complete. The subperiosteal implant and RP-4 transitional prosthesis may be completed within 2 months.

The financial condition of the patient may limit the amount of investment in oral rehabilitation. And yet, the advanced atrophic mandible requires more implants than patients with more bone. The size and surface area of each implant is smaller, so additional implants are required to obtain a certain amount of support needed for long-term survival of the implant. A consistent condition in the advanced atrophic mandible is the need to replace large amounts of vertical dimension in the prosthesis. The incisal edge position is not only greater than 12 mm from the ridge, but also is cantilevered to the anterior in reference to the implant location. Therefore, these patients require at least three, and usually more, implants for the support of the prosthesis. If posterior soft tissue or advanced bone loss is also a problem, five or six implants are needed for a completely implant-supported removable prosthesis. In these patients, the root form implants and reconstruction costs to the dentist are usually more than twice as much as those for subperiosteal implants. Remember, the superstructure bar is included in the cost of the subperiosteal implant, yet must be fabricated by the doctor and laboratory for root form implants. In addition, the "chair time" is greater for root form implants and prostheses than for the subperiosteal implant and prosthetic costs. As a result, the fee to the patient may be less for the subperiosteal reconstruction.

The arch form may be tapered, ovoid, or square. A square arch form requires anterior root forms to be placed in almost a straight line. The anterior-posterior distance (see Chapters 12 and 15) is not adequate for a posterior cantilever and RP-4 restoration. However, a subperiosteal implant uses the ramus region and anterior mandible for the superstructure support. The anterior-posterior support distance is greater than any root form system, regardless of arch shape. Therefore a RP-4 restoration is still indicated for square arch form patients, but contraindicated for patients with only anterior implant support. Therefore, the indications for mandibular complete subperiosteal implants are related to anatomic, financial, and prosthetic considerations.

The contraindications for subperiosteal implants include a dentist's lack of training and inadequate volume of bone. Subperiosteal implants also require adequate volumes of available bone to establish support systems for the prosthesis over the long term. At one time in implant history it was reported that the less bone present, the better the conditions for a subperiosteal implant. However, all implant support systems rely on adequate surface area to resist such forces as occlusion and habit. The Division D anterior mandible only has bone for one labial and one lingual strut for the substructure support. The amount of required surface area is often greater than the conditions permit. Implant failure may severely compromise the remaining bony structures. As such, the anterior Division D region usually requires grafts to provide sufficient bone volume for predictable support, regardless of the prosthesis type or implant selection.

The surgical training required to place subperiosteal implants is more extensive than root form implants. The design of this implant is customized to each patient's anatomic and prosthodontic condition. The short-term and long-term complications of this procedure require unique clinical experience.

TERMINOLOGY

The terminology for the subperiosteal implant includes portions of the implant below and above the tissue. The *substructure* is the portion of the implant that is responsible for the support of the implant and is located below the periosteum, on top of the bone. It consists of many components called *struts*. *Primary struts* are the major components of the substructure and can be either peripheral or abutment. The *peripheral struts* are the outermost regions of the implant and lay upon the most extended areas of the cortical bone. The *abutment struts* connect the labial and lingual peripheral struts and a vertical permucosal post on the crest of the edentulous ridge. *Secondary struts* are placed to help dissipate force from the primary abutment struts and also improve rigidity and casting of the substructure and are extra areas for the tissue support mechanism of the implant. The *permucosal abutment posts* pass through the mucosa, and act as prosthetic retainers.

The *mesostructure* is that portion of the implant designed to be above the tissue and connect the abutment posts. This structure both retains and supports the prosthesis during occlusal loads and distributes these forces to the substructure below the tissue. The mesobar contains the "male" portion of any attachments used to maintain the prosthesis. This portion has also been called a superstructure bar in more recent history.

The *superstructure* is the retentive mechanism or apparatus within the prosthesis, which attaches to the mesostructure. Portions of this structure are designed to be replaced, because friction over time causes loss of material and reduced retention. At one time, the superstructure was a cast framework, similar to a partial denture framework. Today, most RP-4 restorations include only a "female" attachment component.

HISTORY

The mandibular complete subperiosteal implant is approaching 5 decades of clinical application in dentistry. Although the name has remained the same throughout these years, the materials, design, surgery, and prosthetics have been modified and improved. The original implant design and insertion protocol was proposed in 1937 by Gustav Dahl of Sweden.[1-3] Many have modified the technique and design of this implant, primarily in the United States, after its introduction by Gershkoff and Goldberg in 1948.[4-52]

Early Subperiosteal Implants

The first subperiosteal implants were fabricated from overextended soft tissue impressions and interpretation of intraoral periapical radiographs. The casts of the soft tissue were scraped and modified in accordance to the tissue thickness evaluated from the radiographs, to simulate the underlying bone topography. This technique permitted the use of only crestal bone to hold the implant. The cobalt-chrome implant casting which incorporated canine and molar abutments, was made from the adjusted cast. In one surgical approach, the tissues were reflected and the implant inserted. The casting did not fit accurately to the residual bone, so screws were inserted to fixate the appliance. This technique did not obtain predictable longevity.

Gershkoff and Goldberg recognized the instability of the flat metal design and problems with periapical assessment of the soft tissue[4-8]. They began to fabricate a metal superstructure with vertical struts to rest on the soft tissue from the initial study cast. The intraoral radiographs were coordinated to the vertical struts and improved the accuracy of the implant substructure, but it was still not predictable.

Lew and Berman began taking direct bone impressions for the mandibular subperiosteal implant about 1951.[10-17] This required two, separate, almost identical surgical reflections of the tissue, but greatly improved the fit of the implant casting. In addition, lateral regions of the anterior mandible could be used in the substructure design. The 5- and 10-year prognosis of the implant immediately improved. The improved survival of the implants was related to both a more stable, rigid casting, and a greater surface area with lateral support of the implant design.

Evolution of Substructure Design

The substructure design of the complete subperiosteal implant has evolved greatly over the past 40 years. The design changes have primarily occurred in the first 10 years after its introduction, and in the past 10 years. The original design of Dahl was a solid piece of metal on the crest of the ridge. Incision line opening was a common consequence. A heavy lattice design was used by Gershkoff.[5] Berman reduced the thickness of metal in the lattice design.[14–17] Lew also modified the heavy lattice work designs and used much less metal, especially around the permucosal posts.

A group of Americans including Jermyn, Bodine, Cranin, Herschfus, Lee, Linkow, Mentag, and Weber continued to influence the substructure design, which became rather consistent for the next 20 years.[21–50] The primary support struts were extended on the lingual and labial bone between the mental foramina to the most inferior, lateral regions of the bone. The primary strut would ascend over the foramen if more than 5 mm of bone was superior to the mental foramen, and would be discontinued if less vertical bone were present. The primary strut of the posterior section of the complete mandibular subperiosteal implant extended to the external oblique, up on the ascending ramus in the third molar region, and on top of the mylohyoid ridge. The permucosal posts were in the canine and second molar regions and were connected to the primary peripheral struts by two to three secondary struts. A mesobar connected the molar post to the cuspid post if the labial primary strut did not ascend over the mental foramen. This substructure design was predicated on the harder, more dense areas of bone, because it was believed the basal bone did not change and supported the implant.

The survival of the subperiosteal implant with this classic design was very predictable for 5 years, ranging from 90% to 100%. The 10-year survival was reduced to 75% to 80%, primarily as a result of posterior bone loss that often resulted in settling of the implant and soft tissue complications. The 15-year survival further decreased to 60% to 65%. This also related to posterior region problems, as well as to health changes of the individuals.[26, 27, 28, 44]

The classic design subperiosteal implant was supported by a fibrous tissue network. The collagen surrounding each strut was reported by Bodine and Mohammed to encapsulate and run parallel to each strut.[25] This concept considered the fibrous tissue as a protective mechanism to absorb occlusal forces. A dichotomy of beliefs existed. The dense bone was believed to support the implant, yet the implant was completely surrounded by fibrous tissue. In addition, the posterior areas of dense bone would resorb more often if the buccal peripheral strut did not extend over the external oblique ridge.

James reported on the presence of a tissue support mechanism with the blade-vent implant in the mid 1970s.[47] Later, James also reported on a similar suspensory ligament support for the subperiosteal framework.[48, 49, 51] He stated that the geometric configuration of the suspensory sling was determined by the dynamic forces in the various regions of the subperiosteal implant.

Effects of Resorption

Any strut which places compressive forces to the area under the strut may cause resorption. This causes an initial settling of the implant, and can be observed in a clinical environment by occlusal changes on the prosthesis during the first several weeks after implant insertion. Once the implant has settled, the surrounding fibrous tissue can form Sharpey's fibers and bundle bone along the lateral and superior aspect of the crestal struts.[48, 50]

Struts placed on the lateral aspects of the mandible can develop a suspensory sling without bone resorption. Therefore, if the primary struts of the substructure design extend to the lingual and labial lateral surfaces, a primary region of support may be established without bone loss. The majority of bundle bone around the subperiosteal implant occurred on the lateral struts.[51]

The mandible flexes toward the midline upon opening. Therefore a posterior lingual strut will cause pressure on the bone and resorption during this constant medial movement. If the strut is near the crest of the ridge, the tissue around the implant will dehisce and the metal strut will become exposed. This is the cause of posterior lingual metal exposure. The anterior lingual struts rarely become dehiscent, even though the tissue thickness is the same. There is minimal medial movement of the mandible in front of the mental foramina, and the anterior lingual struts are placed more inferior on the lateral plate of bone. If the posterior lingual strut is placed on the lateral regions of bone, resorption may occur to the adjacent bone, but a supportive sling can form above the implant and attach to bone. Therefore lateral struts on the facial or lingual regions of bone may incorporate the tissue support system.[51, 52]

A large region of lateral bone never used before the James support concept for the subperiosteal implant was the lateral aspect of the ramus of the mandible. The masseter muscle does not form primary attachment to this region. This muscle mainly attaches to the zygomatic arch and the inferior border of the ramus. Therefore, James redesigned the subperiosteal implant to capitalize on the identified support system.[48] Slight modifications of this design have been contributed by Linkow,[53] Misch,[54] and Judy.[55]

Evolution of Mesostructure Design

The mesostructure of the subperiosteal implant has also undergone an evolution. The original tooth shaped abutments of Gershkoff and Goldberg were changed to small diameter permucosal posts. The mesobar concept was reported by Bodine and Vakay[29] which connected the molar and canine posts and improved rigidity of the casting, especially if the labial peripheral strut did not ascend over the mental foramen. A continuous mesobar from molar to molar was consistently used and appreciated by Cranin in 1978.[36] The continuous bar concept helped equalize the stresses transmitted to bone in the anterior and posterior region.[56, 57] The mesobar was eventually extended up the ascending ramus, to the lateral ramus support wings in the early 1980s, with six permucosal posts.[51, 53, 54] This not only better utilized the lateral ramus support regions, but also provided a secondary method by which to correct the molar post region when it became compromised. Segments of a casting could be removed in the posterior region if soft tissue complications persisted, and the prosthesis support system remained unchanged.

James and Misch further modified the subperiosteal design because forces are transferred to the substructure through the permucosal posts. Additional permucosal posts in the midline and molar regions connected to the continuous mesobar further equalize the distribution of stress. Additional secondary struts on the labial and lingual aspects of each permucosal post were also added to further permit the dissipation of forces throughout the substructure design.[51, 54]

Improvements in Materials

The subperiosteal implant has been fabricated from cobalt chrome alloy since the early 1940s. Improvement in grain boundaries and size, the elimination of contaminants, and careful handling during the fabrication and surgical phases have all improved the tissue response over the past several decades. The 1980's have seen the popularity of hydroxylapatite (HA) used in conjunction with this implant. Golec used particulate forms or HA in any defect areas between the casting and bone, and placed particulate HA around the implant post to increase tissue thickness and decrease soft tissue movement around the post.[58] Coating the implant with HA to decrease metal sensitivity in some patients, or improve the likelihood of a direct bone-implant interface was also introduced in the early 1980s by Rivera.[59] Clinical studies have been reported regarding the benefits obtained, and indicate the HA trend will continue.[60–62] The coating permits the development of a direct bone-implant interface in significant regions of the subperiosteal implant. The combination of improved biomaterials, stress distribution designs for the substructure and mesostructure, and awareness of the requirements or rigid fixation have increased the occurrence of direct bone-implant contact. A method to obtain the bone model required for implant fabrication using computed tomography and a computer-generated model was developed by Truitt.[63] This permits a one-stage surgical procedure for the subperiosteal implant.[64–66]

A two-stage surgical appointment is usually suggested for the subperiosteal implant, separated by at least 6 weeks. A direct bone impression presents advantages compared with the CT scan model approach. Osteoplasty is always required to improve ridge form for stress transfer. The period between surgeries permits the remodeling of bone, and any deficiency between the bone and casting may be corrected at the second surgery. An osteoplasty at the delivery of the implant (with the CT scan approach) does not allow the evaluation of bone remodeling. Any defect that results is not corrected until complications occur. These complications contaminate the HA and metal, and make surgical correction less predictable.

The ideal implant interface is a direct bone-to-implant contact. A requirement for this condition is contact of the implant to the bone. A direct bone impression is currently more accurate than a computer-generated CT scan model. As a result, more implant surface will contact the bone, especially on the crestal regions.

The first stage bone impression surgery permits a more accurate vertical occlusal dimension and centric recording. Because the mesobar location is important for prosthesis design, a more accurate description is advantageous. CT scanning does not permit as precise a mounting of the opposing cast. In addition, the provisional restoration can be delivered without major alterations, since the bone bite also is used for its fabrication.

Incision line tension is greater when the casting is off the bone, and HA is required to fill any voids. The casting is more likely off the bone on the crest with the CT scan technique. Occasionally the casting does not fit, and is not stable with the CT scan method. A compromised result or the decision to make a direct bone impression depends on clinical judgment, and may require greater clinical experience.

The advantage of a CT scan bone model approach is the elimination of one surgery. However, the cost of the CT scan radiograph and computer-generated model is more than the cost of the time and material to obtain the bone impression with surgery. The implant insertion appointment is usually longer for the CT scan model method, since osteoplasty is required, and grafting is more common, and suturing has more tension which must be reduced.

SURGERY

Preparation

The patient is prepared for surgery in a manner similar to other implant procedures. The amount of local anesthetic is consciously monitored, as more solution is administered than with any other routine implant procedure. Bilateral Gow-Gates or Akinosi injections are given with long-acting anesthetic. In addition, extraoral or intraoral infiltration is used to anesthetize the cervical nerves (C2 to C3) at the inferior border of the mandible, anterior and posterior to the mental foramina. Infiltration is also used to anesthetize the lateral aspect of the ascending ramus. The region of the mandibular foramina is marked on the soft tissue, similar to the technique described for anterior root form surgery (see Chapter 21).

The surgical team prepares for surgery in aseptic conditions. After the surgical scrub for the doctor and assistant, an intraoral and extraoral scrub of the patient is performed with betadine or chlorhexidine, followed by gowning and draping, and the local anesthesia is tested to ensure complete comfort.

The radiograph is evaluated in the posterior regions to determine if bone is covering the inferior alveolar canal. If a radiopaque line is present on the posterior residual crest, the soft tissue reflection will be easy and least traumatic, because fewer gingival fibers will insert in the crest. In addition, less bone recontouring will be required, because a stable crestal region is represented by the thick cortical plate. The region over the mental foramen is also observed. Because this structure is about 2 mm above the canal, the foramen resides near the crest of the ridge more often than the canal is dehiscent (Figs 24–1 and 24–2).

Soft Tissue Reflection

Incisions

The posterior primary incision is similar to the mandibular plate form surgical approach. It begins in the posterior region at the retromolar papilla at the base of the retromolar pad. A full-thickness incision through the periosteum actually scores the underlying bone if the canal is not dehiscent. The incision corresponds to the location of attached tissue on the resorbed ridge. The narrow band of attached tissue remains on the lingual aspect of the crest of the mandible and usually medial to the major portion of the mandibular nerve. If 3 mm or more of attached tissue exists, the incision is made in the middle. If less than 3 mm of attached gingiva is present, the incision is made to the lingual aspect to ensure that at least 2 mm of attached tissue will be facial to the incision line. This places attached gingiva on the facial aspect of the permucosal post and limits the pull of the buccinator muscle. If the mandibular canal is dehiscent, a split-thickness incision is made even further lingually, with caution to avoid the underlying neurovascular canal.

Once the incision progresses anterior to the marked region of the mental foramen, the incision remains on the crest of the ridge. The amount of attached tissue is usually greater, and since there will be a midline permucosal post, care is taken to ensure that attached tissue will reside on the facial aspect.

Accessory incisions are made in the posterior regions bisecting to the retromolar pad and up the ascending ramus, approaching the two heads of the temporalis muscle which attach in this area. An anterior accessory incision is made off the midline, on the labial aspect of the ridge.

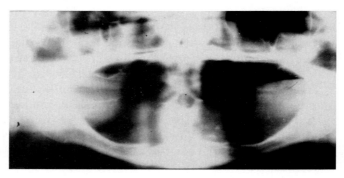

FIG 24–1.
Panoramic radiograph of a Type I Division C mandible. Note the radiopaque crestal region.

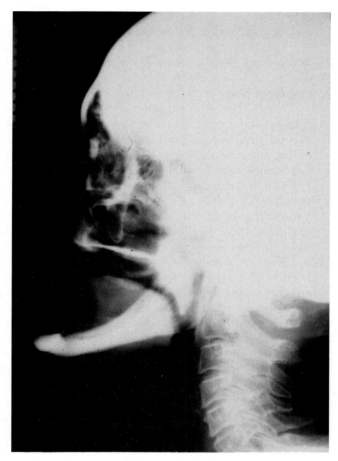

FIG 24–2.
Lateral cephalogram of patient with skeletal Class III. Significant anterior angulation is accentuated by the resorption process.

Reflections

A full-thickness periosteal reflection exposes the underlying residual ridge and lateral regions of the mandible. This reflection is usually started in the canine area and reflects the posterior-lingual portion of the mucosal flap, to the retromolar pad. The anterior lingual reflection is often more difficult, as portions of the periosteum are more often embedded into the residual alveolar crest. The genioglossus muscle remains attached to the superior genial tubercle. The retromolar pad is reflected to the lingual, making sure the periosteal elevator stays below the periosteum. The lingual nerve lies in the soft tissue just medial to the pad, and injury of this structure may cause lingual paresthesia.

Retraction sutures are placed in the lingual elevated soft tissue. An interrupted 2-0 silk suture is placed from the right canine to the left first molar region, and similarly on the contralateral side. This not only reflects the lingual tissue but also keeps the tongue retracted, yet not in the way of the airway.

The anterior portion of the mylohyoid muscle is reflected from the mylohyoid ridge to the second molar region. This permits the lingual strut of the implant substructure to pass from the first molar post more vertical to the lateral aspect of the posterior mandible. Improved force transfer results, while eliminating strut dehiscence from lingual crestal bone resorption.

The anterior lingual region is reflected to the digastric fossa, lateral to the genial tubercles. The index finger is used in this reflection. The finger technique permits palpation of the undercut, permits evaluation of its amount and character, ensures sufficient reflection for the impression material, and prevents tearing of the thin lingual periosteum with sharp elevators.

The top of the superior genial tubercles is reflected. This is often the highest portion of a severely resorbed mandible. The genioglossus muscle tenaciously attaches to the structures. Do not reflect the muscle completely off the tubercles. If this occurs, the tongue retracts to the posterior of the throat and compromises respiration. In addition, this muscle does not easily reattach to the tubercles, so often needs to be tied into position during healing if complete detachment occurs. Remember, the tissue covering the tubercles is the floor of the mouth, not the attached gingiva. Do not design permucosal struts arising from the superior tubercles, as they would be far too lingual for proper prosthetic support and would interfere with deglutition, speech, and normal tongue position.

The lateral posterior molar region is the next region to reflect. The tissues reflect very easily if the elevator remains below the periosteum. The lateral aspect of the ascending ramus is reflected with two elevators. One is positioned under the periosteum, making sure the fibers of the buccinator muscle are elevated at the beginning of the external oblique. The other elevator can visibly be placed under the masseter muscle and periosteum and inserted horizontally at the level of the retromolar pad, along the lateral ramus approximately 25 mm. The elevator may then proceed superior 20 mm and inferior to the attachment of the masseter muscle.

The two elevators may proceed anterior along the lateral aspect of the body of the mandible toward the mental foramen. The mental foramen is often approached from a posterior, then anterior position, while pulling on the lateral flap for access, and reflection. A surgical sponge may be used on the lateral cortical bone and against the periosteum to help in the reflection. This sponge may also be used to rub over the crestal bone surface to remove any fibrous tissue. Do not dissect out the mental nerve or reflect the tissue inferior to the foramen. This only increases trauma to the nerve, and also allows room for impression material to flow under and around the nerve, which impairs the bone impression removal.

The anterior lateral portion of the edentulous mandible is then reflected. This necessitates the reflection of the superior portion of the mentalis muscle. The main portion of this muscle attaches on each side of the mental protuberance, in three regions called the mandibular trigone. The most inferior attachment occurs bilaterally to the symphysis, upon bony protuberances. Do not reflect the most inferior attachment of this muscle. Reattachment of the muscle is sometimes compromised if entirely reflected, and may result in a "witch's chin," which folds under the mandible. It is especially important to evaluate the mentalis muscle before surgery in the patient with an advanced atrophic mandible, because this cosmetic problem may already be present. The patient should be informed of the preexisting condition before any surgical intervention.

Retraction sutures with 2-0 silk are placed on the lateral aspect of the reflected mucosa just anterior to the mental foramen. This helps retraction during the bone impression and helps locate the area of the foramen before impression removal to ensure that entrapment of the nerve is not present. Additional retraction sutures may be placed in the molar areas.

Evaluation of Landmarks

Once the mandibular tissues are reflected, the necessary landmarks for substructure support (Fig 24–3) are evaluated to ensure that a subperiosteal bone impression can be made of each region. These areas include:

1. Crest of the atrophic ridge
2. Mental protuberance

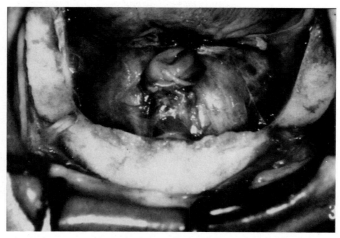

FIG 24–3.
Exposed atrophic mandible with retraction sutures. The lateral aspects of the mandible are reflected as related to the implant design.

3. Anterior mandible
4. Mental foramina
5. Lateral aspect of mandibular bodies
6. Lateral ascending rami
7. Mylohyoid ridges
8. Digastric fossae
9. Superior genial tubercles

The crest of the residual ridge is then evaluated. Ideally, it should be oval and smooth, but this condition is rarely observed. The permucosal site regions are especially important. Thin, knifelike edges resorb shortly after implant insertion, if not before. An osteoplasty should recontour the bone so the crest is broad enough to have a blood supply from the underlying trabecular bone. Broad, flat regions are also recontoured and rounded at the corners. A gothic arch shape is best for the force transfer from the permucosal abutment post to the implant substructure; however, a roman arch form is acceptable (Fig 24–4).

The osteoplasty is performed at the bone impression appointment, rather than the implant insertion date. In this way the interlude of several weeks permits initial remodeling. The change in bone can be observed directly in relation to the implant substructure, and if necessary, corrective measures can be implemented during the same surgical procedure.

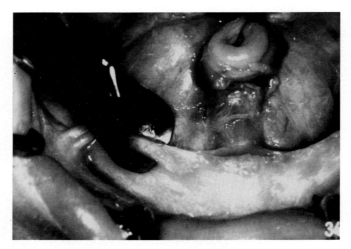

FIG 24–4.
Recontouring of the crest by osteoplasty to improve the biomechanical force transfer of the custom implant.

Vertical Occlusal Dimension

The purpose of the first surgical appointment is to obtain a direct bone impression of the edentulous mandible and an orientation of this structure in relation to the maxillary teeth or prosthesis, at an approximate or slightly decreased vertical dimension. The vertical dimension should slightly err on the short side, because the permucosal abutment post length is related to the vertical dimension. Too great a vertical dimension recorded at this appointment may result in too long a post height for proper prosthodontic management of the mandible. The mesobar also will be incorrectly designed too facial and compromise anterior tooth placement at the correct vertical dimension.

The patient's existing denture is usually at a decreased vertical relation as a result of long-term wear and may be used for the vertical occlusal measurement. However, if the vertical dimension is dramatically reduced, the mandible will appear more like a skeletal Class III. As a result, the mesobar may be designed too lingual in position. An approximate vertical relation is therefore indicated.

A resin duplicate of the mandibular denture is fabricated before surgery. This duplicate is reduced in size so that it does not extend past the first molar region, and the flanges are reduced in peripheral extension. This permits the duplicate denture to be inserted easily under the reflected periosteum on top of the bony ridge. The anterior teeth of the denture are also removed to permit the patient to breathe through the mouth while holding the posterior teeth together and during occlusal record setting. The altered duplicate mandibular prosthesis is hand articulated to the maxillary prosthesis and luted in position with acrylic resin. The tissue surface of the mandibular appliance is then coated with impression adhesive. The whole assembly is soaked in betadine or chlorhexidine until the tissues are surgically reflected.

Addition silicone putty is mixed and rolled into a cigar-shaped structure. The putty is placed on the reflected bone and molded gently beneath the tissue. Another rolled amount of silicone is applied to the tissue surface of the lower duplicate denture, and the maxillary and mandibular denture complex is inserted into position. The mandible is guided into centric relation and rotated into the impression material placed in the denture. The ideal thickness of the impression material is the thickness of the tissue which was previously over the crest of the ridge. After setting, the luted dentures and impression material are removed in one piece and evaluated. The bone and soft tissues are irrigated with saline, and the areas checked for any remaining impression material.

The maxillary denture is separated from the duplicate denture. The maxillary denture is returned to the patient at the conclusion of surgery. The mandibular occlusal record is used with the direct bone impression cast to mount the maxillary denture cast on an articulator. If in any region it was difficult to place impression material, the tissues are further reflected to ensure ease during the final impression phase.

Direct Bone Impressions

Material Considerations

There currently exists two alternatives by which to obtain a laboratory cast for the fabrication of the subperiosteal implant. The more recent technique converts a three-dimensional computed tomographic image to a hard copy or model of the mandible. The classic technique records the surface of the atrophic mandible during a separate surgical procedure, by means of a direct bone impression.

Lew and Berman began taking direct bone impressions for the subperiosteal implant in the early 1950s.[10, 15] Initially, impressions were taken using the rigid materials of plaster of paris or zinc oxide eugenol paste. The first surgery recorded the topography of the bone after soft tissue reflection. A direct bone impression cast was then used to fabricate the implant. A second surgery was required to place the implant after fabrication.

The initial elastic impression material for subperiosteal implants was called "Thiokol,"[67] the trade name of the polymer that was the principal ingredient. This type of material is today classified as a polysulfide, and is still commonly used for direct bone impressions.[68]

Ideal Qualities

The direct bone impression requires a material with several specific features for a successful result for the subperiosteal implant.[69] Most of these properties are similar for all impression procedures and will not be addressed; however, several unique qualities are desired for a direct bone impression. The impression material should be nontoxic. This is important because the casting is made to fit the cast from the first surgical procedure. If the surface of the bone changes because toxic materials cause a remodeling of the bone after repair, the end result will not be representative of the bone at the impression stage. In addition, the material should be accurate and compatible with a stone cast, so it will not distort while the die stone is setting.

The color of the material should be bright and completely different from that of bone or soft tissue. This would permit easy identification if a portion of the impression should tear and be left behind after removal of the impression. The tear strength of the material should be adequate to prevent separation during removal from the mouth. If impression material is left behind, infection, bone resorption, and implant failure may be a consequence. However, if the impression material should surround the contents of the mental foramen, the material should be weak enough to tear, rather than separate the artery and nerve. The ideal impression material would be radiopaque. This permits postoperative radiographs to determine if any material was left behind during the procedure.

The impression material should be without odor and taste. This procedure is often performed on a conscious patient, and large amounts of material are used to capture the topography of the entire reflected mandible. Noxious odor or taste may compromise patient management and may cause unnecessary problems.

The ability to manipulate the impression material with rubber gloves and in a sterile environment permits the aseptic technique to be maintained during the direct bone impression. If bacteria infects the wound, the soft and hard tissue will be compromised and may remodel with a different contour.

The cost of the material and the shelf life should be reasonable. Most practitioners do not perform subperiosteal implants on a daily or even monthly basis. The need to reorder materials every time the procedure is scheduled complicates office management.

Adequate working time for the impression material is also important. It is often difficult to place impression material under the reflected soft tissue and on the lateral aspect of the exposed mandible before the initial setting time. Hence longer working time is required compared to impressions for other prosthetic procedures.

The material must be elastic. There are many undercuts to record in an edentulous mandible. For example, the digastric fossae in the anterior mandibles are always undercut from the crest of the ridge and the mental protuberance. Yet this region must be captured in the impression to allow the primary strut of the implant to engage this area for immediate stability during healing. However, the material should not be too flexible. Large regions of impression material are not supported by a tray (such as the lateral aspect of the ramus). If the material is too flexible, it may distort while dental die stone is poured into the impression.

There is no impression material available which satisfies all the ideal criteria for a direct bone impression. Each material has particular strengths and weaknesses. The more important qualities for direct bone impressions are discussed for each of the elastic impression materials used in implant dentistry.

Types of Impression Materials

Several elastic impression materials are used in dentistry today. However, three major types of elastic materials are used in implant dentistry for obtaining the direct bone impression: polysulfides, silicones, and polyethers. The silicones are composed of two groups with completely different properties that are of concern to the implantologist. The addition silicones (or polyvinylsiloxanes) and the condensation silicones are both used by the profession.

Dimensional Changes

The dimensional change of the material from 2 minutes after it leaves the mouth to 24 hours later is an important property for direct bone impressions. In addition, the amount of change can be used as a yardstick to evaluate other properties of the material. All elastic impression materials shrink once they are removed from the mouth. The rate of shrinkage is not uniform. In general, approximately half the shrinkage occurs during the first hour after removal from the mouth. Therefore, greatest accuracy occurs if impressions are poured soon after they are removed from the mouth. Polyethers absorb water, which increases dimensional change and should not be stored in this medium. In addition, most impression materials continue to change after the 24-hour period. The exception to this rule is additional silicones, which are very stable and may not change for several months.

The greatest dimensional change occurs with condensation silicones. This material exhibits over a 0.5% dimensional change. This is clinically relevant. Subperiosteal implants made from these models will be more difficult to seat on the bone. Polysulfide has approximately half the amount of shrinkage as the condensation silicone. This is not clinically relevant, as implants do well with this technique. However, polysulfide continues to shrink dramatically after 24 hours. Therefore it is strongly advised the impression be poured as soon as possible. The least amount of dimensional change occurs with addition silicones. The amount of change is less than one tenth that of condensation silicones.[70, 71, 72]

Working and Setting Times

A reciprocating rheometer tracing permits the direct comparison of several impression materials relative to working time, setting time, and elasticity. It is composed of two plates which can be temperature controlled. The lower plate oscillates at 10 cycles/min, and the impression material is placed between the two plates. As the viscosity of the material increases, the movement of the lower plate decreases.[73]

The shortest working time is with condensation silicone, which also has the shortest setting time. The next shortest working and setting time is polyether.[74] Both these materials have working times in the range of 2 to 4 minutes. This is not enough time for direct bone impressions.

The working time may often be extended by lowering the temperature of the material before it is placed under the tissue. The longest working time available for elastic impression material is additional silicone. This material is also the most affected by temperature, and the working time can be almost doubled with the heavy body putty if the temperature is reduced from 37° C to 23° C.[73]

Permanent Deformation

Permanent deformation is measured by the 10% compression of an impression for 30 seconds after setting time is complete. The amount of change is a function of the percent compression, the time under compression, and the time after removal of the compressive load. Lower permanent deformation occurs when the compressive load is reduced, the time of compression is reduced, or the time for recovery is increased.[75] This property is most important for the direct bone impression when the impression is removed from bone undercuts, such as the digastric fossa.

All impression materials permanently distort when removed from an undercut causing more than 10% compression. The material with the greatest deformation is polysulfide, with approximately 2.4%. This is 10 times more inaccurate than the dimensional change of polysulfide, and is clinically relevant. A casting made with this much distortion will not fit completely against the bone in the area of the undercut. Polyether has 1.1% permanent distortion, and addition silicone has the least, at 0.1%.[72, 75]

Flow

The flow is measured on a 1-hour-old cylindrical specimen of impression material, and the permanent deformation is observed 15 minutes after a 100-g load is applied.[75] This is clinically relevant especially if the large unsupported bone impressions are wrapped and sent to a laboratory rather than poured beforehand.

The material with the largest flow is polysulfide, with 0.5%, or twice as much as the dimensional change at 24 hours. The least amount of flow occurs with addition silicone or polyether materials, at 0.04%.[70] It is not recommended that an unpoured bone impression be shipped. However, if this becomes necessary, a polysulfide impression is most at risk because of continued dimensional change, permanent deformation, and flow.

Toxicity

Limited information exists on tissue reactions to impression materials. A screening test has been independently devised by Kawahara and Craig to evaluate the toxicity of impression materials of a nondensity-dependent strain of mouse fibroblasts called 3T3 cells.[76]

The 3T3 cells are grown and placed on a petri dish at a density of 10^5/mL. Cylinders of impression materials were sterilized in ethylene oxide and placed in the center of each dish, at 37° C for 24 hours. The toxicity of the impression samples was evaluated by ranking the succinic dehydrogenase activity. The worse impression materials for toxicity were condensation silicone and polyether rubber, which exhibit no cell activity at all on the petri dishes. Polysulfide rubber exhibited a toxic level comparable with dental compound, which showed little toxicity. The only elastic impression material with no toxicity was addition silicone.

Direct bone impressions for subperiosteal implants require that large amounts of material be placed over the entire mandibular bone. Changes in bone contour can exist as a result of trauma to this structure. Hence, non-toxic materials are advised.

Hardness

The Shore A hardness of elastic impression materials, as well as the strain, determines the force necessary for removal of the material from the mouth.[70] This is important for the direct bone impression, especially if teeth are present as with circumferential subperiosteal implants, because severe undercuts may be present.

The hardness increases from 30 for polysulfides to 43 for condensation silicones, to 55 for addition silicone, and to 62 for polyether.[75] Low flexibility and high hardness can be compensated for clinically by providing more space for the impression material between the tray and the bone. In unsupported regions of the direct bone impression (lateral rami region) the thicker the material, the more rigid the impression.

The hardness and flexibility of polysulfide requires a custom tray for the bone impression. This usually necessitates the use of acrylic or polymers on the study cast and/or bone. The properties of heavy body addition silicone permit the use of a stock tray for ease and no adverse effects.

Tear Strength

Tear strength is important for bone impressions because the separation of the material may result in the need to redo the impression, or some material may be left that can cause bone resorption and complications with the implant. Polysulfides have the highest resistance to tearing, followed by the silicones; polyether has the lowest tear strength.[70] Hence, the hardest material has the lowest tear strength.

If some impression material surrounds the neurovascular bundle of the mental foramen, the material should tear rather than the bundle, causing anesthesia to the lip, chin, and adjacent areas. Addition silicone is more likely to tear than polysulfide.

Conclusion

The two-stage surgical approach for the subperiosteal implant used in the past 10 years has resulted in clinical success rates above 95%. The direct bone impression is the primary purpose of the first stage in this technique. The properties of elastic impression materials permit the practitioner to choose a material based on knowledge, rather than tradition. A review of ideal qualities, types of materials, dimensional changes, working and setting times, permanent deformation, flow, toxicity, hardness, and tear strength indicate addition silicone is the impression material of choice.[69]

Making the Impression

Two 4 × 4-inch surgical sponges are moistened with lidocaine 2% with 1:100,000 epinephrine and packed under the tissues, on top of the residual bone. This will permit the rehearsal of impression material placement under the tissue, and enhance vasoconstriction before the bone impression to improve the conditions of the impression. The sponges are moistened and removed immediately before impression placement.

A periosteal retractor is used under the masseter, along the ascending ramus. The gloves of the surgeon are moistened to prevent the impression material from sticking. A small portion of addition silicone putty, the size of a finger, is placed into the tunnel of the reflection and molded for a few seconds onto the ramus and along the lateral body of the mandible. The contralateral side is treated in the exact manner. Another small portion of impression material is then placed into the digastric fossae and mental protuberance regions. A modified prefabricated plastic alginate impression tray is filled with putty and inserted over the mandible. The sections are molded together and upon the bony surface. Any excess is brought over the tray to maintain attachment during impression removal.

Do not spend too much time molding the separate sections before placement of the tray; otherwise, the impression sections will separate upon removal. Also, hold the patient's lower lip down during impression setting, or the mentalis muscle will push the material away from the peripheral extension.

The mandible should be closed in an approximate vertical dimension. Otherwise, the body of the mandible moves toward the midline upon opening and the casting may spring up from position when the patient closes, since it will be too narrow in the posterior.

After complete setting, the mental foramina locations are identified by the retraction suture position. The impression tray is gently lifted and the neurovascular bundles region inspected for impingement of impression material. If found, an instrument is used to tear the impression material away from under the bundle to avoid injury upon removal. If the undercuts in the digastric fossae make removal of the impression difficult, an elevator is placed vertically under the anterior section and on the impression crest of the ridge. A vertical force is used with the instrument in the midline position until the impression springs out of the digastric fossae. The elevator then slides to the distal near the first molar region and is lifted gently until the impression is removed from under the masseter muscle. The impression may then be rotated and removed from the mouth. Saline irrigation is used to rinse and moisten the tissues, and all reflected regions are inspected for remnants of impression material. The direct bone impression is evaluated for all necessary landmarks (Fig 24–5). The retraction sutures are removed, and the tissue reapproximated.

Suturing

The margins of the mid-anterior area are approximated first. This prevents the inaccurate repositioning of these tissues and maintains proper alignment with the rest of the soft tissue flaps. The posterior ramus region is then sutured bilaterally, and suturing continues forward to the original midline suture. Vicryl 3-0 sutures are usually used for this procedure. The sutures may be interrupted, horizontal mattress, or continuous, as the tissue, location, and access indicate.

Postoperative Procedure

The postoperative procedures are similar to other intraoral surgery of the mandible. The mouth is irrigated with sterile saline and inspected for the presence

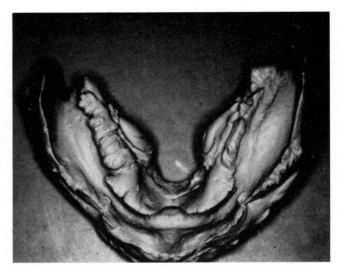

FIG 24–5.
Direct bone impression with addition silicone putty. All necessary landmarks for the implant design are recorded.

of any foreign body. The borders of the patient's lower denture are shortened and relieved. A soft tissue conditioner is used to reline the prosthesis. Moistened 4 × 4-inch gauze is rolled in a tube and placed over the surgical site. The patient is instructed to bite firmly on the gauze for 1 hour, to decrease postoperative bleeding. Because the greatest soft tissue reflection occurs with the subperiosteal surgery, rest and use of ice are more critical for the immediate postoperative instructions. Exercise should be curtailed for at least 3 days, and ice is used at the site as much as practical for 3 days. Postoperative medications include steroids for the 2 days following the procedure, analgesics for the next 5 to 7 days, and an antibiotic for a few days.

More swelling can be expected compared to anterior root forms or posterior plate form surgery. This is a result of extended soft tissue reflection. Steroid dosage given on the morning of surgery is increased to 8 to 10 mg in healthy patients to further decrease postoperative swelling.

MANDIBULAR SUBPERIOSTEAL IMPLANT FRAMEWORK

Master Cast Design

The direct bone impression is boxed and poured in die stone. A die stone that expands at least 0.2% is suggested. After setting and separation from the impression, the cast is mounted on an articulator opposing the cast of the maxillary teeth and/or prosthesis using the vertical occlusal dimension bone recording. In addition, a die spacer may be placed onto the bone region of the cast. Stone expansion and die spacer slightly increase the size of the cast, and account for the thickness of the HA coating on the castings.

The location of the mental foramina and neurovascular bundles are identified and marked with a red pencil. In addition, any area of the cast which is not representative of the atrophic mandible is also marked. These areas of the cast are to be avoided when designing the substructure.

The next step in implant design is to locate the regions of the permucosal posts. The molar post is placed in the area of the mesial half of the first molar, and two ramus permucosal sites are positioned at the superior and inferior aspects of the retromolar pad. The mid first molar site permits the lingual strut to descend more vertical into the submandibular region for more support and less tissue dehiscence, since the mandible flexes less as it is more forward in the arch. The ramus posts permit greater distribution of stress to the lateral ramus support regions described by James.[51] Additional abutment sites are designed in the midline and in the first premolar areas. The permucosal sites are often placed too facial by the inexperienced practitioner. These posts should be as far lingual as practical. The only attached gingiva that remains on an atrophic mandible is to the lingual of the ridge. If the posterior posts are placed in the center of the ridge of the mandibular atrophic body, they will be too lateral once the tissue is approximated. The buccinator muscles will cause constant irritation and breakdown of the mucosa.

The lingual primary struts of the substructure are designed next. The lingual aspect of the substructure extends only in the region anterior to the first molar. A single vertical lingual abutment strut descends from each permucosal site from the first molar forward, to the depth of the bone extension. Wherever possible, an additional two secondary struts are placed in an inverted V shape 2 to 5 mm from the crest of the ridge. This distributes stresses in more directions as it descends. The lingual peripheral strut is placed in the depth of the reflection, making sure it is on the lingual plate of bone and not on a fold of soft tissue recorded in the impression. The peripheral strut extends from the first molar oblique to the submandibular and digastric fossae, then over the top of the superior genial tubercles. If adequate bone permits, secondary struts are placed parallel to the plane of occlusion, 3 to 5 mm apart and no closer than 5 mm to the crest of the ridge.

The anterior lateral portion of the substructure may then be designed. The primary peripheral strut is designed to extend anterior to the mental foramen. If 5 mm or more of bone are above the foramen, the peripheral strut may pass 3 mm or more superior and anterior to its position. This primary strut continues to the inferior aspect of the bone reflection, and proceeds to its mirror image on the other side of the mandible. Two inverted V abutment struts are drawn from the bicuspid region and midline post locations to the peripheral strut. The inverted V-shaped struts are placed with the apex of the V 3 mm to 5 mm from the crest of the ridge. Secondary support struts are added parallel to the plane of occlusion, starting 5 mm from the crest of the ridge and placed 3 to 5 mm apart. An anterior screw hole is placed between the abutment and peripheral strut on the right side (left side for left-handed practitioners).

The modulus of elasticity for cobalt chrome is approximately 11 times greater than bone. If too much metal crosses the foramen region, the casting will attempt to stop the flexure of the mandible upon opening. This may result in pressure and bone loss, possibly with pain, during opening movements. Therefore the number of struts which completely cross over the mental foramen region are reduced to only the primary peripheral strut on the lingual and labial.

The posterior lateral substructure design is considered next. The primary peripheral strut continues 3 to 5 mm distal to the mental foramen, extends along the lateral body of the mandible, and outlines the reflected ramus region. The peripheral strut joins the ramus permucosal posts on the front of the ascending ramus, in two sideways V-shaped struts, about 3 mm from the most anterior border of the ramus. The primary strut continues along the external oblique to the region of the second molar, where it joins the lateral body primary strut. A V-shaped primary abutment strut joins the lateral strut from the first molar post. Secondary struts are placed parallel or angled to the occlusal plane along the lateral ramus and body. These V-shaped struts are placed every 5 mm from the ramus permucosal sites.

The mesobar is designed to connect all nine primary abutments. The ramus portion must swing from its lateral position medial and inferior to join the first molar site. Four O rings,[77] ERA attachments, or Hader attachments are placed in the first molar and canine sites. The anterior bar between the canines is much narrower than the posterior mesobar segment, to accommodate mandibular flexure. The size of the mesobar permits the addition of a dolder bar attachment in the midline and premolar regions. If the canine and molar attachment sites are inadequate because of height, retention, or prosthetic limitations, they may be substituted by the other three dolder clip site options.

Implant Fabrication

The subperiosteal implant is fabricated with surgical cobalt chrome alloy. In the near future we will most likely use titanium or its alloy, once casting procedures are without flaw.[78] It is very important that the metal is not overheated which introduces carbon or contamination during fabrication. The grain size of the casting is also very important. Because this is a custom device, the laboratory should have vast experience, and testing procedures in place to maintain the highest standards. The implant should be thoroughly cleaned, passivated, and sterilized before placement (Fig 24–6).

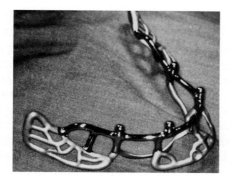

FIG 24–6.
Complete mandibular subperiosteal casting. Nine permucosal abutments, continuous superstructure or mesobar, and improved force transfer substructure are evident.

There are some advantages of HA coating on metal, especially on cobalt chrome. A growing segment of our population is allergic to nickel, and even allergy to chrome has been identified. In surgical cobalt chrome alloy, almost all nickel has been eliminated from the material, but chrome remains a major component. It is difficult to assess chrome sensitivity. The HA coating on the subperiosteal makes this rare complication even more unlikely. In vitro tests illustrate a tenfold decrease in metallic ion release for HA-coated cobalt chrome alloy compared to the uncoated metal. Golec reports the HA added to the substructure design improves the chance for a direct bone-implant interface, may decrease bone loss under the substructure, heals faster if strut dehiscence occurs, and improves the environment for the overlying soft tissue, especially around the permucosal posts.[60,61]

The long-term consequences of HA coatings on endosteal or subperiosteal implants are not known. Resorption of the material may occur, but if the design is adequate this should not be of consequence. The material may flake or break off the metal on implant insertion and cause local foreign body reaction, often short lived. However the material may be contaminated during application or placement, and may not really be HA, but rather calcium phosphate derivatives. Bacterial plaque is more difficult to remove if it is able to form on the material at the permucosal sites. Coatings on the implant increase its size, and difficulty in seating has been observed. Survival reports are very good for implants with or without the HA coating, and the process increases the cost to the patient. In spite of these shortcomings, the early 3- to 5-year reports regarding implants with HA coatings are most promising.[60,61]

Implant Insertion

The surgery to insert the mandibular subperiosteal implant is very similar to the direct bone impression surgery, but is more rapid and causes less swelling and discomfort to the patient. The time frame from the first surgery to the second can be separated by several hours, or several months; however, 6 or more weeks are strongly recommended. The benefits of HA coating warrant its use, and this process requires greater time in fabricating the implant. The soft tissue requires approximately 6 weeks before elastic fibers and mature collagen form in the surgical site. Incision line opening is the most common postoperative complication. Hence, it is rational to wait at least 6 weeks before implant insertion. In addition, osteoplasty results in bone remodeling. It is better to wait for bone remodeling so the fit of the casting may be checked. Shorter interval reentry may appear to give better casting fit, but the remodeling process will still progress and correction requires an additional surgery, often after complication.

The aseptic protocol for patient sedation, anesthesia, and the tissue reflection is exactly similar to the first stage surgical procedure. A common mistake is to underreflect the tissue, because the casting is thinner than the impression material. This not only decreases visibility, but may also cause more tension on the incision line, which in turn leads to incision line opening.

The implant is wider than the orifice of the patient. It must be rotated into position, placing one lateral support wing in the mouth before the other. Once the casting is in the patient's mouth, a retractor pulls one masseter muscle lateral and the corresponding implant wing is placed along the ramus. The contralateral side is approached in a similar fashion. The casting is rotated superiorly and posteriorly in one motion, until the anterior lingual section is distal to the crest of the ridge. The lingual tissue is checked for entrapment between the substructure and bone before final seating. The casting is then rotated down and forward into position, and often snaps into the undercut of the digastric fossa. All peripheral regions are inspected for adaptation of the implant on the atrophic mandible. The casting is tested with vertical and lateral pressures. It must be rigid in position, with no rocking or movement (Fig 24–7).

The retention of the casting is then evaluated. If any movement is noted with upward force, an anterior 5 mm screw is placed in the anterior screw hole. A rotary instrument must first prepare the screw site, because the dense nature of the bone does not permit complete self tapping screws. A cobalt chrome or titanium screw is used, and is rotated one turn forward and one-half turn back as it is placed into final position, to minimize stress buildup in the bone.

The casting is again evaluated for its accuracy in relationship to the bone. If any discrepancies on or near the crest of the ridge exist, grafting material is used to fill the void. This graft material should be a combination of DFDB and dense HA, and/or local autogenous bone from the symphysis, or coronoid process. The greater the void, the more autogenous bone is used in the combination graft.

Suturing

Suturing is the most time-consuming phase of the implant insertion appointment. Suturing is a more difficult step under the mesobar of the casting.

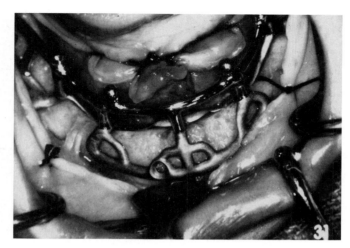

FIG 24–7.
Casting in place at the second surgical appointment. Close adherence to the bone improves the interface.

The tissue immediately mesial and distal to each permucosal site is the most critical to position without separation or voids. The midline tissue is first approximated and sutured, then the most posterior ramus regions proceeding forward. A continuous horizontal mattress suture is the easiest to perform under a bar. However, several interrupted sutures are also placed as required. Another useful technique is to pull the tissue to the facial side of the bar, and place sutures without the bar interference.

Provisional Prosthesis

A transitional restoration is placed onto the mesobar of the implant. It should have abundant clearance over the tissue, so swelling will not impinge and cause pressure necrosis of the tissue. The occlusion is carefully evaluated so no tipping actions are transmitted to the implant. The patient should not remove the lower provisional restoration until the sutures are removed, about 2 weeks after surgery. Instead, the maxillary denture is removed at night to limit parafunction. Once the sutures are removed, the mandibular provisional restoration is removed at night. Postoperative procedures are similar to phase one surgery. The patient remains on a liquid diet the rest of the day and a mechanical soft diet until the final restoration is delivered approximately 8 weeks later. A normal diet can proceed approximately 3 months after implant placement. The goal for the implant substructure is to result in a direct bone interface. Limiting the force applied to the implant for 3 months improves the conditions for rigid fixation (Figs 24–8 and 24–9).

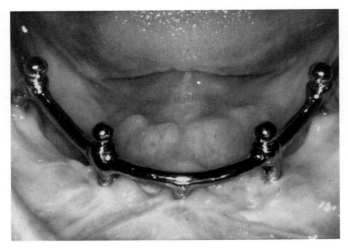

FIG 24–8.
Intraoral view of the implant after soft tissue healing. The O-ring attachments provide retention for the restoration, the bar provides prosthesis support and force transfer advantages to the substructure.

Postoperative Complications

The most common immediate postoperative problem is opening of the incision line. This occurs with greater frequency in smokers, because nicotine can contaminate the epithelium in the incision line and affect the blood circulation to the tissues. The patient who examines his or her mouth after surgery and shows the suture to other people also tends to pull the tissues apart and cause problems. The anterior region above the mentalis, and the posterior region at the second

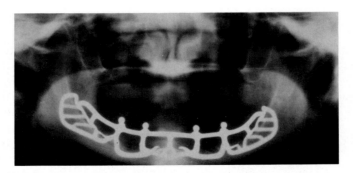

FIG 24–9.
Panoramic radiograph of a complete mandibular subperiosteal implant (3 years after surgery).

molar position of the buccinator muscle are the two most common muscle involvement regions which lead to openings. Postoperative incision opening is a uncommon occurrence if patient compliance is good regarding smoking or stretching the lips, and if the tissues have been closed without tension or too many sutures.

If immediate opening is noted 3 or more days after surgery, the surgeon should not attempt to correct it by resuturing. The cause of the incision opening is rarely corrected, epithelial cells have begun to migrate, the tissue has decreased resistance to tearing, and there is a decreased blood supply. If there is exposed metal in the opening, it should be kept as clean as possible. The patient is taught daily abrasion techniques, with gauze or cotton applicators dipped in chlorhexidine, to prevent plaque and debris accumulation. The area will usually granulate in over several weeks with secondary intention healing.

The most common intermediate problem is swelling of the lateral mandible in the first molar region, just anterior to the masseter muscle. The swelling usually is preceded by an aggressive eating or increased load history. The area is firm to palpation, no temperature exists, no exudate is observed (even if incised), and the incident occurs more often from the 6 months to 3 years following insertion. The treatment of choice is to place the patient on heat and an anti-inflammatory medication as ibuprofen. Make sure the patient is not wearing the prosthesis at night (nocturnal bruxism may also be a cause). The occlusion is evaluated and often reduced on the affected side. The swelling and discomfort lasts about 3 days. It is likely that the cause of the swelling is muscle inflammation from fibers being traumatized between the bone and metal. The mandible flexes with function or clenching, and the casting may not stay adapted completely. The incidence of postoperative swelling has been reduced from 15% to 2% since HA has been added to the castings. The direct bone-implant contact apparently leads to less muscle fiber trauma and swelling.

The most common long-term problem of the mandibular subperiosteal is posterior bone loss, tenderness and/or swelling of the posterior permucosal post(s), and purulent exudate. Initial treatment, if observed early in the process, is with an antibiotic and use of chlorhexidine rinses for 5 to 7 days. If this does not correct the swelling, the presence of an anaerobe bacteria is suspected and Flagyl or appropriate antibiotic is added to the regimen. A culture is taken and sensitivity tests ordered, and the patient is appointed for exploratory surgery the following week. If the culture sensitivity indicates another class of antibiotics would be more effective, they are used as indicated.

If the area is still swollen, or several swelling episodes have occurred, surgery is indicated. The exploratory surgery is often done under intravenous sedation, because the area is often difficult to completely anesthetize. An incision is made similar to the initial surgery, but is compromised because the substructure adheres to the mucosa, the scalpel becomes dull as it passes over the metal, and the infected tissue is very friable.

There are two choices to treat the void between the new bone level and implant substructure. One is to obturate the void with a localized graft procedure. The granulation tissue is curetted and removed. Citric acid or tetracycline is used in the area, to improve the surface of the contaminated implant and to kill the bacteria. The void is filled with graft material using the same concepts discussed in the insertion section. If the HA coating is contaminated, tetracycline is used with pumice to remove the HA coating prior to augmentation.

The second option is exteriorization of the metal over the void. The more difficult and less predictable choice is to place the tissue under the strut and permit it to be exposed or dehisced after healing. This is more predictable in regions of thin tissue. If the metal is coated with HA, it is removed so it does not encourage plaque accumulation.

The more predictable exteriorization management is the complete removal of the offending strut. Diamond burs or metal cutting carbides are used to section the metal. The ends of the metal must be completely smooth, or granulation tissue will constantly form in the area. The cutting procedure is performed before any granulation tissue is removed in the area. The fibrous tissue collects the metal filings and when curetted after metal resection, the grindings are removed at the same time. The wound is debrided and closed by primary intention if possible. The prosthesis is usually not altered, because the problem usually occurs in one area at or behind the first molar site. Therefore, even if a complete permucosal abutment is eliminated, the mesobar remains intact.

The most predictable treatment is the removal of the metal. However this affects the force transfer and support of the substructure. The least predictable long-term result is adding graft material, but this maintains the original substructure design. Since force is a common condition found in bone loss, parafunction is closely evaluated, and the occlusion modified. Chlorhexidine and aggressive tissue cleaning are also indicated on a routine basis.

REFERENCES

1. Dahl GSA: Om Mojlighoten Fur Implantation i de Kaken Av Metallskelett Som Bas Eller Retention for Fastaeller Avtagbara Proteser, *Odontol Tskr* 51:440, 1943.
2. Dahl GSA: Dental implants and superplants, *Rassegna Trimestrale Odont* 4:25–36, 1956.
3. Dahl GSA: Subperiosteal implants and superplants, *Dent Abstr* 2:685, 1957.
4. Goldberg NI, Gershkoff A: The implant lower denture, *Dent Dig* 55:490–493, 1949.
5. Gershkoff A, Goldberg NI: Further report on the full lower implant dentures, *Dent Dig* 56:11, 1950.
6. Goldberg NI, Gershkoff A: Fundamentals of the implant denture, *J Prosthet Dent* 2:1–90, 1952.
7. Goldberg NI, Gershkoff A: Implant lower dentures, *Dent Dig* 5:11, 1952.

8. Goldberg NI, Gershkoff A: Six-year progress report on full denture implants, *J Implant Dent* 1:13–16, 1954.
9. Lew I: Full upper and lower dentures implant, *Dent Concepts* 4:17, 1952.
10. Lew I: Implant and denture: a simplified upper technique using immediate prostheses, *Dent Dig* 58:10, 1952.
11. Lew I: Progress report on full implant dentures, *J Prosthet Dent* 3:571, 1953.
12. Lew I: Case histories and reports: upper and lower implant dentures—fixation with surgical prosthetic splinting, *J Implant Dent* 1:36–38, 1955.
13. Lew I: An implant dentures case study of twelve years duration, *J Implant Dent* 8:41–49, 1962.
14. Berman N: Implant technique for full lower denture, *Wash Dent J* 19:15–17, 1950.
15. Berman N: An implant technique for full lower dentures, *Dent Dig* 57:438, 1951.
16. Berman N: Physiologic and mechanical aspects of the implant technique and its application to practical cases, *Dent Dig* 58:342–347, 1952.
17. Berman N: Methods for improving implant dentures, *Oral Surg* 8:227–236, 1955.
18. Jermyn AC: Peri-implantoclasia: cause and treatment, *J Implant Dent* 5:25–48, 1958.
19. Jermyn AC: Implant dentures, *Dent Radio Photog* 3:34, 1961.
20. Bodine RL: Implant denture, *Bull Nat Dent Assoc* 11:11–21, 1952.
21. Bodine RL, Kotch RL: Experimental subperiosteal dental implants, *US Armed Forces Med J* 4:441, 1953.
22. Bodine RL: Construction of the mandibular implant denture superstructure, *J Implant Dent* 1:32–36, 1954.
23. Bodine RL: Implant denture bone impression: preparations and technique, *J Implant Dent* 4:22–31, 1957.
24. Bodine RL: Prosthodontic essentials and an evaluation of the mandibular subperiosteal implant denture, *J Am Dent Assoc* 51:654–664, 1955.
25. Bodine RL, Mohammed CI: Implant denture histology: gross and microscopic studies of a human mandible with a 12-year subperiosteal implant denture, *Dent Clin North Am* 14:145, 1970.
26. Bodine RL: Implant dentures: follow-up after 7–10 years, *J Am Dent Assoc* 67:352–363, 1963.
27. Bodine RL: Evaluation of 27 mandibular subperiosteal implant dentures after 15 to 22 years, *J Prosthet Dent* 32:188–197, 1974.
28. Bodine RL: Twenty-five years experience with the mandibular subperiosteal implant denture, *J Oral Implant* 8:124–145, 1978.
29. Bodine RL, Vakay LR: Rigidity of implant denture substructure with the mesostructure bar, *J Prosthet Dent* 39:88–94, 1978.
30. Bodine RL, Melrose RJ, Grenoble DE: Long-term implant denture histology and comparison with previous reports, *J Prosthet Dent* 35:665–673, 1976.
31. Herschfus L: Histopathologic findings on vitallium implants in dogs, *J Prosthet Dent* 4:412–419, 1954.
32. Herschfus L: Progress report on implants: histopathologic findings in dogs and a clinical report in a human, *J Implant Dent* 1:19–25, 1955.
33. Herschfus L: A perspective appraisal of the mandibular intraperiosteal implant, *J Oral Implant Transplant Surg* 10:3–14, 1964.
34. Cranin NA: Simplifying the subperiosteal implant denture technique, *Oral Surg* 22:7–20, 1964.

35. Cranin NA: Nomenclature submitted by nomenclature committee, American Academy of Implant Dentures, *J Implant Dent* 2:41–43, 1956.
36. Cranin NA: The Brookdale Bar subperiosteal implant, *Trans Soc Biomater* 2: 1978.
37. Lee TC: Present-day evaluation of implant dentures, *J Calif Dent Assoc, Nev State Dent J* 35:168–172, 1959.
38. Lee TC, Lattig EJ: Mandibular subperiosteal implant technique, *J Calif Dent Assoc* 34:400–405, 1958.
39. Linkow LI: Clinical article—some variant designs of the subperiosteal implant, *J Oral Implant* 2:190–205, 1972.
40. Linkow LI: Theories and techniques of oral implantology, St Louis, 1970, CV Mosby.
41. Linkow LI: *Mandibular implants, a dynamic approach to oral implantology,* New Haven, Conn, 1978, Glarus.
42. Linkow LI: *Implants for edentulous arches: essentials of complete denture prosthodontics,* Philadelphia, 1979, WB Saunders.
43. Mentag PJ: Mandibular subperiosteal implant, *J Oral Implant* 9:596–603, 1979.
44. Mentag PJ: Current status of the mandibular subperiosteal implant prosthesis, *Dent Clin North Am* 24:553–563, 1980.
45. Weber SP: The one-phase subperiosteal implant, *J Am Dent Assoc* 81:3, 1970.
46. Weber SP: Complete bilateral subperiosteal implants for partially edentulous mandibles, *J Prosthet Dent* 20(3):239–241, 1968.
47. James RA: The support system and pergingival mechanism surrounding oral implants, *Biomater Med Devices Artif Organs* 7:147, 1979.
48. James RA: Subperiosteal implant design based on peri-implant tissue behavior, *NY J Dent* 53:407–414, 1983.
49. James RA: Tissue response to dental implant devices. In *Clinical dentistry 4,* Philadelphia, 1983, JB Lippincott.
50. Boyne PJ, James RA: Advances in subperiosteal implant reconstruction, *Dent Clin North Am* 30:259–268, 1986.
51. James RA et al: Subperiosteal implants, *Can Dent Assoc J* 16(1):10–14, 1988.
52. Whittaker JM et al: The suspension mechanism of subperiosteal implants in baboons, *J Oral Implant* 16:190–197, 1990.
53. Linkow LI: Evolutionary trends in the mandibular subperiosteal implants, *J Oral Implant* 11:402–438, 1984.
54. Misch CE: *Design consideration of the complete mandibular subperiosteal implant,* (workbook), 1985, Misch Implant Institute, Dearborn, Michigan.
55. Judy KWM, Misch CE: Evolution of the mandibular subperiosteal implant, *NY J Dent* 53:9–11, 1983.
56. Jones S et al: Load transfer characteristics of mandibular subperiosteal implants, *J Prosthet Dent* 42:211–216, 1979.
57. Travis C, Jones S: A comparison of load transfer characteristics between bilateral and continuous mesostructure bar mandibular subperiosteal implant dentures, *J Oral Implant* 12:270, 1986.
58. Golec T: Hydroxyapatite used in implant dentistry, American Academy of Implant Dentistry Western District Meeting, Las Vegas, 1982.
59. Rivera E: HA castings on the subperiosteal implant, International Congress of Oral Implant, Puerto Rico, 1983.
60. Golec T: The use of hydroxylapatite to coat subperiosteal implants, *J Oral Implant* 12:21, 1985.

61. Kay JF, Golec TS, Riley RL: Hydroxyapatite coated subperiosteal dental implants: design rationale and clinical experience, *J Prosthet Dent* 58:343, 1987.
62. James RA: HA coated subperiosteal implants, 6th Annual Meeting, New Concepts in Prosthetic Surgery and Implant Dentistry, Louisiana State University, New Orleans, 1986.
63. Truitt HP: The application of high technology in contour replication of jaw bones, 32nd Annual Meeting of the American Academy of Implant Dentistry, Washington, D.C., 1983.
64. Truitt HP et al: Non-invasive technique for mandibular subperiosteal implant, a preliminary report, *J Prosthet Dent* 55:494, 1986.
65. James RA, Truitt HP: CT scan models for subperiosteal implants, Proceedings of the International Congress of Oral Implant, San Diego, 1984.
66. Golec TS: CAD-CAM multiplanner diagnostic imaging for subperiosteal implants, *Dent Clin North Am* 30:85–95, 1986.
67. Meyers GE, Wepfer GG, Peyton FA: The thiokol rubber impression material, *J Prosthet Dent* 8:330–339, 1958.
68. Root D: Laboratory techniques and implant dentistry, American Academy of Implant Dentistry, Washington D.C., 1988.
69. Misch CE: Direct bone impression—material and techniques, International Congress of Oral Implant, 1st Subperiosteal Symposium, San Diego, Calif, October 1981.
70. Craig RG: A review of properties of rubber impression materials, *Mich Dent Assoc J* 59:254, 1977.
71. Schnell RJ, Phillips RW: Dimensional stability of rubber base impressions and certain other factors affecting accuracy, *J Am Dent Assoc* 57:39, 1958.
72. Craig RG: Restorative dental materials, ed 6, St Louis, 1980, CV Mosby, pp 179–223.
73. Inoue K, Wilson HJ: Viscoelastic properties of elastic impression materials. II: variation of rheological properties with time, temperature and mixing proportions, *J Oral Rehabil* 5:261, 1978.
74. Mansfield MA, Wilson HJ: Elastomeric impression materials: a comparison method for determining working and setting times, *Br Dent J* 132:106, 1972.
75. Phillips RW, Swartz ML, Norman RD: *Materials for practicing dentists,* St Louis, 1969, CV Mosby, pp 117–135.
76. Craig RG: Characteristics and clinical and tissue reactions of impression materials. In Smith DC, Williams DF, editors: *Biocompatibility of Dental Materials,* vol 3, Boca Raton, Fla, 1982, CRC Press, pp 277–289.
77. D'Alise D: The micro-ring for full subperiosteal implant and prosthesis construction, *J Prosthet Dent* 42:211–216, 1979.
78. Linkow LI: Titanium subperiosteal implants, *J Oral Implant* 15:29–40, 1989.

Chapter 25

Maxillary Sinus Lift and Elevation With Subantral Augmentation

Carl E. Misch

The maxillary posterior edentulous region presents more challenging conditions in implant dentistry than any other region of the jaws. However, treatment modalities designed specifically for this area allow it to be as predictable as any intraoral region. Most noteworthy of these treatments are subantral (SA) augmentation to increase available bone height, modified surgical and treatment approaches that relate to bone density, and progressive bone loading during the prosthodontic phase of reconstruction. Treatment options, clinical criteria, and radiographic assessment of the posterior maxilla were presented in Chapter 13. In this chapter, surgical aspects of treatment plans specific to the maxillary posterior edentulous region, based on available bone, are addressed.

The posterior maxilla represents the most predictable area for synthetic bone grafting procedures.[1] However, it is important to note that a prerequisite to the procedure is the presence of healthy, natural anterior teeth, including at least the maxillary canines, or anterior Division A or B available bone. Patients with C-w premaxillae require osteoplasty or anterior autogenous grafts, or in selected patients a maxillary subperiosteal implant. Patients with Division C-h premaxillae often require subnasal elevation, and those with Division D premaxillae require reconstruction with autogenous bone grafts to the premaxilla. The SA augmentation procedure is then performed simultaneously with the autogenous bone grafts.

ANATOMY

The changes in the anatomy of the maxillary sinus were addressed in Chapter 13. The maxillary sinus is surrounded by six bony walls that contain many structures of concern during surgery and postsurgical complications.[2] The anterior wall of the maxillary antrum possesses the branches of the infraorbital nerve and blood vessels, which innervate the anterior maxillary teeth and surrounding periodontal tissues. It consists of thin, compact bone above the area of the canine teeth. The blood vessels and nerves may run directly below the sinus mucosa. Tenderness to pressure over the infraorbital foramen may indicate inflammation of the sinus membrane from infection or trauma. This anterior access should be used during Caldwell-Luc procedures to correct sinus complications, to prevent complications related to the lateral subantral augmentation approach presented later in this chapter. The infraorbital neurovascular structures may be less than 10 mm from the crest of the severe atrophic anterior maxilla.

The superior wall represents the very thin orbital floor. A bony ridge is usually present which houses the infraorbital canal, with infraorbital nerve and associated blood vessels. Dehiscence may be present, resulting in direct contact between the infraorbital structures and the sinus mucosa. Manipulations of the superior wall are not indicated. Eye symptoms may result from infections or tumors in the sinus region and include proptosis and diplopia.

The posterior wall corresponds to the pterygomaxillary region, separates the antrum from the infratemporal fossa, and contains the posterior superior alveolar nerve and blood vessels. The infratemporal fossa also contains the internal maxillary artery. The posterior wall must be identified on the radiograph. When it is missing, tumors or diseases are suspected. This wall should not be perforated during surgery to limit bleeding complications from branches of the internal maxillary artery.

The medial wall separates the maxillary sinus from the nasal fossa. On the nasal aspect, it supports the lower and middle conchae. Its vertical wall is smooth on the sinus aspect. The lower section of the medial wall corresponds to the lower meatus and floor of the nasal fossa; the upper aspect corresponds to the middle meatus. The maxillary ostium is a 7- to 10-mm-long angular passage several millimeters in diameter located in the anterosuperior aspect of the medial wall. This is the main opening through which the maxillary sinus drains its secretions into the nasal cavity. An accessory opening may be located posterior and inferior to the main opening. Repeated sinus infections may erode an opening through the medial wall. A surgical curette may perforate this structure during the graft surgery. A hole in this wall will cause the loss of graft material through the nares during the healing process.

The floor of the sinus is located up to 10 mm below the level of the floor of the nasal cavity. The sinus is closely related to the apices of the maxillary molars and premolars. These teeth remain separated from the sinus mucosa by a thin layer of bone, but may occasionally be in direct contact with the mucosa. With the loss of teeth, the antrum expands and the sinus floor may ultimately become consistent with the crest of the residual alveolar ridge. Perforations of this wall are common from past infections or trauma associated with teeth or implants.

The lateral wall of the maxillary sinus forms the posterior maxilla and zygomatic process. The wall may be several millimeters thick in the dentate person, especially if parafunction exists. This wall gradually decreases in thickness over time, with the loss of posterior teeth. Reinforcement webs for force transfer exist on the floor and lateral wall. The lateral wall gives access for the Tatum sinus elevation and subantral augmentation procedure.[3]

Vascularization and innervation of the maxillary sinus are shared with the maxillary teeth. The arterial supply originates from the nasal mucosa vasculature (arteries of the middle meatus and ethmoid arteries) and from the osseous vasculature (infraorbital, facial, and palatine arteries). The medial sinus wall drains through the sphenopalatine vein. All other walls drain through the pterygomaxillary plexus. Lymphatic circulation is ensured by means of collecting vessels in the middle meatal mucosa. Innervation is provided by nasal mucosal nerves (lateral-posterior superior branches of V2), the superior alveolar and infraorbital nerves.[4]

Sinus Membrane

The lining of the maxillary sinus is consistent with that of the other paranasal sinuses; however, fewer blood vessels are present, accounting for its paler color. The lining is a mucoperiosteum consisting of three layers. The periosteal portion of this membrane has few elastic fibers.[4] Separation from the bone, thus, is relatively easy.

The perinasal sinuses are normally lined by a mucous membrane composed of pseudostratified, ciliated, cuboidal to columnar epithelium with goblet cells. Its thickness varies but is generally 0.3 to 0.8 mm.[5] In smokers, it varies from very thin and almost nonexistent, to very thick and similar to skin. Most of the serous and mucous glands found in the lining are located near the maxillary ostium. A blanket of mucus is propelled toward the ostia by the beating motion of the ciliated lining cells.

The maxillary sinus ostium and the infundibulum link the maxillary sinus with the nasal cavity. The infundibulum is a narrow passage representing the superomedial extension of the ostium and extends approximately 7 to 10 mm. The maxillary sinus is connected with the nasal cavity through the ostium, infundibulum, and the middle meatus. These structures are referred to as the osteomeatal unit.[6]

Of particular interest is that this opening is near the superior aspect of the sinus. Adequate lateral manipulation of the membrane and placement of graft bone are possible without impeding the drainage of the sinus. In fact, after sinus elevation and bone graft procedures many edentulous patients have noted improved sinus drainage, most likely because the inferior border of the sinus is closer to the ostium. Factors that interfere with ostium patency, mucous production, or ciliary function will increase the risk of developing sinusitis.

Patients with a history of sinusitis may have undergone irreversible mucosal changes such as mucosal fibrosis, polypoid growth, and/or loss of cilia or their function. This group of patients is especially vulnerable to blockage and mucus stasis.

PREMEDICATIONS

Antibiotics

Surgical candidates who require manipulation of the sinus membrane must be given prophylactic antibiotics. The incidence of infection in clean-noncontaminated surgeries using excellent technique and prophylactic antibiotics is approximately 1%.[7] Clinical experience demonstrates that the infection rate in subantral augmentation is closer to a 10% to 15% without antibiotic coverage; the procedure may be classified as a class II or clean-contaminated surgery and requires use of prophylactic antibiotics. Antibiotics reduce the infection rate to approximately 5%. Patients with chronic sinusitis and systemic conditions that decrease healing may have a greater incidence of infection.

The antibiotic should be effective against the bacteria most likely to cause infection, and the vast majority of postoperative infections are caused by endogenous bacteria. The sinus elevation technique has the potential for contamination because of its transoral approach, involvement with the maxillary sinus, and the introduction of synthetic allografts and autogenous grafts. The most likely contaminating organisms following transoral surgery are primarily streptococci, anaerobic gram-positive cocci, and anaerobic gram-negative rods.[7, 8] *Streptococcus pneumoniae* and *Haemophilus influenzae* are the most important isolates of acute maxillary sinusitis; however, over the past several years *Branhamella catarrhalis* has also emerged as a significant pathogen in acute sinus infections.[9] The organisms associated with infection of allografts as demineralized bone in oral surgery include α-hemolytic streptococci, *Staphylococcus aureus, Bacteroides,* and *Streptococcus viridans.*[10, 11]

The antibiotic of choice should be bactericidal, not just one that prevents reproduction of the bacteria. The choice of prophylactic antibiotic for the sinus elevation procedure is amoxicillin, as it is effective against the bacterial spectrum, nontoxic, and bactericidal. Ampicillin is also effective, but amoxicillin is preferred because of its better absorption, better compliance, and comparable cost.

The patient with a history of nonanaphylactic allergic reaction to penicillin, such as a rash, may take a cephalosporin,[7] such as cefaclor, which has higher sinus fluid level than most other oral cephalosporins. Although the structures of penicillins and cephalosporins are similar, the cross-reaction rate is low. For those patients having an anaphylactic reaction to penicillin, clindamycin is a good alternative. Clindamycin possesses excellent activity against anaerobic microorganisms and has a spectrum of activity against gram-positive organisms, *Actinomyces,* and *Bacteroides.*[12]

Maximum effectiveness of prophylactic antibiotics occurs when the antibiotic is in the tissue before bacterial invasion. Therefore, oral antibiotics should be administered at least 1 hour prior to surgery. The antibiotic level must be high to achieve effective plasma concentration and should be given at twice the usual therapeutic dose.[7] For orally administered amoxicillin and cefaclor, this dose is 1 g; for clindamycin, the dose is 300 mg.

The antibiotic concentration within a blood clot of the subantral graft stabilizes, and further antibiotics do not enter the area until revascularization.[13] An allograft is a dead space with minimum blood supply and no protection by the host's cellular defense mechanisms. This leaves the graft prone to infections that would normally be eliminated by either the host defenses or the antibiotic. The osteogenic induction of allografts is greatly retarded when contaminated with infectious bacteria.[14]

To ensure adequate antibiotic levels in a subantral allograft, it is recommended that one add antibiotic to the graft mixture.[15] This local antibiotic may protect the graft from early contamination and infection. Antibiotics such as penicillin and cephalosporins, even in high concentrations, have not been found to be destructive to the bone inductive protein.[14, 16, 17]

The locally delivered antibiotic should be efficacious against the most likely organisms encountered. When possible the clinician should avoid the use of combination drug therapy, to avoid problems such as interactions and allergies. Therefore the same drug category is chosen as the oral prophylactic form.[18] However, the antibiotic should be prescribed in its parenteral form. Orally administered capsules and tablets contain fillers that are not conducive to osteogenesis. Amoxicillin is given orally, but is not available in parenteral form, so ampicillin is mixed with the graft. The graft may be reconstituted with sterile saline solution and single-dose vials of ampicillin, cefazolin, or clindamycin. The volume of liquid added to the graft should be minimized to allow adequate handling of the graft mixture. The amount of antibiotic is related to the size of the graft, but does not exceed half the oral dose. Clinical experience indicates that there is less risk of infection when preoperative and postoperative prophylaxis is used both orally and in the graft. Infection causes considerable problems related to the longevity of the implant. Therefore, for patients undergoing sinus elevation and subantral augmentation procedures, antibiotic coverage is continued for 5 to 7 days. The extended prophylactic dose of antibiotic is either amoxicillin 500 mg three times daily, cefaclor 500 mg four times daily, or clindamycin 150 mg three times daily.

Decongestants

A most important factor in the pathogenesis of sinusitis is the patency of the ostium. If postoperative inflammation and edema of the sinus mucosa obstruct the ostium, it may quickly become secondarily infected by common pathogens. Additional foreign bodies, such as graft particles, may also cause an obstruction.

Sympathomimetic drugs that influence alpha adrenergic receptors have been used as therapeutic agents for decongestion of mucous membranes. Both systemic and topical decongestants are useful in reopening a blocked sinus ostium and facilitating drainage.

Oxymetazoline 0.05% (Afrin or Vicks Nasal Spray) and phenylephrine (Neo-Synephrine) are useful topical decongestants. The vasoconstrictor action of oxymetazoline lasts approximately 5 to 8 hours, compared with 1 hour for phenylephrine, and is preferred. The effectiveness of the topical decongestant is markedly enhanced by proper position of the patient's head during administration of the drug. The patient should lie supine with the head hanging over the edge and turned to one side, and apply the nose drops to that side of the nose. Remaining in this position for a few minutes allows the solution to reach the sinus ostium. The use of topical decongestants is limited to 3 or 4 days to avoid rebound phenomenon and the development of rhinitis medicamentosa.

Phenylephrine, pseudoephedrine, and phenylpropanolamine are sympathomimetic drugs most commonly used in oral preparations to relieve nasal congestion. Sudafed, an oral pseudoephedrine, is a nonprescription decongestant that is not combined with a H_1 antihistamine. Because the vessels of the nasal mucosa have been shown to be sensitive vascular beds, orally administered decongestants are effective, but will also have systemic sympathomimetic actions. Therefore caution is advised in administration to patients with high blood pressure, heart disease, diabetes, thyroid disease, and prostatic enlargement. The use of pseudoephedrine should be avoided in patients taking antihypertension or antidepressant drugs containing a monoamine oxidase inhibitor, because of a potentiation of the action of the sympathomimetic amine. Patients on digitalis may experience an increase in ectopic pacemaker activity. Side effects of the systemic decongestants include nervousness, dizziness, or sleeplessness. Oral and topical decongestants are used three times daily on the day of surgery and for 2 days following surgery. Topical decongestants are preferred before surgery and also postoperatively when the sinus membrane remains intact.

The use of antihistamines following surgery is discouraged because of the increase in the viscosity of mucous associated with their use. This thickened sinus fluid may impair proper sinus drainage.

Glucocorticoids

Many authors have evaluated the use of corticosteroids in cases of postoperative edema associated with oral surgery (see Chapter 19). The clinical manifestations of surgery can also be decreased by use of a steroid on the sinus mucosa.[19] Therefore, the surgical protocol includes a short-term, tapering dose of dexamethasone, which is begun before surgery.[20]

Analgesics

Tylenol 3, or any analgesic containing codeine, is prescribed postoperatively, as codeine is a potent antitussive. Coughing may place additional pressure on the sinus membrane and introduce bacteria into the graft.

SURGICAL TECHNIQUE

Subantral Option 1: Conventional Implant Placement

The first treatment option in the posterior maxilla, SA-1, occurs when 12 or more millimeters of bone height is available to permit the placement of endosteal implants following the usual protocol. With the bone volume of Division A, root form implants are used for prosthetic support (see Chapters 20 and 21). Division B bone may be treated with osteoplasty or augmentation to increase the width to Division A, or with the insertion of smaller surface area implants as plate form implants (see Chapter 23) or small-diameter root form implants. Smaller surface area implants require healthy abutment teeth or additional implants for adequate support. Osteoplasty may change the SA category if the height of the remaining bone is less than 12 mm.

Augmentation for width with osteoinductive and/or osteoconductive materials in Division B bone is accomplished with intrapositional grafts leaving the lateral periosteum intact, or with an onlay graft and small pore membranes. Autogenous grafts may be onlay or intrapositional in nature. Augmentation for width is rarely indicated in the posterior maxilla. Adequate height may be obtained by subantral augmentation, and is more predictable. In addition, rarely is esthetics a major concern in this region.

If less than 2.5 mm of width is available in the edentulous region, the height of the ridge is reduced until a 2.5 mm width is obtained, or onlay oppositional autogenous bone is used to augment the width of available bone. The area is then reevaluated to determine the proper treatment plan classification. The Division A or B approach is similar for all four treatment options.

Although a common axiom in implant dentistry is to remain 2 mm or more from an opposing landmark, this is not indicated in the posterior maxilla. As long as rotary instruments do not perforate the thin cortical plate and membrane lining the sinus, no contraindications exist to preparation or placement of implants at the level of the cortical plate.

Endosteal implants in the SA-1 category are left to heal in a nonfunctional environment for approximately 4 to 8 months (depending on bone density) before the abutment post (or posts) is added for prosthodontic reconstruction. Care is taken to ensure that the implant is not traumatized in any way during the initial healing period.

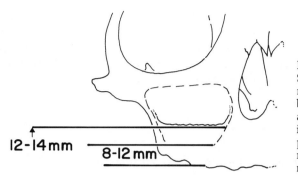

12-14 mm   8-12 mm

FIG 25–1.
SA-2 approach to the posterior maxilla has 8 to 12 mm of bone between the floor of the antrum and the crest of the ridge (which is wider than 2.5 mm). A sinus lift procedure raises the floor and sinus membrane 2 to 4 mm, to a minimum of 12 mm.

Subantral Option 2: Subantral Lift and Implant Placement

The second subantral option (SA-2) is selected when 8 to 12 mm of vertical bone is present between the floor of the maxillary antrum and the crest of the ridge and when more than 2.5 mm of bone width is present. The goal of the sinus lift surgery is to increase the vertical bone height 2 to 4 mm, to a minimum of 12 mm (Fig 25–1).

Antiseptics

The patient is sedated and prepared for surgery. Preparation of the surgical site is important to reduce contamination by the patient's own normal flora. Intraoral preparation prior to surgery may not significantly reduce the bacterial count in the mouth; however, studies reveal a remarkable reduction in bacteremia during extractions following preparation with antiseptic mouth rinse.[7]

Iodophor compounds (Betadine) are a most effective antiseptic. However, because the iodine is complexed with organic surface-active agents, it has been shown to inhibit the osteoinduction of demineralized bone. Therefore, care is taken to avoid contamination of the graft. For intraoral preparation of the surgical site a chlorhexidine (Peridex) scrub and rinse may be used. Extraoral presurgical scrubbing of the skin may be performed with either iodophor or chlorhexidine antiseptics.

Anesthesia

Infiltration anesthesia has been used with success; however, more profound regional anesthesia is achieved by blocking the secondary division of the maxillary nerve (V2). This achieves anesthesia of the hemimaxilla, side of the nose, cheek, lip, and sinus area. When administered with a high-tuberosity approach, there is an increased risk of hematoma of the internal maxillary artery. Too deep administration with a greater palatine approach may result in the penetration of the orbit floor, with periorbital swelling and proptosis; regional block of the sixth cranial nerve and diplopia; retrobulbar block, with dilated pupil; corneal anesthesia and motionless eye; and optic nerve block, with transient loss of vision and retrobulbar hemorrhage. Prevention of these complications is ensured by reduction of the needle depth measurement for smaller patients and the strict application of the technique. Proper angulation during penetration prevents the penetration into the nasal cavity through the medial wall of the pterygopalatal fossa. A long-acting anesthesia (Marcaine or Etidocaine) is preferred. Block anesthesia is longer acting than infiltration in the maxilla.

The surgical scrub follows the usual routine for implant surgery. Draping the patient is performed after the surgical team scrubs. Xylocaine 2%, 1:100,000 epinephrine, is infiltrated in the labial mucosa and the palatal region to decrease initial hemorrhage and evaluate the effectiveness of the regional local anesthesia.

Incision and Reflection

A full-thickness incision is made on the crest of the ridge from the tuberosity to the distal of the canine region. A vertical, lateral relief incision is made at its distal and anterior extension for approximately 1 cm. If there is little attached tissue on the crest of the ridge, which is more often observed in the premolar region, the primary incision is made more palatal, so at least 3 mm of attached tissue is lateral to the primary incision line.

The full-thickness palatal tissue is first reflected. The palatal bone has dense cortical plate, and the tissue is easily reflected. Care is taken either to avoid the pathway of the greater palatine artery or to remain completely subperiosteal so that it remains in the soft tissue.

The labial mucosa is pulled off the edentulous ridge, rather than elevating the tissue off the bone. Do not use the crest to leverage the tissue, as the ridge may not have cortical bone, and gouging the underlying residual ridge is possible.

Once the tissue is reflected, the width of the available bone is evaluated. With a width greater than 5 mm, Division A root form implants are used; for a 4-mm width, Division B root forms are used. For a width of 2.5 to 4 mm Division B plate form implants are most often used. Osteoplasty to increase ridge width is also considered if the reduction in bone height does not alter the subantral option category.

Osteotomy and Sinus Lift

The endosteal implant osteotomy is prepared as determined by the density of bone protocol (see Chapter 22). The depth of the osteotomy is 2 mm below the floor of the antrum. Reduced speed of the handpiece rotation (less than 800 rpm for root form implants) allows more tactile sense and may permit the surgeon to feel the cortical plate of the inferior antral floor and prevent penetration with a rotary drill.

A flat-end trial implant is inserted and tapped firmly into final position 4 to 6 mm beyond the prepared implant osteotomy and 2 to 4 mm beyond the floor of the antrum. A greenstick type fracture occurs in the antral floor during this technique and usually elevates the bone and sinus membrane over the broad-based, flat-ended trial implant. Extraction forceps are used to rotate the trial implant from the osteotomy. Do not luxate the trial implant, as this will increase the width of the final osteotomy. The final implant may then be inserted into the osteotomy at a depth 2 to 4 mm beyond the antral floor.

The success of the sinus lift cannot be confirmed prior to or at the time of implant placement. Attempts to feel the elevation of the membrane from within a 8-mm implant osteotomy may easily tear the sinus lining. Six months after the surgical procedure in D-2 and D-3 bone, or 8 months in D-4 bone, a radiograph indicates the success of the 2 to 4 mm of increased vertical height (Figs 25–2 and 25–3). After this time interval, the patient's prosthodontic treatment is similar to that in the treatment plan 1 category. If sinus mucoperiosteum perforation occurred during the initial implant placement procedure, increased bone height is not likely.

Worth and Stoneman have reported a comparable phenomena called "halo formation."[21] They observed the natural elevation of the sinus membrane around teeth with periapical disease. The elevation of the membrane results in new bone formation below. The sinus membrane has properties similar to periosteum, and bone generation is possible under a variety of circumstances.

FIG 25–2.
Four to 6 months after the sinus lift procedure, a radiograph reveals the increase in bone height. This periapical radiograph demonstrates a 3 mm increase in height from the original antral floor (distance between opaque line of original antral floor and increase in radiopacity).

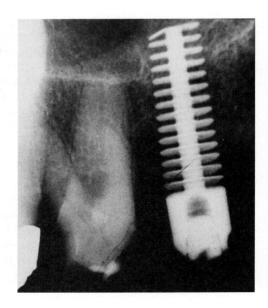

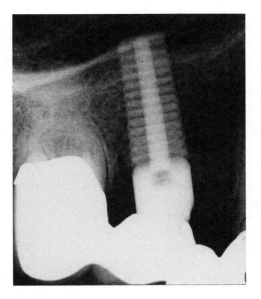

FIG 25–3.
Radiograph of the patient in Figure 25–2 obtained 9 years later, showing reformation of sinus floor.

Subantral Option 3: Sinus Membrane Elevation and Subantral Augmentation With Simultaneous Endosteal Implant Placement

The third option for endosteal implant placement in the posterior maxilla is indicated when 5 to 8 mm of vertical bone height is present between the crest of the ridge and the antral floor, and the width of available bone is greater than 2.5 mm (Fig 25–4). Patient sedation, local anesthesia, preparation, and aseptic environment are similar to those used for the SA-2 approach.

Incision Line and Reflection

A long bevel incision on the palatal aspect of the edentulous ridge from the hamular notch to the canine area with sufficient attached gingiva is the preferred design. However, because ridge resorption occurs toward the midline at the expense of the buccal plate if the incision is made too palatal, especially in Division D ridges, the greater palatal artery, which passes close to the crest of the ridge, may be severed. The pulsating bleeding is rarely of major consequence but is annoying and impairs vision. Pressure in the area, the placement of a hemostat, suture of the vessel above the bleeding point, or electrocoagulation may be used to stop the bleeding.

A relief incision is made buccally in the maxillary tuberosity to enhance access and vision. The anterior vertical relief incision should be at least 1 cm anterior to the anterior vertical wall of the antrum. As usual, the flap is designed with a base wider than the crest to ensure proper blood supply.

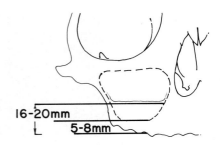

FIG 25–4.
SA-3 approach is used when 5 to 8 mm of bone exists between the antral floor and crest of the ridge. The Tatum lateral wall approach increases the available bone height to 16 to 20 mm.

The reflection of a full-thickness mucoperiosteal flap is performed to expose the complete lateral wall of the maxilla. The flap should be reflected enough to provide vision and access to the totality of the lateral wall. The reflection is usually excessive if the infraorbital nerve (fan-shaped appearance) emerging from the infraorbital foramen is visualized. Aggressive reflection of the flap may cause damage to this exposed nerve structure. However, in Division D maxillae it is necessary to expose this landmark, the lateral wall, and the zygomatic arch. The access window in the severely atrophic maxilla often is designed in the zygomatic arch.

The reflected labial tissue can be tied to the cheek with 2.0 silk sutures. All fibrous tissue should be removed from the lateral wall to avoid soft tissue contamination of the graft. A wet sponge can be used for this purpose. Palatal reflection is not aggressive and is kept to a minimum for the simultaneous implant placement.

Access Window

The outline of the lateral access window is scored on the bone with a rotary drill under copious sterile saline. It is often easier to perform this step at 50,000 rpm, but it is possible even at 2,000 rpm. The most superior aspect of the lateral access window should be approximately 5 mm below the superior aspect of the soft tissue reflection. A soft tissue reflector placed on the superior margin of bone helps retract the tissue and prevents its inadvertent slip into the access window, which may damage the underlying mucoperiosteum of the sinus. The anterior vertical line is scored just distal to the anterior vertical wall of the antrum.

The distal vertical line on the lateral maxilla is approximately 15 mm or more from the anterior and within direct vision of the operator. The vertical score lines should be at least 8 to 12 mm in height, and if the sinus outline is difficult to determine, should err over the antrum rather than over the bone around this structure.

The inferior score line of the rectangular access opening on the lateral maxilla is placed approximately 2 mm above the level of the antral floor. The corners of the access window are usually round, rather than at right or acute angles. If the corner angles are too sharp, the surgical curette cannot be introduced into the corners without risk of tearing the membrane.

Once the labial access window is delineated, the rotary bur continues to scratch the outline with a paintbrush stroke approach and saline rinses, until a bluish hue is observed below the scratched line region, or hemorrhage from the site is observed. Either of these signs may indicate the approaching sinus membrane. This should be observed all around the access window (Fig 25–5).

A flat-ended metal or wood punch and mallet are used to gently separate the lateral window from the surrounding bone, while still allowing its attachment to the thin sinus membrane. The patient is informed he or she will feel some tapping. If the window does not separate easily, the punch is rotated so only a corner comes in contact with the scored line. This decreases the surface area of the punch against the window and increases the force against the bone. Another firm tap with the mallet will cause greenstick fracture of the bone along the scratch site. If this still does not release the window in the area, further bone scratching with the rotary bur is indicated. Do not overprepare the access window with the bur, because touching the membrane during this step causes it to tear immediately.

A soft tissue curette is introduced along the margin of the window. The curved portion is placed against the window, while the sharp edge is placed between the mucoperiosteum and the margin of the inner wall of the antrum. The curette is slid along the bone, completely 360 degrees around the access window margin. This ensures the release of the periosteum without tearing from the sharp bony access margins.

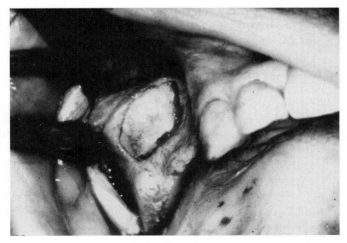

FIG 25–5.
Lateral access window is scored with a bur, and its size is related to the surgical access and size of the antrum.

A larger periosteal or sinus membrane elevator is then introduced through the lateral access window along the inferior border. Once again, the curved portion is placed against the window, and the sharp margin is dragged along the bottom of the antrum, while elevating the mucoperiosteum. The curette is never blindly placed into the access window. The surgeon should see and/or feel the curette against the antral floor or walls at all times. The sinus membrane is evaluated for lack of defects or openings into the antrum.

It is easier to gain direct vision and access to the distal portions of the antrum, than the anterior portions when the sinus area expands beyond the access window. Therefore, whenever the periosteal elevator or curette cannot stay against the bone with good access in the anterior, the access window should be increased in size toward the anterior. A Kerrison rongeur or method similar to the original scratch-and-fracture technique may be used. Resorbable hydroxylapatite (HA) or calcium phosphate is mixed with a few drops of saline, and the dry mixture is placed into the slightly elevated antral floor region. The sinus membrane may be elevated from the antral walls easily, as it has few elastic fibers and is not well attached to the cortical lining. In addition, the lateral access window is as large as practical. This large surface area places minimum stress on the underlying membrane and allows excellent visibility and direct access. The osteoconductive alloplasts further increase the surface area against the sinus membrane. When the elevators push the material along the floor and walls, the membrane is gently lifted off the bone and elevated from its position. In addition, the dry mix of the alloplast absorbs any hemorrhage and further improves vision.

The periosteal elevators and alloplast reflect the membrane off the anterior vertical wall, the floor, and the medial vertical wall to a height of at least 16 mm from the crest of the ridge, or 8 to 11 mm in an SA-3 procedure. It is better to err on the high side, to ensure that maximum implant height may be placed without compromise.

Subantral Augmentation: Graft Material

The components of the subantral augmentation graft have been investigated by the author from animal research, clinical biopsies, reentry observations, and clinical case series studies (Fig 25–6). Several materials have been studied, which include autogenous bone, demineralized freeze-dried cortical bone powder, beta tricalcium phosphate, calcium phosphate mixtures, and hydroxylapatite. Each graft material presents a similar, yet unique, biological approach to the subantral augmentation.

An osteogenic material is capable of producing bone, even in the absence of local undifferentiated mesenchymal cells (see Chapter 20). Autogenous bone predictably exhibits this activity in the subantral augmentation. Clinical case series studies of autogenous bone for subantral augmentation were first developed and reported by Tatum in the 1970s,[3] and first published by Boyne and James in 1980.[22] Misch performed two primate case studies *(Macaca fascicularis),* using iliac crest or

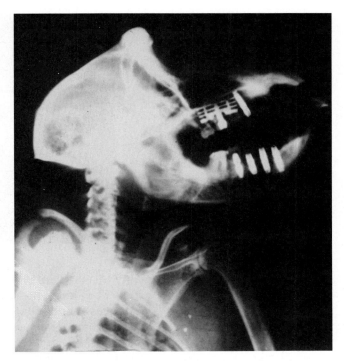

FIG 25–6.
Macaca fascicularis monkey with one of 18 sinus augmentations and implant placements in order to evaluate different graft materials. The mandible demonstrates a root form study in the same animal.

tail bone in subantral grafts, and found bone slightly more dense than typical for the region at a 10-month reentry procedure. Similar findings have been observed during case series studies with patients undergoing subantral augmentation with autogenous bone and from the iliac crest. The time interval used in these patients is 6 months. Six months elapse prior to implantation in the SA-4 approach, and 6 months are typically used for the SA-3 treatment option with subantral autogenous bone and implants before prosthetic reconstruction.

All the grafts studied by Misch include at least some autogenous bone. The Tatum surgical approach, using a portion of the lateral maxilla attached to the mucoperiosteum to gain access to the graft region, results with at least some autogenous cortical bone in the graft. Whether the lateral wall cortical bone is an actual medium for bone growth has not been determined, but is a reasonable speculation. Misch has performed reentry of over 200 human subantral grafts (SA-4 grafts reentered at implant placement) and 18 monkey sinus augmentations. A consistent histologic and clinical finding is that bone growth occurs from the

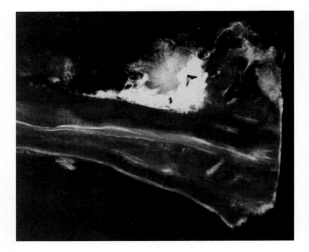

FIG 25–7.
Core of bone taken from a monkey demonstrates calcium phosphate next to the sinus membrane and bone growing from the medial wall and original antral floor. (Histology courtesy of W.E. Roberts).

subantral region, which originally was the floor and walls of the maxillary antrum where the mucoperiosteum was elevated. The last regions to form bone are usually the center of the lateral access window and the region of the new floor of the antrum, under the elevated mucoperiosteum (Fig 25–7).

As a result of these observations, Misch altered the surgical approach and alloplastic and/or autogenous graft placement position in 1987. Since this time, the mucoperiosteum of the medial wall of the antrum is consistently elevated to the height of the subantral augmentation. This provides an additional wall for host bone to help form new bone in this region. The mucoperiosteum of the anterior wall, and usually the posterior wall, are elevated to the expected height of the subantral augmentation. In addition to the lateral access window, as much autogenous bone as practical is used in the subantral graft. Any debris of implant osteotomies is used, and the tuberosity region, exostosis, and so forth, are harvested and added in the graft site. The autogenous bone is placed on the bony floor of the previous sinus location in the area most indicated for implant insertion. This permits a blood supply from the host bone to be established earlier and benefits the osteogenic potential of the autogenous graft.

Demineralized freeze-dried cortical bone (DFDB) is an osteoinductive material capable of inducing undifferentiated mesenchymal cells to form osteoblasts. The mechanism for this process appears to relate to the bone morphogenic protein found primarily in cortical bone.[10, 14] The ideal particle size appears to be between 250 and 750μ (see Chapter 20). In the animal study, use of only DFDB in subantral augmentations did not provide a firm consistency of the graft material, and therefore is not currently used by Misch. Bone was present, but not in as much volume as the graft originally placed. Speculation is that the material could resorb more rapidly than the bone formation process and result in lesser volume of bone. In addition, any bleeding in the surgical site or perforation in the mucoperiosteum easily carried the graft away.

The DFDB portion of the graft used in the Misch graft concept is positioned over the autogenous graft mixture and along the remainder of the previous cortical region. The DFDB is mixed with sterile saline or D5W (5% dextrose in water), not with blood or anesthetic solution. The toxic byproducts of blood catabolism[23] and the acidic pH of anesthetic both decrease bone formation.

Osteoconduction describes the ability of a material to permit bone to grow in its presence. An osteoconductive material does not grow bone in the absence of bone or differentiated mesenchymal cells. Hence, these materials are more bone fillers, and may help form a future bone matrix or maintain volume and consistency for surgical placement. Calcified or mineralized cortical or trabecular bone, beta tricalcium phosphate, calcium phosphate mixtures, and HA are all osteoconductive bone graft materials. In the subantral augmentation, these materials are mixed with DFDB and form the superior portion of the augmentation, under the mucoperiosteum and the restoration of the lateral aspect of the maxilla. A sandwich-type graft is therefore placed into the antrum. The first material introduced into the antrum is osteoconductive calcium phosphate or very porous HA. The next layer (and often the largest) is a mixture of calcium phosphate and DFDB, which has a mixed osteoinductive and osteoconductive property. The next layer is DFDB placed over the autogenous bone graft and the bone previously lining the antrum. The most inferior portion is autogenous bone, usually harvested from implant osteotomies or the tuberosity. This is an osteogenic portion of the graft and is typically placed in the more anterior regions or more critical future implant sites (Fig 25–8).

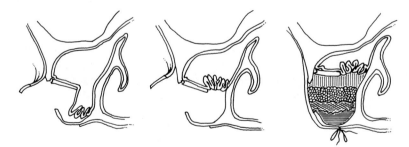

FIG 25–8.
Left, diagram shows the lateral wall of the antrum separated from the original position, but maintaining attachment to the sinus membrane. *Center,* diagram demonstrates the sinus membrane elevated from the medial antral wall to the level of the augmentation. *Right,* layered approach to sinus augmentation is shown. The bottom layer *(horizontal lines)* is autogenous bone. The *cross-hatched* layer represents DFDB. The third layer *(circles; usually the largest)* is a mixture of DFDB and resorbable calcium phosphate. The top layer *(vertical lines)* represents resorbable calcium phosphate and the original lateral access wall of the maxilla. The top layer is placed first, to help elevate the window membrane.

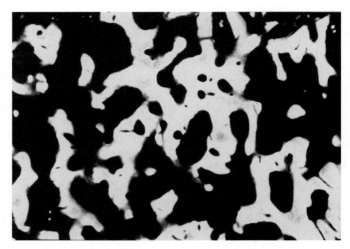

FIG 25–9.
Photomicrograph of a core of bone removed from a patient with the layered graft approach after 11 months. The trabecular bone is completely normal for the anatomic location and is lamellar bone. (Histology courtesy of W.E. Roberts).

These materials are placed in the subantral graft site with a forward and inferior packing motion. Because the membrane has been elevated, the graft can be introduced into the site below it and condensed into position. Do not pack too firmly, because perforation through the medial wall is possible and because blood vessels must be able to grow into the region to form new bone (Fig 25–9).

Implant Placement

The implant osteotomy is performed after the graft has been added for the SA-3 subantral augmentation, to maintain the elevated membrane away from the drill. If a plate form implant is inserted, the horizontal slots are packed with graft mixture to fill any voids and to ensure ideal firmness of the graft. If during its placement, an implant is pushed into the antrum, it may be removed through the lateral access wall. However, this complication usually converts the procedure to the SA-4 approach, because implant stability is at risk. With Division A or B root form implants, the bone is harvested from the twist drills and added to the bottom of the graft. The placement of a root form or plate form implant is dependent only on the width of the available bone, because the height of bone has been augmented to at least 16 mm.

The 5 to 8 mm height of original bone, the cortical bone on the crest, and the cortical bone on the original antral floor stabilize the implant and permit its rigid fixation to the original bone and newly formed bone from the graft. A more delicate insertion technique is indicated for root forms, usually with a handpiece rather than hand ratchet. A resorbable membrane may be placed over the lateral access window. This delays the invasion of fibrous tissue into the graft and permits the lateral wall of the augmentation to be restored with bone.

The tissues are reapproximated so the periosteum on each side of the primary incisions are in contact, with absence of graft material and tension. Interrupted horizontal mattress (3.0 vicryl) sutures or a continuous suture may be used. Suturing is more critical with this procedure than with many other implant placements. The border of the denture is relieved, so pressure is not applied against the lateral access area.

Healing

For implants placed into subantral grafts similar clinical findings have been observed with many different mixtures. The greatest variable appears to be the time interval and amount of new bone formation. It is fastest and most complete with autogenous bone (4 to 6 months), followed by DFDB (6 to 10 months), and tricalcium phosphate (12 to 16 months) depending upon the amount of material, number of bone septa, and systemic condition of the patient. Reentries in diabetics consistently exhibit lesser bone formation than healthy individuals. A subantral graft site may be 5 to 25 mm in depth and 5 to 40 mm in length. The time required to form new bone in this region corresponds with the volume of graft; therefore, the time required before stage two uncovery and permucosal extension placement on the implant is dependent on the amount of autogenous bone, the volume of graft placed, and the health of the patient. The sizes of antrums are variable, not only in height and length but also in width. If all autogenous bone is used for the augmentation, 6 months' healing time is adequate for primary bone healing around the implant. If the bone density is D-4, the subantral graft site large, and little autogenous bone was used in the graft, the time before uncovery of the implants may be as long as 10 months.

Subantral Option 4: Sinus Elevation and Subantral Augmentation for Future Endosteal Implant Placement

In the fourth option for implant treatment of the posterior maxilla, SA-4, the region for future endosteal implant insertion is augmented. This option is indicated when less than 5 mm remains between the residual crest of bone and the floor of the maxillary sinus. There is inadequate vertical bone in these conditions to predictably place an implant at the same time as the subantral augmentation graft (Fig 25–10).

The Tatum lateral wall approach for sinus elevation is performed as in the previous SA-3 procedure. The SA-4 condition results in a larger antrum and less host bone on the lateral, anterior, and distal regions of the graft site, because the antrum generally has more time to expand into these regions. In addition, less autogenous bone is usually present in the tuberosity for the autogenous portion of the graft, and more alloplastic material is required in the graft site. Once the tuberosity is harvested, the resorbable HA and DFDB mixture is placed to restore the contour of the anatomy.

The medial wall of the sinus membrane is elevated at least 16 mm so that adequate height is available for future endosteal implant placement. The combination of graft materials used and their placement are similar to those for the SA-3 technique.

The augmented region matures for 6 to 10 months prior to reentry for placement of endosteal implants. The design of the implant, as in any region, is dependant on the width of bone at the crest of the ridge. Typically, when less than 5 mm is present between the crest of the ridge and the floor of the antrum, the width of crestal bone is wide enough for placement of root form implants after the graft matures. The implant does offer an advantage if coated with HA, because bone density is usually D-3 or D-4 at implant insertion.

The implant surgery at reentry is similar to SA-1 with one exception. The periosteal flap on the lateral side is elevated to allow inspection of the previous access window of the original subantral augmentation. The previous access window may appear completely healed with bone; soft, and filled with loose graft material; or any state in between. If the graft site appears clinically as bone, the implant osteotomy and placement follow the approach designated by the bone density.

If there is soft tissue growing into the access window from the lateral tissue region, a curette should be used to remove it from the bone graft area. The graft region is again packed to a firm consistency with autogenous bone from the previous augmented tuberosity, DFDB, and resorbable HA—similar to the contents of the original graft. The implant osteotomy may then be performed and the implant placed using D-4 bone protocol. When this occurs, additional time is given until the stage two implant uncovery is performed and the progressive loading started.

The time interval for rigid osseous fixation is dependent on the density of bone at the reentry implant placement. The crest of the ridge may be the only

FIG 25–10.
SA-4 option is used when 0 to 5 mm of bone exists between the antral floor and the crest of the ridge. This condition requires the greatest amount of graft material. Implants are not placed until the graft matures.

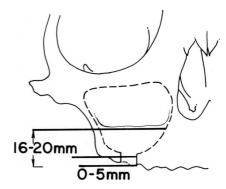

TABLE 25–1.

Healing Times for Various Treatment Categories

Treatment Category	Height (mm)	Procedure	Healing (mo)
SA-1	> 12	Division A root form	4–6
		Division B root form or plate form	
SA-2	8–12	Simultaneous placement:	
		Division A root form	6–8
		Division B root form or plate form	
SA-3	5–8	Simultaneous placement:	
		Division A root form	6–10
		Division B root form or plate form	
SA-4	< 5	Placement after healing:	
		Division A root form	6–10
		Division B plate form	+4–8

cortical bone in the region for implant fixation. The most common bone density observed is D-3 or D-4, but more often it is softer than the region in general. Progressive loading after uncovery is most important when the bone is particularly soft and less dense. Inadequate bone formation after the subantral augmentation healing period of SA-4 surgery is a possible, but uncommon, complication. When this condition is observed, the SA-3 technique may be used to place additional subantral graft prior to implant placement (Table 25–1).

Postoperative Instructions

The postoperative instructions are similar to those for most oral surgery procedures that include sinus manipulation. Smoking is a consideration, as it may compromise the healing from both the intraoral and subantral graft region. Blowing the nose and/or creating negative pressure while sucking through a straw or cigarette, should also be eliminated for the week following surgery. Coughing, if it occurs, should be done with the mouth open to relieve pressure within the sinus. Swelling of the region is common, but pain is less severe than after mandibular implants.

COMPLICATIONS

Surgery

Membrane Perforation

The most frequent complication of the sinus elevation is tearing or an opening in the sinus mucoperiosteum. This has several causes, which include a preexisting condition, tearing during scoring of the lateral window, and attempting to elevate

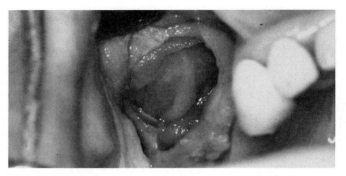

FIG 25–11.
Sheet of collagen has been placed within the access opening and over the superior positioned lateral wall and membrane, which was separated during the procedure. The graft may then be placed once continuity is restored.

the mucoperiosteum. Once the tear or hole is identified, the sinus elevation procedure is modified. The regions distal from the opening are first elevated. The membrane elevation then approaches the opening from all sides, so the torn region may be elevated without increasing the opening size. The antral membrane elevation decreases the size of the defect and creates excess membrane on its inferior aspect. The opening can often be sealed with the excess membrane by laying the margins of the opening over each other. A piece of collagen is placed over the opening to ensure continuity before the graft is placed.

If the sinus membrane tear is larger and cannot be closed off with the circumelevation approach described, a resorbable collagen membrane may still be used to seal the opening. A section of collagen matrix is cut to cover the sinus opening and overlap the margins more than 5 mm. Once the opening is sealed, the graft procedure may be completed in routine fashion (Fig 25–11).

A third option is suturing. This delicate repair should be attempted only by an experienced surgeon. The membrane is elevated to permit its mobilization from all sides. Two or three holes are prepared above the bony access window with a number 2 bur. Ophthalmic sutures (5.0 vicryl) are used to pass through the distal portion of the sinus tissue and through one bony hole. The procedure is repeated until the perforation is closed and the membrane resumes movement with respiration. A collagen membrane may also be placed over the sutures to complete the seal.

When a perforation has occurred in the SA-3 option, no implants are placed, and the treatment follows a SA-4 option; placement of implants is deferred for at least 1 month. Postoperative infection increases with sinus perforation, and this waiting period permits assessment of postsurgical complications before the implants are inserted. The incidence of sinus tear is approximately 10%. If this surgical complication occurs more frequently, reevaluation of the technique is indicated.

A sinus perforation may cause an increase in both short-term and long-term complications. There is a greater incidence of postoperative entry of bacteria into the graft material through the torn membrane; therefore, additional antibiotic is added to the actual graft material. In addition, mucus may invade the graft and affect the amount of bone formation. The sinus membrane tear permits the graft material to leak through from the subantral augmentation into the sinus proper. The material may be transported to and through the ostium and be eliminated from the nose. It may also be lost through an opening in the medial wall caused by the surgery or by long-term sinus infections. As a result, less graft is present to form additional bone. The graft material may also block the ostium after surgery and temporarily obstruct any drainage of mucus. This condition is also possible from swelling of the membrane related to the surgery. These conditions increase the risk of infection.

Webs

A buttress or web formation may be present in the lateral wall of the maxilla (Fig 25–12). These dense projections complicate the surgery in several ways. The lateral wall will not as easily release into its medial position. The strut is also more likely to tear the membrane when the greenstick fracture occurs during the tapping process. The mucoperiosteum is often torn at the apex of the buttress,

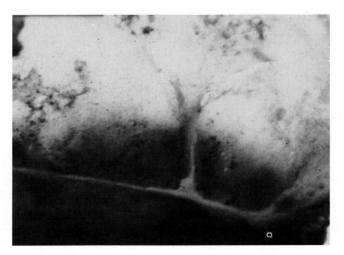

FIG 25–12.
Web or buttress of bone is shown in a dry skull from the superior aspect of the antrum. The sinus membrane elevation often tears in this region.

because there is difficulty in elevating the membrane over the sharp point of the web.

Once the lateral wall is adequately scored and attempts to separate the wall fail, further scoring is indicated. If the lateral wall does not separate again, the presence of a lateral strut is suspected and is often confirmed on the radiograph. The access window is divided into two parts with an additional vertical score line. This permits the release of one section after additional tapping. The elevation of the released section permits investigation into the region more difficult to elevate. Another vertical score line separates a distal access window. The curette may then approach the crest of the buttress web from both directions, up to its sharp apex. This permits elevation of the tissue from this web region without tearing the membrane.

Bleeding

Bleeding from a vessel within the thin lateral bone is rarely a concern. Bone wax can be used to contain the vessel or electrocautery can be used. Crushing the vessel is not the first priority, because further fracture of the thin bone, or sinus membrane tearing, may be a problem.

Short-Term Complications

Incision Line Opening

Incision line opening is uncommon for this procedure because the crestal incision is in attached gingiva and at least 5 mm away from the lateral access window. The consequences of incision line opening are delayed healing, leaking of the graft in the oral cavity, and increased risk of infection. Because the graft is more at risk with failure of the incision line, reapproximating the tissue with additional surgery becomes a concern. If the incision line failure is only on the crest of the ridge and away from the grafted window, the area is allowed to granulate in, as is done in most implant incision line complications.

Infection

Postoperative infection occurs as a complication in approximately 5% of procedures.[15] Chanavaz reports 241 sinus lift and sinus elevation and implant insertions (SA-2 and SA-3) which primarily received the Omni S implant (a 3- to 6-mm-wide submergible plate form).[24] Moderate sinus infection (treated with antibiotics) was observed in 5% of cases, noninfected hemosinus resorbed spontaneously in 3%, infected hemosinus was treated successfully in 3 cases, oral antral or fistulae in 3 cases, loss of implant by infection in 3 cases, and total graft failure in 1 case. The subantral augmentation and later implant placement (SA-4) procedure was performed on 129 antrums, with moderate sinus infection in 6 cases, noninfected hemosinus in 6 cases, infected hemosinus requiring treatment in 2 cases and noninfected oral-antral fistulae in 2 cases. Acute infection which required aspiration of the grafted antrum occurred in 2 cases. Because the surgery field is close to several vital structures, complications may be more serious than for other implant procedures. Therefore, it is recommended that the doctor be trained and knowledgeable and remain available for several days following the operation. It is also recommended to familiarize an ear, nose and throat specialist with the procedure. Although not yet reported, severe complications may lead to eye complications, brain abscess, and oroantral fistulas, which require treatment with an obturator, soft tissue grafts, and other maxillofacial techniques.

Cases of maxillary sinusitis following dental implant surgery have been reported. Linkow has stressed that the sinus membrane should be kept intact and advised caution in placing implants inferior to the sinus.[25] Branemark et al. reported on animal histologic studies and 44 clinical cases of implants penetrating the maxillary sinus. They reported success rates comparable to other maxillary implants and no postoperative signs or symptoms.[26] The assumption was that direct connection between hard and soft tissues to the integrated implant created a barrier to the migration of microorganisms. It appears the incidence of infection associated with DFDB is low but may be increased if contaminated by intraoral or sinus pathogens. Prophylactic antibiotics and sound surgical principles minimize this complication. Autogenous cancellous bone in the subantral graft is also subject to infection, but has the advantage of early revascularization. However, free nonvascularized grafts have a decreased density of viable cells and a compromised blood supply during the initial period of healing. The resistance to contamination is low, and good coverage with viable soft tissue is essential.[26] With both autogenous bone and allografts, the shielding of the graft area from the oral cavity or sinus is an important factor. If a large perforation of the sinus membrane cannot be repaired by suturing or covered by a collagen barrier, the graft should not be placed. Small perforations allow graft placement, but no implants should be inserted at the same time.

Infections have occurred more frequently than any other complication. In case of postoperative infection, it is recommended that one perform a thorough examination of the area by palpation, percussion, and visual inspection to identify the area primarily affected. Drainage follows the path of least resistance, and is observed by changes in specific anatomic sites to which it spreads (Table 25–2). These complications require rapid initiation of aggressive antibiotic therapy.

The most common postoperative complication of concern is intraoral swelling in the region of the access window. Infection is the usual cause, and antibiotics are indicated. If the swelling is localized, an incision and drainage are indicated. If antibiotics do not improve the condition within 3 days, a culture should be obtained as an anaerobic bacteria is suspected. An additional antibiotic (metronidazole; Flagyl) is given to control the suspected anaerobe, and a culture and sensitivity test is ordered. The tissue is reflected, the infected grafted area curetted, and if anything is used to replace the graft material, it is only synthetic alloplasts mixed with an antibiotic. Alloplastic graft materials are less prone to

TABLE 25–2.

Pre-Postoperative Physical Examination

Site	Signs of Infection
Inferior wall	Bulge in hard palate, ill-fitting denture, loose teeth, hypesthesia or unvital teeth, bleeding, palatal erosion
Medial wall	Nasal obstruction, nasal discharge, epistaxis, cacosmia, visible mass in nostril
Anterior wall	Swelling, pain, skin changes
Lateral wall (most common symptoms)	Trismus, bulging mass, exudate from incision line
Posterior wall	Midface pain, hypesthesia of half of the face, loss of function of lower cranial nerves
Superior wall	Diplopia (double vision), proptosis (eye bulging out), chemosis, pain or hypesthesia, decreased visual acuity

infection than autogenous grafts or DFDB. However, in the presence of infection, all materials will resorb rather rapidly as a result of low pH and high macrophage involvement. If the swelling or infection produces any symptoms in the eye, such as diplopia or proptosis, a more aggressive approach is indicated. A curette is needed to remove the infected area and the material not replaced. The graft may be added once the infection has resolved. Although the incidence of infection following the sinus elevation and subantral augmentation is low, the damaging consequences on osteogenesis and the possibility of serious complications requires that any infection be treated aggressively.

Empirical antibiotic therapy is directed against the most common pathogens. The treatment of choice is amoxicillin, and alternative therapy for the patient allergic to penicillin is cefaclor or clindamycin, as discussed earlier. The dose of the antibiotic must be high because the infecting organisms are lying outside the body proper within the graft or sinus cavity. The antibiotic regimen is amoxicillin 1 g three times daily or amoxicillin-clavulanic acid 1 g/250 mg three times daily; cefaclor 1 g four times daily or clindamycin 300 mg three times daily. The course of therapy should continue for 5 to 7 days. Progressive clinical improvement can be expected within a few days. Small oral antral fistulas often close spontaneously following systemic antibiotics and daily rinsing with chlorhexidine. Larger fistulas require additional surgical management. The patient should be followed for any signs or symptoms of uncontrolled infection. Patients with clinical evidence of severe or persistent infection require a direct aspirate for gram stain and culture sensitivity. Emergency consultation should be considered if the patient complains of severe headache, headache not relieved by mild analgesics, persistent or high fever, lethargy, visual impairment, or orbital swelling. Vomiting, aphasia, paresis, seizures, or altered status demand immediate hospitalization. There should be no hesitation to hospitalize patients for intravenous antibiotics and radiographic assessment of complications. Potential complications include orbital cellulitis, osteomyelitis, and cavernous sinus thrombosis.

Long-Term Complications

Few long-term complications have been reported with this technique. Misch reported only two cases of oral antral fistulas that lasted more than 2 weeks, with an uneventful resolution of both.[15] In addition, an allergy-like symptom developed in one patient postsurgically that consisted of "itching of the legs and arms." The condition lasted over 1 year, and was controlled with terfenadine (Seldane).

Chanavaz also described a low incidence of postoperative long-term complications, which included oral antral fistulas. These developed in two patients 4 and 5 years after surgery, and both cases were treated successfully.[24] With implants penetrating the sinus, Branemark et al., in 1984, found no postoperative or long-term signs of disease.[26]

In 1927, Kubo reported a cyst arising in the maxilla as a delayed complication of radical surgical intervention in the maxillary sinus.[27] Since then, many names have been given to describe this lesion including postoperative maxillary cyst,[28] postoperative buccal cyst,[29] postoperative cheek cyst,[30] mucocele,[31] surgical ciliated cyst,[32] and postoperative paranasal cyst.[33] Incidence is reported as common in Japan but rare in other parts of the world. A history of previous Caldwell-Luc surgery is a common finding. The cyst is thought to arise from the entrapment of epithelial remnants in the wound during closure. Misch et al.[34] reported one incidence of a maxillary cyst associated with a sinus augmentation and implant procedure.

The recommended treatment of the postoperative maxillary cyst is a Caldwell-Luc type operation completely removing the cyst wall and forming an intranasal window. However, treatment by marsupialization may be indicated. Enucleation and primary closure, or enucleation and open packing are effective when the cyst is small and unilocular.[35] To prevent reoccurrence, complete enucleation is necessary but may be difficult in multilocular lesions and areas of adhesion to adjacent structures. The cyst cavity may be grafted with allogenic bone in the event the patient elects to have another implant placed.

LONG-TERM RESULTS

The primary method of long-term evaluation of subantral augmentations has been the endosteal implant survival in these regions. Hypothetically, if the graft is composed of good quality bone, the endosteal implant should be maintained in health. Of course, proper implant and prosthetic procedures are required for these implants. Between 1980 and 1990 Misch reported on 385 human subantral augmentations performed using the Tatum lateral wall approach (SA-3 or SA-4). Of the 385 subantral augmentations, two maxillary antrum regions did not grow enough bone for implant placement, and the procedure was aborted after the 8 month healing interval. These patients had DFDB mixed with lincomycin as the major constituent of the graft.

The primary graft compositions during the past 10 years were 100% autogenous or 25% to 50% autogenous plus 25% DFDB plus 25% to 50% resorbable calcium phosphate. The type of implant placed in the region during the first 6 years of the study were plate form implants. The primary endosteal implants placed during the next 3 years were titanium threaded implants, and the primary implants placed in 1990 were HA-coated threaded implants. The most common length of root form implant is 16 mm; the most common diameter approximately 3.8 mm. Implant survival has been more than 98% in the last decade.[36]

SUMMARY

The posterior maxilla has previously been reported as the least predictable area for implant survival. Causes cited include inadequate bone height, poor bone density, and high occlusal forces. Past implant approaches to this region attempt to avoid the maxillary sinus. As a result, excessive cantilevers are often present when posterior implants are not inserted, or excess number of pontics when implants are placed posterior to the antrum. Misch has organized four treatment options according to the height of bone remaining between the crest of the ridge and the floor of the antrum. SA-1 corresponds to abundant bone height (>12 mm) and permits placement of implants. SA-2 has 8 to 12 mm of bone, and endosteal implants are inserted simultaneous to a sinus lift procedure. SA-3 ridges have 5 to 8 mm of bone remaining; a translateral wall approach is used to graft the floor of the antrum, and endosteal implants can be inserted simultaneously. In SA-4 (0 to 5 mm) there is not sufficient bone to place endosteal implants. The area is first grafted using a Tatum lateral wall approach and subantral augmentation. Endosteal implants are inserted at graft maturity.

These options were further modified to reflect the width of available bone once adequate height was obtained. A Division A edentulous site has 5 mm or more width, 5 mm or more length, 10 mm or more height, an angulation of less than 30 degrees load to the implant body, and a crown-implant ratio less than 1. Root form implants are indicated under these conditions.

If the ridge anatomy is 2.5 to 5 mm in width and the length is 15 mm or more, while the remaining factors remain similar, a Division B anatomy is present. These ridges may be treated by osteoplasty or narrow, smaller surface area endosteal implants (plate forms or narrow root forms). Rarely is augmentation for width used in this region, because esthetics is not a factor, and bone height increase is predictable.

REFERENCES

1. Tatum OH: Maxillary and sinus implant reconstruction, *Dent Clin North Am* 30:207–229, 1986.
2. Blitzer A, Lawson W, Friedman W, editors: *Surgery of the paranasal sinuses,* Philadelphia, 1985, WB Saunders.
3. Tatum OH: Maxillary sinus elevation and subantral augmentation, Lecture, Alabama Implant Study Group, Birmingham, Alabama, May 1977.
4. Moss-Salentija L: Anatomy and embryology. In Blitzer A, Lawson W, Friedman W, editors: *Surgery of the paranasal sinuses,* Philadelphia, 1985, WB Saunders.
5. Morgensen C, Tos M: Quantitative histology of the maxillary sinus, *Rhinology* 15:129, 1977.
6. Bell RD, Stone HE: Conservative surgical procedures in inflammatory disease of the maxillary sinus, *Otolaryngol Clin North Am* 9:175, 1976.
7. Pederson LJ: Antibiotic prophylaxis against wound infections in oral and maxillofacial surgery, *J Oral Maxillofac Surg* 48:617–620, 1990.
8. Flynn TR, Tompazian RG: Infections of the oral cavity. In Waite D, editor: *Textbook of practical oral and maxillofacial surgery,* Philadelphia, 1987, Lea & Febiger, p 280.
9. Lebowitz AS: Antimicrobic therapy in rhinologic infection. In Goldsmith J, editor: *The principles and practice of rhinology,* New York, 1987, Wiley, pp 855–868.
10. Mulliken JB et al: Use of demineralized allogenic bone implants for the correction of maxillocraniofacial deformities, *Ann Surg* 194:366–372, 1981.
11. Marx RE et al: The use of freeze-dried allogenic bone in oral and maxillofacial surgery, *J Oral Surg* 39:264–274, 1981.
12. Dajani A et al: Prevention of bacterial endocarditis: recommendations by the American Heart Association, *JAMA* 264:2919–2922, 1990.
13. Gallagher DM, Epker BN: Infection following intraoral surgical correction of dentofacial deformities: a review of 140 consecutive cases, *J Oral Surg* 38:117–120, 1980.
14. Urist MR et al: The bone induction principle, *Clin Orthop* 53:243–283, 1967.
15. Misch CE: Maxillary sinus augmentation for endosteal implants: organized alternative treatment plans, *Int J Oral Implant* 4:49–58, 1987.
16. Mabry TW, Yukna RA, Sepe WW: Freeze-dried bone allografts combined with tetracycline in the treatment of juvenile periodontitis, *J Periodontol* 56:74–81, 1985.
17. Pertri WH: Osteogenic activity of antibiotic-supplemented bone allografts in the guinea pig, *J Oral Maxillofac Surg* 42:631–636, 1984.
18. Misch CM: The pharmacologic management of maxillary sinus elevation surgery, *J Oral Implant* 18:15–23, 1992.
19. Mabry RC: Corticosteroids in rhinology. In Goldsmith J, editor: *The principles and practice of rhinology,* New York, Wiley, 1987, pp 847–853.
20. Misch CE, Moore P: Steroids and reduction of pain, edema and disfunction in implant dentistry, *Int J Oral Implant* 6:27–31, 1989.
21. Worth HM, Stoneman DW: Radiographic interpretation of antral mucosal changes due to localized dental infection, *J Can Dent Assoc* 38:111, 1972.
22. Boyne PJ, James RA: Grafting of the maxillary sinus floor with autologous marrow and bone, *J Oral Surg* 38:613–616, 1980.

23. Marx RE, Snyder RM, Kline SN: Cellular survival of human marrow during placement of marrow cancellous bone grafts, *J Oral Surg* 37:712–718, 1979.

24. Chanavaz M: Maxillary sinus: anatomy, physiology, surgery, and bone grafting related to oral implantology, eleven years of surgical experience (1979–1990), *J Oral Implant* 16:199–209, 1990.

25. Linkow LI: Maxillary implants: a dynamic approach to oral implantology, New Haven, Conn, Glarus Publishing, 1977, p 109.

26. Branemark P-I et al: An experimental and clinical study of osseointegrated implants penetrating the nasal cavity, *Int J Oral Maxillofac Surg* 42:497, 1984.

27. Kubo I: A buccal cyst occurring after a radical operation of the maxillary sinus, *Z Otol Tokyo* 33:896, 1927.

28. Kaneshiro S et al: The postoperative maxillary cyst: a report of 71 cases, *J Oral Surg* 39:191–198, 1981.

29. Nique T et al: Particulate allogeneic bone grafts into maxillary alveolar clefts in humans: a preliminary report, *Int J Oral Maxillofac Surg* 45:386–392, 1987.

30. Kubo I: Postoperative wangenzyste, *Z Otol Tokyo* 39:1831, 1933.

31. Mennig H: Zur Pathogenese der Kieferhohen Mucocelen, *Arch Otorhinolaryngol Suppl* 169:465, 1956.

32. Gregory GT, Shafer WG: Surgical ciliated cysts of the maxilla: report of cases, *J Oral Surg* 16:251–253, 1958.

33. Tamura S: Study on the postoperative paranasal cyst, *J Otolaryngol Jpn* 63:319, 1960.

34. Misch CE et al: Postoperative maxillary cyst associated with sinus elevation procedure: a case report, *J Oral Implant* 19:432–437, 1991.

35. Yoshikawa Y et al: Effective treatment of the postoperative maxillary cyst by marsupialization, *Int J Oral Maxillofac Surg* 40:487–491, 1982.

36. Misch CE: Implants in the partially edentulous patient and subantral augmentation (abst). UCLA Symposium, Palm Springs, Calif, April 19–21, 1990, p 16.

Chapter 26

Premaxilla Implant Considerations: Surgery and Fixed Prosthodontics

Carl E. Misch

Several factors affect the condition of the premaxilla and may result in a decrease in implant survival, an increase in prosthetic complications, or both. The maxillary anterior ridge is often inadequate in available bone for endosteal implants. The facial cortical plate over the roots of the maxillary teeth is very thin and porous. It may be resorbed from periodontal disease or is often fractured during the extraction of teeth. In addition, the labial plate is resorbed during initial bone remodeling after tooth loss, and the anterior ridge loses 40% to 60% of its width within a year after tooth loss and migrates to a more palatal position.[1]

There are frequently labial undercuts of bone in the premaxilla region. The distance between the apices of the maxillary anterior teeth and the floor of the nose, and the height of the alveolar ridge are both variable. When the apices of the roots do not extend to the floor of the nose, an undercut or depressed region of bone is often present between the roots and the piriform rim. The greater the height of bone between these structures, the more depressed the region. Additional causes of labial undercuts are periapical disease of the anterior teeth, trauma, vertical fracture of teeth, and surgical corrective techniques.

A maxillary denture is more acceptable to patients than its mandibular counterpart. A longer time interval often occurs between the complete loss of the teeth and the desire to have additional retention or a fixed restoration. As a consequence, bone loss is greater in width and height than in the mandibular anterior region.

In the majority of patients, the bone is less dense in the anterior maxilla than in the anterior mandible. In the mandible, a dense cortical layer is present on all surrounding dimensions. The maxilla presents porous bone on the labial aspect, very thin dense compacta in the nasal region, and thick cortical bone on the palatal aspect. The coarse trabecular bone is often similar in nature in the anterior regions of the maxilla and mandible.

In the premaxilla, esthetics and phonetics dictate that the replacement teeth be placed near their original position. Because the anatomic ridge is now more palatal and superior, an anterior cantilever is necessary. The crown-implant ratio is an important consideration in the anterior maxilla, where the natural crown height is greatest of any region. The arc of closure is anterior to the remaining bone; as a consequence, the moment force is greatest against the maxillary anterior crowns supported by implants. All mandibular excursions place horizontal forces on the maxillary anterior teeth. These rotation forces increase the amount of stress on the crestal bone, especially on the labial aspect of the implant. Because the cortical bone is thin and less dense in this region, it is less resistant to these moment loads.

The most common indication for a single-tooth implant is in the maxillary anterior arch. Implants to replace a single tooth are one of the more difficult treatments to perform in implant dentistry. They are often overused, in the belief that replacing a single tooth will be easy and a good entry into the learning curve of implant dentistry. The average number of implants used per patient for the past few years in the United States has been less than two implants per patient. This emphasizes the overuse of the single tooth implant.[2]

There are many disadvantages of single tooth implants. Contradictions for anterior single-tooth implant abutments include the following:[2]

1. Inadequate mesial-distal length
2. Inadequate bone width
3. Inadequate bone height
4. Inadequate intraocclusal space
5. Moderate mobility of adjacent teeth
6. Time requirement
7. Cost
8. Difficult esthetics
9. Removable transitional appliance

The time period for a rigid fixated implant to heal and be restored is approximately 5 to 7 months. A traditional three-unit fixed prosthesis may often be completed in less than 3 weeks. The transitional restoration of a three-unit bridge is an acrylic fixed prosthesis, fabricated the day the procedure is started. The transitional restoration for a single-tooth implant is usually a removal prosthesis. These acrylic restorations lack stability and retention, hence the name "flipper" is applied to them. If a resin-retained transitional restoration is fabricated to permit a fixed transitional condition, the inability to prepare the adjacent teeth properly leads to an increase in debonding.

The reason the single tooth was lost is almost always related to poor surrounding bone. The two most common examples of single-tooth loss are lesions of endodontic origin related to root fracture and periodontal disease. The root fracture destroys the facial bone and, after extraction, the lack of bone causes the implant to be inserted more lingual and apical to ideal placement. The final crown appears longer than adjacent teeth, and prosthetic management is often compromised. When a tooth is lost to periodontal disease, there also is a longer clinical crown on an implant abutment. In addition, the adjacent teeth of an anterior edentulous implant site should be healthy and exhibit minimum mobility. If anterior implants are placed between mobile teeth, the entire occlusal force in all excursions will be solely on the implant(s). Three or more implants are necessary to distribute all the anterior lateral loads effectively over the long term. Single tooth implants with anterior mobile teeth are not indicated unless the occlusion is relieved so most all forces are distributed to the natural teeth.

The cost of a three-unit fixed prosthesis should be less than that of a single-tooth implant. The laboratory fee for three crowns is approximately $300. The implant body, abutment, analog, and final crown fee usually is $400. The scheduled room time to set up, prepare, impress, temporize, insert, and clean up for a three-unit prosthesis is less than 2 hours. The setup and cleanup time alone for an implant surgery is more than 30 minutes. The surgery, transitional restoration, uncovery, abutment selection, preparation, impression, transitional stage two restoration, and insertion is 3 hours. The training to perform a three-unit fixed prosthesis is acquired in dental school; the training for a single tooth implant is acquired only after graduation. The equipment to perform a fixed prosthesis is present in any general dentist office. The electric motor, handpiece(s), and inventory to place a single-tooth implant is additional expense. Malpractice insurance may be greater for some practitioners when implant surgery is included in the practice. As a result, the cost to the patient of a single-tooth implant should be several hundred dollars more than a three-unit prosthesis.

The esthetics of a maxillary anterior single crown is often one of the most difficult challenges in restorative dentistry. The challenge on an implant abutment is much more difficult. The implant is only 4 mm in diameter and round in cross-section. A natural tooth is 6 to 12 mm in cross-section and never is completely round. As a result, the cervical esthetics of a single implant crown must compromise standard hygiene contours to improve esthetics. Many additional prosthetic applications are required to improve the appearance of the crown.

The premaxilla requires the most varied surgical approaches to improve success and is the most critical region for esthetics and phonetics. As a result, an additional bone Division, B-w, is introduced. Options for Division B, B-w, and C-w more often include augmentation, rather than the usual osteoplasty performed in other intraoral regions. The opposing landmark is the floor of the nose, and this structure may be slightly modified to improve implant support in the C-h and D bone divisions. In this chapter the unique surgical and prosthetic aspects of implant dentistry in the premaxilla are addressed.

TREATMENT OPTIONS

The treatment options for the restoration of a maxillary anterior missing tooth (or teeth) include a fixed partial denture, removable partial denture, acid-etched resin-retained bridge, implant-supported prosthesis, or a combination of implant- and tooth-retained restoration. When possible the fixed partial denture is the treatment of choice. The three- to six-unit fixed restoration can be fabricated in shorter time, is more predictable, and satisfies the criteria of normal contour, comfort, function, esthetics, and health. However, there are contraindications for the fixed bridge. The patient with poor abutment teeth support, inadequate edentulous bone for proper pontic contour, anterior diastemas which the patient desires to maintain, or a young patient with incomplete formation of the root apices and/or large pulp horns in the clinical crowns are dental limiting factors.[2]

The second option to replace the maxillary anterior tooth is a removable partial denture. A common axiom in restorative dentistry is to use a fixed prosthesis whenever possible.[3] The usual indication for the removable option is when patient's economics are a factor. Rarely does a patient desire a removable prosthesis to replace anterior teeth. However, the easiest interim treatment modality for replacing a tooth during implant submerged healing is the removable appliance. The transitional procedure should be factored into the cost of the implant restoration. If a bone augmentation is necessary, this appliance may need to be used for longer than 1 year before the final prosthesis is inserted.

The third option to restore the edentulous site is a resin-bonded prosthesis. This procedure is often a compromise for the fixed partial denture. Improvements continue in this restoration; however, a common complication is uncementation or debonding. This most often occurs during function, and because eating is a social experience, may cause the patient embarrassment and insecurity. This option is occasionally selected during the graft and/or implant healing process for patients not willing to wear a removable prosthesis.

The most common indication of tooth- and/or implant-supported restorations is inadequate periodontal support of abutment teeth, long spans of edentulism, and/or additional support required as a result of force factors or occlusion. Anterior teeth often demonstrate mobility. As a result, when implants and anterior teeth are joined in the same restoration, splinting several teeth together or adding enough implants to make an independent restoration or living pontic of the natural tooth is usually required.

The most common observed contraindication for a traditional fixed prosthesis with natural tooth abutments is psychological. Typically, an anterior tooth was damaged by decay or trauma and was restored with a full crown. The tooth later required endodontic therapy. Subsequent endodontic failure lead to an apicoectomy. A vertical fracture was discovered, and the tooth was extracted. Because this whole chain of events started with an anterior single crown, the patient may not accept a three-unit conventional fixed partial denture. In addition, patients are more concerned regarding the esthetic aspects of anterior teeth and do not desire tooth preparation of these structures. Unfortunately, these same events have usually resulted in inadequate width of bone for ideal implant insertion. The implant dentist must then consider bone augmentation before implant placement. This delays treatment and requires additional training.

Another indication for anterior single tooth implants is the congenitally missing tooth. The bone in the region of the missing tooth will continue to resorb and affect the pontic contour of the future fixed prosthesis. The patient's parents often feel the need to replace the anterior congenital missing tooth with an implant. However, the adjacent roots of the natural teeth often impinge on the edentulous bone, or the mesial distal length is inadequate for proper final esthetics. Orthodontic therapy prior to implant placement should be considered to improve the local situation. The implant should not engage the opposing cortical bone, and the fixed prosthesis should not cross the midline in young, growing patients.

The ideal location of a single tooth implant is usually anterior to the maxillary sinus or mandibular foramen. The amount of force generated in the anterior region of the mouth is less than in the posterior sections. In front of these anatomic landmarks the bone is more often adequate in height for implant placement. The free-standing implant in less dense bone commonly observed in the maxilla should be at least 12 mm in height and 3.75 mm in diameter, and the crown-implant ratio should be less than 1.

PREMAXILLA SURGERY

The surgery for the intradental anterior tooth root form surgery is similar to that described in Chapter 21 and 22, with some variations. The implant abutment selected is usually for a cemented restoration. Single anterior crowns do not require screw-retained crown procedures and, unlike bridge abutments, can turn or rotate. A cement-retained crown finish line may end anywhere on the abutment post and when possible on the body of the implant, provided it is 2 mm or more above the bone. This further contributes to secure the abutment post to the implant and helps prevent crown rotation, abutment fracture, or unsecured restorations. Because the intra-tooth implant is guarded by the adjacent teeth, micro movement during healing from premature loading is less likely, even if the implant body remains permucosal. The transitional partial removable denture must be relieved to avoid any contact between the gingival surface and the implant body.

An implant that is not placed ideally also has more corrective options with a cemented-in prosthesis. The straight abutment for cement may be prepared, or an angled abutment may be utilized. The screw-retained crown requires more exact surgical placement, because the screw location must fit within the cingulum of the tooth for ideal esthetics. The height of the cingulum must be adequate to provide screw retention length.

The implant is positioned in the lingual two thirds of the natural tooth location. The straight abutment for cement will be directly below the incisal edge position. The implant is typically 4 mm in diameter, whereas the natural tooth was 6 to 9 mm. Because the labial bone is most at risk and the crown profile is in two planes, with the incisal edge more lingual than the cervical portion, the lingual position is ideal for implant placement (Fig 26–1). In addition, if necessary the final crown may be fabricated with a modified ridge lap design if the abutment post is too lingual. This permits the labial contours to be esthetically pleasing; however, dental floss and hygiene procedures are more difficult.

There is no ideal way to restore proper esthetics when the implant body exits the soft tissue above the facial cervical region of the tooth. At best, the final crown appears too long, and the tooth usually appears too facial. Soft tissue grafts and/or bone augmentation do not improve the condition. In addition, when this condition is observed, the implant body is more than 30 degrees from the axial load. As a result, implants placed too facial should be considered for extraction, rather than inventive prosthetic manipulations.

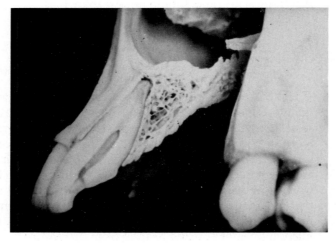

FIG 26–1.
Anterior tooth has little facial bone over the root. The natural crown has two planes on the labial contour. The implant abutment for cement has one plane and is more narrow than the tooth. The abutment for cement should be placed 2 mm under the incisal edge and in line with the lingual two thirds of the tooth.

Implant Extraction Site

The goal of the maxillary tooth and anterior implant is to simulate the clinical aspect of a natural crown extending from the implant body. Available bone width must be present for ideal contours. Implant placement soon after initial alveolar bone healing or bone grafting is usually advantageous. The placement of an implant in an immediate extraction site should consider the socket dimension and the defect between the labial plate of bone and the implant. Usually, immediate implant placement in the anterior region requires the osteotomy and implant insertion to contact the lingual wall of the alveolus, and penetrate halfway down to two thirds down the extraction site into the remaining lingual apical bone. Because the implant is usually 4 mm in diameter and the extraction socket is often greater than 6 mm, a surgical defect of 2 mm remains on the facial aspect. Typically, techniques include countersinking the implant 2 mm or more, and placement of calcium phosphate or hydroxylapatite (HA) to fill the labial defect.

The implant will obtain rigid fixation with this technique. However, the anatomic crown height is increased. Also, synthetic grafts placed over titanium do not grow bone as well as regions where a blood supply may be easily established. Primary closure may be difficult with the immediate extraction technique. The labial tissue is often reflected to close the defect. This further compromises the blood supply to the labial cortical bone and also decreases the amount of attached gingiva. The labial bone usually remodels, and a soft tissue pocket greater than 5 mm often remains at the midfacial tooth position. Tissue recession or the presence of anaerobic microorganisms in the greater depth pocket are more likely, and result in long-term esthetic or soft tissue complications. There is also an increased risk of postoperative infection around the implant by the bacteria associated with the cause of tooth loss.

An improved bone interface may be obtained if the large-diameter extraction site is grafted with demineralized freeze-dried bone (DFDB) and autogenous bone and/or resorbable alloplasts at the time of the extraction. If the labial plate is compromised, additional intraoral harvested bone, DFDB, and guided tissue regeneration using a laminar bone strip, collagen, or Teflon membrane are indicated (see Chapter 20). Hence the result of the augmentation should be evaluated *before* implant placement, rather than risking an increase in compromises (Fig 26–2).

Division A Premaxilla

First-Stage Surgery

When ideal anterior bone is present, a surgical template is fabricated to identify the incisal edge of the final prosthesis. The soft tissue incision may be made on the crest of the ridge, permitting minimum reflection. The anterior

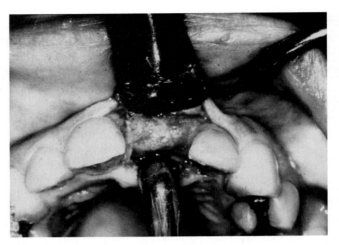

FIG 26–2.
Edentulous site was augmented at the time of extraction 6 months earlier with DFDB and calcium phosphate. The site is Division A and ideal for proper implant placement.

implant site should be ideally greater than 5 mm in width, so Division A root forms may be placed. The greater the diameter of the implant, the more esthetic the cervical portion of the anterior crown. Because many implants are 4 mm in diameter and maxillary teeth are 6 to 9 mm, a prosthetic challenge is to make the cervical region appear natural. The mesiodistal contours must expand rapidly from the gingiva margin to appear as a natural tooth. The crown margin may begin 1 to 2 mm above the crest of bone, preferably on the implant body rather than on the abutment for cement.

The implant should be placed slightly distal to the center of the final crown's mesiodistal length. In this way, the height of contour of the crown may be slightly distal as in natural anterior teeth. The distal placement of the central incisor implant offers an additional advantage. The incisive foramen often expands laterally within the palatal bone. The central incisor implant osteotomy may inadvertently encroach upon the soft tissue in this structure. As a result, fibrous tissue may grow at the interface in the region. Therefore a more distal placement helps avoid this area (Fig 26–3).

The bone loss from a previous extraction site occurs at the expense of the thinner facial plate of bone. As a result, the implant body often needs to be placed more lingual than the natural root predecessor. The implant position should be in the same angulation as the lingual two-thirds of the natural tooth.

The anterior implant osteotomy is evaluated with a probe, especially on the facial before implant placement, because labial undercuts may result with facial fenestrations during the osteotomy. The labial tissue is palpated during the actual bone preparation, to feel if the drill can be detected. When in doubt, the labial tissue should be reflected and the area evaluated. If the labial tissue has been reflected, the blood supply to the labial porous compact bone is diminished. Calcium phosphate and DFDB over the region may prevent loss of bone after labial bone remodeling and resultant implant thread exposure.

A dense HA ridge augmentation may be placed on the facial aspect of the implant. This will increase the tissue thickness, so an interdental papilla may be carved at the second stage implant body uncovery, improve ridge contour, and also prevent the titanium implant body from showing through the labial mucosa if future crestal bone loss occurs (Fig 26–4).

A single-tooth implant body is placed above the crest of the bone approximately 2 mm, if the abutment for cement is the same diameter as the implant body. Some systems have a wider abutment post than implant body, and because the crown margin cannot extend beyond the resultant undercut, the implant body is placed even with the crest of bone. The provisional restoration is aggressively recontoured so no contact with the implant occurs during healing. The adjacent teeth easily protect the implant from early loading. When possible, the final cemented crown margin is placed 0.5 to 1 mm on the implant body. This helps prevent post rotation, improves the cervical contour, and increases the strength of the abutment-to-implant connection. Multiple implants or combination implant and tooth restorations associated with long edentulous spans have the implant placed level with the crest of the bone. The soft tissue–supported

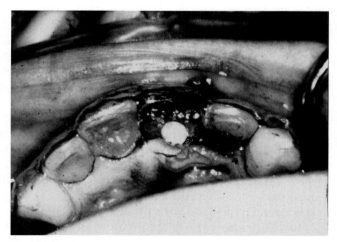

FIG 26–3.
Surgical template in position which determines the incisal edge position. The implant and healing cover is in the mesiodistal position, which corresponds to the facial height of contour of the crown.

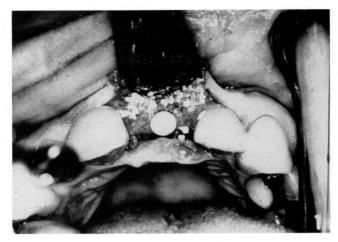

FIG 26–4.
Dense HA is placed on the facial aspect of the bone, which increases the tissue thickness to form interdental papilla, improves labial contour, and can mask facial implant body exposure with long-term bone loss.

provisional restoration is more likely to load the tissue, and implant movement during healing is more a concern.

Second-Stage Surgery

The uncovering of the implant body should be accomplished with a gingiplasty procedure. There will be a lack of an interdental papilla next to the implant post. This results in a V-shaped defect lateral to the crown neck, in between the implant(s) and adjacent teeth. A gingiplasty with a coarse diamond recontours an interdental papilla with proper labial gingival contour, and eliminates this cosmetic defect (Fig 26–5).

The crestal bone-implant interface should be closely evaluated to ensure an absence of crestal bone loss before the abutment post is added to the implant body. If bone loss is suspected, the tissue should be reflected for direct observation. Correction of a cervical horizontal defect includes local autogenous grafts mixed with dense HA, since bone growth is not predictable. The dense HA does not resorb, but acts as a cosmetic filler for the final restoration. A vertical defect may use autogenous bone with DFDB and/or resorbable calcium phosphate, because actual bone growth is more probable in presence of a lateral wall of bone.

The incisal edge position of the abutment post should be 2 mm directly inferior to the actual incisal edge position of the abutment crown. An abutment post labial to the incisal edge position will compromise the final facial esthetics of the restoration. The implant body too facial may use a porcelain butt joint preparation on the abutment post. The neck of the implant body may be prepared below the gingival margin prior to the final impression. The butt joint–crown preparation then includes the implant body and abutment post (Figs 26–6 and 26–7). The implant abutment and body may have a labial slot when placed above the bone. The crown margin on the implant body and facial seating groove prevent abutment rotation. The mesial and distal contact areas on each side of the single tooth crown are shaped on the lingual aspect to be ovoid, and extend toward the gingiva. The facial crown contour remains the same, but the lingual contour is wider than normal. This technique decreases the need for the intedental papilla to extend into the region, and eliminates a triangular opening. The wider contact also resists rotation of the abutment and/or crown. The use of a lateral finger rest is not indicated since the adjacent teeth move away from the rest during initial tooth movement. Decay is a common consequence of a finger rest, because plaque is able to form in the region and hygiene is not possible. The wider lingual contour and contact is able to be cleaned with dental floss and yet provides resistance to lateral forces.

Division B Premaxilla

The Division B maxillary bone is 3.5 to 5 mm in width, and the ideal implant is a Division B root form, 3 to 3.5 mm in diameter. The implant is placed in the position of the lingual half of the natural tooth. The lingual contour of the final crown is not compromised, and will not affect phonetics. Greater interarch clearance is needed under these conditions as the permucosal post exits the tissue in a more lingual position. The opposing natural teeth are more likely to be in

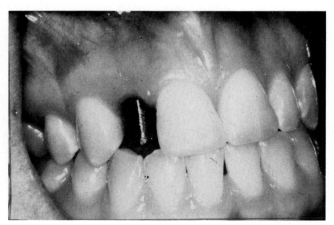

FIG 26–5.
Abutment for cement in proper position, and healed interdental papilla formed.

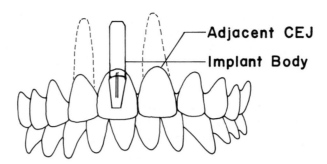

FIG 26–6.
Diagram which demonstrates the implant body is placed above the bone. The abutment for cement has a labial groove which extends onto the implant body. The crown secures the abutment for cement and implant body and follows ideal crown contour above the crest of bone. *CEJ,* cementoenamel junction.

direct line with the lingual implant abutment. Inadequate interarch space may exist in Angle Class II Division II patients for a single-tooth implant.

Richmond Crown Technique

Occasionally, the implant body is too facial or the interarch space is too limited for proper post design for esthetics or retention. A Richmond crown fabricates both crown and post in one restoration. The extended length of crown cement

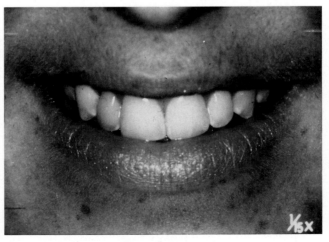

FIG 26–7.
Maxillary right lateral implant (from Figure 26–5) 5 years following surgery. The height of contour and interproximal region has been maintained for esthetics.

area with the attached post improves crown retention. The crown-post substructure should be made of precious metal, to limit corrosion from post contact with the internal titanium implant body (Figs 26–8 and 26–9).

Modified Ridge Lap Crown

For restoration of the implant abutment crown to ideal esthetic contour, the cervical portion of the tooth often needs to be repositioned to the facial. The restoring dentist is confronted with this same esthetic decision for pontics of a fixed prosthesis. The modified ridge lap (MRL) pontic fulfills the esthetics and contour requirements of the missing teeth. In addition, the relief of the palatogingival region provides a means of acceptable hygiene.

The same pontic design may be used for an implant abutment in a palatal situation. An abutment hole on the lingual aspect of the "pontic" connects the implant abutment to the designed crown. Dental floss may be passed under the modified ridge lap crown to remove plaque. A common mistake is to place the labial of the implant abutment coping or substructure margin subgingival or below the pontic contour. This creates unaccessible areas for homecare maintenance at the level of the MRL crown contours. Therefore, supragingival margins on the labial metal substructure are indicated unless crown retention must be increased.

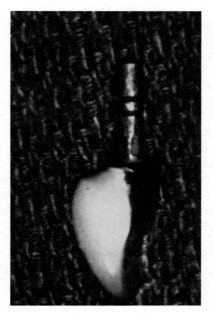

FIG 26–8.
Richmond crown, which connects the post and crown. The crown contour is similar to that of a modified ridge lip pontic.

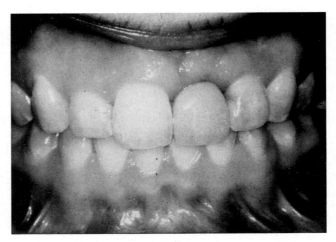

FIG 26–9.
Left maxillary centrical incisor from Figure 26–8, 3 years postoperatively.

The restorative material of choice for a FP-1 prosthesis or crown is porcelain to precious metal. Precious metal allows the substructure to be separated and soldered if a passive fit does not exist at the metal try-in for multiple units. The noble metals are also less likely to cause metal corrosion, especially when subgingival margins on a metal implant are present. Any history of exudate around a subgingival base metal margin will dramatically increase the corrosion effect.

Division B-w

A common situation presents 2.5 to 3.5 mm of bone width, with the long-term missing tooth, yet adequate height for implant placement. Several options are available to the practitioner. A host bone and DFDB intrabony graft after bone expansion may increase the width of bone. The ideal approach limits periosteal reflection and does not alter blood supply to the labial plate of bone. Bone spreading is accomplished with a bone wedge used after a narrow osteotomy is made with a surgical bur, similar to a plate form osteotomy. The edentulous ridge is expanded facially, to a width of 6 mm or more, and packed with the DFDB and autogenous bone graft mixture (Fig 26–10). Four to six months later, the area is reentered, and a root form implant may be ideally placed (Fig 26–11). A second alternative of treatment is to place a plate form implant. The plate form implant should be at least 16 mm in height and 7 mm in length to compensate for the reduced width. A HA coating on the implant also enhances the initial bone-implant contact. The plate form implant most always requires a modified ridge lap crown. Hygiene is more a problem, as the implant post has a considerable undercut region where it attaches to the body of the narrow implant.

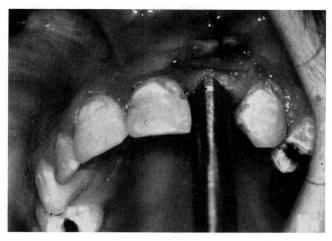

FIG 26–10.
Division B ridge, which is expanded with a tapered bone spreader (Omni International) after initial osteotomy.

A third option is to use a small-pore membrane with an onlay graft technique. This requires a labial periosteal reflection and autogenous bone and or DFDB on the labial aspect. Small-pore membranes permit guided hard tissue regeneration in the region. However, fibrous tissue within the bone and/or infection has been reported in 25% or more of clinical trials. As a result, greater success has been reported with other techniques.

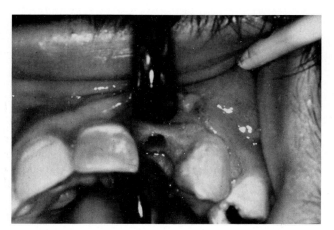

FIG 26–11.
Reentry of the patient shown in Figure 26–10 4 months after bone spreading and augmentation with an implant osteotomy.

Division C-w

Division C with advanced width atrophy (C-w) requires an onlay graft, as bone spreading is not as predictable. Based on clinical experience, the ideal dimensions required in anterior bone include a ridge width of greater than 5 mm, allowing at least 1 mm of bone for the lateral aspects of the implant and a minimum vertical height of 12 mm.[4, 5] Several surgical procedures have been described to regenerate this volume of bone, including autogenous grafts or bone substitutes and small-pore membrane techniques. Although autogenous bone is preferred in maxillofacial reconstruction, the nature of the surgery and morbidity from bone harvest[6] has led to the development of allogenic[7, 8] and alloplastic materials[9, 10] and guided tissue regeneration techniques.[11, 12]

Results with DFDB are best when placed within the bone site, rather than an onlay graft. It does not have the healing capabilities and predictability of autogenous bone. Alloplastic bone substitutes are safe and effective for a variety of clinical applications, but also lack histologic studies to prove onlay grafts provide predictable results, especially in the premaxilla. Reports on the use of guided tissue regeneration techniques for ridge enlargement reveal unpredictable and variable gain in width, potential for acute infections associated with the membrane, and a healing of 6 to 10 months.[13, 14] The variable gain in width and the favorable results reported with the use of chin bone in the repair of alveolar cleft defects,[15–18] prompted evaluation of this procedure for reconstructing severe alveolar defects prior to placing dental implants in the maxilla. Applicable cases include alveolar defects of a C-w edentulous ridge involving a span of one to four teeth requiring an increase in width (see Fig 26–10).

Clinical and radiographic examinations are performed to evaluate if sufficient bone is present at the mandibular symphysis to reconstruct the defect. A panoramic radiograph and lateral cephalogram are suggested to evaluate the presence of at least 12 mm of mandibular bone height below the apicies of teeth and 7 mm of bone width in this region. If future implants are planned in the anterior mandible, the graft is harvested months before the insertion of implants in the region.

Symphysis Grafts

Following local anesthesia of the maxillary alveolar defect with 2% lidocaine with 1:100,000 epinephrine, a crestal incision on the palatal aspect is made with a subsequent mucosal flap elevation and incision of the periosteum on top of the crest. Divergent relieving incisions adjacent to bordering teeth are then made, and a full-thickness flap elevated to expose the defect. The recipient graft bed is prepared by removing any fibrous tissue or foreign body material from previous endodontic treatment (Fig 26–12). The lateral aspect of the moderately resorbed C-w ridge is scored with a handpiece to allow trabecular blood supply access to

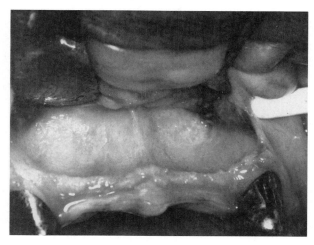

FIG 26–12.
Reflection of soft tissue demonstrating a C-w ridge in the maxillary anterior. The lingual soft tissue has not been elevated from the bone, and maintains blood supply to the thin cortical bone.

the graft. This also increases the regional accelerated phenomena reported by Frost, which increases the rate of repair and bone modeling.[19]

The bone graft is then obtained from below the apices of the mandibular incisors and canines by way of an intraoral approach. Local anesthesia is accomplished with bilateral mandibular blocks of 0.5% bupivacaine with 1:200,000 epinephrine and local infiltration of 2% lidocaine with 1:100,000 epinephrine in the labiobuccal vestibule to improve hemostasis. An anterior incision is made in the alveolar mucosa 5 mm or more below the mucogingival junction between the premolars. After the symphysis and location of the mental foramina are exposed, the external contour of the block graft for the maxillary defect is outlined with a surgical bur under copious sterile saline irrigation at approximately 50,000 rpm. The superior aspect of the graft harvest is at least 5 mm below the apices of the teeth, and the lower border of the graft is predicated on the location of the chin and mentalis muscle attachments, which are maintained. The depth of the osteotomy depends on the width of the anterior mandible. Osteotomes are then used to free the block graft, and harvest cancellous bone (Fig 26–13). The block harvest includes the facial cortical plate and the attached trabecular bone to the depth of the lingual cortex. A mixture of DFDB and resorbable calcium phosphate restores the defect at the donor site, and a collagen membrane is placed over the mixture.

The block graft is recontoured to fit the maxillary defect, firmly inserted into the prepared bed, and held in place with titanium screws or ligature wire (Fig

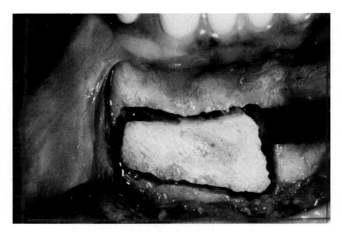

FIG 26–13.
Block graft of cortical and trabecular bone is harvested from the mandibular symphysis.

26–14). Final recontouring is performed after rigid fixation has been achieved. The harvested cancellous bone is placed into any defects, and DFDB is used to cover and fill any discrepancies. Additional graft material may be added over the adjacent region and covered with a small pore membrane. A final reconstructed and recipient ridge should be 6 to 7 mm in width to allow for possible resorption of the graft. Prior to suturing, the periosteum of the mucosal flap covering the graft is horizontally scored with a scalpel to achieve tension free wound closure. The incisions are closed using 3-0 vicryl with interrupted and mattress sutures.

The provisional removable partial denture is adjusted to avoid contact with the grafted area. Pressure is applied to the chin for several hours to ensure an

FIG 26–14.
Symphysis block graft is fixated to the C-w ridge with titanium screws.

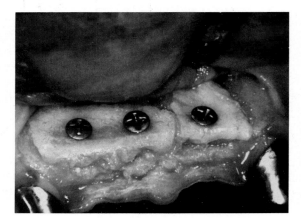

absence of bleeding and close adaptation of the mentalis muscles. Chlorhexidine mouth rinse twice daily is used for about 2 weeks to reduce risk of infection. Two weeks and 16 weeks postoperatively, the recipient site is evaluated for morphology of the reconstructed alveolus and soft tissue healing. The donor site area is examined clinically for vitality of teeth, soft tissue healing, injury to the mental nerve, and a radiograph assessing bone repair and possible damage to the roots. The soft tissue profile and function of the lower lip are also evaluated and should not be altered compared to the previous condition. Complaints of postoperative pain from the donor site are mild to moderate and controlled with analgesics.

Studies in animals indicate that membranous bone illustrates faster revascularization than endochondral bone.[15, 16] The rapid development of a vascular bed in membranous bone grafts (as obtained from the chin) allows reentry for implant placement at 4 months, compared with a recommended 6 to 9 months in free nonvascularized bone grafts of endochondral origin. At the re-entry procedure the grafted area is evaluated and fixation elements are removed prior to the insertion of endosteal implants. A resorption of 0% to 25% has been observed and reported using chin bone.[17, 20] The bone quality determined by surgical preparation has been favorable, and the quantity of bone regenerated allows the placement of Division A root form implants. These factors give an improved prognosis to the restoration of the edentulous premaxilla (Fig 26–15).

A problem of incision line dehiscence at the donor site area was observed in patients with vigorous chin musculature. This may be avoided with a marginal

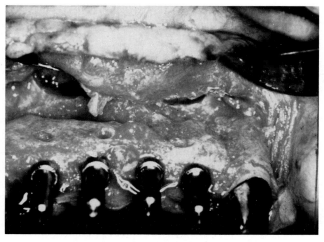

FIG 26–15.
Four direction indicator pins in prepared implant osteotomies after the titanium screws were removed 4 months after Figure 26–14. (Courtesy of J. Crawford)

incision in the gingival sulcus along the lower incisors.[21] Maxillary frenectomies may be performed on patients at the initial surgery receiving grafts in the central incisor region. Secondary soft tissue procedures in the maxilla may be required and can usually be done during the implant uncovering procedure. Failure to preserve the mentalis muscle attachment during reflection could result in chin ptosis.[22] Previous studies on symphyseal grafts revealed radiographic evidence of healing at the donor site within 6 months after surgery.[15, 16] Past techniques did not augment the donor site with alloplast and/or allograft. To restore the chin profile immediately after surgery, the donor area is augmented with a resorbable calcium phosphate and DFDB, which may act as a scaffold and induce bone formation.[5, 23]

The inherent advantage of mandibular bone grafts compared with other extraoral donor sites is the easier access. Operating in the same field as the recipient site decreases operating time. Other advantages of chin grafts include diminished postoperative morbidity, minimal postoperative discomfort, no alteration in ambulation, and avoidance of a cutaneous scar. Operating intraorally is also perceived as a less extensive surgery by the patient as compared with extraoral donor sites. Compared with other intraoral sites such as the tuberosity, zygoma, palate, and coronoid process, the symphyseal region provides a block graft of cortical and trabecular bone with greater quantity of bone. Unlike the initial osteoid-like bone formed by guided tissue regeneration, the chin graft bone quality is similar to alveolar D-2 bone.

The disadvantages of the mandibular symphysis as a donor site include a limited availability of bone and the risk of damaging the mandibular tooth roots or mental nerve. Mandibles exhibiting long anterior tooth roots, inadequate anterior height or width, and/or maxillary defects requiring a graft for a span of more than four teeth or gross vertical bone loss may require alternative donor sites.

Division C-h

The partially edentulous anterior maxilla which is deficient in height and requires a fixed restoration often needs an extraoral autogenous bone graft and possible elevation of the floor of the nose and/or lateral piriform rim. However, on occasion the C-h premaxilla, which requires a RP-4 or 5 restoration, may benefit in the canine region from a symphyseal graft. The C-h maxilla has resorbed from the labial aspect. Implants placed on the crest of the ridge will be several millimeters lingual to the natural tooth position. An overdenture has more room to set the anterior teeth as a result. However, patients requesting a fixed prosthesis require bone on the crest and labial position, and/or LeFort osteotomy, and/or anterior block grafts of extra-oral origin.

The primary incision is split-thickness on either the labial or palatal aspect, approximately 1 cm from the crest of the ridge. The size of the symphyseal bone block is limited in length, height, and depth. As a result, it is often placed on a bed of trabecular bone harvested from the tuberosity, or the ascending ramus. The symphyseal block may require full thickness in the anterior canine region; however, the genial tubercle area in the midline and associated genioglossus muscles are maintained in position. Both DFDB and resorbable calcium phosphates are used to fill the chin harvest and any voids as previously described for Division C-w. On occasion, one block may be placed on the crest of the ridge, while another one placed on the labial aspect. Rarely is enough bone found in the symphysis for more than two implant sites requiring height, or one site of height and width.

Subnasal elevation may also be necessary with the symphysis graft in the C-h anterior premaxilla. The canine region of the C-h patient is resorbed to the lingual and approaches the lateral piriform rim of the nose. Hence implants in this region may perforate the bone on the lateral aspect of the nose. The labial periosteum of the maxilla is reflected to expose the inferior and/or lateral piriform rim. The inferior piriform rim is level with the floor of the nose in half of individuals with natural teeth.[24] However, the long-term loss of maxillary anterior teeth often causes a depression of bone behind the inferior aspect of the piriform rim of the nose. A nasal undercut region is also typically formed at the junction of the lateral inferior piriform rim. This region, often corresponds to implant placement in the canine area. The nasal mucosa in this region may be elevated by a soft tissue curette, similar to the mucoperiosteum elevation in the subantral augmentation. The nasal mucosa is thicker and easier to elevate without tearing. However, more firm pressure is required because elastic fibers are present and firmly attached to the bone.

The nasal mucosa may be elevated approximately 2 to 4 mm, depending on the depth of the depression behind the piriform rim, and augmented with a graft. The subnasal augmentation may use DFDB and resorbable calcium phosphate.[25]

The lateral piriform augmentation is allowed to heal for 4 to 6 months along with the symphysis graft. The fixation screws are removed from the block graft and endosteal implants may be inserted. The final prosthesis is removable because implants cannot be placed in the ideal fixed prosthesis position and the symphysis graft is limited in volume. If this is not acceptable, autogenous bone grafts of extraoral origin are considered.

Division D

The Division D premaxilla requiring an implant-supported restoration requires an autogenous bone graft of extraoral origin (see Chapter 26). A subnasal elevation is also often indicated, if anterior implants are required for the restoration.

CONCLUSION

The replacement of teeth in the premaxilla is the most critical region of the mouth because esthetics, phonetics, function, occlusal pattern and patient awareness blend to provide very specific incisal edge and contour position. Anterior tooth loss usually compromises ideal bone volume and position for proper implant placement. Implant diameter, compared with that of natural teeth, result in challenging cervical esthetics. Unique aspects of surgery and prosthetics are interrelated for proper results.[26]

REFERENCES

1. Pietrokowski J: The bony residual ridge in man, *J Prosthet Dent* 34:456–462, 1975.
2. Misch CE: Single tooth implants: difficult, yet overused, *Dent Today* 2:46–51, 1992.
3. Shilingburgh HT: In Hobo S, Whitsett LD, editors: *Fundamentals of fixed prosthodontics,* Chicago, 1981, Quintessence, p 17.
4. Lekholm U, Zarb GA: Patient selection and preparation. In Branemark P-I, Zarb G, Albrekstsson T, editors: *Tissue-integrated prostheses,* Chicago, 1985, Quintessence, pp 199–209.
5. Misch CE: Divisions of available bone in implant dentistry, *Int J Oral Implant* 7:9–17, 1990.
6. Marx RE, Morales MJ: Morbidity from bone harvest in major jaw reconstruction: a randomized trial comparing the lateral anterior and posterior approaches to the ilium, *Int J Oral Maxillofac Surg* 48:196–203, 1988.
7. Deeb ME, Hosny M, Sharawy M: Osteogenesis in composite grafts of allogenic demineralized bone powder and porous hydroxylapatite, *Int J Oral Maxillofac Surg* 47:50–56, 1989.
8. Nique T et al: Particulate allogenic bone grafts into maxillary alveolar clefts in humans: a preliminary report, *Int J Oral Maxillofac Surg* 45:386–392, 1987.
9. Jarcho MJ: Biomaterial aspects of calcium phosphates: properties and applications, *Dent Clin North Am* 30:25–47, 1986.
10. Council of Dental Materials, Instruments, and Equipment, Council on Dental Research, and Council on Dental Therapeutics: Hydroxylapatite, beta tricalcium phosphate, and autogenous and allogenic bone for filling periodontal defects, alveolar ridge augmentation, and pulp capping, *J Am Dent Assoc* 108:822–831, 1984.
11. Nyman S et al: Bone regeneration adjacent to titanium dental implants using guided tissue regeneration: a report of two cases, *Int J Oral Maxillofac Implants* 5:9–14, 1990.
12. Dahlin C et al: Generation of new bone around titanium implants using a membrane technique: an experimental study in rabbits, *Int J Oral Maxillofac Implants* 4:19–25, 1989.
13. Buser D et al: Regeneration and enlargement of jaw bone using guided tissue regeneration, *Clin Oral Implant Res* 1:22–32, 1986.

14. Balkin B: Guided tissue regeneration and implant dentists, American Academy of Implant Dentistry National Meeting, Washington, D.C., 1988.
15. Zins JE, Whitaker L: Membranous vs. endochondical bone: implications for craniofacial reconstruction, *Plast Reconstr Surg* 72:778, 1983.
16. Kusiak J, Zins J, Whitaker L: The early revascularization of membranous bone, *Plast Reconstr Surg* 76:510, 1985.
17. Sindet-Pederson S, Enemark H: Mandibular bone grafts for reconstruction of alveolar clefts, *J Oral Maxillofac Surg* 46:533–537, 1988.
18. Linkow LI: Bone transplants using the symphysis, the iliac crest and synthetic bone materials, *J Oral Implant* 11:211–247, 1983.
19. Frost HM: *Bone remodeling and its relationship to metabolic bone disease,* vol III, *Orthopedic lectures,* Springfield, Ill, 1973, Charles C Thomas, pp 54–85.
20. Misch CM, Misch CE: Mandibular symphysis bone grafts for placement of endosteal implant, in press.
21. Koole R, Bosker H, Noorman van der Dussen F: Secondary autogenous bone grafting in cleft patients comparing mandibular (ectomesenchymal) and crista iliaca (mesenchymal) grafts, *Cranio Maxillofac Surg* 17(suppl J):28, 1989.
22. Rubens BC, West RA: Ptosis of the chin and lip incompetence: consequences of lost mentalis muscle support, *Int J Oral Maxillofac Surg* 4:359–366, 1989.
23. Block MS et al: Mandibular augmentation in dogs with hydroxylapatite combined with demineralized bone, *Int J Oral Maxillofac Surg* 45:414–420, 1987.
24. Blitzer A, Lawson W, Friedman W, editors: *Surgery of the paranasal sinuses,* Philadelphia, 1985, WB Saunders.
25. Misch CE: Surgical treatment of the premaxilla, Implantology and Biomaterials, abstract, First World Congress, Rouen, France, March 22, 1991.
26. Misch CE: Single tooth implants, abstract, *Int J Oral Implant* 7:121, 1991.

Chapter 27

Autogenous Bone Grafts for Endosteal Implants: Indications, Success, and Failures

Carl E. Misch
George Sotereanos
Francine Dietsh

The ideal goals of modern dentistry, to restore a patient to complete contour, comfort, function, esthetics, speech, and health, have become closer to reality with the help of dental implants. In ridges with abundant bone, all factors converge, providing an ideal long-term prognosis for the implant-supported prosthesis. These factors include high and wide endosteal implants in adequate numbers, favorable crown-implant ratio and ridge relationships, adequate bone density, and favorable orientation of occlusal forces toward the support system. In addition, patients with this advantage have less demanding needs than those in the condition of advanced bone atrophy who are in dire need for prosthetic support and retention.

When confronted with cases of extreme alveolar and basal bone resorption or discontinuities, the usual treatment modalities fall short of the intended result.[1-3] Autogenous bone grafts in conjunction with implants are often required to restore these patients.[4-7] In addition, patients with moderate resorptive conditions and ideal prosthetic goals may also require augmentation. The usual goal of autogenous bone grafts is to provide sufficient available bone to permit the placement of endosteal implants in severely resorbed or compromised maxillae and mandibles or to meet the prosthetic and/or esthetic needs and desires of the patient with moderate resorption. Autogenous grafts permit the placement of endosteal implants of increased surface area, height, width, number, and improved location. The type of final prosthesis can be upgraded to a more natural appearance by enhancement of the soft tissue support and possible correction of ridge relationships. The placement of the implants in ideal locations improves stress distribution patterns, interarch relationships, and esthetics of the final prosthesis. As a result, benefits to the patient include implant longevity and improved prosthetics.[7]

HISTORY

Throughout the evolution of oral implantology, several approaches have been proposed to address the problems of the severely resorbed jaw. The lack of support for traditional endosteal implant designs has led to the development of the subperiosteal implant, resting on the remaining bone of the ramus and symphysis in the mandible.[8, 9] The endosteal ramus frame design also takes advantage of these areas.[10] In the maxilla, extension to the pterygoid plates, maxillary tuberosity, and lateral aspect of the zygomatic process are attempted with endosteal and subperiosteal implants.[11, 12] However, the extremely atrophic conditions and the resultant poor biomechanics of the implant system have led to many complications. The violation of fundamental prosthodontic principles in the final restoration, as insufficient implant support (in size, number, and location) and excessive number of pontics, has encouraged the development of more predictable techniques.

The concepts of jaw reconstruction with varied autogenous and alloplastic materials has been used for many years.[13, 14] However, jaw reconstruction with autogenous bone alone has been characterized by rapid, advanced bone resorption during the 3 to 5 years following the procedure.[15, 16] In addition, augmentation of atrophic ridges for conventional complete dentures often requires secondary surgery and still does not return a patient to normal mastication and comfort. Implants in conjunction with autogenous grafts have been reported in the literature with improved success in relation to prosthetic support and maintenance of the graft.[5, 6, 17]

When the placement of rigid fixated endosteal implants is advantageous for prosthodontic support, it is beneficial to reconstruct the anatomy of the atrophic jaw with bone or a material that will resorb and be replaced by living bone. The posterior maxilla can be augmented predictably by subantral augmentation to permit the placement of endosteal implants, using synthetic bone substitutes combined with demineralized freeze-dried bone (DFDB) and intraoral harvested autogenous bone.[18] No other region of the mouth permits as predictable augmentation for endosteal implants in the severe atrophic state. The placement of endosteal implants requires autogenous bone for long-term predictable reconstruction in other regions. Thus in most regions of the mouth the treatment of choice for oral reconstruction and implant rehabilitation for implant supported prostheses in the moderate to severe atrophic condition is autogenous bone grafting.

An extraoral origin for autogenous bone grafts is necessary for large regions of the jaws. The preferred extraoral donor sites of autogenous bone are the ilium, tibia, scapula, cranium, and the rib. Smaller regions of the atrophic state may be augmented with intraoral harvested bone. The most common locations are the mental protuberance, ascending ramus, coronoid process, tuberosity, exostoses, or edentulous regions where implants are not indicated.

INDICATIONS

The prosthetic goal and the patient's needs and desires are the primary determinants for implant-related treatment option selection. The patient's oral status and expectations are first compared. If these two aspects do not predictably correlate, the practitioner should modify the mouth to improve conditions, or should modify the mind of the patient to lower expectations as needed for the treatment goal. Demanding esthetics or functional desires and expectations of the patient may mandate the augmentation of the bony structures even when other treatment alternatives are available. Therefore, when there is any discrepancy of hard tissues, which cannot render predictable implant prosthesis treatment, the implant dentist has three options:

1. Select a traditional prosthodontic rehabilitation without implants.
2. Modify the patient's mind by lowering expectations and plan a prosthesis requiring less implant support.
3. "Improve" the available bone to the amount and form needed to achieve the expected result.

Indications for autogenous grafts for the placement of endosteal implants are presented using the Misch/Judy Available Bone and Misch Prosthetic Options Classifications (see Chapters 4 and 7).[19–21] In addition, Bone Division E has been added to the original four divisions (A through D) to encompass those conditions where trauma, disease state, surgery, or genetics have resulted in a discontinuity defect of the jaw.

GENERAL CONSIDERATIONS

Autogenous bone grafts are osteogenic and able to form bone in the absence of undifferentiated mesenchymal cells. The grafted bone forms new bone in three different phases (Table 27–1). The first step involves the surviving cells from the transplanted bone, which are responsible for proliferation and formation of new osteoid by osteogenesis. They are most active within the first 4 weeks after transplantation. Phase one dictates the amount of new bone that will form beyond the original dimension and is directly proportional to the density of cells transplanted.[22, 23] To accomplish this goal, the overall volume of the graft is packed into a syringe and compressed to provide as many bone cells per area as possible. Fresh autogenous cancellous bone provides the maximum number of transplanted cells survival and undifferentiated cells of the marrow,[14] and for large grafts is usually harvested from the ilium.[22, 24] However, it should be noted that only the osteocytes within 300 μm of a blood supply will survive, while all others die before adequate nutrition can reach them by diffusion.[25] The graft success therefore depends on early vascularization.[26]

The second phase of bone growth is similar to the osteoinduction phenomenon. It begins 2 weeks after grafting and peaks at 6 weeks to 6 months, then progressively decreases. The cells from the host connective tissue invade the graft. Bone cells from the host tissue follow and remodel the graft by resorption. The bone morphogenetic protein (BMP) derived from the mineral matrix of the transplanted bone (especially from cortical bone) acts as a mediator and permits a blend of both osteogenesis and osteoinduction to form new bone.[23] Fonseca and Davis recommended the addition of chips harvested from the lateral iliac cortex to increase the BMP concentration.[27] The addition of DFDB over the grafted bone attempts to further stimulate the second phase of bone formation, and in theory may start the process earlier.[7] The third phase occurs as the inorganic component of the grafted bone acts as a matrix and source of minerals during creeping substitution of the surrounding bone, and resembles an osteoconductive mechanism.

Advantages of the corticotrabecular block or composite graft is the solid block appearance, which permits contouring and adaptation of the graft to the recipient bed anatomy.[28] The block composite graft maintains greater volume of bone compared to only particulate grafts, because resorption is delayed and rigid fixation is possible. The compact cortical graft illustrates osteogenesis from the surviving cells within 1 week of the grafting procedure.[14] The cortical portion of

TABLE 27–1.

Autogenous Bone

Bone blood supply
    Phase 1: Osteogenesis
        Surviving cells 4 wk → Osteoid
    Phase 2: Osteoinduction
        BMP release 2 wk–6 mo; peak at 6 wk
    Phase 3: Osteoconduction
        Inorganic matrix–space filler
        Cortical plate, guided tissue regeneration

the graft provides increased BMP for the second phase. The cortical bone on the outside of the graft also acts like a membrane for guided tissue regeneration (see Table 27–1). The fibrous tissue is prevented from invading the graft site, and this provides additional time for blood vessels and autogenous bone to develop below the cortical layer. The rigidity and stability of the graft can be achieved by the use of endosteal implants to stabilize the graft, eliminating the need for wiring, pins, or the use of a crib.[5, 6]

RECONSTRUCTIVE OPTIONS: NONVASCULARIZED

Facial Bones

The facial bones may be used for the autogenous graft. The most common source used for implants is the mental symphysis graft or in larger graft sites the cranium. Animal studies indicate that membranous bone illustrates faster revascularization than endochondral bone.[29, 30] This permits greater viability of the graft with better volume results than endochondral bone. Advantages reported by advocates of the technique using the cranium are minimal resorption and morbidity of the graft, early revascularization, early ambulation of the patient, no visible scar, abundant material, no secondary deformity, and decreased pain.[31–33] Thickness can be obtained by stacking of thinner strips of bone. Membranous types of bone grafts have been reported for various applications and reconstruction of craniofacial defects, including onlay augmentation to the maxilla, and onlay and inlay grafting intraorally combined with endosteal implants.[31, 32, 34, 35] Minimum bone loss is a consistent report when used with endosteal implants. However it is cautioned that although the cranium has become the most often donor for facial repair, it may not always be satisfactory to graft in the alveolar regions.[36]

Ilium

According to several publications, autogenous bone harvested from the ilium is the location of choice for bone grafts to the jaws.[14, 37, 38] Harvesting the medial cortex of the anterior aspect of the ilium has been advocated by many authors.[39–41] Advantages of the iliac crest graft are less resorption compared with donor sites such as the rib. The outer portion of the graft is almost entirely cortical, yet has abundant cancellous bone underneath. Easy shaping, easy access, and easy removal have made it a safe and well-accepted procedure. The volume of bone harvested permits shaping up to half a mandible or maxilla, or filling osteotomy voids.

Rapid bone resorption of 30% to 90% of the iliac crest bone grafts are reported when conventional dentures are placed on top of the reconstruction.[15, 16, 42–45] However, the placement of implants into the grafted bone has dramatically modified this resorption rate. Once the implants are placed and in function, the rate of bone resorption is similar to host bone of similar quantity and density and under the same conditions.[46, 47]

An improper incision at the harvesting site may cause neurologic problems, with injury to the femoral cutaneous nerve. The complication can be avoided by making the incision medial or lateral to the crest and ensuring proper exposure of all structures. The lateral incision is preferred. The risk of wound breakdown, abdominal and urologic problems if there is loss of bony contact at time of incision, detachment of lateral thigh musculature, hernias, meralgia paresthetica, adynamic ileus, hematomas, seromas, pain and infection have all been reported.[14, 43, 44, 48]

In the past decade, there have been reports of concomitant use of grafted bone from the iliac crest with implants placed simultaneously or in a second step.* The bone graft procedure was originally reported by Kratochvil and Boyne in 1972 with subperiosteal implants.[17] The reported success rates of autogenous bone grafts and dental implants are highly variable (Table 27–2). Breine and Branemark placed implants in 18 atrophic jaws in conjunction with autogenous marrow and cancellous bone.[6] Only 25% of the implants remained integrated. Most jaws required additional implants, and 20% of the maxillary jaws never achieved permanent bridge stability. As a result, Breine developed a two-step graft operation. First, implants were placed in the tibia or ilium of nine patients and allowed to fixate. After 3 to 6 months, a block section containing the implants was transplanted to the intraoral site, where it was fixated with longer implants. This two-step graft approach resulted with most patients having 55% initial implant

*References 5–7, 35, 38, 39, 46, 47, 49, 51–52.

TABLE 27–2.

Summary of Reported Success Rates of Autogenous Bone Grafts and Dental Implants

Study	Arches	Maxilla	Mandible	Implants in Graft − Lost = Total	%	Implants added − L = Total	%
Breine and Branemark (1980)	18	14	4	129 − 95 = 34	25	63 − 18 = 45	73
Breine and Branemark (1980)	9	8	1	53 − 24 = 29	54.6	19 − 7 = 12	60
Keller and Triplett (1987)	5	5	—	28 − 4 = 24	85	—	—
Listrom and Symington (1988)	10	?	?	7 − 1 = 6	85	43 − 13 = 30	77
Kahnberg Nystrom and Bartholdsson (1989)	10	10	—	57 − 8 = 49	85	—	—
Hall (1990)	10	2	8	—	—	41 − 0 = 41	100
Adell et al (1990)	23	23	—	124 − 30 = 94	75.8	16 − 9 = 5	31
Jensen et al (1990)	4	4	—	—	—	29 − 17 = 12	41
Keller and Tollman (1992)	7	—	7	32 − 4 = 28	87.5	—	—
Misch (in press)	36	21	15	58 − 4 = 54	93.1	173 − 2 = 171	98.8

success, and 60% success of additional implants placed at least 3 to 6 months after the second graft operation.[6]

Keller et al.[49] reported on 5 patients with 28 implants and bone grafting, with 4 failing to fixate (85% survival) and 4 patients with 76% survival (16 of 21 implants) when placed after LeFort I osteotomy and grafts. Listrom and Symington reported on implants inserted in grafted bone as a secondary procedure with a 77% implant survival (43 implants were placed after healing and 30 survived) in 10 patients.[38]

On the other hand, Jensen et al. reports the procedure should still be considered in an evaluation stage. Twenty-nine implants were placed in 4 patients who received iliac crest grafts, and 12 remained fixated and in function, or 41% implant success.[50] Kahnberg et al.[51] reported on patients having received 57 implants simultaneously with a graft from the iliac crest, with eight implants lost (85% survival). Complications reported included graft exposure in 3 patients. The use of a splint to protect the graft was reported to significantly improve the procedure. In a study of 23 consecutive grafted maxillae over a 10-year period, Adell et al.[52] reported on 124 fixtures placed simultaneously with the grafts, 16 implants added in a second stage. The survival rate of fixtures placed with the graft was 75.3% in 4 years after grafting. However, 16 implants placed at a secondary procedure resulted with 9 implant failures (a 31% implant survival). Keller also reported on seven mandibles with iliac crest graft and simultaneous implant placement, with 32 implants and 2 failed, while 2 were left as sleepers resulting in 87.5% success rate.[52a]

A retrospective case series study of 32 patients from 1984 to 1990 was performed by Misch and Dietsh.[47] A total of 36 arches received autogenous bone grafts from the iliac crest to the jaws. There were 25 women and 7 men in the study group, and the primary intention was to improve available bone for implant placement. There were 58 implants placed to stabilize a block graft in 20 patients, of which 35 implants were in the mandible and 23 in the maxilla. Six months later, the implants were evaluated by direct observation for rigid fixation and quantity of bone around the implant. One implant was mobile and three implants had rigid fixation, but two had poor placement and one had more than one third crestal-facial bone loss. These four implants were removed (three of four were in the maxilla). Thus, 97% of mandibular implants were maintained, while 87% of maxillary stage 1 implants were maintained (overall success 93.1%). The nerve was repositioned bilaterally in the mandibular reconstruction in six patients with no paresthesia observed after 3 months.

There were 173 endosteal implants placed 5 to 8 months after the autogenous bone graft. The maxilla received 121 implants and the mandible an additional 52 endosteal implants. Two implants did not achieve rigid fixation and were removed at the next second stage surgery (one each occurred in the anterior mandible and maxilla). The survival of the implants placed after 5 to 8 months into autogenous bone graft sites was 99% (120 implants) in the maxilla and 98% in the mandible (51 implants), overall success 98.8% (see Table 27–2).

All 32 patients and 36 arches were restored with a final implant retained prosthesis. There were 8 fixed prostheses and 7 completely implant-supported removable prostheses in the mandible. In the maxilla, 14 fixed prostheses were fabricated, while 7 completely supported implant overdentures were the final restoration. Therefore, the bone graft is more often used to provide implants for a fixed restoration in the maxilla than the mandible (Table 27–3).

The premaxillae were diagnosed with six C-w, five C-h, and seven Division D arches, and three patients required only posterior Division D augmentation. In the mandible, nine patients had Division D, four patients had C-h available bone, and two posterior ridges were division C-h bone (Table 27–4).

The cause of the six implant losses included poor implant position (two patients); parafunction and trauma from the overlying removable prosthesis against natural teeth (two); and incision line opening after the autogenous graft (two), related to smoking and to past cocaine abuse (suspected poor blood supply). All "sleepers" in this study were removed and counted as failures.

The patients have been in function with their final restoration from 81 months to 10 months. The amount of crestal bone loss observed during this time frame on implants placed after graft maturity is similar to that for implants placed in full arches which did not receive a graft. There was an average of 1.0 mm bone loss around successful implants which were used to stabilize the anterior autogenous block graft segments at the augmentation surgery in Division D and C-h patients at 5 to 7 months, with more bone loss in the maxilla than mandible. The range of bone loss after 10 to 12 months augmentation at the second stage surgery of implants placed after graft maturity was 0 to 2.5 mm, with an average loss of less than 1 mm. Bone loss on implants was directly visualized at the second implant insertion surgery and again recorded by direct observation at the second stage surgery abutment installation.[47]

Hall had similar implant success (100%) after graft maturity in ten patients and also reported bone loss similar to non grafted bone sites where implants were inserted.[46] Therefore, the placement of implants after the graft bone has matured for 5 to 8 months provided a higher implant survival for Breine, Hall, and

TABLE 27–3.

Number of Fixed and Removable Prostheses in Maxilla and Mandible

	FP-2 or FP-3*	RP-4*	Total
Maxilla	14	7	21
Mandible	8	7	15
Total	22	14	36

*FP = fixed prosthesis; RP = removable prosthesis.

TABLE 27–4.

Types of Bone Available in Maxilla and Mandible in 36 Patients

Site	Bone Division			Total
	C-w	C-h	D	
Maxilla	6	5	10	21
Mandible		6	9	15
Total	6	11	19	36

Misch.[6, 46, 47] However, lower implant success with this approach was reported by Listrom and Adell.[38, 52]

SURGICAL APPROACH

Autogenous grafts for endosteal implants have indications and surgical approaches related to the final prosthetic design and original bone anatomy. The surgical approach and related treatment is addressed for each anatomic condition.

Division B

Division B available bone may be treated by osteoplasty, small-diameter root form implants, plate form implants, or augmentation. Osteoplasty increases the crown height of the restoration, and decreases the implant height. Small-diameter implants may result in fixed prosthodontic contours that are narrow and/or placed more lingual to the original missing tooth contour. Excessive occlusal forces may require additional surface area of support and warrant more and greater diameter implants. Ideal prosthetic goals in esthetic regions may necessitate an increase in available bone width by augmentation and improve cervical contours of the associated crown. Ridge location may also require improvement for ideal prosthetic support (Plate 9). The augmentation of a Division B ridge also permits an increase in the implant height, compared to osteoplasty procedures. The longer implant resists moment forces and increases overall surface area of support. Therefore, prosthetic requirements and stress factors may indicate autogenous bone grafts for Division B available bone. The donor site may be the symphysis if small regions are augmented, or extraoral grafts when larger areas are involved.

An incision is usually made on the crest of the ridge. A full-thickness reflection exposes the moderately resorbed ridge. The side to be augmented is determined by the prosthetic end result. The most common region is the labial aspect of the narrow ridge. The cortical plate on the lateral aspect of the ridge is scored with a handpiece to allow trabecular blood supply access to the graft. This also increases the regional accelerated phenomena reported by Frost, which increases the rate of repair and bone modeling.[53]

A block of bone is harvested from the intraoral or extraoral donor site (Plate 10). This block is fixated to the lateral aspect of the ridge with titanium screws or wires. Demineralized freeze-dried bone is applied over the graft and the tissue is approximated without tension, with horizontal mattress sutures. Four to 6 months later, the autogenous graft may be reentered, the fixation screws removed, and endosteal root form implants inserted (Plates 11 and 12). The density of bone is typically D-2, and the ideal surgical protocol is followed.

Division C-w

The inadequate bone in width (Division C-w) can be modified by osteoplasty and the resultant C-h bone may have subperiosteal or endosteal implants if the resulting bone is greater than 5 mm in width and 10 mm in height. The final prosthesis has to compensate for the loss of additional bone height from the osteoplasty (often between 3 to 8 mm) and may be a RP-5 or RP-4 in either jaw or even a FP-3 prosthesis in the mandible, depending on the related dental evaluation and the number and position of implants. Implants placed in the C-h ridge result with greater crown-implant ratios. The esthetics and biomechanics compromise should be explained to the patient prior to the surgery.

If patients desire a fixed maxillary restoration, or if after osteoplasty the width deficient ridge does not increase adequately (also occurs more often in maxilla), the patient may require autogenous bone grafts to permit the placement of endosteal implants. Autogenous grafts in the C-w ridge have a primary intent to increase the width of the atrophic bone, but also often requires some vertical increase for ideal bone volume.

An incision is placed on the crest of the ridge in the C-w ridge when no additional height is required, and a full thickness periosteal reflection exposes the moderately resorbed residual ridge. When additional height is desired, a labial split thickness incision may be used as in the C-h approach (Plate 13). A block graft is harvested from the ilium or mandibular symphysis, depending on the amount of bone required. The overlaying cortical plate is scored to permit quicker revascularization. The block bone graft is fixated with titanium screws to the side of the host bone to restore the final ridge form in a more ideal position for future implant placement. The most usual placement is on the facial aspect of the C-w bone (Plate 14). However, an Angle Class III mandible may indicate lingual fixation. The block graft may also be extended above the crest of the atrophic ridge to increase bone height.

Once the block is fixated into position, a blend of DFDB and cancellous bone is placed around the blocks and fills in any defects. This blend may also be placed under the block before fixation if any irregularity exists. The tissue is approximated without tension with horizontal mattress sutures. The posterior maxilla usually requires a SA-3 or SA-4 sinus elevation and subantral augmentation. This procedure is performed as in Chapter 25.

Autogenous grafts and implants improve long-term predictable results and provide the soft tissue support necessary for acceptable esthetics for a fixed prosthesis. The autogenous grafts eliminate the need for pink porcelain or acrylic as replacement of the soft tissues, especially indicated for loss of bone with a high smile line. Furthermore, the biomechanics of the system are considerably improved with shorter crown height and larger implant height, which enhances the long-term prognosis of the treatment. The final decision for a FP-1 result should not be made before reevaluation of the bone available after the grafting procedure, and depends on the amount of bone grafted and/or modeled, and the position of the lips with the high smile line (Plates 15 to 18).

Division C-h

The patient presenting with a Division C-h ridge has moderate bone in height for endosteal implants and implant prosthetic treatment. In selected cases, short endosteal implants can be used for a stable, removable restoration which may be a RP-5 or, with greater implant number, a RP-4 prosthesis. Patients with moderate desires can still be treated adequately by these implant modalities, provided the crown-implant ratio and factors of stress are compatible with the planned prosthesis. However, for the more demanding patient expecting a fixed restoration, the addition of autogenous bone is often necessary to obtain sufficient height and width of bone (especially in the maxilla). Most patients with C-h ridges requiring grafts are for improved prosthodontic conditions for the maxillary arch.

The initial incision for C-h available bone is split thickness starting approximately 10 to 15 mm anterior to the crest of the ridge from each first premolar. The superior tissue should be thick enough to maintain a blood supply after suturing. This requires a depth of about 1.5 to 2 mm. A full-thickness incision is made through the periosteum when the reflection reaches the labial aspect of the atrophic maxilla (mandible). A full-thickness reflection reveals the anterior section. A tunnel procedure is used to expose the lateral maxilla when SA-3 or SA-4 subantral augmentation procedures are also required, or the posterior mandible when onlay augmentation is desired.

An alternative approach in the maxilla is to place full-thickness vertical incisions distal to the canine eminence. A partial thickness incision extends posterior and then across the palate and anterior to the crest of the ridge. A full thickness incision is then made on the crest of the atrophic residual crest. The full thickness tissue reflection then exposes the facial bone to the nasal spine and piriform rim. The advantage of this approach is an increase of attached gingiva on the crestal and labial aspects of the ridge when the tissue is reapproximated short of its original incision.

The C-h edentulous available bone is usually augmented with a block graft on the superior aspect of the atrophic bone. It often extends to the facial of the bone in the maxilla, whereas it is positioned more lingual in the mandible. Cephalometric analysis is required for the predetermined ideal graft placement in most patient conditions. Endosteal implants (two to four) often are used to fixate the block graft of autogenous bone. These implants should be positioned as far distal as possible, preferably in the first premolar region. The additional implants are placed 5 to 6 months later, after the final graft amount and position is determined. In this way the anterior esthetic positions are not compromised and may be determined after healing and a prosthetic template determines their placement. In addition, using second stage implant placement has a higher implant survival compared to the initial implants placed to stabilize the graft.

Cortical and trabecular bone are ground in a bone mill and then compressed in a 5- to 10-ml modified syringe. The particulate bone may be added to the posterior regions (subantral augmentation and/or onlay tunnel procedures) and on the labial regions above the block of autogenous bone. This permits further soft tissue support in the anterior and greater bone volume for future implant placement. The DFDB is placed over the grafted site, especially on the mixed cortical and trabecular bone. The tissue approximation may be short of the original incision with either the anterior or posterior initial incision approach. This technique also reduces the tension on the incision line.

The greater available bone permits the placement of higher and wider implants, improves the surface area of support, improves the stress distribution, recreates a more favorable crown-implant ratio and returns the soft tissue contours to a more natural appearance. Autogenous grafts of extraoral origin are not necessary where only posterior segments of the maxilla necessitate augmentation, because alloplastic/allograft bone grafts are effective. However, the premaxilla Division C-h permits the placement of endosteal or subperiosteal implants in only very carefully selected cases and usually requires a RP-5 or RP-4 prosthesis.[54] Many C-h premaxilla treatment plans which desire a fixed restoration mandate augmentation with autogenous bone grafts prior to the placement of implants.

Division D

The completely edentulous Type I Division D patient presents with a flat maxilla, or pencil thin mandible with dehiscent mandibular canals, occasionally accompanied by paresthesia of the lower lip. The Division D maxillae and mandibles require special considerations because of unfavorable biomechanics, surgical, prosthetic and esthetics factors. Although these patients have greater needs to satisfy their oral condition, the severe bone loss creates an unfavorable crown-implant ratio (>5:1), lack of soft tissue support, poor bone quality with decreased blood supply, and the complexity of surgical procedure, poor tongue position, unfavorable ridge relationship, increased moment forces and unfavorable stress distribution patterns for predictable endosteal implant support (see Plates 10, 16, and 17).

Autogenous grafts represent the treatment of choice prior to most any implant restoration in the Division D maxilla or mandible. The risks associated with the aggressive placement of implants of any type in the severely atrophic mandible have been recently reported.[73, 74] Regardless of past training in any surgical or prosthetic discipline, these patients require many unique surgical and prosthodontic treatment modifications. The patient's condition may worsen rather than improve if treatment plans are not specific and well coordinated. Implant survival of 90% in Division D conditions is more dangerous for these patients, as the 10% failure may result in fractures, oro-antral fistulae, and more extensive complications requiring many surgeries to restore them to their original poor Division D condition. Therefore, augmentation is indicated for most patients.

The primary incision is 10 to 15 mm anterior to the crest of the ridge, as described in the C-h patient. The full-thickness incision scores through the periosteum once the labial aspect of the ridge is determined. Care is taken in the maxilla to avoid incision through the nasal mucosa, which may increase the risk of infection. The severe atrophic maxilla may not have a nasal spine, and location of the labial bone below the nares is more difficult. A small rotary drill may perforate the crest of the mandible, or slightly score it or the maxilla if less than 5 mm in height, to improve blood supply and the regional accelerated phenomena.[53]

Mandibular nerve repositioning may be indicated when patients desire a fixed prosthesis, because additional implants and shorter cantilevered restorations result (Plate 19). The thin cortical covering and/or dehiscent anterior mandibular nerve and artery are decorticated and repositioned 1 cm distal to the mental foramen. This improves the anterior-posterior dimension of implant placement, places the most distal implant in the second premolar or first molar region, therefore decreasing dramatically the length of the cantilever, and modifies the arch form to an overall more favorable condition for long-term survival of the prosthesis.

As in the C-h patient, the crest of the ilium is sectioned along with the inner or outer table, so that the cortical bone may be shaped to augment the anterior segment of the mandibular width and height and extend at least 1 cm past the original foramen (Plate 20). The inferior portion of the block of bone is compressed to increase the cells per area.

In the mandible the block is positioned on the anterior region and over the foramina. A surgical template is selected that corresponds to the arch form.[6] The graft is placed and contoured with awareness of the final form for the proposed restoration. The autogenous block graft is positioned on the atrophic mandible, with the cortical bone on its most superior aspect. Two to four endosteal implants are placed through the block of bone and fixated into the inferior border of the atrophic mandible.

If the residual ridge is wide enough and nerve repositioning was indicated, one implant is placed in the original positions of the mental foramina. The cortical bone around these structures usually maintains better width and height of remaining bone than the regions adjacent to it. If a third implant is needed, it is placed about 7 mm distal to the midline. This allows implant insertion in a region that still has adequate width from the genial tubercles and muscle attachments and corresponds to the position of a lateral incisor. An additional implant may also be placed in the contralateral side of the midline if further fixation is required (Plate 21).

Care is taken to direct the implant osteotomy to the center of the atrophic ridge. The osteotomy is prepared as for D-1 bone, using smaller increments in drill diameter and a final size slightly larger than the manufacturer suggests. This further decreases the risk of fracture during bone tapping of the implant osteotomy. The inferior border is not completely penetrated to maintain cortical integrity for additional strength during the initial healing process. The implant is passively inserted into the prepared implant site after bone tapping, rather than using force which may fracture the thin regions of bone. The grafted bone block is contoured for smooth borders and any remaining bone harvested is ground in a bone mill, compressed in a 5- to 10-mm syringe to increase the cells per volume, and placed into a distal periosteal tunnel. If additional volume is required, DFDB and resorbable calcium phosphates may be added to the cortical and trabecular particulate mixture. After 6 months, three to five additional implants may be placed between the existing two to three implants. Seven endosteal implants may support a final fixed prosthesis, and no soft tissue support is required over the autogenous graft (Plate 22).

The maxillary Type I, Division D severely atrophic ridge may also use autogenous iliac crest of cortico-cancellous and particulate grafts for endosteal implant placement. A split-thickness incision is made 10 to 15 mm anterior to the residual ridge. A split-thickness soft tissue approach is used until the anterior border of the atrophic maxilla is identified. An incision through the periosteum is made bilaterally, anterior and just distal to the canine eminence. A full-thickness tissue reflection exposes the bony landmarks of the anterior and palatal portions of the maxilla. A tunnel procedure is then used to reflect the lateral aspects of the maxilla and zygomatic process. A rotary drill scores the lateral maxilla for the Tatum lateral wall approach for the sinus membrane elevation. The membrane is elevated after the medial rotation of the lateral maxilla window, approximately 15 to 20 mm in the superior direction. Care is taken to keep the sinus membrane intact.

Subnasal elevation of the soft tissue for approximately 2 to 4 mm may be indicated in the lateral aspect of the piriform rim for canine implants, or the inferior piriform rim elevated for lateral or central implants. Once this procedure is also accomplished on the contralateral side, a template is used to determine the arch form of the premaxillary block graft. The harvested iliac crest and inner or outer table which corresponds in size to the template is shaped for proper contour (Plate 23).

The block is usually placed 5 to 8 mm anterior to the residual ridge, to improve the facial contour of the maxillary hard and soft tissue. The inferior surface of the block is compressed to increase the cellular component per area (Plate 24). A template of the denture is used to locate the first premolar region in the block of bone (Plate 25). This often corresponds to the remaining canine eminence region of the atrophic maxilla. An endosteal screw implant is inserted in this region. The final implant osteotomy is undersized, and no bone tap is used to improve fixation. A countersink bur may be used if the cortical plate of the iliac crest is thick and prevents the implant from being seated level with the graft. The remaining harvested bone is placed in the bone mill, and along with DFDB and resorbable calcium phosphate may be used to augment the subantral region.

After block fixation a rotary drill is used to smooth the contours of the cortico-cancellous particulate graft covered with DFDB used to fill the void above the block positioned anteriorly (Plate 26). A tissue barrier may be used over the particulate bone graft in areas not covered with cortical bone to prevent soft tissue invagination. The tissue is approximated with interrupted horizontal mattress sutures without tension (Plate 27). After 6 months, a total of six to eight implants may be placed in the anterior and posterior regions for a RP-4 restoration, or 8 to 10 implants for a fixed prosthesis (Plate 28).

Division E: Vascularized Grafts

Discontinuity defects of the jaw may require use of autogenous bone grafts to restore a patient to normal contour and function. The cause of the discontinuity may be from trauma, disease, surgery, or genetics. Pathologic causes for discontinuity may include many conditions, of which carcinomas are most frequent. The most common site for intraoral carcinomas is the lateral aspect of the tongue (20%); this affects mainly males. Carcinomas of the floor of the mouth account for 10% to 15% of all intra-oral malignancies. Alcohol and tobacco abuse are the main etiologic factors.[37] The prognosis depends greatly on the size of the tumor, location, extent, and differentiation. Treatment is accomplished by surgical removal of the lesion, radiation therapy, and/or combined chemotherapy. The surgical excision of the lesion often requires extensive resection of the floor of the mouth, variable portions of the mandible and regional lymph nodes. Preoperative radiation therapy increases postoperative complications, infection being the most common. Nerve damage with eventual shoulder drop, hemorrhage, and necrosis of the flaps are also possible complications. The patient is left with severe physiologic, cosmetic, and psychological deficits. The remaining mandibular segment is retruded, then deviated medially and upward. The deviation is often increased during opening up to 1 or 2 cm. The loss of mandibular continuity impairs mastication, deglutition, phonation, and respiration. The patient presents a concave facial asymmetry because of the loss of tissues and the adherence of the skin to the deep tissues of the neck. The deviation and partial loss of innervation around the commissures result in drooling of saliva.[27, 55, 56]

Optimum treatment of mandibulectomy patients is achieved with coordinated surgical, prosthodontic and speech therapies. The decision to reconstruct the mandible immediately or in a second phase depends on the amount and character of the remaining tissues (more than 55 gray irradiation reduces the healing capacity of hard and soft tissue), the prognosis of the treatment, the age and general health of the patient, and whether any residual tumor remains.[57–59] Mandibular reconstruction with various types of materials has been attempted since the early 1800s, including transplantation, grafting allogenic, alloplastic materials, and autogenous materials.[60]

Vascularized bone grafts are more often indicated when blood supply is severely compromised to the graft site or when the recipient bed is scarred. The most common conditions are the cancer patient who has undergone radiation therapy, or the Division E bone anatomy (no bone as a result of genetics, trauma, or disease conditions (Plate 29). Therefore, complex three-dimensional bone defects are also indications for this type of restoration.

The success of bone grafts depends on the survival and proliferation of the osteogenic cells. Special consideration should be given to the recipient tissue bed irradiated above 5,000 rads. The risk of avascular necrosis is higher in the presence of a soft tissue bed of poor quality (hypoxic, hypovascular, and hypo-cellular).[57–59] Surgical reconstruction of the mandible with large defects may also require replacement of soft and hard tissue. Additional soft tissue to cover the defect may use myocutaneous flaps combined with hyperbaric oxygen, and may be indicated in patients to induce angiogenesis and fibroblastic activity (Plate 30).[53, 61] The results of osteomyocutaneous grafts using a vascular pedicle are variable due to technical difficulties and problem of venous drainage.[62, 63]

Microvascular autogenous bone grafts permit the restoration of composite tissue defects after trauma or tumor resection. The technique combines the advantages of free grafts and pedicled grafts and offers greater resistance to infection and more rapid vascularization of the bone. The procedures use osteomyocutaneous flaps with an associated artery and veins. They permit the immediate reconstruction after tumor correction in areas where the recipient bed would otherwise be deficient in vascularity and cellular content. The bony part of the graft heals by callus formation. Complications may arise with non viable soft tissue problems which may cause the loss of the graft.

Different donor sites for microvascular grafts have been utilized to restore the patient with cancer and radiation therapy or for immediate reconstruction.[64, 65]

The most common are the ilium, tibia, and scapular grafts. An ilium microvascular graft consists of a portion of the iliacus and gluteus medius muscles, the anterior and medial aspect of the iliac crest and the deep circumflex iliac artery and variable veins. Ryan[66] reported on the morbidity complications when grafted to the mandible, and Stone and Franklin on the relevant blood loss.[67] Groin grafts are limited in bone shaping and three-dimensional positioning of the skin, especially in palatal and mandibular reconstruction, and therefore are not indicated for hemimandibulectomy patients past the canine region. Riediger concluded that the advantages are the stability, and size of the graft, which consists of excellent cancellous bone.[68] In the report on 41 grafts (36 to the mandible and 5 to the maxilla), 19 were in preirradiated bone. Thirty-eight aluminum oxide implants were added to the grafts and were reported all successful.

The scapula is also a source of bone in microvascular grafts for jaw reconstruction and endosteal implants because of the volume and geometry of the bone available. Teot et al.[69] and Swartz et al.[70] reported on the potential of the lateral scapular border with blood supply by branches of the circumflex scapular artery. The scapula is a favorable donor site because of its geometry, which allows the design of multiple cutaneous panels on separate vascular pedicles to facilitate three-dimensional reconstruction. Complications are those common to the microvascular grafts and restricted elevation for the arm if scarring occurs.

Once the vascularized grafts are healed, the soft tissue and bone may be receptive for endosteal implants following the usual protocol based on prosthesis type, amount of available bone, and density of bone (Plates 31 to 34).

COMPLICATIONS: RECEPTOR SITE

The general causes of failure for autogenous grafts or of the donor site are variable, and well documented.[14, 27, 44, 48] The primary cause of failure of bone grafts in conjunction with endosteal implants include improper diagnosis, treatment planning, and/or sequencing; poor soft tissue management; too many implants placed at surgery; improper implant position at surgery; and esthetic requirements ignored during augmentation.[7]

Improper diagnosis includes sinus pathology prior to subantral augmentation, periapical pathology, or advanced periodontal disease which may cause disease of remaining teeth and compromise the graft as a result of infection, and systemic or local disease which compromise hard and soft tissue healing.

Improper treatment planning includes an attempt to restore a patient to a FP-1 prosthesis, when their intraoral condition is Division D. These patients may result with a fixed restoration after the autogenous graft, if adequate amounts of bone, soft tissue coverage at surgery, and bone modeling occurs, but a natural appearing prosthesis can not be promised. Patients requesting this specific result are prone to unrealistic expectations. Poor treatment plans also include too few and too short implants to support the final prosthesis. For example, a maxillary fixed prosthesis almost always opposes a fixed restoration or natural teeth. The moment forces are greater, the esthetics demands are greater, the bone density is poorer, and the subantral augmentations are more critical to success. To obtain over 95% implant and prosthetic survival in the grafted maxilla, eight to ten implants may be required, with limited posterior cantilever of the prosthesis.

Poor treatment sequencing may include attempting to place all the implants at the time of the autogenous graft. Division C-h and most Division D mandibles are best treated with only selected implants placed for fixation of the block graft. Division C-w atrophic conditions usually have fixation of a block of bone with a lateral screw or a particulate graft and small pore membrane with a tunnel approach and no implant placement. Only place implants at the graft surgery which can be positioned without compromise to the position, angulation, contour, hygiene considerations, and direction of load for ideal conditions. The more implants placed at the time of the graft, the greater the risk for implants incorrectly placed, the risk of mandibular fracture increases, splitting of the graft block is possible, the loss of one implant may spread to two or three, and the risk of prosthetic compromise dramatically increases. In addition, the progressive bone loading concepts used during prosthetic reconstruction are very important in patients with autogenous augmentation.[71, 72]

Poor soft tissue management has the most devastating effect during the immediate postoperative phase of the autogenous graft and is reported most often. Improper flap design may result in compromised blood supply to the underlying graft. Trauma from the opposing teeth, or excessive tension on the incision line results with the incision line opening and graft exposure with loss of significant height and/or width of bone. Soft tissue management also includes the second stage uncovery of the implants. Adequate width of attached gingiva of minimum thickness is the tissue of choice around the implants and autogenous tissue grafts and gingiplasty techniques are commonly required for graft patients.

A Division D mandible is often less than 7 mm in width. An implant placed through the block graft and into the underlying host bone may not go through the center of this atrophic ridge. Instead, the osteotomy may be off center, and have removed all the lateral cortical plate and half the inferior plate at the implant site. When the implant is threaded into position, or shortly there after, the mandible may fracture.[73, 74] This compromises the rigidity of the implant graft and the mandibular bony healing.

An implant design for block graft fixation should be wider at the top of the implant than at the body. This permits the implant to fixate the block to the atrophic bone. The countersink drill should not be used to full depth if the cortical bone of the graft is less than 3 mm thick. The implant should be placed level with the crest of the block graft. Countersinking the implant may result with poor block fixation, which will compromise success.

The primary reason to place implants in conjunction with the graft is to ensure the stability of the grafted bone. Wires may stretch and allow graft movement during healing. In addition, they may erode the graft on the surface regions where they are tied with pressure. Most wires are stainless steel, and fibrous tissue often forms at the interface. As a result, a fibrous tissue trail forms through the bone and may result with soft tissue next to the implant placed in the site. The implants act as fixation screws to rigidly position and maintain the block. The fact that they are rigidly fixated after healing is an additional benefit.

The implants placed to stabilize the graft should be thoroughly evaluated when the additional implants are placed 6 months later. If an implant-bone defect exists, the area may be repaired with autogenous bone, or the implant is removed and another reinserted deeper into position, or removed and another placed in a different site.

The patient requiring autogenous grafts is usually compromised from the lack of soft tissue support. The maxilla resorbs toward the medial aspect in the posterior and anterior regions. The mandible resorbs towards the lateral in the Division C-h and D conditions. As a consequence, the autogenous grafts should be placed in position for the required esthetic result, not the current position of the atrophic bone. This requires maxillary grafts to be cantilevered to the facial plane, or to perform a Lefort osteotomy in conjunction with the graft placement. Mandibular grafts should be placed with a lingual inclination, but with implants at a more vertical inclination. If these requirements cannot be accomplished, implants should be placed 6 months after the grafting procedure.

CONCLUSION

The use of autogenous grafts for or in conjunction with implants has been reported for over 15 years. During this period, predictable techniques and refinements have occurred. The grafting procedures may be indicated for the moderately resorbed jaw with demanding prosthetic requirements. The autogenous grafts are usually indicated for severe resorption, in order to improve anatomic conditions for long-term survival of implants and the related prosthesis. The Misch/Judy Bone Classification may be used as a diagnostic guide for surgical approach and prosthetic concerns. An additional Division E is added for discontinuity defects of the jaws. This chapter addresses these indications, survival rates, and failures of autogenous grafts in conjunction with endosteal implants.

REFERENCES

1. Raveh Y et al: New concepts in the reconstruction of mandibular defects following tumor resection, *J Oral Maxillofac Surg* 1:3–16, 1983.
2. Boyne PJ, Zarem H: Osseous reconstruction of the resected mandible, *Am J Surg* 132:49–53, 1976.
3. Lawson W, Biller H: Mandibular reconstruction bone graft technique, *Otolaryngol Head Neck Surg* 90:589–594, 1982.
4. Misch CE, Zaki H, Dietsh F: Osteointegrated implants in a microvascular graft to restore a subtotal mandibulectomy—case report, *Int J Oral Implant* 7:25–29, 1990.
5. Branemark P-I et al: Repair of defects in the mandible, *Scand J Plast Reconstr Surg* 4:100–108, 1970.
6. Breine U, Branemark P-I: Reconstruction of alveolar jaw bone, *Scand J Plast Reconstr Surg* 14:23–48, 1980.
7. Misch CE, Dietsh F: Autogenous bone grafts for endosteal implants, indications and failures, *Int J Oral Implant* 8:13–20, 1991.
8. Dahl GSA: Om Molijhoten fur Implantation: karen au meitalskett som bas eller fur fasta eller autagbara proteser, *Odont Tidskr* 51:440, 1943.
9. Judy KWM, Misch CE: Evolution of the mandibular subperiosteal implant, *NY J Dent* 53:9–11, 1983.
10. Cram DL, Roberts HD, Baum: Ramus endosseous frame implant for use with patient's dentures, *J Am Dent Assoc* 84:156–162, 1972.
11. Linkow LI: The pterygoid extension implant for the totally and partially edentulous maxillae, *Dent Concepts* 12:17–28, 1973.
12. Tulasne JF: Implant treatment of missing posterior dentition. In Zarb G, Albrektsson T, editors: *The Branemark implant,* Chicago, 1989, Quintessence.
13. Blackstone CH, Parker ML: Rebuilding the residual alveolar ridge, *J Oral Surg* 14:45, 1965.
14. Converse JM: *Reconstructive plastic surgery, principles and procedures in correction, reconstruction and transplantation,* ed 2, Philadelphia, 1977, WB Saunders.
15. Curtis T, Ware W: Autogenous bone grafts for atrophic edentulous mandibles, a review of 20 patients, *J Prosthet Dent* 49:212–216, 1983.
16. Burwell RG: The fate of bone grafts. In Apley AG, editor: *Recent advances in orthopaedics,* London, J and A Churchill, pp 115–207.
17. Kratochvil FJ, Boyne PJ: The combined use of a subperiosteal implant and bone marrow grafts in deficient mandibles, *J Prosthet Dent* 27:645–653, 1972.
18. Misch CE: Maxillary sinus augmentation for endosteal implants: organized alternative treatment plans, *Int J Oral Implant* 4:49–58, 1987.
19. Misch CE: Available bone influences prosthodontic treatment, *Dent Today* 7(1):44–75, 1988.
20. Misch CE: Divisions of bone in implant dentistry, *Int J Oral Implant* 7:9–18, 1990.
21. Misch CE: Prosthodontic options in implant dentistry, *Int J Oral Implant* 7:17–21, 1991.
22. Marx RE: Principles of hard and soft tissue reconstruction of the jaws, abstract ML 315, *J Oral Maxillofac Surg* (special issue), Sept 1990.
23. Friedenstein AJ, Piatetsky-Shapiro II, Pietrakova KV: Osteogenesis in transplants of bone marrow cells, *J Embryol Exp Morphol* 16:381–386, 1966.

24. Boyne PJ: Autogenous cancellous bone marrow transplants, *Clin Orthop* 73:119–209, 1970.
25. Bright RW, Friedlander GE, Sell KW: Tissue banking: the United States Navy tissue bank, *Milit Med* 142:503–510, 1977.
26. Holmstrand K: Biophysical investigation of bone transplants and bone implants, an experimental study, *Acta Orthop Scand* 26(suppl): 1957.
27. Fonseca RJ, Davis WH: *Reconstructive preprosthetic oral and maxillofacial surgery,* Philadelphia, 1986, WB Saunders.
28. Pedersen GW: *Oral surgery,* Philadelphia, 1988, WB Saunders, pp 119–147.
29. Zins JE, Whitaker L: Membranous vs. endochondral bone: implications for craniofacial reconstruction, *Plast Reconstr Surg* 72:778, 1983.
30. Kusiak J, Zins J, Whitaker L: The early revascularization of membranous bone, *Plast Reconstr Surg* 76:510, 1985.
31. Topper DC: Modified approach for use of cranial bone in facial augmentation grafts (abstr). *J Oral Maxillofac Surg* (special issue) 1990; 71.
32. Markowitz NR: Reconstruction of severely atrophic mandibles with cranial bone grafts and Branemark implants (abstr). *J Oral Maxillofac Surg* (special issue) 1990; 138.
33. Markowitz NR, Allan PG: Cranial bone graft harvesting, a modified technique, *J Oral Maxillofac Surg* 47:1113–1115, 1989.
34. Misch CM, Misch CE, et al: Reconstruction of maxillary alveolar defects with mandibular symphysis grafts for dental implants: a preliminary procedural report, *Int J Oral Maxillofac Implants* 7(3):360–361, 1992.
35. Jensen J: Reconstruction of the atrophic alveolar ridge with mandibular bone grafts and implants (abstr). *J Oral Maxillofac Surg* (special issue) 1990; 125.
36. Jackson I, Helden G, Marx RE: Skull bone grafts in maxillofacial and cranio-facial surgery, *J Oral Maxillofac Surg* 44:949, 1986.
37. Beumer J III, Curtis TA, Firtell DN: *Maxillofacial rehabilitation, prosthetic and surgical considerations,* St Louis, 1979, Mosby–Year Book.
38. Listrom RD, Symington JM: Osseointegrated dental implants in conjunction with bone grafts, *J Oral Maxillofac Surg* 17:116–118, 1988.
39. Keller EE, Triplett WW: Iliac bone grafting, review of 160 consecutive cases, *J Oral Maxillofac Surg* 45:11–14, 1987.
40. Levy RN, Siffert RS: Inner table iliac bone graft, *Surg Gynecol Obstet* 128:705, 1969.
41. Hall MB, Smith RG: The medial approach for obtaining iliac bone, *J Oral Surg* 39:462, 1969.
42. Leake PL: A new alloplastic tray for osseous contour defects, *J Oral Maxillofac Surg* 2:164, 1974.
43. Converse JM, Campbell RM: Bone grafts in surgery of the face, *Surg Clin North Am* 39:365, 1974.
44. Keathlay CJ: Postoperative morbidity of iliac crest donor site in preprosthetic surgery (abstr). Presented at the 64th Annual Meeting, American Association of Oral and Maxillofacial Surgery, Oct 1988.
45. Swart JN, Allard RHB: Subperiosteal onlay augmentation of the mandible, a clinical and radiographic survey, *J Oral Maxillofac Surg* 43:183–187, 1985.
46. Hall MB: Marginal bone loss around Branemark fixtures in bone grafts used for augmentation (abstr). *J Oral Maxillofac Surg* 1990; 117.

47. Misch CE, Dietsh F: An 8-year evaluation of 231 endosteal implants inserted into 36 arches with iliac crest bone grafts between 1984 and 1990, submitted for publication.

48. Laurie SWS et al: Donor site morbidity after harvesting rib and iliac bone, *Plast Reconstr Surg* 73:933, 1984.

49. Keller EE et al: Prosthetic surgical reconstruction of the severely resorbed maxilla with iliac bone grafting and tissue integrated prostheses, *Int J Oral Maxillofac Implants* 2:155–165, 1987.

50. Jensen J, Simonsen EK, Pedersen SS: Reconstruction of the severely resorbed maxilla with bone grafting and osseointegrated implants, a preliminary report, *J Oral Maxillofac Surg* 48:27–32, 1990.

51. Kahnberg KE, Nystrom E, Bartholdsson L: Combined use of bone grafts and Branemark fixtures in the treatment of severely resorbed maxillae, *Int J Oral Maxillofac Implants* 4:297–304, 1989.

52. Adell R et al: Reconstruction of severely resorbed edentulous maxillae using osseointegrated fixtures in immediate autogenous bone grafts, *Int J Maxillofac Implants* 5(3):233–246, 1990.

52a. Keller EE, Tolman DE: Mandibular ridge augmentation with simultaneous onlay iliac bone graft and endosseous implants–a preliminary report, *Int J Oral Maxillofac Implants* 7(2):176–184, 1992.

53. Frost HM: *Bone remodeling and its relationship to metabolic bone diseases,* vol III, *Orthopaedic lectures,* Springfield, Il, 1973, Charles C Thomas, pp 54–85.

54. Misch CE: The maxillary subperiosteal implant, dental evaluation, *Dent Today,* 9(4): 44–47, 1990.

55. Murphy J, Weisman R, Kent K: The use of stabilization plates in the immediate repair of defects following mandibular resection, *Oral Surg Oral Med Oral Pathol* 68:380–384, 1989.

56. Buchbinder D et al: Functional mandibular reconstruction of patients with oral cancer, *Oral Surg Oral Med Oral Pathol* 68:499–502, 1989.

57. King M, Casarett G, Weber D: A study of irradiated bone: histopathology and physiological changes, *J Nucl Med* 20:1142–1149, 1979.

58. Marx RE, Johnson R: Studies in the radiobiology of osteoradionecrosis and their clinical significance, *Oral Surg Oral Med Oral Pathol* 64:379–390, 1987.

59. Conley JJ: A technique of immediate bone grafting in the treatment of benign and malignant tumors of the mandible, a review of 17 consecutive cases, *Cancer* 6:568, 1973.

60. Perel SM, Drane JB, Williams EO: Mandibular replacements, a review of the literature, *J Am Dent Assoc* 94:120, 1977.

61. Marx RE, Ames JR: The use of hyperbaric oxygen therapy in bony reconstruction of the irradiated and tissue deficient patient, *J Oral Maxillofac Surg* 40:412–420, 1982.

62. Snyder CC, Bateman JM, Davis CE: Mandibular facial restoration with live osteocutaneous flaps, *Plast Reconstr Surg* 45:14, 1970.

63. Canalis RF et al: The fate of pedicle osteocutaneous grafts in mandible and facial restoration, *Laryngoscope* 87:895, 1977.

64. Mc Cullough DW, Fredrickson JM: Neovascularization rib grafts to reconstruct mandibular defects, *Can J Otolaryngol* 2:96, 1973.

65. Ostrup LT, Fredrickson JM: Distant transfer of a free living bone graft by microvascular anastomoses, *Plast Reconstr Surg* 54:274, 1974.

66. Ryan DE: Microvascular free transfers of ilium for mandibular reconstruction, Pro-

ceedings Sty of Air Force Clinical Surgeons Meeting, San Antonio, Texas, May 1983.
67. Stone JD, Franklin JD: Immediate mandibular reconstruction using free osseous myocutaneous groin flaps, 1980, Proceedings of the 62nd Annual Meeting of the American Association of Oral and Maxillofacial Surgery, 1980.
68. Riediger D: Restoration of masticatory function by microsurgically revascularized iliac crest bone graft using enosseous implants, *Plast Reconstr Surg* 81:861–876, 1988.
69. Teot L et al: The scapular crest pedicled bone graft, *Int J Microsurg* 3:257, 1981.
70. Swartz WM et al: The osteocutaneous scapular flap for mandibular and maxillary reconstruction, *Plast Reconstr Surg* 77:530–545, 1986.
71. Misch CE: Density of bone: effect on treatment plans, surgical approach, healing and progressive bone loading, *Int J Oral Implant* 6:23–31, 1990.
72. Misch CE: Progressive bone loading, *Pract Periodont Esthet Dent* 2(6):27–30, 1990.
73. Mason M et al: Mandibular fracture through endosseous cylinder implants, *J Oral Maxillofac Surg* 48:311–317, 1990.
74. Tolman DE, Keller EE: Management of mandibular fractures in patients with endosseous implants, *Int J Oral Maxillofac Implants* 6:427–436, 1991.

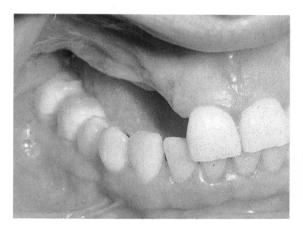

PLATE 9.
Division B ridge medial to the opposing mandibular arch. Offset loads and difficult hygiene considerations mandate augmentation rather than other treatment options.

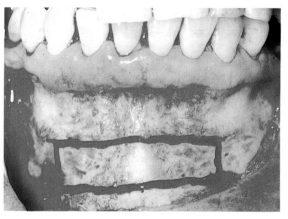

PLATE 10.
Intraoral block of bone is designed to be harvested from the mandibular symphysis region.

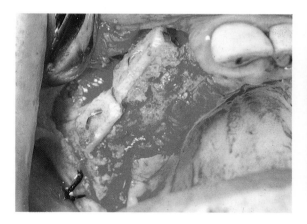

PLATE 11.
Membranous block is fixated to the lateral aspect of the Division B ridge, after sinus elevation and subantral augmentation in the posterior region. (Surgery performed by Dr. C.M. Misch.)

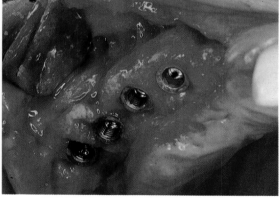

PLATE 12.
Reentry 4 months later permits the placement of endosteal implants in the proper location for axial loading, esthetics, and hygiene.

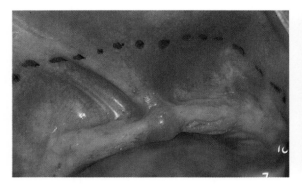

PLATE 13.
C-w ridge that requires height and width for the final restoration. A split-thickness anterior incision is designed.

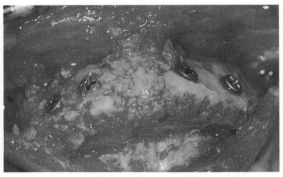

PLATE 14.
Block graft is fixated to the facial of the C-w ridge with titanium fixation screws.

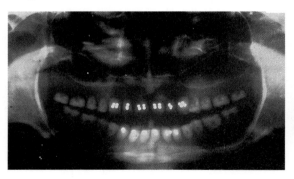

PLATE 15.
Division D mandible in a patient requesting a fixed prosthesis.

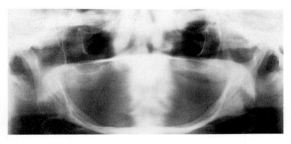

PLATE 16.
Division D maxilla and mandible in a patient requesting a fixed prosthesis.

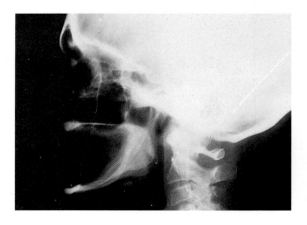

PLATE 17.
Lateral cephalometric radiograph of the patient in Figure 27–8.

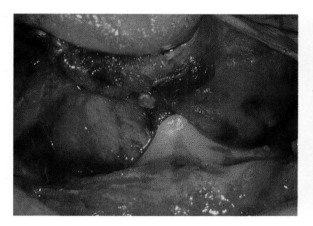

PLATE 18.
Patient in Figure 27–7 with an anterior split thickness incision to anterior of ridge, and then a full thickness reflection exposing the anterior mandible. Note the height of the genial tubercle.

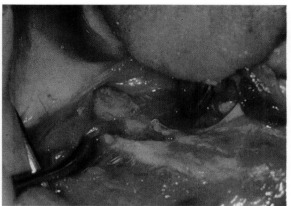

PLATE 19.
Mandibular nerve repositioning at 1 cm permits a more distal implant when the anterior arch form has limited anterior-posterior distance and the patient desires a fixed prosthesis.

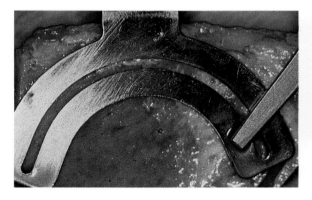

PLATE 20.
Surgical template (Nobelpharma) is used to contour the block graft so it will extend beyond the mental foramen region.

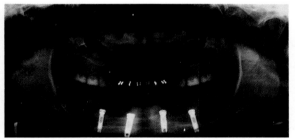

PLATE 21.
Panoramic radiograph of the block graft in position with four endosteal implants as fixation devices.

PLATE 22.
Panoramic radiograph of seven endosteal implants and a FP-3 prosthesis in the patient in Figure 27–7 following augmentation. Note the formation of the new mental foramen distal to the implants placed in the original foramen position.

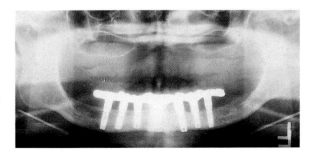

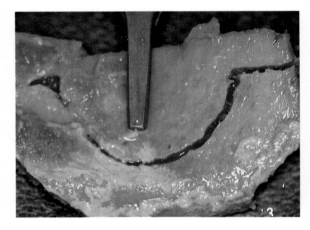

PLATE 23.
Iliac crest and outer table is contoured to the final arch design.

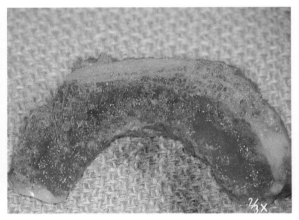

PLATE 24.
Block graft is designed so the corticle region extends to the facial 5 mm, and the trabecular region is compressed to increase the cellular component per area.

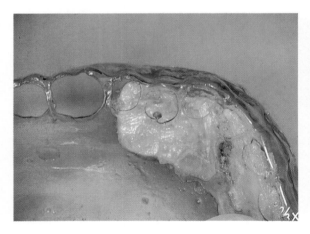

PLATE 25.
Clear surgical template of the final prosthesis wax-up determines the block form and the location of the first premolar region.

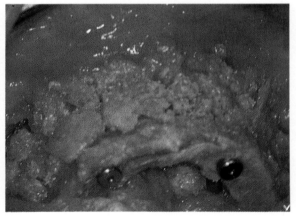

PLATE 26.
Remaining harvested bone is placed in a bone mill and placed in the subantral regions and in any void regions of the block graft.

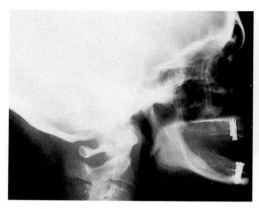

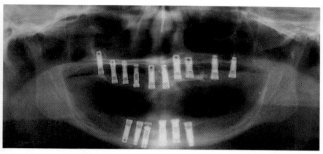

PLATE 28.
Panoramic radiograph 6 months later with 10 endosteal implants in the maxilla for a fixed prosthesis.

PLATE 27.
Lateral cephalogram radiograph of the block grafts fixated in the mandible and maxilla with 15 mm root forms. (Original lateral cephalogram is shown in Plate 17.)

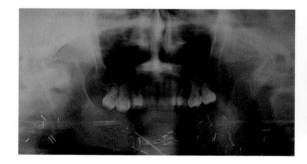

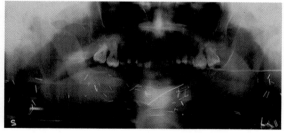

PLATE 30.
Panoramic radiograph of the restored mandible with a vascularized bone graft using the scapula and branches of the circumflex scapular artery. (Surgery performed by Dr. G.C. Sotereanos.

PLATE 29.
Panoramic radiograph of a Division E mandible, which was resected as a result of cancer.

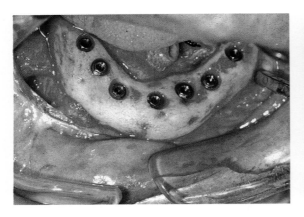

PLATE 31.
Endosteal implants placed into the scapular vascularized bone graft and remaining mandible.

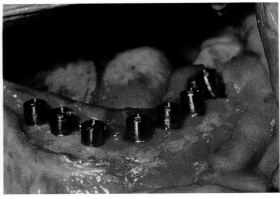

PLATE 32.
Stage-2 surgery and abutment for screw placement 6 months after the original implant surgery. Note no bone loss is observed during this initial 6 months.

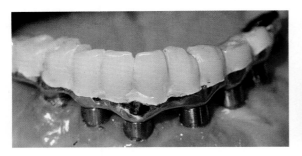

PLATE 33.
Final FP-2 prosthesis.

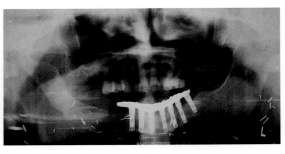

PLATE 34.
Panoramic radiograph of the fixed restoration in the mandible with a vascularized bone graft and seven endosteal implants.

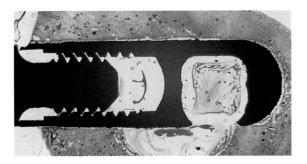

PLATE 35.
Implant placed in the anterior mandible at 1 month, which contacts thick dense compact bone on the crest, lingual, and apical regions. The D-1 bone provides the highest bone-implant interface and ranges more than 80%. (Courtesy of Dr. Richard A. Kraut, Bronx, N.Y.)

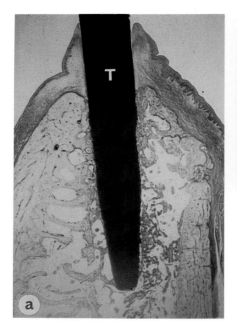

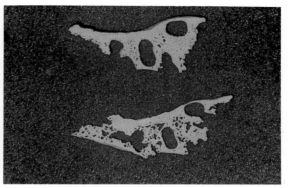

PLATE 37.
Cross-section of two different maxillae that still had natural teeth. The *top section* is D-2 bone with coarse trabecular, and the *inferior section* is D-3 bone with fine trabecular. There will be less contact with the implant in D-3 bone. (Courtesy of Dr. O. Hilt Tatum, St. Petersburg, Fla.)

PLATE 36.
Implant inserted into D-2 bone that has cortical bone at the crest and coarse trabecular bone around the majority of the implant. The actual bone-implant contact is approximately 75%.

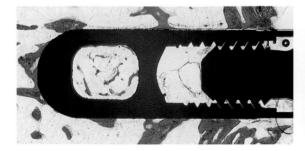

PLATE 38.
Implant after 4 months healing in a posterior maxilla with fine trabecular bone (D-4). The least amount of bone contact is present and ranges around 25%. (Courtesy of Dr. Richard A. Kraut, Bronx, N.Y.)

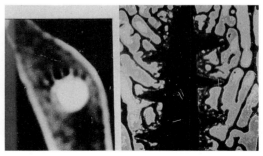

PLATE 39.
Computed tomographic scan of an implant that has undergone progressive loading in a sheep. (Courtesy of A. Pierazzini, Mesa, Italy.)

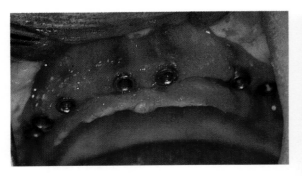

PLATE 40.
Maxillary arch at stage two uncovery, at which bone loss and rigidity are assessed.

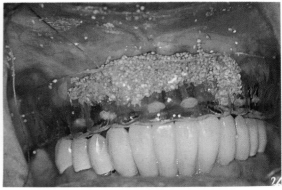

PLATE 41.
Surgical template in position after the low-profile permucosal extensions are in place. This template permits the correct amount of dense HA on the labial aspect to provide proper lip support above the prosthesis; the template also evaluates the placement of the implant bodies related to angulation of load and prosthesis contours.

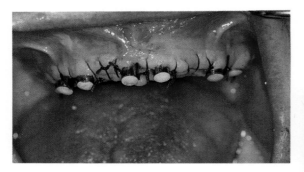

PLATE 42.
Tissue is approximated and sutured. The 4-mm extension should exit the tissue at least 1 mm to ensure that sulcus depth will be 3 mm or less.

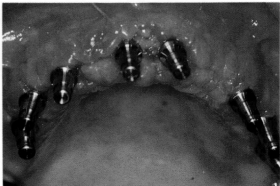

PLATE 43.
Straight abutments for cement are added to the implant bodies after 2 or more weeks.

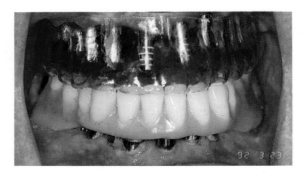

PLATE 44.
Clear template of the diagnostic wax-up is placed over the implant abutments for cement. Height correction is often required to completely seat the template.

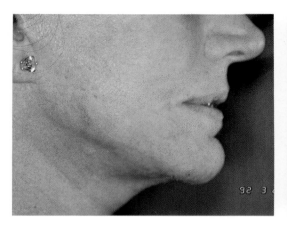

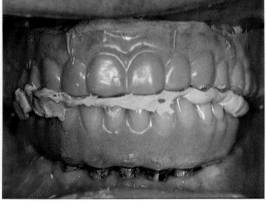

PLATE 45.
Clear template is evaluated for lip position, vertical, and incisor edge position. If no template is available, a wax-rim may be fabricated to provide this information.

PLATE 46.
Silicone putty is placed into the clear template and serves as a preliminary impression. An occlusal registration allows the maxillary cast to be mounted to a cart of the lower arch.

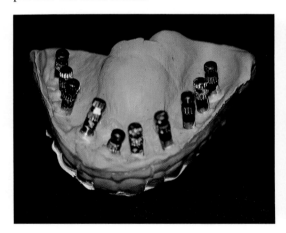

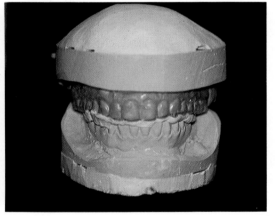

PLATE 47.
Abutments for cement are unthreaded from the implant bodies, threaded into an implant body analog, and repositioned into the preliminary impression in the prosthetic template.

PLATE 48.
Preliminary impression with implant abutments for cement and implant body analogs are indexed with the occlusal registration into the mandibular cast on an articulator.

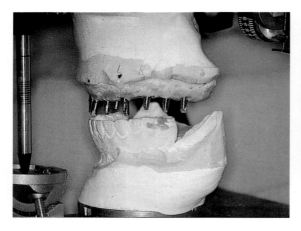

PLATE 49.
Preliminary impression and prosthetic template are removed from the maxillary cast, and the implant abutments for cement are evaluated for length and angulation.

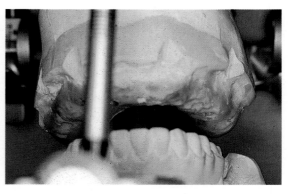

PLATE 50.
Abutments for cement are removed, and the maxillary arch is evaluated for interarch space and position.

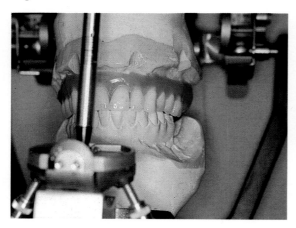

PLATE 51.
Ideal wax-up with denture teeth is performed on the maxillary arch without the abutments for cement in position.

PLATE 53.
Abutments for cement are replaced into the maxillary working cast, and the clear prosthetic template is closed into position. The abutments may now be evaluated for placement within the contours of the final restoration. Preparation of the abutments is possible in the laboratory, related to length and angulation.

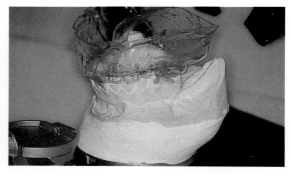

PLATE 52.
Vacuum form is made of the ideal denture tooth wax-up and attached in the appropriate position on the mandibular cast.

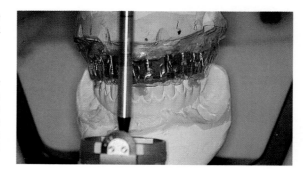

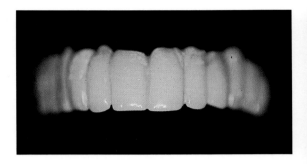

PLATE 54.
Transitional restoration is fabricated on the laboratory-prepared abutment with the clear prosthetic template. There are no posterior cantilevers, and only crowns over axial positioned implants are pinpoint loaded.

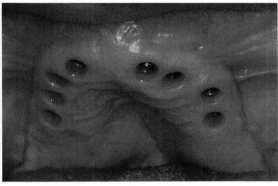

PLATE 55.
Low-profile permucosal extensions are removed in this patient 3 weeks after the previous appointment (the bone was D-3). The soft tissue is completely healed and keratinized, to allow proper evaluation before the final impression.

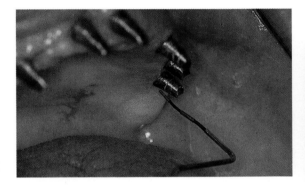

PLATE 56.
Perio-probe evaluates the sulcus depth around each implant before the final impression. A gingivoplasty was performed on the most posterior abutment, since the pocket depth approached 4 mm.

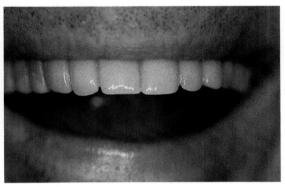

PLATE 57.
Provisional restoration is seated after the abutments for cement have been evaluated and prepared. The incisal edge position is important to determine before the superstructure is fabricated to ensure that unsupported porcelain will not occur.

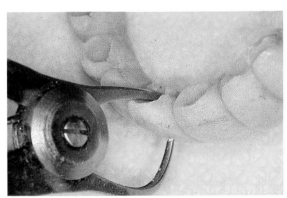

PLATE 58.
Thickness of the acrylic over the facial of the abutments for cement is measured to ensure that 2 mm or more is present for the metal and porcelain required for esthetics and strength.

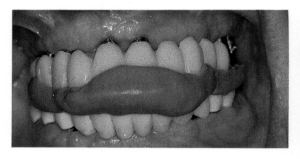

PLATE 59.
Additional silicone putty is placed onto the roof of the mouth and rolled onto the occlusal and facial surfaces of the provisional restoration.

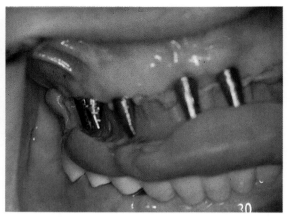

PLATE 60.
Transitional appliance is removed from the occlusal index and reinserted into the mouth. The position of the abutments for cement may be evaluated once more prior to making the final impression. When correct, the space is filled with additional silicone material for bite registration, so the master cast may be mounted at the correct vertical and centric prior to superstructure fabrication.

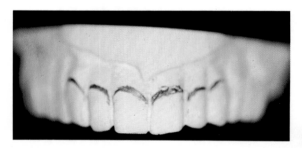

PLATE 61.
Impression is made of the transitional appliance, along with occlusal registration. The impression is poured and the lip line position marked on the cast to transfer this information to the laboratory. The midline may also be noted if different from that on the temporary restoration.

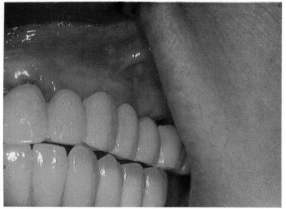

PLATE 62.
Occlusion on the provisional restoration should not load any cantilever, pontics, or implants that are not within 20 degrees of the axial load. No offset loads, no balancing, and no working contacts are present.

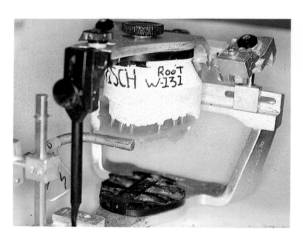

PLATE 63.
Facebow is used to mount the master cast of the maxilla on an adjustable articulator. The mandibular cast will be mounted using the additional silicone putty and occlusal index.

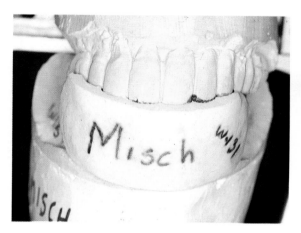

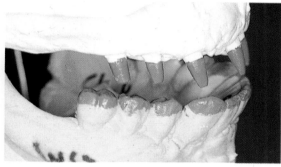

PLATE 65.
Maxillary working cast of the transitional appliance is removed from the articulator, and the master cast of the prepared abutments for cement are replaced.

PLATE 64.
Maxillary master cast is removed from the articular, and the cast of the temporary restoration is mounted with a different base plate on the maxillary bow of the articulator with the occlusal registration of the temporary appliance. An index is then made of the incisal edge position related to the mandibular arch.

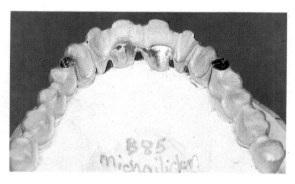

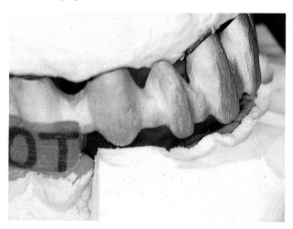

PLATE 67.
Superstructure is fabricated on the maxillary master cast. This casting has two rigid attachments between the canine and first premolar, without a gingival seat. This allows the posterior and anterior castings to be seated or removed independently of each other.

PLATE 66.
Index of the transitional appliance is used so the superstructure is fabricated 2 mm from the incisal edge position and labial contours.

PLATE 68.
White wax anterior tooth contour is made on the superstructure. Posterior acrylic indexes are made on the metal work which represented the index at the previous clinical appointment.

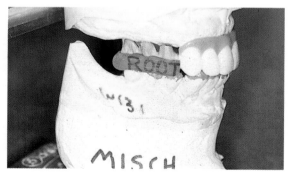

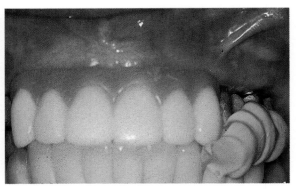

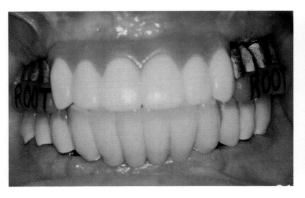

PLATE 69.
Metal try-in with acrylic index. Esthetics, phonetics, and occlusion are evaluated.

PLATE 70.
Final occlusal registrations are recorded, including protrusive and lateral excursions after the incisal edge position is determined.

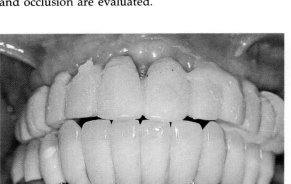

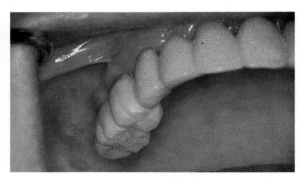

PLATE 72.
Occlusion of the transitional restoration is modified so no working or balancing contacts are present.

PLATE 71.
Transitional prosthesis is inserted and acrylic is added to the posterior occlusal surfaces; there is occlusion in the centric and all excursions by the patient.

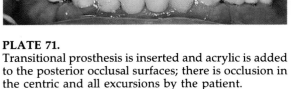

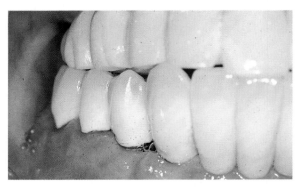

PLATE 73.
Centric relation occlusion axially loads the implants in ideal position. Lighter contacts are present on pontics or implants beyond 20 degrees of axial load.

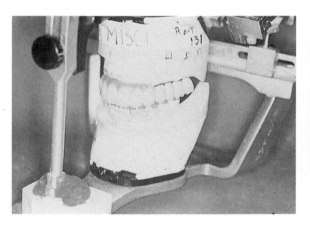

PLATE 74.
Laboratory mounts the maxillary try-in restoration, and with the protrusive and lateral excursive registrations builds a customized incisal guide table with cold cure acrylic. The posterior occlusion may then be fabricated without working or balancing interferences.

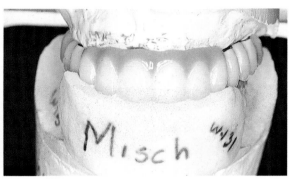

PLATE 75.
If the white wax was modified at the try-in appointment a new index is fabricated. The index allows the porcelain to be shaped similar to the contours determined in the clinical setting.

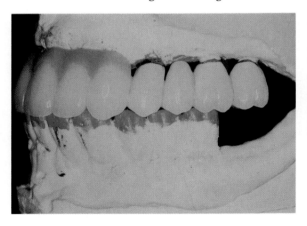

PLATE 76.
Final restoration mounted on the articulator has modified ridge lap crowns and pontics in the anterior for speech and esthetics and open embrasures in the posterior for hygiene considerations.

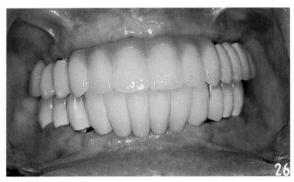

PLATE 77.
Initial try-in restoration should fit passively, yet be stable and retentive.

PLATE 78.
Occlusion is evaluated in centric relation occlusion. The implants should have axial load. A "medial positioned lingualized occlusion" established by Misch is most often observed in implant prostheses.

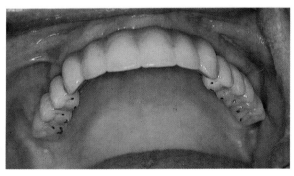

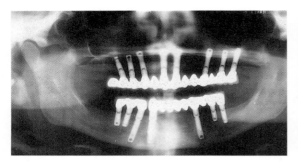

PLATE 79.
Panoramic radiograph is taken at this appointment and compared with the bone study used at surgery. The new radiograph will be the baseline for future evaluation of bone loss, especially during the first year of implant use.

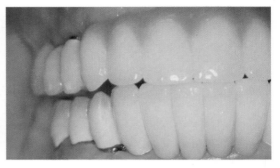

PLATE 80.
Protrusive movement which demonstrates no posterior contacts.

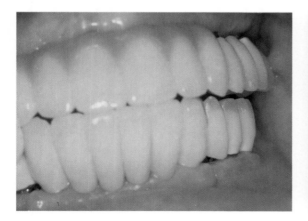

PLATE 81.
Right working movement demonstrates no balancing contacts on the left posterior sections.

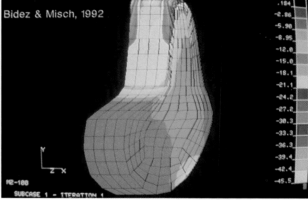

PLATE 82.
Finite stress analysis of volume of bone (Divisions A, B, and C-w) interrelated to bone density (D-1, D-2, D-3, and D-4) demonstrated a relationship between the two macroscopic entities.

Chapter 28

Progressive Bone Loading

Carl E. Misch

The surgical and prosthetic protocols for a predictable direct bone-implant interface with root form implants was developed and reported by Branemark.[1] Success with this protocol is reported to be 10% greater in the anterior mandible than the anterior maxilla and 25% to 50% greater than the posterior maxilla following similar surgical and prosthodontic modalities for all regions and bone densities.[2-4] A major difference in these regions is bone density.[5-7] Modification of the surgery and healing time based upon bone density, not location within the jaws, was addressed in Chapter 22. These principles achieve similar surgical success rates in all jaw regions.

Once an initial direct bone-implant interface has been obtained and confirmed at the post-healing second-stage surgery, the implant is most at risk of failure within the first year.[1] This occurs primarily as a result of excessive stress. If the treatment plan is satisfactory for adequate support, the three most common causes of prosthetic-related implant failure are nonpassive superstructures, partially unretained restorations, and too rapid loading of the implant support system.[8] In this chapter the rationale and protocol to gradually load the implant after the initial bone interface has been established are addressed.

BONE-IMPLANT INTERFACE

Four different densities of bone have been identified in the jaws,[5, 9] and relate to Wolff's law and generalized bone loss in regions that lack stress.[10] This phenomenon occurs throughout the skeletal system as evidenced by a 15% decrease in the cortical plate and extensive trabecular loss to bone immobilized for 3 months.[11] Cortical bone decrease of 40% and trabecular bone decrease by 12% have also been reported with disuse of the bone.[12, 13] The density decrease in the jaws is related to the length of time the region has been edentulous, the original width of bone, muscle attachments, flexure and torsion, parafunction before and after tooth loss, hormonal influence, and systemic conditions.[14–16]

Bone also increases in density if an increase in stress occurs within physiologic limits.[17] The deformation of the alveolar bone by mechanical forces is even related to the thickness of the bony plate.[18] Dahlin and Olsson report an increase in both cortical bone thickness and overall mineral content under stressful stimuli.[19] Clinical evaluation confirms an increase in the amount of trabecular bone and cortical plate thickness in patients with natural teeth exhibiting parafunction.

Computer-aided assessment of fixated implants have used digital subtraction radiographic image analysis and an interactive image-analysis system to demonstrate an increase in density of peri-implant bone structures over a 6-month to a 2-year period after the implant was placed into function.[20, 21] Bone density increase is primarily reflective of the local stress factors, and endosteal implants are the major method to alter the stress and increase bone density in the edentulous jaws.

The macroscopic ranges in jaw bone density demonstrate a physical difference in the amount of cortical and trabecular bone. The actual amount of bone in initial contact with the surface of the implant is related to the bone density. In D-4 bone only 25% of the implant may be in contact with bone, D-3 bone has approximately 50% bone contact, D-2 bone about 70% bone interface, and D-1 bone around 80% (Plates 35 to 38). The implant transforms a load to the surrounding bone, primarily where bone contacts the implant surface. The greater the bone contact, the better the force distribution, and the less stress transmitted to any one region on the implant body. Hence the same load can give less stress to the interface of an implant in D-1 bone than in D-4 bone.

The histologic type of bone in contact with the implant is variable and can affect the amount of stress the bone can support within physiologic limits. The ideal bone for implant prosthetic support is lamellar bone.[16] It is highly organized, but takes approximately 1 year to completely mineralize after the trauma induced by implant placement. At 16 weeks the surrounding bone is only 70% mineralized and still has woven bone as a component. Woven bone is the fastest and first type of bone to form around the implant interface; however, it is only partly mineralized and demonstrates an unorganized structure unable to withstand full-scale stresses.[16] Computer-aided radiographic densitometry studies confirm that bone-implant interface decreases the first several months following a procedure. Therefore, the percentage of bone contact and the type of supporting bone both influence whether a load to the implant may remain within physiologic limits.[22] Because the greatest stress around a fixated implant occurs at the crest, a premature or too great functional load may overstress the system and cause bone resorption in this region.

The macroscopic coarse trabecular bone heals approximately 50% faster than dense cortical bone.[23] Therefore, the length of time elapsed between the initial and the second stage surgeries is 5 months for D-1 bone, and 4 months for D-2 bone, because the latter has a much greater trabecular component. The D-1 bone has greater bone contact, so even though it heals slower, the interface percentage is great and the histologic type is lamellar. A longer time is suggested for initial healing of D-3 and D-4 bone. Because the percentage of bone contact is less and the amount of cortical bone is decreased, the extra time permits formation of more lamellar bone with a higher mineral content. Hence 6 month's healing is permitted for D-3 bone. A period of 8 month's healing is suggested for D-4 bone. The implant interface has minimum contact with bone, with little to no cortical bone on the crest or apex. An implant may increase the amount of bone in the region, even though it is not loaded. For example, bone will grow completely around a submerged titanium screw inserted into an open marrow chamber of the femur.[22] The extra time also permits more lamellar bone to form in the trabeculae that contact the implant, and the presence of hydroxyapatite (HA) or titanium can increase the surface contact with bone. The second stage surgery evaluates the rigid fixation, ideal crestal bone situation, implant body location, tissue thickness, and attached gingiva. A 2-week healing period is suggested before suture removal and the beginning of the prosthetic gradual bone loading.

The combined observations of the macroscopic amount of bone in contact with a nonloaded implant and the microscopic type of bone at the second stage surgery of the implant demonstrates the wide difference in D-1 to D-4 bone densities. In addition, the bone responds to physiologic forces, and a gradual increase in loads stimulates a reaction of increased density. The principles and methods of progressive bone loading were established by Misch in 1980 on the basis of empirical information. Over the years these guidelines have matured and are founded upon observations in both animal and human clinical trials (Plate 39).[24, 25] Clinical assessment of progressive load guidelines were evaluated over a 2-year period using a Periotest.[26] This instrument evaluates the mobility and damping effect of implants, prostheses, and teeth. As a general rule, the implants recorded a positive number when first uncovered, and the number became more negative with time. Most all implants presented a negative number after they had been in function for more than 1 year. There is not a linear curve relationship between load, time, and bone density. However, a clinical protocol has been established that errors on the side of safety.[5, 24]

Two surgical appointments are used for the initial implant placement and second stage uncovery; these are separated by 4 to 8 months depending on the bone density at the initial surgery. Five prosthodontic steps are suggested for reconstruction of the partially or completely edentulous patient, using an endosteal implant support system with a cemented prosthesis. Each of the five major prosthodontic appointments are also separated by a period of time related to the bone density observed at the initial time of surgery. In addition, an attempt is made to gradually increase the load to the implant at each prosthetic step. The progressive bone loading appointment sequence for cement retained prostheses is as follows:

1. Initial healing
2. Stage two uncovery
3. Initial abutment selection and preliminary impression
4. Final impression and transitional prosthesis I
5. Try-in (teeth and/or metal) and transitional prosthesis II
6. Initial insertion
7. Final delivery

D-1 bone has the greatest amount of bone contact and lamellar bone at the beginning of the restoration. As a result, the prosthodontic appointments may be separated by 1 week, and gradual loading of the implant interface is least important. D-2 bone is ideal in its ability to respond to physiologic loads. The five prosthetic appointments in which the implant body is sequentially loaded are separated by 2 weeks. As a result, the longer healing time of D-1 combined with a shorter interval prosthetic time results in a similar overall time compared to D-2 bone, and is approximately 6½ months for the overall treatment. D-3 bone has little cortical bone and fine trabecular bone primarily contacts the implant body. The prosthodontic appointments are separated by 3 weeks and overall treatment takes almost 10 months to complete (including the stage two uncovery procedure). During this time frame the bone contact percentage can increase, the size of the fine trabeculae can increase to coarse trabeculae, and the mineral content of the bone increases. The progressive loading process is more important for D-3 bone than for D-2 or D-1 because of the decrease in initial bone contact. In D-4 bone, the progressive bone loading program is most critical. The restorative appointments err on the side of safety, and are separated by 4 weeks or more. The overall treatment time for D-4 bone is twice the period for D-1 or D-2 bone. As a consequence the total treatment time is at least 12½ months. This allows sufficient time for mature mineralized bone to develop at the interface and increases the amount of trabeculae in direct contact and within the network region of the implant. Comparison of the time intervals is provided in Table 28–1.

TABLE 28–1.

Treatment Times for Progressive Bone Loading for Cement-Retained Prostheses

Bone Density	Initial Healing (mo)	Reconstruction (wk)	Interval Between Appointments (wk)	Total Time (mo)
D-1	5	6	1	6.5
D-2	4	10	2	6.5
D-3	6	14	3	9.5
D-4	8	18	4	12.5

The principles of gradual loading are best demonstrated in the cement-retained prosthesis and least applicable for the screw-retained bar of a mandibular RP-5 restoration. In addition, it is difficult to gradually load a removable RP-4 or RP-5 prosthesis that uses a screw-retained superstructure bar because the transitional prosthesis often remains removable during the final reconstruction. The screw-retained FP-1 to FP-3 fixed prosthesis is most critical, because excess forces from nonpassive superstructures and unretained restorations occur most often with this prosthesis type. As a result, a different protocol that requires additional prosthetic appointments is used to restore this patient, which increases the overall treatment time in order to improve the bone interface.

COMPLETE ARCH CEMENTED FIXED PROSTHESIS

Stage-2 Uncovery

The stage 2 uncovery procedure for a cement or screw-retained restoration evaluates an absence of clinical mobility, bone loss (horizontal and vertical), proper placement in reference to prosthetic design and angulation to load, zones of attached gingiva, and gingival thickness (see Chapter 21). A low-profile permucosal extension is added to the implant body. This component extends through the tissue approximately 2 mm and is protected from early loading. The patient with a posterior implant in a partially edentulous arch is instructed not to wear any removable restoration (Plates 40 to 42). If anterior teeth are part of the removable prosthesis, a 7-mm hole is placed through the partial denture framework around each permucosal extension. In completely edentulous patients the tissue surface of the denture is relieved at least 5 mm over and around the implants, and replaced by a tissue conditioner. The conditioner is also relieved a few millimeters after it is cured in the mouth. The patient returns in 2 weeks for the suture removal. The tissue is reassessed, and gingivoplasty may be indicated. Uncovery is discussed in detail in Chapter 21.

Initial Abutment Selection and Preliminary Impression

At the first prosthetic appointment, initial selection is made of the final abutment for cement. When the doctor performs the surgery and prosthesis placement, this appointment may occur as soon as during the suture removal appointment after the second stage surgery. In the team approach, the suture removal is scheduled by the doctor placing the implant, so the tissue may be reassessed and gingivoplasty or other procedures performed as required. A sulcus depth greater than 5 mm requires correction. A 3 mm sulcus depth is evaluated relative to esthetics and crown height. The patient is referred to the restoring dentist once the tissue health is proper for long-term health. The second-stage permucosal extensions are removed by the restoring dentist and straight abutments for cement are inserted. The abutment for cement is placed with two thirds of the final torque force because the interface is still not mineralized completely and the abutment will be removed. If a choice of lengths is available, the longest abutment is selected first (Plate 43).

A clear template of the final prosthesis wax-up fabricated from the study model prior to the appointment is placed in position over the straight abutments for cement (Plate 44). The length of the abutments is evaluated. Minor corrections may be performed intraorally with a high-speed handpiece and cross-cut fissure bur, with copious amounts of water and intermittent cutting of the abutment. A 2-second pause after every 3 seconds of cutting with continuous water coolant errs on the side of safety. One should correct the too long abutments first, so the clear prosthetic template can fit into final position.

Once the clear prosthetic template is seated in correct position, it is evaluated for lip position, esthetics, and vertical and centric occlusion (Plate 45). The abutments are checked for maximum length, crown contour, and path of insertion. The abutments for cement should have a flat side to prevent shear forces on the cement and allow the abutment to be placed into the impression in the correct threaded position with the implant body analog. The clear prosthetic template is filled with an addition silicone putty and reinserted in final position. A bite registration material is placed on the occlusal surfaces, and the mandible is guided into centric occlusion (Plate 46). The template impression and bite registration are removed and serve as a preliminary impression of the abutments for cement. An impression is then made of the opposing arch.

If the prosthetic template was not fabricated beforehand, a roll of addition silicone putty is placed onto the abutments for cement and the mandible is guided to centric relation occlusion at the approximate vertical. A preliminary impression is then made of the abutments for cement and the opposing arch.

The abutments for cement are removed, threaded into the implant body analogue, and placed into the corresponding location of the impression (Plate 47). The second-stage permucosal extensions are reinserted into the implant bodies. The tissue conditioner of the removable prosthesis is removed and replaced by a soft liner. The liner is relieved over the permucosal extensions. The patient is instructed to limit the diet to mastication of very soft foods and remove the denture at night to prevent nocturnal parafunction. The patient returns in 1 to 4 weeks or more, depending on the bone density.

Laboratory Steps After First Phase

Laboratory steps following this appointment include pouring the preliminary impression with the implant abutment and implant body analog in dental stone. The cast is mounted against the opposing arch model on an articulator with the template and occlusal registration (or roll of addition silicon putty) before it is separated from the template (Plates 48 and 49).

Once the cast is mounted in the appropriate vertical and centric registration, the abutment posts may be removed and denture teeth and wax used to wax-up the proposed form of the final prosthesis (Plates 50 and 51). A clear template is fabricated over this wax-up. The occlusal surface of the template may be sticky waxed on the occlusal of the opposing arch and the articulator closed into position (Plate 52). The abutment posts initially selected are evaluated on the mounted study cast. The abutments may be reevaluated to the new wax-up related to length, angulation, and proper clearance for crown contours (Plate 53). Additional recontouring of the abutments or replacement with another straight abutment is possible. A dental surveyor may evaluate the path of insertion. If an abutment cannot be corrected by drilling, it is noted to replace the abutment with a more favorable post at the next appointment. It is not predictable to remove and place a correct angled abutment in the study model, because the implant body analog thread rarely exactly corresponds to the actual implant body. As a result the angled post is often incorrectly aligned when selected in the laboratory and reinserted in the mouth.

A transitional acrylic prosthesis may be fabricated on the study cast once the abutments for cement are modified, when the clear prosthetic template was correct regarding lip position, vertical dimension, and occlusion (Plate 54). No posterior cantilever should be present. No opposing contact on any pontic regions should exist. Only those teeth over implants that can be loaded with axial forces within 20 degrees should contact. No posterior contact in excursions exist if adequate anterior implants are present and the restoration opposes a fixed or natural dentition. Posterior occlusal tables should be very narrow and correspond to the abutment for cement. A clear prosthetic template is fabricated from the transitional prosthesis.

If the vertical and incisal edge position cannot be determined at the initial appointment, a modified base plate and wax-rim may be fabricated over the abutments to determine these recordings similar to a complete denture fabrication at the next appointment.

A custom impression tray may also be fabricated on this working model. The transitional restoration or wax-rim is removed, and a 3 mm wax spacer is placed around and between the implant posts, with 1 to 2 mm space for impression material over the soft tissue, and soft tissue stops on the palate or retromolar pads. An acrylic custom tray is then fabricated around the entire arch at least 24 hours before the next appointment, to reduce the effect of dimensional change.

The steps are provided in detail by the sequence shown in Table 28–2.

Final Impression and Transitional Prosthesis I

The second restorative appointment removes the permucosal extensions (Plate 55) and places the final abutments for cement into position. A perio-probe evaluates the implant sulcus depth (Plate 56). More than 3 to 6 weeks have elapsed

TABLE 28–2.

Sequence of Steps in Initial Abutment Selection

Cement-retained prosthesis
    Evaluate soft tissue thickness
    Place straight abutment for cement
    Insert clear prosthetic template into position over abutment
    Correct length first, then angulation for crown contour and path of insertion. Flatten one side
    Make sure template fits regarding lip position, vertical, and centric occlusion
    Place addition silicone putty into the template and insert over abutments. Bite registration material records centric
       relation occlusion

Or

If no template was fabricated
    Insert straight abutments for cement (with a flat side)
    Place a roll of addition silicone putty over abutments and guide mandible into approximate vertical at centric rela-
       tion occlusion
    Make a preliminary impression of the abutments for cement and surrounding soft tissue

Then

    Remove abutments for cement, thread into implant body analog, and insert into corresponding site into prelimi-
       nary impression
    Make impression of opposing arch
    Replace permucosal extensions
    Remove soft tissue conditioner, place soft tissue liner and relieve
    Limit diet to very soft food

since the surgical uncovery, and the tissue can be evaluated at its final position without estimate. If the pocket depth is greater than 3 mm, especially in nonesthetic regions, a gingivoplasty or apical position flap is performed (depending upon the amount of attached gingiva present). This procedure does not usually delay the rest of the appointments or delay the final prosthetic delivery; however, it does improve soft tissue conditions and helps limit long-term complication.

The clear template of the final prosthesis wax-up is placed into position and the abutments evaluated for ideal placement. When the abutments for cement are correct, they are cemented into final position with a final crown and bridge cement. The cement prevents bacteria from growing in the implant body abutment receptor site and releasing endotoxins into the gingival sulcus. In addition, it permits final preparation of the abutment with rotary burs without the post unthreading or the abutment unthreading during the progressive loading period.

A rough diamond is used to gently roughen the abutments for cement above the gingiva, to further improve retention. This is especially necessary for the most posterior and anterior abutments, when abutment posts have a tapered preparation more than 20 degrees or are shorter than ideal (2 mm less than the occlusal plane). The first transitional prosthesis is also fabricated at this appointment. A most important step for the temporary is the evaluation of incisal edge position for esthetics and phonetics. This position should be established before the superstructure is fabricated, to ensure ideal support of porcelain and/or acrylic in the final restoration (Plate 57). This position also greatly influences posterior occlusion relationships in any excursive position. The thickness of the acrylic provisional prosthesis facial to the abutments for cement can be measured to ensure adequate space for metal and porcelain on the final restoration (Plate 58).

Once the first temporary restoration satisfies the criteria established in the laboratory and confirmed at the clinical try-in, occlusal recordings are made of the approximate vertical and centric along with a facebow registration. Addition silicone putty may be mixed and placed over the occlusal and incisal surfaces of the temporary restoration and on the hard palate and/or soft tissue regions (or teeth not involved in the prosthesis). The patient closes into centric relation occlusion though the putty (Plate 59). Once set, the registration and transitional appliance is removed from the mouth and separated. The putty is reinserted into the mouth, and the tissues and/or teeth hold the jaws into the recorded position (Plate 60). Injectable rigid additional silicone may be placed into the void created from the prosthesis removal. The abutments for cement are embedded into the bite registration material at the appropriate vertical and centric positions. The final occlusal recordings will be registered on the metal framework at the next appointment. A facebow recording is made of the maxillary arch.

An impression is also made of the temporary restoration in place. This, together with a centric occlusion registration, allows the laboratory to determine the incisal edge and midline position for the final restoration. The high smile line position is noted on the temporary prosthesis and will be drawn on the cast of the temporary restoration to also transfer this information (Plate 61). The shape of the anterior teeth may be selected using a denture mold guide to help the technician determine the final esthetic result.[27]

The occlusion on the first transitional prosthesis should be similar to that of the final restoration in mandibular excursions. In centric relation occlusion the implants should be loaded with only axial implant body loads. No offset loads or cantilevers should be present. In addition, the first temporary prosthesis has no contact on the pontics and very narrow posterior occlusal tables. Do not hesitate to adjust the opposing dentition to improve the direction of occlusal loads (Plate 62). The transitional restoration may be cemented with a soft access cement with no eugenol, because eugenol may prevent adherence of future acrylic relines to the restoration. Modifier or vaseline is often added to the soft access cement when many abutments are present to ensure removal without complication. The diet of the patient at this time is still very soft. It is wise to explain to the patient the need to remain on this very soft diet. The first time the implants are being loaded with a restoration is at the conclusion of this appointment. Too aggressive a force may cause implant overload or break the cement seal of the provisional restoration, which will cause cantilever and moment loads on the remaining implant(s). The patient is warned that any implant loss from this point may require implant removal, bone graft, implant placement, and long healing times.

Laboratory Steps for Second Phase

The laboratory staff pours the final impression in die stone. A die spacer is used on the abutments to help ensure a passive superstructure. The facebow and occlusal registrations allow the master casts to be mounted on the articulator. The implant cast is removed, and the temporary model is mounted on the articulator (Plate 63). An index is taken of the incisal edge and facial tooth position (Plate 64). The die model is replaced on the articulator and the superstructure is fabricated 2 mm from the index and occlusal planes (Plates 65 and 66).

A white wax model of the six anterior teeth may be made on the metal superstructure. This permits a clinical evaluation of the actual casting, and wax may be added or carved quickly if any changes are indicated. Acrylic indices may be used in the posterior at the recorded centric and vertical to check this registration at the next try-in appointment (Plates 67 and 68).

Try-In and Transitional Prosthesis II

At the third prosthodontic appointment, the passive, yet accurate marginal fit of the superstructure is evaluated. The casting should not be tapped into position if too tight. Instead, there are three alternatives. The most frequent and easiest is to slightly modify the abutment for cement, using a diamond and copious amounts of water. The second option is to grind the internal aspect of the superstructure. The third, and least used, option for a cement-retained prosthesis is to separate the casting and lute it with acrylic and a plaster index prior to soldering. The first two options are rarely possible for a screw-retained restoration.

Decay is not a problem around an implant abutment, so the marginal seal is not as important. However, poor margins may affect soft tissue health or lead to cement wash-out. Therefore, margins are an important aspect of the superstructures evaluation.

Once the superstructure is passive and the margins correct, the posterior acrylic indices are checked for centric occlusion and vertical dimension (Plate 69). The white wax models of the anterior teeth are evaluated for lip position, length, phonetics, and esthetics. The white wax may be modified to represent the ideal form. The high lip line is determined and scored in the cervical region of the wax. The final decision relative to FP-2 or FP-3 restoration options is determined at this step. The patient is not anesthetized, has been wearing a transitional prosthesis with no interferences, has only been opening the mouth for a short time, and has a very rigid, stable structure in place. As a result, an accurate jaw relationship record can be obtained. If any variance is noted in the original occlusal registrations, a new recording is indicated. The protrusive bite registration is more related to the incisal edge position than the angle of the eminentia in the disc-fossa relationship.[28] Once the incisal edge is determined, the protrusive and lateral excursions of the mandible may be recorded on the framework (Plate 70). The final shade selection for the gingiva and/or teeth are determined during this session.

The first transitional restoration is then modified. Monomer is added to the occlusal aspect, and petroleum jelly is placed over the opposing teeth. Acrylic is added on the occluding surfaces of the temporary restoration and the patient occludes into the material and moves in all excursions (Plate 71). After setting, the unwanted balancing and working occlusal contacts are then removed (Plate 72). The pontic areas are brought into light centric occlusion. Implants not perpendicular to the occlusal plane are slightly loaded. Heavier contacts exist on the implants in ideal position than on pontics or angled abutments (Plate 73). No cantilever is added to the restoration. The transitional prosthesis should have an occlusal pattern similar to the final prosthesis in excursions.

The restoration is cemented with a soft access cement. The cement used in the first transitional prosthesis is evaluated as to difficulty in removal and maintenance during the interim appointments. If too rigid, a softer cement may be used at this appointment, and vice versa. The patient may begin to include some slightly harder foods into the diet (such as cooked meats). Hard foods (such as raw carrots) are still avoided. Patients with parafunction may remain in an acrylic transitional registration for as long as 6 months. A laboratory processed restoration is usually indicated for this extended period. If the patient has excessive forces, especially with restorations of more than two pontics, a composite fixed bridge with metal superstructure may be indicated during the extended transition period (Plates 74 and 75).

Initial Delivery

The fourth restorative appointment (1 to 4 weeks later) marks the initial delivery of the final restoration (Plates 76 and 77). The casting must fit passively. On occasion, porcelain added to the metal superstructure may change the casting fit. If this occurs the correction is similar to that on the third appointment. Oral hygiene regimens are demonstrated and stressed. The final occlusion is evaluated and corrected as indicated. This is the first time cantilevers appear on the restoration. The occlusion is designed to axially load the implant wherever possible (Plate 78).

A soft access cement is used in the restoration. The cement material of choice is variable and depends on the number of abutments, the stability and retention of the casting, and the parafunction of the patient. The diet of the patient still does not include hard foods, but most foods can be enjoyed. A panoramic radiographic may be taken to establish the baseline values of bone for future comparison and compared with the bone level at implant placement surgery (Plate 79).

Final Delivery

At the fifth prosthetic appointment, the final restorative result is evaluated. The patient's soft tissue health and hygiene regimen are scrutinized. Peri-implant probing is indicated to establish soft tissue baseline measurements at this appointment, because soft tissue health is often improved with the final restoration compared with the acrylic transitional appliance. The occlusion is refined. No posterior contacts are present in any excursion when opposing natural dentition or a fixed prosthesis (Plates 80 and 81). The retention and the difficulty in removal of the restoration are evaluated. A soft access cement is preferred, but a partially unretained restoration places considerable risk on the remaining attached abutments. It is usually better to err by having slightly too much retention. Once the restoration is removed, the pontic contours are checked for hygiene and physiologic tissue contact. Difficult access areas for hygiene are improved.

The diet of the patient is normal at this time. However, hard foods are still avoided, when working with D-4 bone. Parafunction may dictate use of an acrylic night guard for bruxism or a soft occlusal appliance for clenching. The patient is asked to return every 3 to 4 months during the first year of prosthesis use so that bone changes and occlusal patterns may be evaluated. Hygiene appointments are often every 6 months after the first year, depending on patient conditions (see Fig 28–21).

COMPLETE ARCH, SCREW-RETAINED FIXED PROSTHESIS

The prosthetic steps for the completely screw-retained fixed prosthesis are very similar to the cement-retained prosthesis. An abutment for cement may be used for the progressive loading with an acrylic transitional prosthesis, or a screw-retained temporary may be fabricated. However, more bone loss is observed during the first year. This is related to more common problems related to nonpassive superstructures[29] and unretained restorations (approximately 20% to 50% of the prostheses the first 6 months[30]). Progressive loading is more difficult for overdentures with screw-retained bars. As a result, more steps are taken to limit these complications and improve the quality of bone around the implant abutments. The differences between cement-retained and screw-retained prostheses will be emphasized in this discussion, rather than completely reviewing the previous material.

Initial Abutment Selection and Preliminary Impression

At the first restorative appointment the permucosal extensions are removed and the abutment for screw is placed into the implant bodies. The abutment is not completely tightened into position if it is subgingival, because it will be removed at the conclusion of the appointment. For screw-retained FP-1 fixed prostheses in gingival esthetic regions, the abutment should be 1 to 2 mm below the soft tissue.

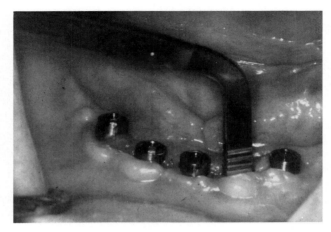

FIG 28–1.
Abutments for screw are inserted into the implant bodies and extend 2 mm above the tissue in the mandible in unesthetic regions. A measuring probe (Nobelpharma) is used to determine the ideal abutment height.

In conditions where gingival esthetics are not involved, the abutment for screw usually is placed 2 mm above the tissue in the mandible for hygiene considerations and level with the tissue in the maxilla to prevent interference with speech as a result of air escaping between the abutments (Fig 28–1). The interarch space is evaluated and must be adequate for placement of the final coping and fixation screw. An indirect impression coping is first inserted and evaluated for correct position regarding implant body loading and the confines of the restoration. An angled abutment for screw may be used if the restoration will be compromised. If this is still inadequate, consideration is given to implant removal and insertion of another implant in the correct position.

An indirect impression transfer aids in visualizing implant body angulation, choosing the final prosthetic abutment, and fabricating a custom tray (Fig 28–2). A preliminary elastic impression is made with irreversible hydrocolloid. To accurately set the teeth for optimal esthetics and location of occlusal plane height, the preliminary impression should capture the soft tissue landmarks for denture construction (retromolar pads, tuberosities, the location of the surrounding unattached mucosa, and the morphology of the residual arch). Syringing the alginate around the impression transfers and tissues facilitates the recording of these landmarks. The preliminary impression is very similar to those for full dentures.

The preliminary impression is inspected. The indirect impression transfers are unscrewed from the abutments and attached to the abutment for screw analogs. No discrepancy should be present. Each indirect impression transfer with analog

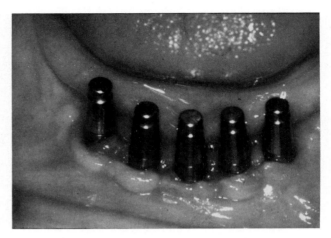

FIG 28–2.
Indirect impression copings are placed into the abutments for screw. If proper load and prosthesis contours can be fabricated, a preliminary impression is made.

is placed carefully into the corresponding hole in the impression. Resistance will be felt, then a snap, which indicates proper seating. The final abutments for screw selected may stay in the patient's mouth when above the tissue. Subgingival abutments are removed and replaced with the permucosal extension. Hygiene covers are placed to protect the threads from calculus and debris. The preexisting tissue conditioner is removed and replaced by a soft liner which is relieved around the abutments. The patient's diet at this time is very soft, and the patient is instructed to leave the prosthesis out of the mouth as much as possible, especially during sleep. The impression is properly trimmed, boxed, and poured in dental stone for fabrication of a working cast.

Laboratory Steps for First Phase

The laboratory step for a complete arch screw-retained prosthesis uses a modified open tray design.[31] The preliminary impressions, with indirect impression copings and abutment analogs, are poured in dental stone (Fig 28–3). The indirect impression transfers are replaced with direct impression transfer copings and screwed on the working cast (Fig 28–4). The impression transfers are blocked out around and between with baseplate wax for approximately 3 mm, except for the top 7 mm of the fixation screws. A 1 mm wax spacer is placed over the residual ridge, with first molar tissue stops. The cast and wax is lightly lubricated with petroleum jelly to prevent the wax from melting to the custom tray (Fig 28–5).

A custom acrylic tray is fabricated on the working cast. The fixation screws protrude 5 mm or more through the top of the tray, yet the tray is intact between and around each screw. The tray does not extend to the soft tissue border, but is

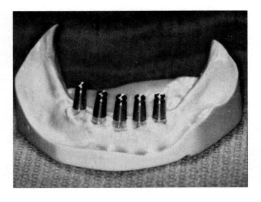

FIG 28–3.
Working cast. Indirect impression copings and abutment for screw analogs are demonstrated.

designed similar to those used for a complete denture impression tray. The impression tray can be removed and inserted without difficulty around the screws (Fig 28–6).

Final Impression

The second prosthetic appointment occurs 1 to 2 weeks after the first appointment, depending on whether soft tissue correction was indicated. Longer periods of time are not indicated, because incremental loading of the implant interface is not possible at this time. Extended periods may even put the implants at risk because they are not splinted but are independent and may have local forces placed upon them. The primary purpose of this appointment is to make the final impression for the master cast. The soft tissue is completely healed at this time. The final abutment may ideally be selected and verified as to fit and position. A peri-implant probing confirms a pocket depth of 3 mm or less. The final

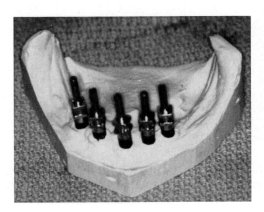

FIG 28–4.
Indirect impression copings are removed from the working cast, and direct impression transfer copings and fixation screws are inserted.

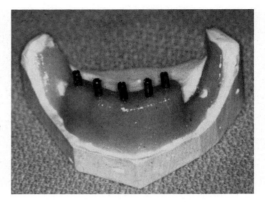

FIG 28–5.
A 3-mm wax spacer is placed around the direct impression transfer copings. The long fixation screws extend 7 or more mm above the wax. A 1 mm wax spacer is used over soft tissue, and first molar tissue stops are designed.

abutment for screw is cemented into the implant body, and care is taken not to trap any soft tissue. If a matching external hex is present on the implant body, the abutment should especially be checked for a complete seat. A radiograph confirms proper placement before the impression is fabricated.

The direct impression transfer copings and fixation screws are placed into the final abutments for screw with firm pressure (Fig 28–7). The custom tray is examined intraorally to ensure that there is adequate space for impression material and that the fixation screws of the direct transfers are accessible, yet do

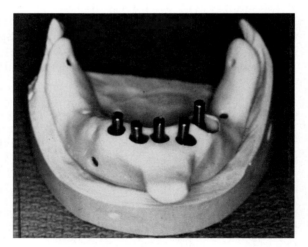

FIG 28–6.
Custom acrylic tray is fabricated on the working cast shown in Figure 28–5. The impression tray can be easily removed from the cast, and the fixation screw extends 5 mm or more above the tray.

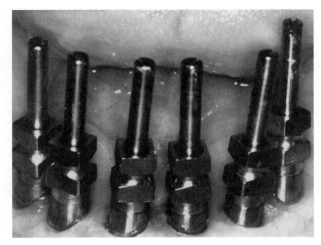

FIG 28–7.
Abutment for screw is cemented into the implant body after ensuring that the patient's soft tissue is healthy. A direct impression transfer coping is placed into the abutment for screw with firm pressure.

not impede the tray placement. Tray adhesive is painted on the internal surface and borders of the tray (Fig 28–8). A very rigid addition silicone is injected around the transfers and into the tray. The custom tray is seated, and any excess is removed from the holes around the screws. The impression tray may be border

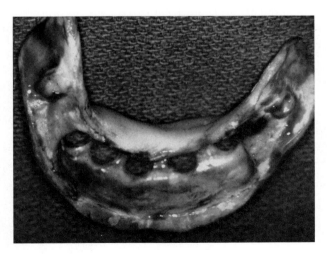

FIG 28–8.
Tray adhesive is painted on the tissue surface and borders of the custom impression tray.

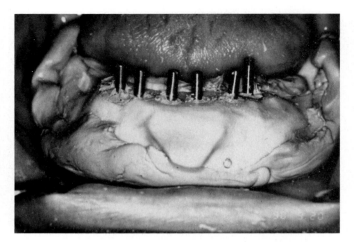

FIG 28–9.
Final impression is made with an addition rigid silicone after border molding the tray similar to a denture fabrication.

molded before the final impression and combines the techniques for denture impressions (Fig 28–9).

After complete setting of the material, the fixation screws are unthreaded and pulled several millimeters to check they are disengaged from the abutments for screw. The direct impression copings are trapped within the impression. The impression and transfer copings are removed and evaluated. No impression material should be present between the impression coping and abutment (Fig 28–10). Hygiene covers are inserted into the abutments for screw to protect the internal threads.

FIG 28–10.
The fixation screws are unthreaded, and the impression is inspected for accuracy. Final impression traps the direct impression transfer copings within the impression.

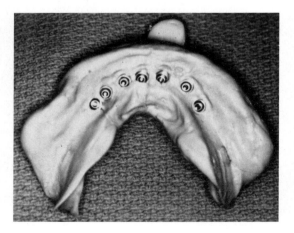

Laboratory Procedure

The corresponding abutment for screw analog is carefully threaded onto the direct impression transfer coping in the impression. The impression is trimmed and boxed with plaster and pumice. Manufacturer guidelines specify the proper amount of dental stone and distilled water. The dental stone is vacuum mixed and vibrated into the impression. Once the stone has set completely, the long screws are removed from the direct impression transfers, and the impression is taken off the master cast (Fig 28–11). The rigid impression transfer copings may be recovered from the impression, sterilized, and reused.

The record base and wax-rim may then be fabricated. The rigid impression transfer copings are secured into position on the master cast. If vertical height is limited, the transfers may be cut in half, or the final precious metal copings may be used. Using 8-gauge sprue wax, the areas around and between the butt joint of the rigid impression transfers and abutment analogs are blocked out to the cast, so only the top two thirds of each coping is visible. The master cast is lightly lubricated with petroleum jelly and incremental portions of acrylic are placed over the posterior residual ridge, incorporating the impression transfer copings. The relief wax prevents acrylic from obscuring the direct vision of the transfer fit to the analogs on the model, or the abutments for screw in the mouth (Fig 28–12). This allows intraoral verification of the accuracy from the final impression at the next appointment. To reduce distortion during shrinkage of the record base, increments of acrylic or light cured resin are applied or a salt and pepper technique used around the copings. Cold-cured acrylic is allowed to set for 24 hours, and light-cured acrylic for 8 to 10 minutes, followed by air barrier coating and cured an additional 3 minutes. The record base is removed, and the borders are finished and polished. A pink baseplate wax rim is applied to the record base, the rim adjusted to approximately 20 mm from the occlusal plane to the vestibule

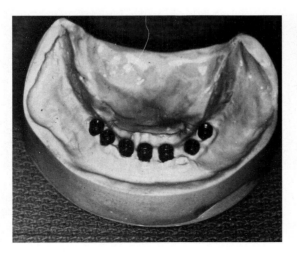

FIG 28–11.
Final impression is boxed and poured in dental stone (see Chapter 30). The separation of the cast demonstrates the master cast and abutment analogs for screw.

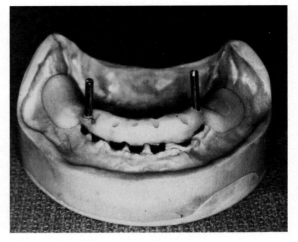

FIG 28–12.
Direct impression transfers are incorporated in the baseplate. The baseplate is fabricated so the abutments for screw and transfer copings are clearly observed. The baseplate is rigid in place while records are established, and the baseplate acts as a verification jig to ensure the accuracy of the master model before the casting is fabricated.

in the labial frenum area. The posterior rim is adjusted to two thirds up the height of the retromolar pad. Openings in the wax are made for the canine or premolar fixation screws on each side of the arch (Fig 28–13).

Wax Try-In and Records

The third prosthetic appointment is scheduled for approximately 1 week later. This appointment is used to verify the fit of the baseplate to the intraoral abutments for screw. Always check the abutments for screw to ensure that they are completely seated. The cement seal may leak (metal to metal does not adhere)

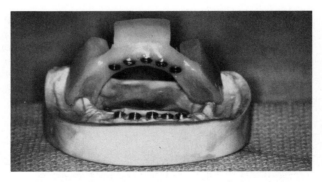

FIG 28–13.
Wax-rim is added to the baseplate, and designed as if it were a final denture. An opening is placed over the canine or premolar region so two fixation screws may firmly seat the baseplate in proper position.

and the abutment unthread a few turns during the week. If any rock or discrepancy exists the baseplate is separated and tried in sections. and/or the incorrect abutment identified. If a stable, accurate fit may be obtained, the laboratory is instructed to cast the superstructure in two (or more) sections separated in the same region(s) as the baseplate, at the proper distance for soldering. At the metal try-in appointment at a future time, the metal superstructure may be joined with acrylic and indexed for soldering in order to provide a passive fit. An alternative approach is to separate the offending impression transfer coping from the baseplate and remake a final impression and master cast.

Once the maxillary base plate or dentition is within the correct position, the vertical maxillo-mandibular relations are established. Centric bite registrations are obtained, as is a facebow recording. Anterior tooth selection regarding size, shape, and shade is made. Protrusive and border movements are also recorded (see Chapter 31).

The diet remains very soft and the patient cautioned to remove the dentures as much as possible, especially at night. A soft protective night splint may be required opposing natural dentition which can be relieved over the implant abutment. The next appointment is in 1 week.

Laboratory Phase

The master casts are mounted on the articulator to the records on the wax-rim. The anterior denture teeth are set for esthetics, phonetics, function, and lip support. The incisal guidance should be as flat as esthetics and phonetics will permit when opposing a denture; this correlates with a protrusive record which enables the condylar guidances of the articulator to be set to an approximation of the condylar path. This record is necessary to develop a balanced occlusal registration for an opposing denture. During this laboratory step, any anterior teeth are modified as required and the posterior teeth are positioned for a medial positioned lingualized occlusion (see Chapter 31). This occlusal scheme incorporates a lingualized occlusion of Payne and Pound and a medial position, bilateral balance, and elevated occlusal plane of the posterior teeth described by the author.

Teeth Try-In

The fourth restorative appointment is 1 week later for a complete screw-retained or supported (FP-1 to RP-4) prosthesis. The baseplate wax model of the teeth is evaluated for esthetics, phonetics, and lip support (Fig 28–14). If these are correct the occlusion is verified for accuracy in centric and excursions. The baseplates are removed, and the hygiene covers are reinserted. The patient's diet remains as soft as possible, and the prostheses are removed at night. The next appointment is in 1 to 2 weeks, depending on the laboratory schedule.

The laboratory fabricates an index of the teeth position on the master cast. The mandibular teeth may also be attached by sticky wax to the maxillary cast. The

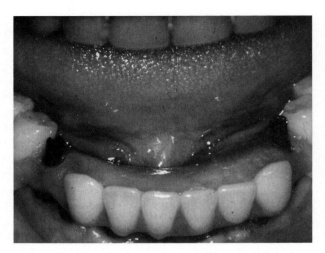

FIG 28–14.
At teeth try-in appointment for the baseplate, esthetics, speech, and occlusion are evaluated.

method of choice uses a vacuum form template made over the facial, occlusal, or incisal, and lingual contours of the try-in restoration. The teeth may be removed from the wax try-in and inserted into the occlusal and incisor portion of the template. The clear template may then be fixed to the opposing cast with sticky wax in the correct occlusal position. In this way the articulator may be opened to permit access to the working cast with analogs, or be closed to relay the position of the contour of denture flange and teeth facial and lingual for the final restoration. In this manner, the bar or superstructure may be affixed to these structures at the proper distance to ensure proper contour, strength, and position (Fig 28–15). Copings are used in the wax-up. Retentive posts, loops and beads are also incorporated. The superstructure is sprued, invested and cast in one piece or in sections, as indicated by size, technique, and verification fit of the base plate jig.

Metal Try-In

The fifth prosthodontic appointment has two purposes. The first is to try-in the superstructure casting and make sure the fit is passive and accurate. Since the acrylic and teeth have not been added at this time, the casting may be more easily evaluated. In addition, if separation and soldering is indicated, it is much easier and more likely to be correctly performed (Fig 28–16). The fixation screws are not completely tightened at this time, especially in D-3 or D-4 bone. Castings are rarely perfectly passive, even though everything appears proper. The copings often are tipped more on the facial or lingual and small openings are evident between the

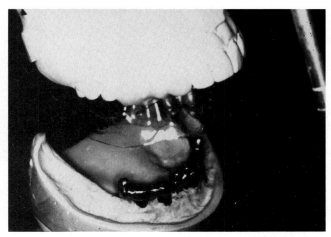

FIG 28–15.
Clear vacuum template is fabricated over the denture teeth and baseplate after verification in the mouth for ideal form (see Figure 28–14). The template is attached to the opposing cast on the articulator. The metal superstructure may be waxed and cast with appreciation for the teeth, facial, and lingual contours of the restoration.

coping and abutment on one side. The first time the implants have received a significant increase in load is during the attachment of the superstructure. The casting is removed, and if any changes were required of the last teeth try-in, a final wax try-in is made of the restoration. The occlusion is evaluated in addition to esthetics and phonetics.

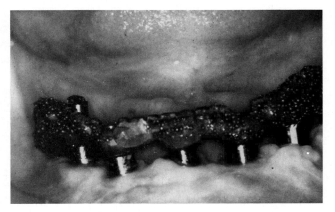

FIG 28–16.
Metal try-in on the abutments for screw. If the copings do not fit all abutments for screw exactly, the casting is separated and luted together in the correct position.

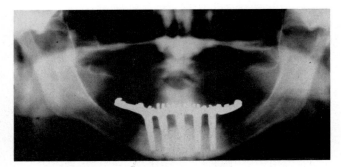

FIG 28–17.
Panoramic radiograph of a FP-3 restoration with anterior root forms in the A, B, C, D, E positions in Division A bone.

Initial Insertion

The sixth prosthetic appointment marks the initial delivery of the prosthesis to the patient. The teeth over the cantilever portions of the restoration are not attached to the superstructure at this time (the bar and retentive elements are visible without teeth). The coping screws are tightened to approximately 10 to 15 newton/cm or two thirds the final amount of force to be applied. Because the superstructure is rarely completely passive, bone must remodel around regions of tension and compression. The occlusion is carefully evaluated to make sure as much vertical load as possible is distributed to the implant body. A panoramic radiograph is taken and compared with surgical placement to establish new baseline information for future evaluation (Fig 28–17). Hygiene protocol is stressed, and the recommended diet is of a soft masticatory nature. This is the first time the implants have been loaded for an extended period. The holes over the coping screws may be filled with addition silicone or a tissue liner. This occludes the opening in the prosthesis, but permits easy removal with an explorer at future appointments. The patient is asked to return in a few days so that tightness of the screws and the occlusion can be evaluated.

Upon the patient's return, the screws are evaluated. Any loose screws require greater application of torque than at the last appointment. If any screws are loose the patient is asked to return again in a few days. If the screws are still firm, the patient is asked to return in 4 weeks.

Short-Term Evaluation

At the seventh prosthetic appointment 4 weeks later the tightness of the screws are evaluated, then the prosthesis is removed. Evaluation of the implants for tissue health, pocket depth, rigid fixation, and any tenderness under vertical or lateral force is performed. The prosthesis is inspected for calculus and plaque retention. The prosthesis is reinserted and the screws tightened with a torque wrench to 20 newtons/cm. The texture of the patient's diet may be increased to a normal consistency. Hard foods are still avoided, especially in cases of D-3 or D-4 bone. Parafunction must be addressed and eliminated by prosthesis removal or decreased with acrylic guards. The patient with D-1 bone is asked to return in 4 weeks, with 2 months for D-2 bone, 3 months for D-3 bone, and 4 months for D-4 bone.

Final Delivery

The eighth prosthetic step is to cold cure the teeth to the distal cantilever portions of the casting (Fig 28–18). The abutments are evaluated as before while the restoration is removed. The screws are evaluated for loosening or breakage. If either is present, the occlusion is carefully evaluated; rocking forces often cause screws to vibrate loose. The patient is instructed to return if any changes in occlusion, movement of the restoration, or tenderness occurs. The patient may use a normal diet. Preventive maintenance appointments are scheduled for every 3 to 4 months during the first year that the implants are in place. The eight prosthetic appointments require 3 to 4 months for D-1 bone and 6 to 7 months for D-4 bone. As a result, total treatment time is approximately 8 months for patients with D-1 bone and 15 months for those with D-4 bone. Total treatment time for those with D-2 bone is 8 months; and for those with D-3 bone, 11 months. The

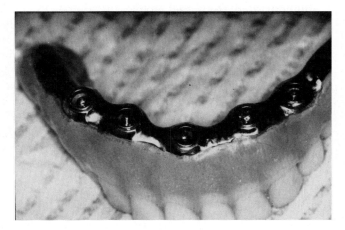

FIG 28–18.
FP-3 restoration in a patient with five anterior root forms in a Division C mandible. The anterior-posterior distance is 10 mm, and the posterior teeth are cold cured to the restoration after 2 months when the bone density is D-2. Note that the position of the teeth permit an axial load on the implants whenever possible.

additional time permits remodeling around the screw-retained superstructures, evaluation of screw retention security, and gradual increase of loads to the implants during the last aspects of the reconstruction.

PARTIALLY EDENTULOUS FIXED PROSTHESES

Variations of the previous described progressive loading sequence may be used for fixed prostheses in the partially edentulous patient. The protocol for prostheses retained by cement may be used in all regions of the mouth with little modification. A screw-retained restoration on occasion requires a fixed transitional restoration. This is easily accomplished by removing the abutment(s) for screw and replace abutment(s) for cement for the interim restoration. However, it is usually easier in these patients to use a cement-retained restoration as the final prosthesis (see Chapter 29).

RP-5 PROSTHESES

The progressive loading concept is used least in placing the RP-5 restoration, which has a combination of soft tissue and implant support. The superstructure is most always screw retained to decrease the crown height and reduce the moment load from the mobile prosthesis. In addition, more space over the low-profile superstructure permits placement of denture teeth without modification. The treatment plan is modified so that there are fewer implants, and thus less implant support and more prosthesis movement. The prosthesis may be removed before the patient sleeps, which decreases the amount of parafunction. In addition, the fewer the implants used, the less variables there are for the superstructure fit, and the casting is more likely to be passive. Distortion of the casting during acrylic or porcelain processing is also eliminated. Overdentures primarily use anterior implants which more often have an ideal D-2 density of supporting bone. As a result of these factors, progressive loading is least necessary for RP-5 restorations with two to four implants.

SUMMARY

Rigid fixation after initial bone healing is primarily the result of the surgery and no movement at the interface during healing. Maintenance of rigid fixation during the first year of prosthesis construction and function with minimum bone loss is related to the formation of lamellar bone and the bone remodeling process. The progressive bone loading approach provides load-bearing bone at the implant interface in two ways. An extended time period is permitted before functional forces are transmitted. During the extended period vertical force is the dominant component. In addition, a gradual increase in loads permits the physiology of bone to respond to the additional load. The increase in bone may be evidenced by radiography, decreased mobility, increased implant survival, and improved crestal bone conditions around the implant compared to an immediate loading protocol. Bidez and Misch[32] performed a three-dimensional finite stress analysis on the bone volumes of Division A, B, and C-w patients. Each volume of bone had cortical and trabecular bone models with four macroscopic densities of bone which correspond to D-1 (100%), D-2 (75%), D-3 (50%), and D-4 (25%). The anatomic ridge form impacted the strength of bone, and a correlation of bone volume and bone density was observed. Clinical failure was mathematically predicted in D-4 bone and some D-3 densities, related to bone volume. Hence, progressive loading is strongly suggested in poor bone density and/or less than ideal anatomic ridge forms (Plates 82 and 83).

REFERENCES

1. Branemark P-I, Zarb G, Albrektsson T: *Tissue integrated prostheses,* Chicago, 1985, Quintessence.
2. Adell R et al: A 15-year study of osseointegrated implants in the treatment of the edentulous jaw, *Int J Oral Surg* 6:387–416, 1981.
3. Schnitman PA et al: Implants for partial edentulism, *J Dent Educ* 52:725–736, 1988.
4. Jaffin RA, Berman CL: The excessive loss of Branemark fixtures in type IV bone: a 5-year analysis, *J Periodontol* 62(1):2–4, 1991.
5. Misch CE: Density of bone: effect on treatment plans, surgical approach, healing and progressive bone loading, *Int J Oral Implant* 6:23–31, 1990.
6. Misch CE: Bone character: second vital implant criterion, *Dent Today* June/July 1988, pp 39–40.
7. Niznick G, Misch CE: The Core-Vent system of osseointegrated implants, in Clark JW, editor: *Clinical dentistry,* Philadelphia, 1988, Harper and Row, pp 1–11.
8. Misch CE: *Protect the prosthesis* (manual). Misch Implant Institute, 1990.
9. Lekholm U, Zarb GA: Patient selection and preparation, in Branemark P-I, Zarb GA, Albrektsson T, editors: *Tissue integrated prostheses: osseointegration in clinical dentistry,* Chicago, 1985, Quintessence, pp 199–209.
10. Geiser M, Treua J: Muscle rarefication and bone formation, *J Bone Joint Surg* 40:282, 1958.
11. Kararian LE, Von Gierke HE: Bone loss as a result of immobilization and chelation: preliminary results in *Macaca mulatta, Clin Orthop Rel Res* 65:67, 1969.
12. Minaire MC et al: Quantitative histological data on disuse osteoporosis: comparison with biological data, *Calcif Tissue Res* 17:57, 1974.

13. Allisson N, Brooks B: An experimental study of the changes in bone which result from non-use, *Surg Gynecol Obstet* 33:250, 1921.

14. Parfitt AM: Investigation of the normal variations in the alveolar bone trabeculation, *Oral Surg Oral Med Oral Pathol* 15:1453–1463, 1962.

15. MacMillan HW: Structural characteristics of the alveolar process, *Int J Orthod* 12:722–730, 1926.

16. Roberts WE et al: Bone physiology and metabolism, *J Calif Dent Assoc* 15:54–61, 1987.

17. Aloia JF et al: Prevention of involutional bone loss by exercise, *Ann Intern Med* 89:356, 1978.

18. DeAngelis V: Observations on the response of alveolar bone to orthodontic force, *Am J Orthod* 58:284–294, 1970.

19. Dahlin N, Olsson KE: Bone mineral content and physical activity, *Acta Orthop Scand* 45:170, 1974.

20. Braggen U et al: Digital substraction radiography for the assessment of changes in peri-implant bone density, *Int J Oral Maxillofac Implants* 6:160–166, 1991.

21. Strid KG: Radiographic results of tissue integrated prostheses, in Branemark P-I, Zarb GA, Albrektsson T, editors: Chicago, 1985, Quintessence, p 191.

22. Roberts WE, Garetto LP, DeCastro RA: Remodeling of demineralized bone threatens periosteal implants with threaded or smooth surfaces, *J Indiana Dent Assoc* 68:19–24, 1989.

23. Plenk H Jr et al: Experimental comparison of Branemark and Ledermann type titanium dental screw implants in sheep, abstract, First World Congress of Implants and Biomaterials, Paris, 1989.

24. Misch CE: Progressive bone loading, *Pract Periodont Esthet Dent* 2:27–30, 1990.

25. Pierazzini A et al: Peri-implant histological reactions: preliminary observations and experimental research, *Int J Oral Implant* 8:33–41, 1991.

26. Misch CE: The Periotest evaluation of progressively loaded implants, a two-year evaluation (submitted for publication).

27. Misch CE, Dietsh F: Maxillary anterior tooth contour for fixed partial dentures to the dental technician, *J Prosthet Dent* 67(2):120, 1992.

28. Dawson PE: *Evaluation, diagnosis, and treatment of occlusal problems,* ed 2, St Louis, 1989, CV Mosby.

29. Assif D et al: Comparative accuracy of implant impression procedures, *Int J Periodontol Rest Dent* 12:113–121, 1992.

30. Jemt T, Linden B, Lekholm U: Failures and complications in 127 consecutively placed fixed partial prostheses supported by Branemark implants: from prosthetic treatment to first annual checkup, *Int J Oral Maxillofac Implants* 7:40–44, 1992.

31. Hobo S, Ichida E, Garcia LT: *Osseointegration and occlusal rehabilitation,* Chicago, 1990, Quintessence, pp 153–162.

32. Bidez M, Misch CE: Bone anatomy and density as determined by finite stress analysis, Lecture, Alabama Implant Study Group Congress XVI, Birmingham, Alabama, May 1991.

Chapter 29

Principles of Cement-Fixed Prosthodontics and Implant Dentistry

Carl E. Misch

PROTECTION OF THE PROSTHESIS

Implant dentistry requires a complex blend of diagnosic, treatment planning, surgical, prosthetic and maintenance skills in order to achieve maximum success rates. A predictable surgical protocol for endosteal rigid fixation was developed and reported by Branemark and associates in a report by Adell et al.[1] However, on occasion, an implant may fail during the initial healing process from poor surgery, poor case selection, or unknown reasons. The patient understands that medicine is not an exact science, and believes that human bodies may have individual variation in response to similar procedures. As a result, they are inclined to accept the implant failure.

Once the implant is uncovered, and the patient told it is acceptable, any short-term complications that lead to implant loss or compromise become unacceptable. Overcontoured restorations or future bone loss on poorly angled implant bodies are rarely attributed to the implant surgeon. The additional time and laboratory costs of inventive prosthetics required on incorrect implant placement are not appreciated by the patient. Patients may feel that bone loss or implant loss resulted because the screws were too tight, the casting did not fit adequately, the occlusion was incorrect, or a screw became loose from other implants. All these factors make patient management more difficult for the restoring dentist.

The discipline of implant dentistry has continued to mature under the guidance of practitioners and researchers who interface with this special segment of medicine. New or improved approaches and concepts are often initially overutilized or overstated as to their specific niche to the overall scheme of patient treatment. Often these new concepts center around the surgical aspect of oral implantology. However, while short-term evaluation of surgical protocols are beneficial, all attempts should be made to protect the long-term results affecting the restoring dentist and prosthesis. The patient can rarely evaluate the cause of implant surgical failure. However, the patient can evaluate all aspects of the prosthetic treatment. The esthetics, occlusion, function, speech, and hygiene considerations of the final restoration are able to be closely scrutinized by many patients and/or their friends.

The time required to remove a failed implant and place an additional implant is often minimal, and this may often be accomplished at the second stage surgical appointment. The time required to restore a patient is usually five or more prosthetic appointments. An implant that fails after the final prosthesis is fabricated may result in five more additional appointments and an additional laboratory fee.

The restoring dentist should not use a malpositioned tooth for a prosthesis without the patient's awareness of the compromise of such a treatment. Orthodontic treatment or extraction is often suggested rather than compromise the final prosthesis. Yet, all too often implants are considered successful when they are not mobile, and proper placement, angulation, attached tissue, sulcus depth, and surface area requirements are not appreciated. Acceptable conditions should be established or the limiting factors appreciated prior to the prosthetic reconstruction, to decrease the occurrence of restoration, maintenance, or patient management complications. As stated in Chapter 1, the goal of implant dentistry is to return a patient to normal contour, comfort, function, esthetics, speech, and health. The implants and prosthesis are responsible for this goal. Time and consideration should be addressed to both vital components.[2]

CEMENT- VS. SCREW-RETAINED ABUTMENTS

Advantages of Cement-Retained Prostheses

A cement-retained implant prosthesis offers several advantages over a screw-retained fixed partial denture (Fig 29–1; Table 29–1). The superstructure is more passive, because the 40-μ cement space may even extend to the margin of the restoration, as decay is not a problem with implants. A space around the screw portion of a retained restoration does not permit rigid fixation and is contraindicated. A screw is a combination of inclined planes and wedges and is one of the most efficient machine designs. A torque force of 20 newtons/cm applied on a screw can move two railroad cars. This same force on a nonpassive casting has a tendency to distort the implant, the superstructure, the bone, or a combination of these. An implant does not predictably move within the bone, yet retained

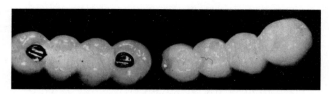

FIG 29–1.
Screw-retained restoration and cement-retained prosthesis each has unique advantages and disadvantages.

stresses from nonpassive castings must be alleviated by a bone remodeling process. This is a considerable advantage for cemented prostheses, because unpassive castings are a prime cause of unretained restorations, crestal bone loss, implant component fracture, and implant mobility.

Metal superstructures are often thicker and larger in implant prosthetics than in traditional prosthetics because the implant abutment is only 4 mm in diameter. As a result, dimensional changes during metalwork fabrication are greater. Large areas of porcelain may also distort the superstructure through shrinkage during the firing process. The final impression; placement of the abutment analog; and dimensional changes of dental die stone, wax, metal, and porcelain all become critical factors for a passive casting.

TABLE 29–1.

Advantages of Cement-Retained Vs. Screw-Retained Restorations

Cement-Retained	Screw-Retained
More passive superstructure	Passive superstructure difficult
Easy correction of nonpassive superstructure (same appointment)	Correction of nonpassive casting difficult (another appointment and laboratory fee required)
Axial load over implant easier	Axial load on implant is over screw; requires more chair time and material that wears (or more expensive, two-piece superstructure)
Traditional prosthetic techniques and laboratory skills used; decreased cost of components, lab fees	Special training, doctor and laboratory; expensive special components; additional fees
Easier esthetics control; progressive loading more gradual; abutments may be splinted to decrease overload	Screw loosening in about 20% to 50%; increased forces on remaining abutments, gradual loading more difficult
Less fracture of acrylic or porcelain; cement failure or partial retained restoration uncommon	Screw holes provide weakened area for fracture of porcelain or acrylic; long-term screw fatigue fracture and component loosening from wear
Easier access to posterior abutments	Access may be difficult in posterior of mouth with limited opening
Fewer appointments and less time to restore patient	More time and appointments required to restore patient

If a cemented prosthesis is not passive, the casting or abutment may be slightly modified at the try-in appointment. High-speed carbides with copious amounts of water may alter the abutment, the internal aspect of the casting, or both, and may provide an immediate solution. A screw-in prosthesis that is not passive requires separation and soldering of the casting or a new impression. The separation of the metal superstructure must be within correct dimensions. Too much space causes shrinkage and a weak joint; too little space may cause distortion from expansion during heating of the metal. Indexing the separate pieces also requires more time. The patient must return for another appointment after the laboratory process of soldering, which includes an additional laboratory fee in most offices. The more abutments in a prosthesis, the more difficult it is to fabricate passive screw-retained restorations.

Because the occlusal surface is intact in a cement-retained prosthesis, the implant body may be loaded in an axial direction in order to decrease crestal bone loads. However, to load an occlusal screw-retained restoration in an axial direction, the screw region must be loaded. Acrylic or composite resin is placed and loaded over the top of the screw, or a two-piece superstructure design is fabricated. Acrylic fillers require more chair time and wear more rapidly, and two-piece superstructures are costly.

The esthetics of a cemented prosthesis are easier to manage. A post too facial may be prepared as a natural tooth. A screw-retained restoration to the facial requires a more costly angled abutment or a substructure, each of which requires additional time, cost, and effort. The occlusal holes in the posterior screw-retained restorations may affect the occlusion and esthetics. Prosthesis redesign, required in about 10% of the restorations, includes an abutment for screw that is too angled or too far above the tissue for ideal esthetics. This must be exchanged for a different abutment component and a new final impression obtained.[4] A margin may be extended further apical on an abutment for cement, without an additional component or impression, when an abutment analog is used in the master model.

A progressive loading of the prosthesis requires modification of the transitional prosthesis and is easier to perform for cement-retained restorations. Often an interim abutment for cement is used in screw-retained prostheses for the transitional restorations and the gradual bone loading process. If this is not performed, the implant is not loaded until the final prosthesis is screwed into place. Progressive loading is more difficult and, in addition, the implant abutments remain independent during the prosthesis fabrication and may be subjected to excessive forces from parafunction on the transitional overdenture.

Partially unretained restorations are reported for approximately 20% to 50% of screw-in prostheses during the first 6 months they are in place.[3, 4] Every time a screw vibrates loose, the rest of the abutments bear an additional force. The forces include increased moment and offset loads, and additional forces on the remaining abutments. Increased loads may lead to implant loss, implant component fracture, and bone loss. However, in clinical trials, reports of an unretained cemented implant prosthesis have occurred in fewer than 5% of cases. In traditional prosthetics, uncemented prostheses result in less than 3% restoration failure.[5] Therefore the cement-retained restoration has reduced associated risks.

More fracture of porcelain or acrylic portions of the prosthesis occur with screw-retained restorations because the screw hole increases stress concentration to the restoring material. A cement-retained prosthesis does not have the weak link through the surface of the materials, and the superstructure is more passive when inserted. Once the material fractures, the repair site is weaker than the original strength, and additional fractures are more common. Patient concerns and psychologic comfort with the prosthesis often are affected.

Fewer and shorter prosthetic appointments are required to restore a patient with a cemented prosthesis than with a screw-retained restoration. Passive castings, progressive loading, appointments to evaluate or redo retention, and esthetics management are less complex for cemented prostheses. Additional appointments are required for the screw-retained restorations.

Access is more difficult in the posterior regions of the mouth for insertion of screw-retained restorations, especially with limited jaw opening. Because titanium and gold are not magnetic, the manipulation of small screws and screwdrivers is more challenging than preparing and cementing a restoration.

A complication that occurs with screw-retained prostheses over the long term is fatigue failure of the screw components. The diameter of the prosthesis retention screws are so narrow that long-term strength is reduced. Wearing of the threads in the abutment for screw also occur when the restoration is repeatedly removed, and reinserted over several years. As a result, screw fracture and component loosening increase in frequency for long-term restorations. Because cemented prosthesis have no small-diameter components and no metal-to-metal wearing, such complications are rarely observed.

Advantages of Screw-Retained Prostheses

The primary advantage of a screw-retained superstructure is the possible lower profile abutment system. Cemented prostheses require a vertical component to increase retention and provide resistance form. The screw-retained system is more resistant to forces than the cement abutment when the abutment height is less than 5 mm. The low-profile abutment offers significant advantages for RP-4 or RP-5 restorations. The lower height of the superstructure permits easier placement of denture teeth. The greater volume of acrylic also increases the strength of the acrylic portion of the restoration.

The moment force is reduced with a low-profile abutment, when stress breakers on the superstructure separate the prosthesis from the implant support. These elements decrease the effect of lateral loads on the implant body. Therefore, greater retention, reduced moment force, and more space for denture teeth and acrylic are indications for screw-retained superstructures for most overdenture prostheses supported by implants and low-profile abutments.

A perceived advantage of a screw-retained restoration is ease of retrieval; however, a cemented restoration on implant abutments does not require use of a permanent cement. A soft access or temporary cement may be satisfactory and provide adequate retention and resistance. Provisional cemented restorations on natural teeth are retrievable. It is often easier to remove, clean, and reinsert a cemented restoration, compared with a screw-retained restoration, especially when the access holes over the screws have been restored.

Fixed partial dentures on natural teeth have a 10-year survival rate of 75%.[5] Implant-supported fixed prostheses have a 10-year survival rate above 95%.[1, 6, 7] Clinical observation suggests that when an implant is joined to a natural tooth, the natural tooth is the most common site of complications. Natural teeth may decay and require endodontic therapy or restoration, and have greater incidence of periodontal problems. Therefore, the question arises why an implant restoration must use screws to be retrievable, yet natural abutments may be cemented? Why should a prosthesis be cemented on the natural tooth, require a precision attachment in the pontic, and require an occlusal screw on an implant? If a screw-in restoration is indicated to help solve the most common source of complications, it should be screwed into the natural tooth. Treatment plans that require all implant prostheses to be screw retrievable, yet continue to use permanent cement on natural abutments, are inconsistent in approach and should be reevaluated. In fact, the need for prosthesis removal is often justified by the need to address problems that have evolved from a screw-retained procedure. Clinical experience, case series studies, and implant registries indicate higher complication rates and lower implant survival with screw retained fixed partial dentures.[6–8]

Each prosthesis should be evaluated for the retention system of the prosthesis *before* surgery. In a screw-retained fixed prosthesis, implants should be placed more lingual than in a cement-retained restoration because correction of facial implants and axial loading over the access hole is more difficult. Considerable advantage of fixed prostheses are observed with cement-retained restorations, including passive castings, direction of load, cost, time, esthetics, access, progressive loading, and reduced complications. Removable restorations do not require modification of surgical placement for the abutments for screw or cement because the height of the superstructure often requires that the implant be slightly more lingual to the anterior incisor edge with either type abutment.

CEMENT-RETAINED FIXED PROSTHESES

The long-term survival of fixed prostheses on natural teeth is well documented. Fixed prostheses on implants in partially edentulous patients have provided equal or superior survival rates during the past 10 years. The causes leading to the replacement of the restoration may primarily be classified into poor diagnosis or treatment planning, poor preparation or fabrication of the restoration, and poor patient cooperation or maintenance after delivery of the prosthesis. Retrospective studies that list the causes for fixed prosthesis failure permit fine tuning of the fundamental principles of fixed prosthodontics and highlight the areas where more attention to detail is required.

The three most common causes of failure of fixed prostheses on natural teeth are caries of abutment teeth, uncemented restorations, and porcelain fracture.[5] The most common causes for failure of cement-retained implant supported restorations include fracture of prostheses or implant components, bone loss, and unretained restorations. Therefore, force factors account for the most common complications for implant prostheses and two thirds of fixed restorations on natural teeth. Once the diagnosis and treatment plan are properly established, the most common cause of excessive forces for the cemented prosthesis may be too rapid loading, faulty occlusal scheme, and partially retained restorations. The combination of natural teeth and implants within the same prosthesis further complicates the biomechanical conditions.

Caries and Abutments

Implant dentistry often requires complete oral rehabilitation. Natural teeth are prepared for abutments, the restoration of the proper occlusal plane, occlusion, or a combination of these. Periodontal disease or extrusion is common, and the cemental surfaces of these teeth are often exposed after periodontal therapy and soft tissue management. The exposed cemental areas of teeth decay easier than the enamel surface, especially if used for a crown margin.

The most common cause of natural abutment failure is caries. Therefore, methods that reduce decay on restored teeth should be addressed. Factors include margin location, medicaments, and uncemented restorations. A common axiom in restorative dentistry is to establish supragingival margins whenever possible. Subgingival restorations are indicated for preexisting caries, replacement of preexisting restorations, esthetics, retention, root fracture, improving hygiene considerations in furca or crowded teeth, and root sensitivity.[9] If the crown margin does not belong in at least one of these seven categories, a supragingival margin design is indicated. The main goal is to decrease the risk of gingival inflammation.[10] The indication for subgingival margins on implant abutments include only esthetics and retention.

If the supragingival crown margin concept is slightly modified to design margins on enamel, the risk of caries is also reduced. Therefore, the supragingival axiom may be replaced by the enamel margin criterion in patients with cementum above the gingiva. In addition, the lingual aspect of any tooth is rarely involved in esthetics, caries, or root sensitivity. If additional retention is not needed or previous restorative margins are not below the enamel, the lingual margin may be both supragingival and on enamel. Additional advantages of margins on enamel include the elimination of hemorrhage during tooth preparation and impression procedures, and improvement of homecare procedures, as the interproximal regions allow greater access for direct, mechanical methods of plaque removal. In addition, lingual tooth sensitivity is reduced because a common cause for sensitivity is cementum removal for margin preparation and final crown margins short of the prepared margin, with dentine exposure (Fig 29–2).

Caries may be further reduced by the topical applications of fluoride by a professional and as a part of daily homecare. The progressive bone loading process involves five clinical appointments during which prepared teeth are covered by provisional restorations. All five appointments require removal of the provisional restoration and represent an opportunity to apply fluoride directly on the surfaces of the prepared tooth. These applications also minimize tooth sensitivity. A daily application of the neutral fluoride and fluoride in toothpastes to crown margins helps prevent caries on the abutment teeth and is prescribed as part of the normal homecare regimen. Because decay is the primary cause of fixed prosthesis replacement, fluoride, rather than chlorhexidine, is used on natural restored teeth. Fluoride may also be found in the glass ionomer cements used for final cementation, which may provide an increased fluoride uptake in the tooth structure around the margins.

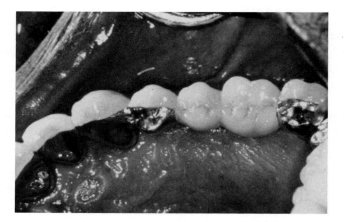

FIG 29–2.
Anterior teeth have the lingual finish line on enamel to reduce decay and tooth sensitivity. The lingual metal permits less tooth preparation, which decreases tooth sensitivity, and if endodontics is required in the future, reduces porcelain fracture around the access hole. The independent posterior implant prosthesis with occlusal rest on the mesiad has metal on the occlusal aspect to permit greater abutment height to improve retention (the patient desired porcelain occlusal, but modified opinion when the uncemented complication was explained).

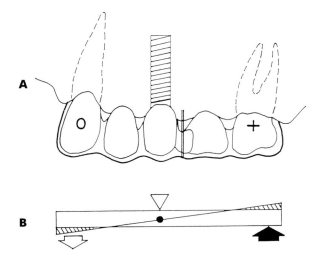

FIG 29–3.
Implant as a pier abutment between two natural teeth is more likely to cause an unretained abutment, especially if one of the teeth has clinical mobility. **A,** precision attachment that permits some movement (rod and tube) may be placed between the implant and the mobile abutment. For example, in this figure the posterior tooth (+) is mobile. The attachment is placed on the distal aspect of the implant, so molar movement will not be transmitted to the implant. This not only stops the implant from acting as a fulcrum but decreases the load to the implant, because the molar abutment may act as a cantilever pontic during occlusal loading. **B,** implant acts as a fulcrum, and the nonmobile tooth will become uncemented.

Caries are also a consequence of a partially uncemented prosthesis. Natural and implant abutments in the same prosthesis may develop biomechanical complications and result in an uncemented restoration on the implant abutment. However, when an implant serves as a pier abutment, the natural tooth may become uncemented, because the implant may act as a fulcrum (Fig 29–3). Retention of the restoration is critical to avoidance of this complication.

Abutment Retention

Partially retained restorations are a cause of failure of teeth and of implant-supported prostheses. The principles of retention and resistance may be addressed specifically for implant abutments. The retention of a fixed-cemented restoration prevents the removal of the retainer along the path of insertion. The resistance opposes movement of the abutment under occlusal load and prevents removal of the restoration by forces applied in an apical or oblique direction. Cements have lower retention strengths compared with their resistance strengths.

The geometric configurations of the implant abutment for cement or prepared tooth are requisites to avoid uncementation.

Taper

The retention of a crown rapidly diminishes as the taper is increased from 6 to 25 degrees.[11] A typical tapered diamond bur shows a taper of approximately 3 degrees on each side. Ames et al. found that actual clinical cases possess a tapered range of approximately 20 degrees.[12] A manufactured implant abutment for cement often has a taper in excess of 25 degrees. As a result, the retentive surfaces of unprepared implant abutments may provide less retention than natural abutments. Therefore, the preparation of implant abutments is usually necessary, even when the path of insertion is proper (Fig 29–4).

Surface Area

The surface area of a crown or implant abutment influences the amount of retention.[13] A molar abutment offers greater retention than a premolar. The diameter of an implant abutment for cement is often less than 4 mm, which is comparable to that of a prepared mandibular incisor. Therefore, the decreased surface area results in poorer retention than most natural abutments. As a result, other criteria that affect retention should be employed.

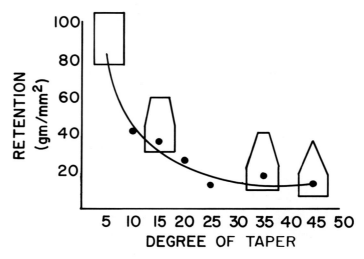

FIG 29–4.
Degree of abutment taper significantly alters the amount of retention. This is more important for implant abutments, because most are only 4 mm in diameter. (Modified from Shillinburg HT, Jacobi R, Brackett SE: Fundamentals of tooth preparation. Chicago, 1987, Quintessence, pp 19–23.)

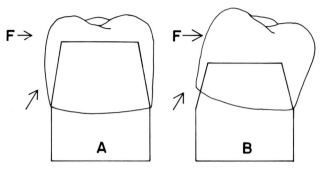

FIG 29–5.
Height of the preparation affects retention and the resistance to lateral forces.

Height

The height of preparation is an important factor in the amount of retention.[14] A long preparation offers more retention than a short abutment. The additional height not only increases the surface area, but also places more axial walls under tensile stress rather than shear stress. Also, the height of a preparation is closely related to the amount of resistance (see Fig 29–2). The higher the abutment, the greater the cement resistance to lateral forces. A higher abutment also decreases the amount of crown above the implant abutment, and also provides increased cement resistance and less torque on the cemented region (Fig 29–5). The lever arm above the abutment for cement is magnified in a fixed partial denture with a cantilever. The height of the implant abutment farthest from the cantilever is the major factor for resistance when a load is applied in the cantilever region. Premanufactured implant abutments are often 5, 7, or 9 mm in height. Some manufacturers only supply 5-mm-high abutments. Although this is usually adequate in the posterior regions of the mouth, a FP-3 anterior prosthesis often may require longer implant abutments. An additional 2 mm height may increase retention 40%, especially when the abutment is only 4 mm in diameter.

Roughness

The surface roughness increases the retention of a restoration, because the cement creates a mechanical microretention by projecting into the irregularities.[15] Cements do not adhere to an implant abutment as with enamel or dentinal adhesive cements on natural teeth; therefore, a course diamond is used over the surface of the implant abutment to increase the amount and depth of these microscopic scratches on the surface to more than 40 μm. A cross-cut fissure bur and water spray are used to reduce the height and gross reduction of the metal abutment post. A coarse diamond is used afterward to increase roughness above the abutment margin. Several manufacturers provide abutments for cement with retention lines 1 mm apart, which increase mechanical retention and also help determine the proper abutment height. A microetcher may be used within the crown for additional retention before cementation.

Shear Forces

Since the introduction of implant-supported cantilevered prostheses for the completely edentulous arch, the cantilever has become a more accepted modality in implant dentistry, and has entered treatment plans for the partially edentulous patient. Implants are often placed more medial than the occlusal or incisal contacts of the attached prostheses. Both conditions place offset loads to the implant abutments and result in greater tensile and shear forces on cement or screw fixation.

The surface area of an abutment submitted to shear forces is more critical than the total surface area for tensile stress.[9] It is therefore critical to limit sheer stresses by reducing the directions in which the crown may be removed from the abutment to as few as possible. A tapered implant abutment post may have multiple paths of insertion or removal. The addition of two or more parallel-sided grooves to an abutment limits the withdrawal path of the crown to one direction.[16] Therefore, whenever possible, retentive elements such as grooves parallel to the path of withdrawal should be added to a narrow, tapered implant abutment for cement (Fig 29–6).

Manufactured implant abutments for cement are often smooth and circular in cross section. There is very little resistance to shear forces, especially on individual, unsplinted crowns. Grooves parallel to the path of insertion mechanically resist rotational forces, place compressive forces on the cement in these regions, and dramatically improve cementation.

The moment of a force produces rotation or bending. The moment is defined as a vector, *M,* whose magnitude equals the product of the force magnitude

FIG 29–6.
Tapered implant abutment may have many paths of removal. Addition of parallel grooves limits the path of removal to one direction. (Modified from Shillinburg HT, Jacobi R, Brackett SE: Fundamentals of tooth preparation. Chicago, 1987, Quintessence, pp 19–23.)

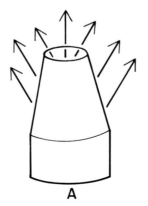
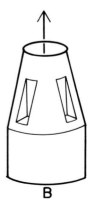

A   B

multiplied by the perpendicular distance (also called "moment arm") from the point of interest to the line of action of the force (see Chapter 15). The imposed moment load is also referred to as torque or torsional load and may be quite destructive with respect to implant systems. Torque or bending moments placed on implants as a consequence of, for example, cantilever bridges or bar sections, may result in interface breakdown, bone resorption, prosthetic screws loosening, and/or superstructure fracture. Proper restorative designs must necessarily include considerations for both forces and moments due to those forces (torque). The tensile and shear forces on the abutment retention system from posterior cantilever bar/pontics may be reduced by placing vertical grooves on the buccal and lingual of the posterior abutments. As a result, the arc of the force on the restoration is mechanically altered.[9]

Resistance and Abutments

The resistance opposes the uncementation of the prosthesis against forces directed in an apical, oblique, or horizontal direction.[9] Resistance is usually greater than retention by the abutment. Cement failures are rare in compression, as compared with shear or tensile stresses. Forces most likely to cause uncemented restorations related to resistance are associated with long spans, cantilever forces, mobile natural abutment teeth joined to implants, offset loading, horizontal loads from occlusal design, and parafunction.

When a force is directed within the margins of the abutment crowns, no leverage or tipping forces exist. However, for implant-supported prostheses, forces often are projected away from the abutment, usually toward the facial in the anterior or posterior direction. In addition, excursive forces on anterior teeth also create a leverage force, especially on maxillary anterior abutments. The forces affect not only the bone-implant interface, but the cemented abutment crown. The arc of rotation of the crown is affected by the direction of forces. The surface of the preparation opposite the fulcrum (or direction of the cantilever) provides the resistance for uncementation. The resistance of the abutment for cement to a moment of force is enhanced by minimal tapering and maximum height, especially on the side opposite to the fulcrum point.

Facial offset loads on a cement-retained prosthesis may be reduced by vertical grooves on the mesial and distal of the restoration.[17] The same locations are beneficial when horizontal forces are introduced from a mutually protected occlusion and/or bruxism.

A wider diameter implant abutment has more retention, but may offer *less* resistance to leverage than a narrow post, even when the height and taper are similar. The wider abutment for cement has a longer axis of rotation, and the resisting area at the opposite side of the preparation is reduced. The resistance form of a short, wide implant abutment, in a molar region, for example, is significantly increased by placing boxes or grooves perpendicular to the arc of rotation, provided the path of insertion is preserved.[17]

Path of Insertion

The path of insertion of the restoration should not be the same as the direction of the load during mastication. Whenever the fixed partial denture path of insertion is the same as the direction of the occlusal forces there will be less retention while chewing sticky foods. Therefore, it is suggested the path of insertion should be approximately 15 degrees different from the axial load of the implant during occlusion, to improve resistance to bridge uncementation when chewing sticky foods. An advantage of a similar path of insertion and occlusal directions permits the placement of straight implant abutments, and helps the laboratory to design prosthesis that direct the forces along the long axis of the implant body, which is favorable for crestal bone loads. The laboratory technician should be instructed regarding the actual implant body direction, as this information is not available on the master cast when an angled abutment post is used. The posterior abutment post for cement should be angled mesial to the vertical load, similar to a crown with slight mesial drift. The forward path of insertion permits easier preparation, impression removal, and prosthesis seating, as it corresponds to the approach of the operator to the mouth. The loads may be vertical to the implant body, yet the prosthesis path of insertion more medial to these loads.

Nonparallel Abutments

The implant abutment diameter is narrower than the natural teeth; thus, there is not as much latitude in correction of unparalleled abutments. For a cement-retained prosthesis, the unparallel posterior implant abutment has several prosthodontic options. The abutment may be initially prepared with a cross-cut fissure bur, copious amounts of water, and intermittent contact. The resulting abutment should not be round in cross-section, and should remain as long as possible. The abutment then is finished with a coarse diamond to increase the surface roughness. A cross-cut fissure bur is then used to add grooves parallel to the path of insertion. A knife-edge margin is usually indicated for all posterior implant abutments for cement, because the abutment is already of limited diameter. This technique is most often used when minimal parallelism adjustment is indicated. Although it is the easiest option, the disadvantage is the additional decrease in diameter of the implant abutment.

A second option for an unparallel abutment for a cemented prosthesis is to place an angled implant abutment. There are several designs available, depending on the manufacturer. This option is most often selected for anterior implants too facial or too lingual for posterior implants.

A third option to improve the path of insertion of a posterior implant abutment is the use of a coping. The implant abutment remains unparallel to the other abutments. It is roughened, and grooves are added parallel to its own path of insertion but different from the path of insertion of the prosthesis. A coping is then designed to be cemented on the abutment, parallel to the common path of

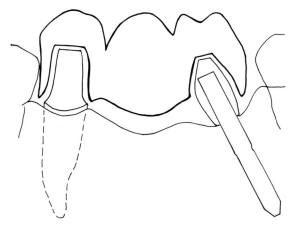

FIG 29–7.
Coping on an angled implant abutment may be cemented with a similar path of insertion to the nonparallel abutment.

fixed-prosthesis insertion. There are several advantages to this technique. The diameter of the coping is larger than that of the original abutment. In addition to the greater surface area, the laboratory may prepare the coping with an ideal taper to simultaneously improve the retention and resistance forms. Parallel grooves may also be designed and added as a laboratory step. The coping is cemented with a resin cement onto the abutment with a different path of insertion than that of the final prosthesis. Soft access or temporary cement may be used on the fixed prosthesis for retrievability, and the coping will stay in place during removal of the prosthesis because its path of insertion is different. This procedure is indicated least often when an anterior abutment is too facial, and most often when a posterior abutment is inclined to the distal (Fig 29–7). A fourth option is to design a custom abutment. It may be fabricated at most any length or angulation. Precious metal should be used to limit corrosion, since it will be cemented within the implant body.

A resin cement is used to cement metal to metal whenever the intent is to permanently retain a coping or prosthesis. The properties of resin cement illustrate the greatest compressive and tensile strengths of any current cement. This is especially warranted when custom implant abutments are cemented within the implant body.

Knife-Edge Margins

There are four indications for a knife-edge margin preparation in cemented implant prosthodontics, because minimum reduction is required. Traditional preparations do not use a knife edge with minimum tooth preparation, to avoid overcontouring of the final restoration.[9] However, whenever minimum implant

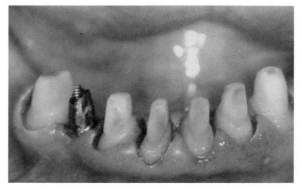

FIG 29–8.
Knife-edge margin is indicated in regions where minimum reduction is desired. Interproximal regions of lower incisor natural teeth close to the pulp chamber or an implant abutment less than 5 mm in diameter are two indications.

abutment or tooth preparation is indicated, a knife-edge finish line should be considered.

Implant abutments are the most common indication for minimum reduction, as they are usually less than 5 mm in diameter. Reduction of the abutment diameter to achieve a beveled margin would further decrease its dimension and

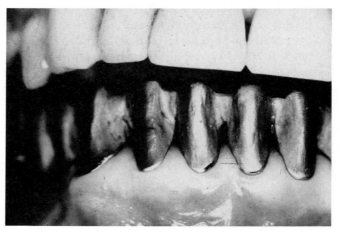

FIG 29–9.
Metal try-in for mandibular incisors should evaluate the amount of space in the interproximal for the addition of porcelain. Too little tooth reduction and/or too much metal does not permit proper contour of porcelain for hygienic maintenance. It is often better to cast the anterior incisors as one unit, with the rigid connectors in the incisal third, than attempting to solder each connection.

the surface area for retention. A second indication is for past periodontal bone loss. Periodontal diseased molars as well as healthy mandibular incisors are often included in implant prosthodontics, because past periodontal disease is a direct cause for replacement teeth, and splinting of anterior teeth is more common than in traditional restorative dentistry. The furcation area of a molar is often closer to the pulp chamber. Excessive removal of dentine in this region increases the chance for endodontic therapy. Third, the same pulpal problem exists for the interproximal areas of mandibular incisors. A knife edge in these areas reduces the risk of pulp exposure (Figs 29–8 and 29–9). The fourth indication for a knife-edge finish line concerns implant or natural abutments tilted more than 15 degrees.[9] The amount of material removed for parallelism jeopardizes the width of the implant abutment or encroaches on the pulp horn of the tilted tooth.

SUMMARY

Fixed prostheses are the most common restorations required of an implant dentist. Over 60 million partially edentulous people in the United States are missing posterior teeth in at least one quadrant, or have long spans between natural teeth. A common axiom used in dentistry is to perform a fixed restoration for partial edentulous patients whenever possible. Implant dentistry permits placement of additional abutments, so this axiom may be expanded to include most patients, especially when adequate bone is available. A cemented restoration has many advantages for a fixed prostheses. The most common complications include decay on natural abutments, fracture of prosthetic material, and partially retained restorations. The concepts of retention, resistance, and fundamentals of abutment preparation include taper, surface area, height, roughness, shear forces, path of insertion, nonparallel abutments, and knife-edge margins. Particular attention addresses the limitations of abutment diameter in implant dentistry.

REFERENCES

1. Adell R et al: A 15-year study of osseointegrated implant in the treatment of the edentulous jaw, *Int J Oral Surg* 10:387–416, 1981.
2. Misch CE: Protect the prosthesis, *Int J Oral Implant* 8(2,3):9, 1991.
3. Jemt T et al: Osseointegrated implants for single tooth replacement: a 1-year report from a multicenter prospective study, *Int J Oral Maxillofac Implants* 6:29–35, 1991.
4. Jemt T, Linden B, Lekholm U: Failures and complications in 127 consecutively placed fixed partial prostheses supported by Branemark implants: from prosthesis treatment to first annual checkup, *Int J Oral Maxillofac Implants* 7(1):40–44, 1992.
5. Walton JN, Gardner FM, Agar JR: A survey of crown and fixed partial denture fixtures: length of service and reasons for replacement, *J Prosthet Dent* 56(4):416–421, 1986.

6. O'Roark WL: Improving implant survival rates by using a new method of at risk analysis, *Int J Oral Implant* 8:31–57, 1991.

7. McKinney RV Jr, editor: *Endosteal dental implants,* St Louis, 1991, Mosby-Year Book.

8. Misch CE: Implant registry of graduates from the Misch Implant Institute. Manual of Misch Institute for Implant Dentistry, Dearborn, Mich, 1991.

9. Shillinburg HT, Jacobi R, Brackett SE: *Fundamentals of tooth preparation,* Chicago, 1987, Quintessence, pp 19–23.

10. Waerhaug J: Histologic considerations which govern where the margins of restorations should be located in relation to the gingiva, *Dent Clin North Am* 4:161–176, 1960.

11. Jorgensen KD: The relationship between retention and convergence angles in cemented veneer crowns, *Acta Odontol Scand* 13:35–40, 1955.

12. Ames WB et al: Techniques to improve seating of castings, *J Am Dent Assoc* 96:432, 1978.

13. Lorey RE, Myers GE: The retentive qualities of bridge retainers, *J Am Dent Assoc* 76:568–572, 1968.

14. Kaufman EG, Coelho DH, Collin L: Factors influencing the retention of cemented gold castings, *J Prosthet Dent* 11:487–502, 1961.

15. Felton DA, Kanoy BE, White JT: The effect of surface roughness of crown preparations on retention of cemented castings, *J Prosthet Dent* 58:292–296, 1987.

16. Rosenstiel E: The retention of inlays and crowns as a function of geometrical form, *Br Dent J* 103:388–394, 1957.

17. Gilboe DB, Teteruck WT: Fundamentals of extracoronal tooth preparation, retention and resistance form, *J Prosthet Dent* 32(6):651, 1974.

Chapter 30

Principles for Screw-Retained Prostheses

Carl E. Misch

With screw-retained prostheses, the most common causes of short-term implant failure and of complications after initial rigid fixation has been ideally achieved are nonpassive superstructures,[1] partially unretained restorations,[2] and too rapid loading of the implant interface.[3] These conditions produce forces on the implant and lead to bone loss, implant mobility, and component fracture. Progressive loading on screw-retained prostheses and the implant interface was addressed in Chapter 28. In this chapter, methods to decrease the frequency of nonpassive superstructures and partially retained restorations are presented.

Passive screw-retained restorations are more difficult to fabricate than cement-retained restorations. A cement space does not exist, and the inclined planes of the screw can develop significant forces when threaded into position. The superstructure may distort and appear to fit the implant abutment for screw. However, the superstructure does not bend beyond the elastic limit, and compression and tensile forces are dissipated to the bone-implant interface. The bone must remodel to eliminate these forces. If the forces are beyond limits, fracture of the bone-implant interface or an implant component occurs.

The most common causes for screw loosening and partially unretained restorations are related to nonpassive castings and uneven occlusal forces. The repeated compressive and tensile forces result in vibration and unthreading of the components. The more passively the casting attaches to the implant abutment for screw, the more secure the fixation device. Hence, accuracy in design and fabrication of the metal superstructure is a major factor for the reduction of forces at the implant and bone interface.

Poor esthetics, discomfort, and poor prosthesis design are observed in approximately 10% of screw-retained restorations.[2] These problems also occur with cement-retained restorations (at a 5% occurence) and are not addressed in this chapter.

PROSTHETIC CONSIDERATIONS: PASSIVE SCREW-RETAINED PROSTHESES

Passive screw-retained prostheses are difficult to fit because there are many variables to accuracy in the fabrication of the prosthesis. Because there is no space between the screws and implant abutment when the screws are in final position, and compressive and tensile forces hold the screw in place, the casting must fit completely passively and accurately before the screw is inserted. Elastic deformation of impression materials, dimensional shrinkage of elastic impressions, wax shrinkage, analog variance, die stone and investment expansion, metal shrinkage, acrylic or porcelain shrinkage, clinical methods of casting verification, soldering, variable torque on screws, and the number of implant components all interrelate in the fabrication of completely passive superstructures. One can only attempt to decrease the range of variance which is directly controlled by the restoring dentist. This need forms the basis for the discussions in this chapter.

Impression Materials

There are four categories of elastic impression materials: polysulfide, condensation silicone, addition silicone (vinyl polysiloxane), and polyether. Permanent deformation and dimensional shrinkage of impression materials were addressed in Chapter 24. The discussion here addresses these aspects related to screw-retained restorations.

Permanent Deformation of Impression Materials

Permanent deformation is measured by a 10% compression of an impression for 30 seconds after setting is complete. Permanent deformation of impression materials in implant dentistry is a concern when the impression distorts from the undercut region of the indirect impression transfer coping during the removal of the impression from the mouth (Fig 30–1). The material distorts out of the undercut, but may not return to the original position next to the transfer pin. It is permanently larger than the original dimension. The range of distortion is approximately 3% for polysulfide impression materials and 0.07% for addition silicone[4–6] (Table 30–1).

The indirect impression transfer copings are replaced into the transfer impression prior to pouring in stone for the working or master cast. The greater the permanent deformation, the less retentive the impression pin and the more variable its position in the distorted receptor site. As stone is vibrated around the

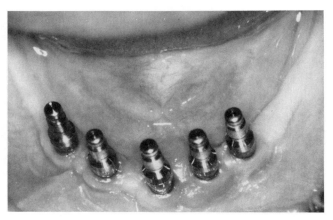

FIG 30–1.
Indirect impression transfers placed into mandibular anterior implant bodies. Preliminary elastic impression material will record location for construction of a custom tray.

indirect transfer, the attached abutment analog moves, and the final position is not accurate relative to the intraoral abutment position.

The effect of permanent deformation may be eliminated by using a direct impression transfer coping for the final impression (Fig 30–2). The impression transfer is not removed from the final impression before the master cast is fabricated. The direct impression transfer coping is also designed to be more rigidly held in place while the stone is vibrated into the impression.

Dimensional Change of Impression Materials

Dimensional change of elastic impression materials occurs when the impression is removed from the mouth. All four elastic impression materials shrink in dimension over a 24-hour period. Almost half of this shrinkage occurs

TABLE 30–1.

Setting Properties of Elastic Impression Materials

Material	Permanent Deformation (%)	Dimensional Change at 24 Hours (%)
Polysulfide	3.0	0.22
Silicone		
Condensation	0.4	0.58
Addition	0.07	0.06
Polyether	1.1	0.10

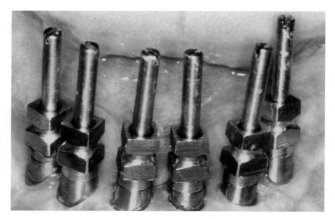

FIG 30–2.
Direct impression transfers placed into mandibular anterior implant bodies. They will be removed in a final impression with a custom tray to record location without the effect of permanent deformation.

in the first hour. Condensation silicones shrink the most often, and over 0.5%. Polysulfide shrinks 0.2%, while addition silicone changes the least, at 0.06%.[5, 7, 8] Therefore, addition silicone is used for the final impression, and the master cast is poured in the office, rather than being mailed to a laboratory. The dimensional change at 24 hours of addition silicone is not only the least, but is also less for long-term dimensional change. For example, a change of 0.2% occurs in polysulfide over a 24-hour period, but 1 week later there is more than twice this level of change. Addition silicone does not change after 24 hours or during the following week (Fig 30–3).

FIG 30–3.
Impression was made of the female portion of these dies in polysulfide impression material and addition silicone. After 24 hours the master models were poured. The addition silicone model fits with no visual discrepancy. The polysulfide model did not fit together *(above),* and represents the 0.2% dimensional change of the material. This illustration clarifies the significance of even small percentage changes for screw-in prostheses.

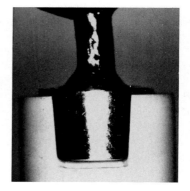

Custom Impression Tray

Dimensional changes have the greatest clinical significance for many implants in complete arch, screw-retained prostheses. A custom impression tray results in smaller error in both interabutment distance and cross-arch distortion, compared with stock impression trays.[9-11] A working cast is fabricated from the indirect impression transfer copings with a preliminary irreversible alginate impression at the first prosthetic appointment. The indirect impression transfer copings are connected to the abutment analog and reinserted into the preliminary impression. A working cast is poured with dental stone. The indirect impression transfer copings are removed from the working cast and replaced with direct impression transfers and long fixation screws (where vertical clearance permits) (Fig 30–4).

Base plate wax is used to block a 3-mm space around the rigid impression transfer copings, and a 1-mm space over the soft tissue regions required in the final working model. These include the landmarks used for final denture construction, as many of these structures help determine the tooth position with regard to esthetics, phonetics, and function. A tissue stop may be added in the molar region and retromolar pad or palate. Petroleum jelly or separating medium is placed over the wax, so it will not adhere to the acrylic placed to fabricate the tray.

Cold or light cure acrylic is placed over the regions of the wax spacers and permits the long fixation screws to protrude through the top of the tray. The tray

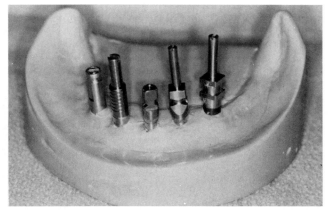

FIG 30–4.
Preliminary impression is made with indirect impression transfers (see Fig 30–1). Indirect transfers are removed from the mouth, inserted into implant abutment analogs, reinserted into the preliminary impression, and poured in dental stone. The indirect impression transfers are removed and replaced with direct impression transfers. *Left to right,* Swede-vent, Screw-vent, Calcitek, IMZ, and Steri-Os direct impression transfers.

is removed, trimmed, and polished. The holes for the fixation screws are increased until the tray is easily inserted and removed from the cast[12] (Fig 30–5).

The custom impression tray fabricated of cold cure acrylic must be made 24 hours or more before the final impression. During this time the tray will distort and dimensionally change because of monomer evaporation. If the custom tray cannot be fabricated longer than 24 hours before the final impression, two options are available. The custom tray may be inserted into boiling water for more than 15 minutes to remove the excess monomer and eliminate the distortion, or a light cured acrylic or thermoplastic material is used to fabricate the impression tray.[13]

The opening around the long fixation screws allows the custom impression tray to be consistently seated in the same position. An adhesive is used in the custom impression tray for retention of the elastic material. A very rigid addition silicone is the impression material of choice for the final direct transfer impression (Fig 30–6).

Analog Variance

The abutment for screw is usually fabricated in titanium or titanium alloy. The laboratory analog is often made of aluminum or brass. The direct impression transfer pin should be firmly screwed in the patient's mouth to ensure complete seating, and the same pressure should be used to fixate the abutment analog. Threads in brass or aluminum can distort, and the transfer pin will not be in the same position. This is especially noted during transfer attempts to locate an indirect angled abutment. Care is taken to ensure that the analog is flush and properly seated with the direct impression transfer coping before the stone is vibrated into position.

FIG 30–5.
Custom tray is made over a wax spacer placed on the direct impression transfers and surrounding soft tissue. Long fixation screws protrude through the top of the tray.

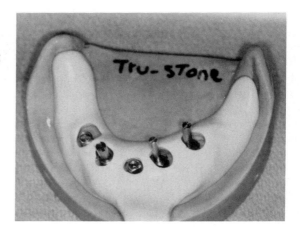

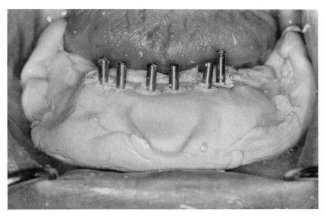

FIG 30–6.
Final impression with a rigid addition silicone records the direct impression transfer locations. The long fixation screws are unthreaded, and the body of the direct impression transfer remains in the impression material to eliminate permanent deformations.

The analog used should represent the abutment for screw, not the implant body. Some implant manufacturers suggest that indirect impression transfers be inserted into the implant body. In this plan, an implant body analog is transferred to the master model, and the abutment for screw is placed in the laboratory. However, this procedure would introduce another factor for error, without providing a proved benefit.

Stone Expansion

Because all impression materials shrink, the die stone should expand to compensate. Inasmuch as addition silicone shrinkage is approximately 0.06% and dimensionally stable at this point in the process, the expansion of the die stone should be in a similar range. The master cast for a screw-retained restoration should have different considerations and properties than a cement-retained restoration. A space is desired in a cemented prosthesis between the abutment for cement and the coping. The space is occupied by cement and permits complete seating of the prosthesis when cement is placed into the coping. The amount of this space is approximately 40 μm but may be larger, especially in regions above the margins. The cement-retained restoration is usually fabricated on dies composed of the actual die stone. These factors require a very hard material, and expansion properties should be greater. In addition, a die spacer is added to the surface of the die, especially above the margins.

The master cast for a screw-retained restoration uses metal analog components to represent the abutment for screw. As a result, surface hardness of the die

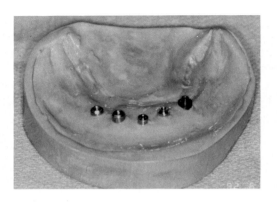

FIG 30–7.
Screw-retained restorations use metal analogs; thus expansion properties are more important than stone hardness. As a general rule, the harder the stone the more the expansion.

stone is not an issue. Instead, the expansion percentage is very important, as it may alter the interabutment distance.[9] The master cast should be poured with a small expansion stone. The expansion of dental stone (ADA product classification III) is product variable, but as a general rule has less expansion than die stone (ADA product classification IV). However, die stones are harder than dental stone, and are less likely to break or be altered during the laboratory process. Die stone (ADA product classification IV) expansion usually ranges from 0.1% to 0.25%, depending on the brand. The addition of hardeners increase the setting expansion. Epoxy resin shrinks at a range of 0.2%,[14] and because impression material also shrinks, should not be used for screw-retained master casts. The doctor and laboratory should be aware of the brand name properties of the impression material and stone in order to obtain results which compensate each other.[15] Of course the doctor must follow manufacturer suggested guidelines for the weight of material and amount of distilled water used in mixing the material. Decreasing the amount of water causes increase in expansion.[16] A vacuum mix provides a more consistent, denser master cast (Fig 30–7).

Esthetics of the final prosthesis is one of the more common complications and may be reduced when the soft tissue around the implants is represented on a duplicate master cast with tissue liner or impression material, when subgingival margins are required on the cemented or screw-retained restoration. Polyether or soft tissue liners do not stick well to addition silicone. These materials may be injected for several millimeters around the abutment analogs and metal clips placed in the tissue substitute before setting. Dental stone is vibrated into position, and when the impression is separated, the soft tissue will be represented by the polyether or tissue liner. Cervical contours of the final restoration may be fabricated with an appreciation for the soft tissue location, even in subgingival esthetic regions. A duplicate cast is not exactly the same as the master cast, as the properties of impression materials and stone also affect this process. Therefore, all laboratory procedures are performed on the master cast, and the metal and porcelain work is evaluated on the soft tissue model.

Acrylic Shrinkage

Processed methyl methylate shrinks approximately 7% in volume,[17] and as much as 18% with cold cure acrylic, especially with excess monomer. The actual change in final dimension is related to the amount of material cured at one time. Therefore, the salt-and-pepper technique is often used for baseplates, so small volumes cure at one time and the effect of dimensional change is limited.

In the laboratory the abutment analogs are placed in a stone model. The acrylic connecting these metal analog units is unable to change the abutment position, even though acrylic shrinkage occurs around them. As a result, baseplates and verification jigs may be fabricated from acrylic (Figs 30–8 and 30–9). However, implants are not rigid in the mouth, and are able to move in a mesiodistal dimension as much as 100 μ with 5 g force.[18] The use of intraoral acrylic to join implants prior to direct impressions is a popular technique, yet this may move the abutment from its original position during setting. No direct studies have been performed to evaluate this specific step. However, clinical experience demonstrates that patients are able to feel the shrinkage pressures on natural teeth during the intraoral setting of an acrylic provisional restoration. Light cured materials shrink 4%, while addition silicone shrinks 0.06% and places less force on abutments during setting than acrylic resin. The dimensional change in addition silicone is least likely to move an intraoral abutment during the final impression stage.

Acrylic shrinkage is also important to consider when the final fixed prosthesis is fabricated of acrylic resin and metal. Acrylic gains strength with bulk, and considerable amounts of resin may be used in the prosthesis. The processing of the denture resin to a metal substructure may actually distort and change the

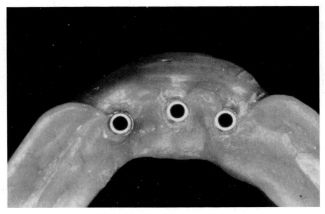

FIG 30–8.
Base plate is made around the direct impression transfer on the master model. This permits the base plate and wax rim to also serve as an implant verification jig in the mouth.

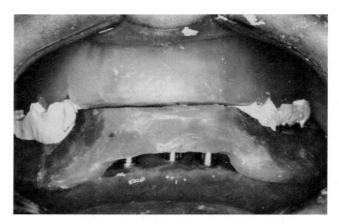

FIG 30–9.
Base plate/wax rim/verification jig is evaluated for accuracy of the final impression before metal superstructure fabrication.

metal. As a result, even though the casting was passive at the metal try-in appointment, the initial delivery of the final restoration may not be the same. Long spans and/or narrow metal superstructures are more at risk of change because the flexibility of metal is related to the cube of the distance.[19] For example, a 10-mm span of metal may flex 12 μ, but a 30-mm span will flex 330 μ if all other conditions are similar. Less acrylic in the region of a distal cantilever results with less shrinkage and distortions, as it is related to volume.

Porcelain Shrinkage

Porcelain shrinkage of approximately 20% occurs during the firing process and may distort the metal superstructure. The stress distribution in porcelain fused to gold crowns covering the facial and lingual surface is increased and even more likely to cause metal distortion.[20] Therefore, metal occlusals on screw-retained restorations result in less material fracture and less risk of nonpassive castings.

Metal Casting Shrinkage

The problems associated with metal shrinkage during the casting process has been a concern for many years in traditional cement-retained fixed prosthetics.[21] The range of precious metal shrinkage is variable, depending on manufacturer and technique, but approximates 1.5%, while shrinkage of semiprecious alloys may be twice that amount[22] (Fig 30–10). Therefore, an investment material with thermal or hygroscopic expansion is used to compensate for the shrinkage related

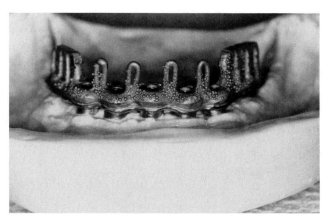

FIG 30–10.
Precious metal shrinkage (1.5%) is half that of nonprecious metals, and precious metals corrode less with implant abutments or screws.

to superstructure fabrication. The expansion of the investment material is highly technique sensitive. The size, shape, temperature, and manufacturer type of the casting ring, and the position of material within the ring also affect the final dimensions of the metal casting. As a result, the final product may be either greater or smaller than the original wax pattern (which may also distort). Precious metal is used for the superstructure casting because metal corrosion with titanium is reduced, accuracy of the casting is improved, and separation and soldering—if required—are less technique sensitive.

SUPERSTRUCTURE EVALUATION

Intraoral superstructure evaluation is more critical for a passive casting than for a marginal seal. However, these two criteria are related. The abutments for screw are first evaluated to ensure that they are completely seated and threaded into position. Any mobility or tenderness is noted and mandates evaluation of both the implant body–hard tissue interface and the soft tissue which may be present between the implant body and loose abutment. The casting is initially placed and evaluated for stability. End-to-end tipping indicates that a most distal abutment(s) does not fit correctly. If end-to-end tipping is not present, the most terminal abutment coping screws may be inserted with minimum torque. Lateral rocking is then noted, and when present indicates that a pier abutment is not correct. Direct vision and/or dental explorer often identifies an open margin between the coping and abutment. The marginal opening may only be on one side and represent the coping tipped on the abutment. If no lateral rocking is evident and all margins approximated, the remainder of the coping screws are inserted. The screws are only moderately tightened first, using a counterbalance approach. A common scenario is to insert the centermost coping screw and thread it with similar force to the previous two terminal coping screws. The intermediary screws are then inserted, one on each side, with more torque force. Once all screws are inserted the center screw is completely fixated, followed by each terminal component, followed by the intermediary coping screws (Fig 30–11).

Patient discomfort during this procedure is particularly noted. Local anesthesia is not indicated. Any tension, pressure, pulling, tenderness, or pain signals a nonpassive casting, incorrect placement, looseness of the abutment for screw, poor bone-implant interface, or casting impingement of the soft tissue.

Soldering

During superstructure evaluation, separation is periodically required in order to obtain a passive casting. The superstructure is separated around the offending abutment(s). Once separated, each component is tested, as previously discussed. The distance of separation is 0.005 to 0.008 inch (0.13 to 0.20 mm) or the thickness of two sheets of paper.[23–25] Too small an opening will cause dimensional change when the casting is heated and expands, while too large an opening may provide a stronger or weaker joint, but casting distortion and warp occur because of shrinkage of the solder during solidification. A one-piece casting may be larger by 2%, whereas a soldered casting is often smaller in mesiodistal dimension.[26–30] A one-piece casting may be indicated if the span is short and thermal expansion for the investment is used, as fewer soldering steps produce fewer errors. However, large castings in volume or distance should be fabricated in sections, because the

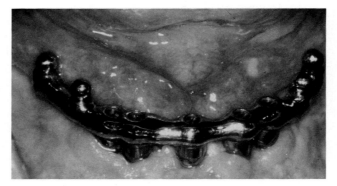

FIG 30–11.
Superstructure try-in is a critical step, because a nonpassive casting can distribute overload stress to the implant abutments.

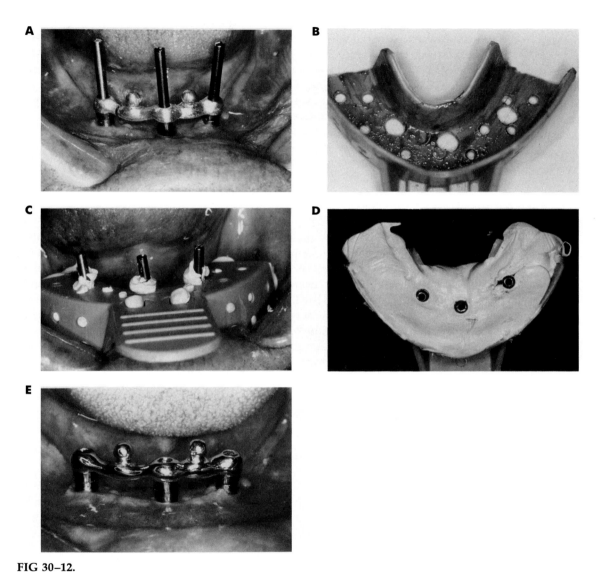

FIG 30–12.
A, non passive casting is separated by the thickness of two sheets of paper and reinserted. Long fixation screws are used to fixate the superstructure. **B,** stock tray is modified to fit over the long fixation screws. **C,** rigid addition silicone impression material is used as a pickup impression of the superstructure. **D,** transfer impression with superstructure within the impression material at the correct position. **E,** superstructure is soldered, polished, and checked for passive placement.

dimensional changes during fabrication and casting are so variable. Once separated the ideal distance, the casting may be rigidly connected while in place intraorally with a composite-filled acrylic applied incrementally. The composite-filled resin or light cured acrylic reduces the amount of shrinkage compared to cold cure products. A rigid addition silicone (designed for occlusal recordings) may be injected around the superstructure to help index the pieces.

An alternative technique uses a stock tray, or the original custom tray may be modified after the final impression material is removed. Long fixation screws are placed in the copings and protrude through the open holes originally for the direct impression transfer fixation screws. A pick-up impression of the super-structure with addition silicone may then be obtained. The new master cast is prepared in similar fashion to the original (Fig 30–12,A–E).

Screw Fixation

The amount of torque used to place a coping screw is considerable. Superstructures are often not completely passive at initial delivery. The bone must remodel and eliminate zones of tension and compression around the implant body. At initial delivery the coping fixation screw is tightened to approximately two thirds to three fourths of the final torque force. The patient returns a few days later so that tightness of the screws can be verified and clinical signs such as tenderness or discomfort can be reported. The patient remains on a soft diet, and after approximately 4 weeks the screws may be tightened to the full 20 newtons/cm torque force. A torque wrench permits equal tension on each screw.

PARTIALLY RETAINED RESTORATIONS

Partially unretained restorations are more common with screw-retained superstructures than with cement-retained prostheses. The screw is most likely to loosen during the first few weeks, in amounts approaching 50% in the maxilla and 20% in the mandible.[2] This complication is observed more often in the partially edentulous restoration, and far less often with overdentures retained by implant abutments with stress relievers on the superstructure. The coping screw is usually the weakest link in the prosthetic chain. Any occlusal, casting, or force discrepancy may result in vibration and screw loosening or breakage where the force is greatest. This protects the implant body from more severe complications; but once it occurs, the other implant abutments are more at risk for overload and complication than the offending implant, because a cantilever and magnification of the load results. The amount of increased force is variable, but may be extreme. For example, moment forces can multiply stress on the crest of the bone-implant interface in direct relation to the distance of the next retained abutment. As a result, a 0 moment force can increase to a 250 lb/mm moment load with a 25 lbf, although the next abutment is only 10 mm away.

Most conditions that cause screw loosening also affect a cement-retained restoration, but the cement seal is often not the weakest link. As a result, unlike the threaded restorations, the overload results in the region of the first complication. However, the overload is not magnified by moment loads created from a partially retained restoration.

The most common conditions under the control of the dentist that cause an unretained abutment for screw include a nonpassive superstructure, uneven occlusal loads, and material fatigue. The nonpassive superstructure has been previously addressed. Uneven occlusal loads cause repeated compression, then tension, of implant components. Because the screw is an inclined plane, the continued vibration causes it to unthread. Methods to decrease this effect include preloading the screw, screw design, screw placement location, and decrease in moment forces.[31]

Preload of the screw places the components under enough tension to create elongation of the material within its elastic limit. As a result, the components stretch and maintain fixation in spite of vibration and external forces. The elongation of metal is related to the modulus of elasticity, which is dependent on type of material and stress per area. Thus, a gold screw has greater elongation but lower yield strength than a screw made of titanium alloy (see Chapter 15).

Coping screws designed with tapered (rather than flat) heads are to be avoided. The tapered head distorts a nonpassive superstructure but gives the appearance of proper fit. A 10 newton/cm torque force applied to an inclined plane and screw can distort a superstructure and result in significant stress at the crestal bone region. In addition, most of the force within the tapered screw is distributed to the head rather than to the fixation screw component. A flat-head screw places a more even force within the threads and the head of the screw.[32]

SUMMARY

A screw-retained prosthesis attaches to the implant abutment with significant compressive forces (10 to 20 newtons/cm torque). The coping screw should not place tension, compression, or shear forces on the superstructure. To accomplish the goal of a passive superstructure, all aspects of prosthesis reconstruction should be as accurate as possible, or should compensate for each other during the process. Variables are evaluated at the casting evaluation appointment. Fabrication variables most important to the clinician include impression material shrinkage and permanent deformation, custom vs. stock impression trays, variance among manufacturers in analog parts, stone and investment expansion, metal shrinkage, acrylic and porcelain shrinkage, soldering, and torque force amount of each coping screw once the process has initially been verified. The step-by-step clinical protocol for superstructures was presented in Chapter 28 in the discussion of progressive bone loading.

REFERENCES

1. Assif D et al: Comparative accuracy of implant impression procedures, *Int J Periodont Res Dent* 12:113–121, 1992.
2. Jemt T, Linden B, Lekholm U: Failures and complications in 127 consecutively placed fixed partial prostheses supported by Branemark implants: from prosthetic treatment to first annual checkup, *Int J Oral Maxillofac Implants* 7:40–44, 1992.
3. Misch CE: Density of bone: effect on treatment plans, surgical approach, healing, and progressive bone loading, *Int J Oral Implant* 6:23–31, 1990.
4. Hosada J, Fusayama T: Distortion of irreversible hydixcollord and mercaptan rubber base impressions, *J Prosthet Dent* 11:318–333, 1961.
5. Stockhouse JA: A comparison of elastic impression materials, *J Prosthet Dent* 39:305–313, 1975.
6. Craig RG: A review of properties of rubber impression materials, *J Mich Dent Assoc* 59:254, 1977.
7. Stauffer J, Meger J, Vally J: Accuracy of six elastic impression materials used for complete-arch fixed partial dentures, *J Prosthet Dent* 35:407–415, 1976.
8. Williams PT, Jackson DC, Bergman W: An evaluation of the time-dependent dimensional stability of eleven elastomeric impression materials, *J Prosthet Dent* 52:120–125, 1984.
9. Schaffer H, Dumfarht H, Gausch K: Distance alterations of dies in sagittal direction in dependance of the die material, *J Prosthet Dent* 61:684–687, 1989.
10. Gordon GE, Johnson GJ, Drenron DG: The effect of tray selection on accuracy of elastomeric impression materials, *J Prosthet Dent* 63:12–15, 1990.
11. Eames WB et al: Elastomeric impression materials: effect of bulk on accuracy, *J Prosthet Dent* 41:304–307, 1979.
12. Hobo S, Ichida E, Garcia LT: *Osseointegration and occlusal rehabilitation,* Chicago, 1990, Quintessence, pp 153–162.
13. Christensen G: Dental materials used in dentistry, Lecture, Chicago Dental Society Mid Winter Meeting, Feb 1990.
14. Toreskog S, Phillips RW, Schnell RJ: Properties of die materials—a comparative study, *J Prosthet Dent* 16:119–131, 1966.
15. Schelb E et al: Compatibility of type IV dental stones with polyvinylsiloxane impression material, *J Prosthet Dent* 58:19–22, 1987.
16. Leinfelder KF, Lemons JE: *Clinical restoration materials and techniques,* Philadelphia, 1988, Lea & Febiger.
17. Phillips RW: *Skinner's science of dental materials,* ed 8, Philadelphia, 1982, WB Saunders.
18. Komiyama Y: Clinical and research experiences with osseointegrated implants in Japan, in Albrektsson T, Zarb G, editors: *The Branemark osseointegrated implant,* Chicago, 1989, Quintessence, pp 197–214.

19. Smyd ES: Mechanics of dental structures: guide to teaching dental engineering at undergraduate level, *J Prosthet Dent* 2:668–692, 1952.
20. Craig RG, El-Ebrashi MK, Peyton FA: Stress distribution in porcelain-fused to gold crowns and preparations constructed with photoelastic plastics, *J Dent Res* 50:1278–1283, 1971.
21. Hollenback GM, Skinner EW: Shrinkage during casting of gold and gold alloys, *J Am Dent Assoc* 33:1391–1399, 1946.
22. Gourley JM: Current status of semi-precious alloys in restorative dentistry, *J Can Dent Assoc* 41:453–455, 1975.
23. Shillingburg HT, Hobo S, Whitsett LD: *Fundamentals of fixed prosthodontics,* ed 2, Chicago, 1981, Quintessence.
24. Ryge G: Dental soldering procedures, *Dent Clin North Am* 2:747–757, 1958.
25. Stackhouse JA: Assembly of dental units by soldering, *J Prosthet Dent* 18:131–139, 1967.
26. Willis LM, Nicholls JI: Distortion in dental soldering as affected by gap distance, *J Prosthet Dent* 43:272–278, 1980.
27. Bruce RW: Clinical application of multiple unit castings for fixed prostheses, *J Prosthet Dent* 18:359–364, 1967.
28. Stade AH, Reisbick MH, Preston JD: Pre-ceramic and post-ceramic solder joints, *J Prosthet Dent* 34(5):527–532, 1975.
29. Gegauff AG, Rosenstiel SF: The seating of 1-piece and soldered fixed partial dentures, *J Prosthet Dent* 62:292–297, 1989.
30. Fusayama T, Wakumoto S, Hosada H: Accuracy of fixed partial dentures made by various soldering techniques and one-piece casting, *J Prosthet Dent* 14:334–342, 1964.
31. Branemark P-I, Zarb G, Albrektsson T: *Osseointegrated fixtures for the completely edentulous,* Chicago, 1985, Quintessence.
32. Nobelpharama Newsletter, vol. 4, 1991.

Chapter 31

Maxillary Denture Opposing an Implant Overdenture or Fixed Prosthesis

Carl E. Misch

Lack of stability and lack of retention are the most common complications related to complete removable prostheses. The mandibular denture has more associated problems than an opposing maxillary prosthesis. Patients often feel that retention and stability of maxillary dentures is acceptable. As a result, a common treatment plan for an edentulous patient uses implants to support the mandibular restoration and a traditional soft tissue–supported maxillary denture.[1-3]

Postinsertion complications of the removable maxillary restoration may be anticipated. The patient complains of maxillary denture sore spots and instability of the restoration. The causes for the complications are related to the implants supporting a mandibular prosthesis, which provide improved forces, function, proprioception, and stability. The sore spots under the maxillary denture result because patients with rigid fixated oral implant prostheses are able to generate masticatory forces approaching that of natural teeth,[4] while complete denture wearers have been shown to exert only 25% of this amount.[5]

Maxillary denture instability is related to increased patient awareness and the conditions of a more stable mandibular prosthesis. A conventional soft tissue––borne complete removable mandibular prosthesis moves to accommodate prematurities or inaccuracy of occlusion, and occlusal position is often anterior to recorded centric relation occlusion.[6] In addition, the patient is accustomed to the mandibular denture lifting up in the posterior when the mandible goes into excursions, and no posterior teeth are in contact. On the contrary, with a rigid mandibular restoration, the maxillary prosthesis moves to accommodate to the mandibular occlusion so the occlusal concepts must be more accurate. This predisposes to maxillary denture instability, soreness, mucosal changes, and ultimately to resorption of the ridge. The maxillary prosthesis will even lose the valve seal retention and be dislodged when the mandibular implant restoration proceeds into excursive movements without posterior contact. This not only occurs with the incision of food, but also during parafunction. Inadequate valve seal and instability of the maxillary denture can also contribute to gagging.

Mandibular implant overdentures provides greater proprioception, and the mandible occludes in a more consistent centric relation occlusion position than would a traditional denture. The occlusal forces are directed in a more consistent direction and location. This requires a more exact occlusal scheme and registration. In many ways the combination of a complete maxillary denture against a lower mandibular implant–supported prosthesis resembles a single complete maxillary denture opposing mandibular natural dentition.

To decrease maxillary denture complications opposing a mandibular implant restoration, several concepts have been developed. These include raising the posterior plane of occlusion,[7, 8] more medial placement of the maxillary and mandibular posterior teeth,[7, 9] and establishing bilateral balanced occlusion in the final restoration. A functionally generated path for maxillary denture occlusion has also been recommended when opposing a combination of natural teeth and implant-supported fixed prostheses, or a combination of prostheses. The purpose of this chapter is to highlight these areas of special concern when fabricating a maxillary denture opposing an implant-supported restoration.

MAXILLARY TISSUES EVALUATION

The foundation of the maxillary denture is bone, the overlying submucosa, and the mucosa.[10] The blood vessels and nerves are located in the submucosa and bony architecture. Denture support should be placed on the regions where fibrous connective tissue is firmly attached to bone, namely, the edentulous ridge. Under ideal circumstances, the residual ridge is the primary stress-bearing region for a maxillary denture.[6] In addition, the teeth are set closer to this structure than to any other supporting region. Placing the denture teeth directly over the edentulous crest reduces moment of force and improves stability under vertical forces. The concept can rarely be exploited in the anterior region, but can be used in the premolar and molar areas with Division A or B available bone.

The tissues of the maxillary ridge must be firm, to limit denture movement during occlusion. If excessive mobility of the anterior on posterior ridges is observed, consider soft tissue surgery.

The premaxillary segment of the edentulous maxilla is a most important structure. The rugae area of the premaxilla is the secondary stress-bearing region.[11] This region helps resist the forward movement of the denture in excursive mandibular movements. The denture is severely compromised without a vertical component to the premaxilla.

Augmentation of the premaxilla with demineralized freeze-dried bone and hydroxyapatite is described in Chapter 20. The graft is firmly inserted into a lingual tunnel to decrease tissue mobility and to square the ridge shape, while simultaneously enhancing the vertical component of the anterior segment. The labial vestibule is also evaluated, and when poor height is present, a vestibuloplasty is considered with or without the anterior augmentation procedure.

The posterior aspect of the hard palate is an area of secondary retention, not support, for a maxillary denture.[6] The submucosa is rich in mucous glands and blood vessels, granting greater resiliency under vertical forces. This region is loaded less with the denture compared to the crest of the ridge or premaxilla.[11]

The tissues over the midpalatal suture are usually thin and nonmobile, whereas the surrounding mucosa can be displaced under minimal pressure. The denture base can be selectively relieved in this region to prevent it from acting as a fulcrum, with resultant instability and soreness when vertical forces are transmitted through the maxillary prosthesis[6] (Fig 31–1). The maxillary denture opposing an implant-supported restoration receives more forces, and should therefore be relieved more in this area (Fig 31–2). Denture relief should also be provided to the incisive papilla to avoid compression of the associated blood vessels and nerves during function. If this is neglected, the patient may experience a burning sensation after delivery of the denture. This structure is usually 5 to 7 mm behind the maxillary central incisors. If no bone exists anterior to the papilla, the presence of a vertical premaxilla is even more important, because the anterior teeth will be cantilevered off the bony support.

The maxillary tuberosities should be firm and placed several millimeters superior to the posterior plane of occlusion. Surgical removal of hyperplastic tissue is indicated. The hamular notch is located halfway between the maxillary

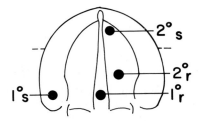

FIG 31–1.
Maxillary edentulous ridge uses a firm keratinized crest as primary support (1°s). A secondary region of support is the premaxilla, especially required to resist lateral excursions of a mandibular overdenture (2°s). A prime area of relief is the midpalatal suture region and incisive papilla (1°r). The additional force of an implant supported overdenture often causes a greater incidence of sore spots or burning in the mouth. A secondary region of retention (not support) is the posterior palate (2°r). The submucosa is rich in blood and mucous glands, which give resiliency to vertical load. It is also a relatively flat region, which is good for retention.

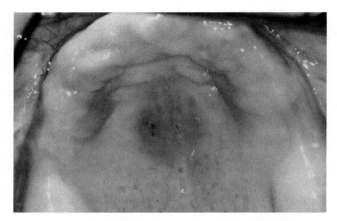

FIG 31–2.
Midpalatal suture region has thin tissue and may act as a fulcrum for maxillary denture instability when loaded with the additional force of a mandibular overdenture. Note the erythemic tissue and ulcer in the center of this palate.

tuberosity and the hamulus of the medial pterygoid plate. The posterior palatal seal is positioned through this area of loose connective tissue to improve tissue contact and retention. The pterygomandibular raphe attaches from the hamulus to the retromolar pad and should not be impinged upon. The posterior limit of the prosthesis is correlated with the soft palate vibrating line, which is more an area than a definite line.[10]

Kydd et al. demonstrated that tissues loaded for 10 minutes may be compressed to 60% of their original thickness and remain at 65% to 85% for extended periods, with 4 hours necessary for complete recovery.[12] Therefore, final denture impressions and delivery follow certain guidelines. The denture should be removed at least 4 hours before the final impression. This often means the appointment for the final impression should be in the early morning before the patient eats, and the patient should leave the prosthesis out the night before the appointment. A tissue conditioner can improve the tissue health and help maintain the final tissue thickness while the prosthesis is worn before the final impression. The day the denture is delivered, a similar routine is repeated. Otherwise, tissue thickness may be compressed, and the retention at initial delivery may prove to be less than ideal.

PROSTHETIC CONSIDERATIONS

Maxillary Incisal Edge Position

For the final impression, a custom impression tray and selective pressure technique are used. The baseplate is made with minimum distortion to evaluate retention and aid in the wax try-in measurements. The baseplate and wax rim are inserted into the patient's mouth and the labial contour of the maxillary lip is determined first, as modification at a later step may alter all other measurements. The position of the maxillary incisal edge is determined next. This position primarily reflects a blend of esthetics and phonetics. A significant decrease of maxillary tooth length exposure is relative to age, especially between the ages of 30 and 40 years.[13] The younger patient exposes more than 2 mm of maxillary vertical incisor. The geriatric patient rarely accepts an incisal edge position above the resting maxillary lip position.

The high smile line is consciously observed. In general, patients do not like to show the pink acrylic above the maxillary teeth. A high lip line may indicate longer teeth, exposure of the cervical portion of the teeth, or on occasion elevation of the incisal edge.

A conventional denture on a Division D maxilla may require the incisal edge position slightly superior and/or inward, closer to the edentulous ridge, to improve anterior stability. In these patients, the labial gingival contour can be slightly increased to improve lip support and slightly elevate the lip.

The anterior width of the wax rim is made similar to that of the final teeth, so phonetics may be evaluated. Speech sounds help refine the position of the maxillary anterior teeth for the individual patient. The length and labiolingual position of these teeth may be evaluated by the "F" and "V" sounds.[14]

Plane of Occlusion

The plane of occlusion has three dimensions: occluso-gingival, anterior-posterior, and bucco-lingual. The occluso-gingival direction is established by the anterior incisal edge. The bucco-lingual dimension is parallel with a line drawn through the pupils of the eyes. The anterior-posterior dimension establishes the height of the posterior occlusal plane.

Once the anterior lip position and incisal edge location are initially determined, the posterior maxillary plane of occlusion is designed. It is often determined in the laboratory from the canine incisal edge position to a point halfway up the retromolar pad.[6, 10] The end result is an occlusal plane inferior to the natural teeth position. In principle, this improves the stability of a lower denture. The lowered plane of occlusion helps decrease moment forces on the lower denture, and the tongue rest position is above the posterior teeth. But when the mandibular restoration is implant supported, this same technique is not indicated, as it places the posterior maxillary teeth lower than the original tooth position and makes the maxillary denture more unstable.

Camper's plane connects the lower border of the alar process of the nose to the middle or most distal portions of the tragus of the ear. The occlusal plane is reported to be parallel to this reference plane. Misch evaluated the existing occlusal plane from the canine to first molar in 50 patients with natural maxillary teeth. In half of the patients, the parallel posterior reference point on the tragus was in the upper third, in 46% it was parallel to the mid tragus, and 4% it was below this reference on the right side of the patient's head. The position was different on the contralateral side in almost 25% of the patients. Therefore, it can be suggested that the posterior plane of occlusion with natural teeth is either parallel to or above Camper's line.[8, 9]

When a maxillary denture is fabricated, the maxillary wax rim is made parallel to Camper's plane for a Type I Division A or Type I Division B maxilla with good retentive form. The posterior reference point is raised to a position near the upper third of the tragus, slightly raising the occlusal plane, to make the maxillary denture more stable for the Division C or D maxillary arch. Thus the anterior occlusal plane is correlated to the length and support of the maxillary lip; ridge shape, height, and position; phonetics, and esthetics. The posterior occlusal plane corresponds to the bone Division, the retentive form of the arch, and to a plane from the middle to upper portion of the tragus of the ear to the inferior portion of the alar of the nose.

If the posterior occlusal plane is too high, the maxillary denture base can be driven forward on the tissues during the mandibular arc of closure.[6] In addition, the posterior plane of occlusion may compromise the action of the tongue when placing food on the occlusal table. The ideal plane of occlusion for a denture opposing an implant denture is similar to that found with the natural teeth, and most often corresponds to the mid to upper third of the tragus.

Once the posterior occlusion plane is established in relation to the alar of the nose and tragus, the bucco-lingual plane is determined. The anterior plane is usually parallel to the pupils of the eyes. However, on rare occasion the eyes are not parallel to the horizontal plane and a reevaluation is required.

The vertical occlusal dimension is then established with a mandibular base plate and wax-rim. The superstructure bar for an RP-4 prosthesis over anterior root forms is not fabricated until the actual tooth position has been established. On the other hand, a mandibular subperiosteal RP-4 restoration already has the superstructure in place at this time, and the baseplate and wax rim may be firmly attached to the bar. This permits a very stable and rigid recording of the vertical occlusal dimension.

Tooth Selection and Position

Selection of the shape, size, and color of the anterior tooth is as much an art form as any part of restorative dentistry. The patient's preexisting denture or natural teeth may serve as a guide. The patient's feeling toward color and contour is noted, as his or her attitude often affects the acceptance of the final restoration.

Once the maxillary and mandibular anterior teeth are positioned according to the wax rims, the posterior position is determined. The amount of incisal guidance will determine the steepness of the compensating curve for a balanced occlusion. The greater the guidance, the greater curve is necessary. It is functionally advantageous to keep this curve minimal, by setting as shallow an angle of the incisal guide as phonetics, esthetics, and function of the anterior teeth will permit.

Anterior natural teeth usually have centric stops or tongue positions to prevent continued extrusion. On the contrary, the maxillary denture usually does not have anterior incisal centric stops. This helps protect the premaxilla from excess forces in centric occlusion relation and initial excursions of the mandible, as the premaxilla is vulnerable to resorption from external stresses. Maxillary anterior teeth are forward of the anterior supporting bone. Moment forces result from contact with the anterior teeth, which may cause instability of the maxillary prosthesis. The tips of the maxillary canines are in a plane related to the middle of the incisive papilla in 92% of cases,[15] which makes their position more over the position of the resorbed residual ridge, compared with the maxillary anterior incisors. Therefore, anterior centric occlusion may begin at the distal aspect of the canine, with reduced anterior moment force. The maxillary six incisors are positioned for esthetics and phonetics first. Accordingly, the implant-supported mandibular anterior incisors are primarily set for phonetics and maxillary denture stability.

Posterior Tooth Position

The maxillary edentulous posterior ridge resorbs in a medial direction as it transforms from Division A to B, Division B to C, and Division C to D bony support. Therefore, the maxillary denture tooth gradually becomes more cantilevered off the bone support, even when positioned in the same spatial location. The mandibular edentulous posterior ridge also resorbs in a medial direction as it transforms from a Division A to B, but then resorbs lateral from a B to C Division, and more lateral as it resorbs from C to D. In posterior tooth position for complete dentures, the position of the mandibular posterior tooth is often first determined. Bone support concepts of occlusion often position the mandibular teeth perpendicular to the edentulous ridge.[6, 10] This positions the central fossa of the posterior mandibular teeth more medial than that of their natural predecessors in Division B, but more facial in Division C and very facial in Division D compared to the natural tooth placement. Mandibular dentures in the neutral zone record the tongue position and also result with posterior teeth more buccal in resorbed arches than the natural tooth placement.[16] This results in the maxillary teeth placed farther facial in the Divisions C or D bone category, if normal cusp-fossa relation is maintained. Consequently, maxillary denture teeth are always placed lateral to the resorbing bony support, and the condition is compounded when the resorption is in Division C or D bone and the mandibular teeth are positioned over bony support or neutral muscular zones (Fig 31–3). The maxillary posterior tooth is also involved in esthetics, especially the premolar region. The more lateral tooth placement affects esthetics when compared with the position of the natural teeth.

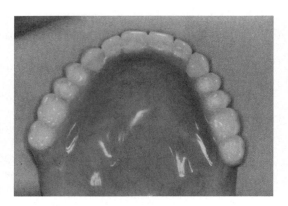

FIG 31–3.
This maxillary denture had the posterior denture teeth set in relationship to a mandibular overdenture on a division C-h ridge using traditional concepts. Note how far buccal the posterior teeth are relative to the bone support. The position does not give proper stability in mastication or unilateral occlusal loads.

The basic concepts of lingualized occlusion were first suggested by Payne.[17] Pound discussed a similar concept and introduced the term "lingualized" occlusion.[18] Pound placed the lingual cusp of the mandibular posterior teeth between lines drawn from the canine to each side of the retromolar pad. The buccal maxillary cusps were ground off by Payne, while the buccal cusps of the mandibular teeth were removed by Pound. Consistent in their philosophy was the belief that the lingual cusp was the only area of maxillary tooth contact. These occlusal schemes were designed to narrow the occlusal table and improve mastication, reduce forces to the underlying bone, and help stabilize a lower denture. The techniques of Payne and Pound may be modified further to a *medial positioned lingualized occlusion,* developed by the author.[8, 9]

Misch observed 30 patients with natural mandibular posterior teeth and compared the lingual cusp position to the position stated by Pound. In all patients the position of the posterior lingual tooth extended *medial* to a line drawn from the canine to the medial aspect of the retromolar pad. In the majority of patients, the lingual cusps extended 2 mm beyond the line, while in approximately 10% they extended to 3 mm, and in another third, were 1 mm beyond the line[8, 9] (Fig 31–4). Therefore, denture teeth set more medial to the retromolar pad are more similar in position to natural teeth than the region established by Pound. The tooth position suggested by Pound helps stabilize a mandibular denture. An implant-supported overdenture does not require tooth position as the primary stability factor. In addition, the more medial the posterior denture teeth, the more vertical are the occlusal forces over the maxillary bone, which reduces tipping forces and makes the upper denture more stable during occlusal contacts.

The position of the posterior line is drawn from the mandibular canine to the lingual side of the retromolar pad. The mandibular posterior teeth are placed so that the central fossa is over this line and the lingual aspect of the tooth extends medial to the most lingual line. The greater the maxillary posterior resorption, the more medial are the lingual cusps. However, the lingual aspect of the mandibular tooth does not extend beyond 3 mm of a line drawn from the lingual aspect of the retromolar pad to the canine tooth. This positions the denture tooth more medial than previous techniques, yet the lingual aspect of the denture tooth is in similar location to that of the natural tooth.

The occlusal centric contacts follow the guidelines of lingualized occlusion from Payne and Pound.[7, 18] Only the lingual cusps of the maxillary posterior teeth are in contact during centric occlusion (Fig 31–5). A maxillary denture occlusion cannot separate the left and right component, or the anterior and posterior influence. Because all teeth are joined to a rigid baseplate, the occlusal contacts in one region affect the entire restoration. A tripod occlusion to stabilize a tooth, or anterior contact to prevent overeruption of teeth, is not required. Because the primary contact is the lingual cusp of the maxillary teeth rather than the buccal cusp of the mandibular teeth, an additional stabilizing factor for the maxillary denture teeth relative to the underlying bone is evidenced (Fig 31–6). In addition a narrower occlusal table is observed, which decreases the force required to penetrate food and simplifies the occlusal adjustment process (Fig 31–7). The

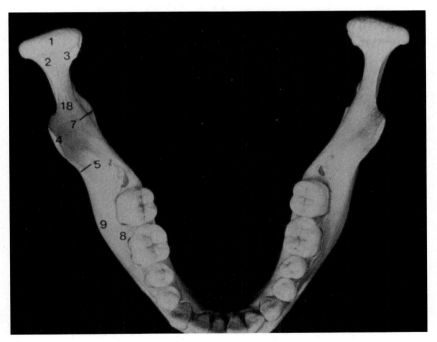

FIG 31–4.
Pound stated that a line drawn from the canine to each side of the retromolar pad was the region where the mandibular lingual cusp should be placed. This does not correspond to the natural tooth position, which always is medial to the retromolar pad region.

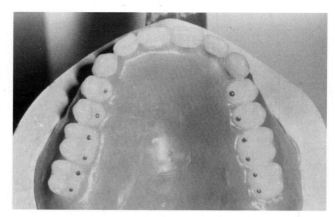

FIG 31–5.
Only the lingual cusps of the maxillary teeth occlude with the mandibular central fossa region. This further helps stabilize the maxillary denture, and reduces the occlusal table.

maxillary posterior teeth are positioned closer to the natural tooth position, as they follow the more natural positioned mandibular teeth. The more medial position of the maxillary buccal cusp also permits the polished labial surface of the denture to slope from the vestibule toward the occlusal surface, so the buccinator muscle may help improve denture base retention.

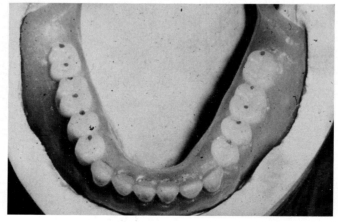

FIG 31–6.
Contact of the maxillary lingual cusp is in the central fossa region of the mandibular implant supported overdenture. The lingual cusps of the teeth are medial to the retromolar pad, similar to natural teeth.

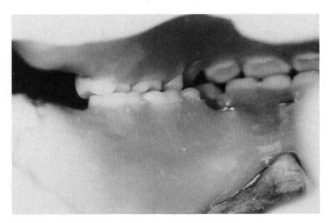

FIG 31–7.
Maxillary lingual cusp to mandibular central fossa contact reduces the occlusal table and makes penetration of food more efficient.

Bilateral balance is suggested to improve denture stability during parafunction. Once food is introduced between the teeth, the balanced occlusion is of less benefit for stability. Payne and Pound did not suggest a bilateral balance occlusion. However, since the lower implant denture is more stable than its maxillary counterpart, the maxillary denture may rotate and become dislodged during parafunction. This causes additional stress on the premaxilla and may result in more anterior resorption. Constant dislodgement of the posterior seal may also cause additional gagging in the patient. Therefore, the stable mandibular denture warrants additional stability of the maxillary prosthesis. It is more important to balance the occlusion within the functional range of mandibular movement, rather than to the extremes of lateral border positions.

The curves of Spee and Wilson, or a compensating curve, may be used in the posterior occlusion. An occlusal analyzer follows the curves of a 3 ⅞-inch, 4-inch, or 4 ⅛-inch sphere. The patient's skull size is estimated to be small, average, or large and determines the size of occlusal analyzer. Posterior block teeth which follow these spheres may also be fabricated to permit the technician to follow the occlusal plane.[19]

A moment force or torque is applied to the maxillary teeth set facial to the residual ridge, and becomes greater as the crown height is increased. This condition is difficult to prevent in the anterior maxilla, because this position is required for proper esthetics and phonetics. However, setting the teeth and the occlusal contacts in the posterior region toward the midline and raising the posterior plane of occlusion reduces moment forces and associated instability. The maxillary second molar may even be set in cross-bite to further improve the vertical force component over the severe atrophic Division D posterior maxilla.

The resultant factors of raising the posterior occlusal plane, "medial position" of the teeth, "lingual occlusion," and bilateral balance help stabilize the weakest member of the removable prostheses, the maxillary denture.

In summary, the following sequence governs posterior tooth position:

1. Position the mandibular teeth. These central fossae are placed over the line from the medial retromolar pad to the canine. The greater the resorption of posterior maxilla, the more medial the mandibular lingual cusp location (the lingual tooth position does not extend beyond 3 mm lingual of retromolar pad to canine cusp tip line).
2. Rotate the maxillary posterior buccal cusp so only lingual cusps occlude with mandibular central fossa in centric relation occlusion. The maxillary second molar may be set in cross-bite for Division D arches.
3. Bilateral balance occlusion in limited mandibular excursions

FUNCTIONALLY GENERATED PATH TECHNIQUE FOR MAXILLARY REMOVABLE PROSTHESES

The functionally generated path (FGP) technique enables the restoring dentist to accurately capture the mandibular eccentric movements of a patient without the use of complicated or expensive instrumentation.[20–23] The eccentric movements are recorded after the vertical dimension and anterior guidance are established. The technique has been used for all types of occlusal schemes, but is most useful when a bilateral balanced occlusion is the occlusal scheme selected (H. Zaki, personal communication). The FGP concept may be used to fabricate the initial prosthesis, or for resetting posterior teeth in conjunction with rebase or reline procedures.

The most common indication for the FGP in the implant practice is a maxillary complete or RP-5 overdenture opposing natural or previous fixed restorations. Bilateral balanced occlusion is especially difficult to establish when one of the arches presents natural dentition. Compounding the problem are patient treatments that do not permit complete occlusal rehabilitation of the natural arch. Implant dentistry often presents treatment options that combine the restoration of the maxillary arch with a traditional complete denture, with the mandibular arch restored with an implant-supported fixed prosthesis.

A less common treatment option is a maxillary complete subperiosteal implant with a RP-4 prosthesis opposing a fixed or removable mandibular prosthesis. Because the weaker premaxilla must be protected during mandibular excursions, the maxillary subperiosteal overdenture is designed with premolar bilateral balanced occlusion and modified protrusive contacts. Therefore, FGP concepts are also slightly modified for a maxillary subperiosteal RP-4 restoration opposing a natural or previously restored fixed prosthesis.

The eccentric movements of the mandible are dictated by the condylar disc assembly paths and the anterior incisal guidance. Because the FGP technique first establishes the vertical and anterior guidance, all necessary information is already available for an accurate customized recording of mandibular movements.

The position of all the teeth are very important for bilateral balanced occlusion. Mutually protected and canine protected occlusion may error in the posterior determinant of occlusion because the posterior teeth do not touch in balancing or working jaw movements. However, bilateral balance is a more difficult occlusal scheme to establish, because posterior and anterior teeth are in constant contact at the closed vertical dimension in all excursions.

The first step in the FGP technique for a maxillary removable prosthesis is the determination of maxillary anterior tooth position, after final impressions and stable base plate records are fabricated. Guidelines previously discussed are employed for esthetics, contour, and phonetics. The mandibular arch is then addressed.

If the mandibular arch is an overdenture and the position of the teeth is selected by the restoring dentist, the maxillary occlusal plane is determined in the occluso-gingival, bucco-lingual, and anterior-posterior directions. If the mandibular arch is already restored with a fixed prosthesis and/or natural teeth, the mandibular anterior teeth are recontoured as necessary to eliminate irregularities in height or labial position. The buccal contours of the mandibular posterior teeth are recontoured to permit more medial position of the occlusal contacts, and the lingual cusp height is often reduced to prevent lateral prematurities. An occlusal plane guide is used to correct the plane of occlusion on study casts, then intraorally on the natural dentition.

The vertical dimension of occlusion is established using established guidelines.[6] A record of vertical centric occlusion relation is obtained after anterior teeth position and vertical dimension are determined. A facebow registration may or may not be used to mount the maxillary cast baseplate with anterior teeth in final position. The opposing cast of the natural fixed mandibular teeth is mounted with the centric registrations. A "verticulator" or articulator with condylar protrusive settings greater than 60 degrees is used as the articulator for FGP techniques.

A maxillary denture opposing an implant overdenture first sets the mandibular posterior teeth, using the medial positioned concepts developed by the author. The maxillary posterior wax-rim is designed to occlude with the opposing cast or denture teeth on the articulator. A narrow slot is cut into the maxillary posterior occlusal rim directly over the central fossa of the mandibular posterior teeth. This slot extends to the acrylic baseplate, and forms a 3-mm-wide groove. Monomer is added to the baseplate in the groove, and the area is filled in with acrylic. The opposing cast is coated with petroleum jelly or separating medium,

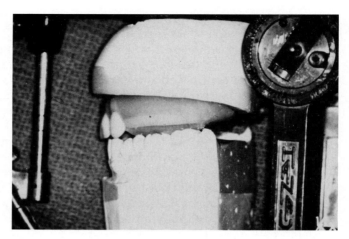

FIG 31–8.
Maxillary wax rim has the incisal edge position and the vertical occlusal dimension determined. An acrylic fin in the posterior occludes with the central fossa region of the opposing arch.

and the casts articulated. The remaining wax rim is removed after the acrylic polymerizes. This results in an acrylic fin occluding with the central fossa of the posterior cast at the recorded vertical occlusal dimension (Fig 31–8).

The maxillary baseplate is placed in the mouth, and the anterior tooth position and vertical occlusion are confirmed. Iowa wax is added around the posterior acrylic fin. The patient is guided first into centric occlusion, and a record of the occlusal surfaces of the mandibular teeth is made with the wax. The wax is softened in warm water and the patient is instructed to bite in centric occlusion and then guided into a left lateral movement until the maxillary and mandibular canines are in the same plane. Once the extent of the movement is registered, the patient opens the mouth and occludes back into centric occlusion. This recording is repeated a second time. The maxillary base plate is removed and examined. The posterior wax should not be unsupported at the base. If the wax extends wider on the occlusal table than on the base, additional wax is added below the occlusal registration table until it is supported.

The maxillary baseplate is reinserted. The patient is guided into centric relation occlusion, and the mandible is guided into a right lateral border movement. The patient opens when the mandibular movement has aligned the maxillary and mandibular canine facial surfaces and closes back into centric occlusion. The movement is repeated. The maxillary base plate is removed and examined for accurate occlusal patterns and supported occlusal wax contour.

The baseplate is inserted once again. This time, the patient is guided into centric relation occlusion and is asked to make one protrusive movement until the maxillary and mandibular anterior teeth are aligned. The patient then opens his or her mouth, and the baseplate is removed. Protrusive movements are not border movements, and may slightly vary with repeated records. Therefore, only one protrusive movement is recorded in the posterior occlusal wax.

A moist, cold towel is placed around the posterior wax to prevent distortion. The region is boxed and poured with dental or die stone. The towel helps prevent distortion of the wax when heat is generated by the stone during setting.

Once the stone is set, the maxillary baseplate is repositioned on the articulator. The mandibular cast of the teeth or dentures is removed from the mandibular component. The posterior stone patties are joined to the mandibular articulator frame with plaster. The mandibular occlusal casts are then separated from the maxillary base plate. The occlusal aspect of the mandibular cast does not appear as teeth; instead, it is the representation of the border movements of the mandibular cusps (Fig 31–9).

The articulator vertical relation pin is increased 1 mm. The maxillary posterior fully anatomic acrylic or composite denture teeth are positioned in the maxillary baseplate. The premolars are placed for esthetics and function. The first molar is often more medial in position in Division C and D, and the maxillary second molar may be set in cross-bite if the posterior ridge has severe resorption. The posterior teeth are set 1 mm too high at the present step, because the articulator vertical incisal pin was increased.

The vertical relation pin is then repositioned to the original vertical dimension. The articulator is used only in the vertical position. No excursions are made. Articulating paper marks the portions of the teeth in occlusion, and they

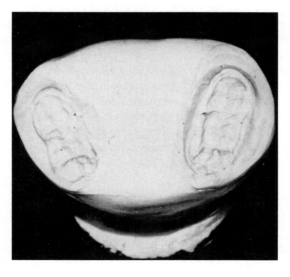

FIG 31–9.
Mandibular occlusal cast does not appear as teeth; rather, it is the representation of the occlusal portion of the mandibular teeth in all excursive movements.

are recontoured until the original vertical dimension is obtained. This results with a bilateral balanced occlusal scheme.

The maxillary prosthesis with waxed-in teeth is tried in the patient's mouth. The left and right border movements are made, along with a protrusive movement. The occlusion is evaluated and adjusted as needed. The esthetics and phonetics are also evaluated. The final denture may then be processed and delivered at the following appointment.

An alternative technique for a FGP denture may be used if the mandibular arch may also be restored. This technique first finishes the maxillary denture to ideal esthetics, contour, comfort, and occlusal plane depending on the amount of maxillary ridge resorption. The mandibular arch will then be restored to the final maxillary prosthesis.

The final maxillary denture is positioned in the patient's mouth. The mandibular anterior teeth are first positioned and evaluated for esthetics and phonetics at the desired vertical dimension. Anterior contact in centric relation occlusion is not usually indicated for a maxillary removable prosthesis. An incisal stop or index is placed on the anterior teeth to record the vertical dimension at centric condylar position. A centric vertical occlusal recording permits the mounting of the maxillary denture cast and mandibular base plate on an articulator.

Once the maxillary cast and mandibular occlusal records are mounted on an articulator, the acrylic fin connected to the mandibular base plate is fabricated in a manner similar to the previous technique. During the next patient appointment, intraoral wax recordings are made similar to those of the previous procedure. The setting of the posterior teeth, occlusal grind-in procedure, and delivery of final prosthesis are also similar.

The occlusal scheme for a maxillary complete subperiosteal RP-4 prosthesis is slightly different from other maxillary overdenture reconstructions. Opposing a RP-5 mandibular prosthesis or traditional denture, a bilateral balanced occlusion is developed. However, in protrusive and lateral movements the maxillary lateral and central incisors do not contact. This helps protect the bone in the premaxilla, which is most critical for maxillary subperiosteal support.

For a maxillary RP-4 overdenture opposing natural teeth, a unilateral balanced occlusion may be used when no central or lateral implants are placed. An FGP concept may also be used for this occlusal scheme. However, after processing, the occlusal nonworking contacts are selectively removed to eliminate all interferences. A mutually protected occlusion is designed when several anterior implants are placed in the canine and anterior position.

SUMMARY

The maxillary denture becomes a source of complaint when opposing natural teeth or a stable mandibular overdenture. Many removable denture concepts have been developed to make the mandibular prosthesis more stable. Once implants are placed in the mandible and attached to a superstructure, the maxillary denture becomes the least retentive and stable member. Methods to improve stability include careful evaluation and treatment of the maxillary soft tissue, raising of the posterior occlusal plane in relation to the bone support, and establishing a balanced "medial positioned lingualized occlusion." As a result, moment forces are reduced, and maxillary denture stability is improved.

REFERENCES

1. Branemark PI et al: Osseointegrated implants in the treatment of the edentulous jaw: experience from a 10-year period, *Scand J Plast Reconst Surg* 1977;suppl 16.
2. Adell R et al: A 15 year study of osseointegrated implants in the treatment of the edentulous jaw, *Int J Oral Surg* 10:387, 1981.
3. Albrektsson T et al: Osseointegrated oral implants: A Swedish multi-center study of 8139 consecutively inserted Nobelpharma implants, *J Periodontol* 59:287, 1988.
4. Haraldson T, Carlsson GE, Ingervall B: Functional state, bite force and postural muscle activity in patients with osseointegrated oral bridges, *Acta Odontol Scand* 37:195–206, 1979.
5. Helkimo E, Carlsson GE, Helkimo M: Bite force and state dentition, *Acta Odontol Scand* 35:297–303, 1977.
6. Winkler S: *Essentials of complete denture prosthodontics*, Philadelphia, 1979, WB Saunders.
7. Misch CE: Classifications and treatment options of the completely edentulous arch in implant dentistry. *Dent Today* 9:26, 30, 1990.
8. Misch CE: Maxillary denture opposing a mandibular implant overdenture, Dearborn, Mich, Misch Implant Institute Manual, 1988, Session I.
9. Misch CE: Maxillary implant opposing a mandibular implant prosthesis, abstract, American College of Oral Implantology National Meeting, Dearborn, Mich, 1991.
10. Hickey JC, Zarb GA, Bolender CL: *Boucher's prosthodontic treatment for edentulous patients,* ed 9, St Louis, 1985 CV Mosby.
11. Boucher CO: A critical analysis of mid-country impression techniques for full dentures, *J Prosthet Dent* 1:472–491, 1957.
12. Kydd WL, Daly CH, Wheeler JB: The thickness measurement of masticatory mucosa in vivo, *Int Dent J* 21:430–441, 1971.
13. Vig RG, Brundo GC: The kinetics of anterior tooth display, *J Prosthet Dent* 39:502–504, 1978.
14. Robinson SC: Physiological placement of artificial anterior teeth, *Can Dent J* 35:260–266, 1969.
15. Schiffman P: Relation to the maxillary canine and the incisive papilla, *J Prosthet Dent* 14:469–472, 1964.
16. Fahmi FM: The position of the neutral zone in relation to the alveolar ridge, *J Prosthet Dent* 67:805–809, 1992.
17. Payne SH: A posterior set-up to meet individual requirements, *Dent Dig* 47:20–22, 1941.

18. Pound E: Utilizing speech to simplify a personalized denture service, *J Prosthet Dent* 24:586–600, 1970.
19. Misch MPLO concept teeth, Root Laboratory, Leawood, Kansas.
20. Zimmerman M: Modifications of functionally generated path procedures, *J Prosthet Dent* 16:1119–1125, 1966.
21. Mann AW, Pankey LD: Concepts of occlusion—the p.m. philosophy of occlusal rehabilitation, *Dent Clin North Am* 4:621–636, 1963.
22. Meyer FS: The generated path technique in reconstruction dentistry: complete dentures, *J Prosthet Dent* 9:354–366, 1959.

Chapter 32

Occlusal Considerations for Implant-Supported Prostheses

Carl E. Misch

The choice of an occlusal scheme for implant-supported prostheses is broad and often controversial. Almost all concepts are based on those developed with natural teeth, and are transposed to implant support systems with almost no modification. No controlled clinical studies have been published comparing the various implant occlusal theories. Implant survival rates reported by different practitioners are often within similar ranges, even though the restoring guidelines differ. However, these statements are not meant to decrease the importance of occlusion and a quest for accurate and precise relationships. Once rigid fixation, angulation, crestal bone level, contour, and gingival health are achieved, stress beyond physiologic limits is the primary cause of initial bone loss around implants. The restoring dentist has specific responsibilities to reduce overload to the bone-implant interface. These include proper diagnosis, leading to a treatment plan designed with adequate support based on individual variation (Chapters 6 to 13); methods to obtain a passive casting with adequate retention and form (Chapters 29 and 30); and progressive loading to improve the amount and density of the bone and further reduce the risk of stress beyond physiologic limits (Chapter 28). The major remaining factor is the development of occlusal concepts in harmony with the rest of the stomatognathic system.

Occlusal factors are a primary requisite for long-term survival, especially when parafunction or marginal support of the foundation are present. A poor occlusal pattern increases and localizes the forces, and in these regions more frequent complications of the prosthesis, bone support, or both occur. In this chapter, clinical case series evaluations are blended and interrelated with finite element analyses, basic prosthetics, and bone biomechanical principles which reduce localized forces, and establish a consistent occlusal philosophy.

OCCLUSAL CONSIDERATIONS

Transosteal Forces

The precursor signs of occlusal trauma on natural teeth are usually reversible and include sensitivity, hyperemia, or an increase in mobility.[1] The presence of a periodontal membrane on natural teeth significantly reduces the amount of stress to the bone, especially at the crestal region.[2] Clinical evidence for this is the overall increase in the periodontal membrane region from occlusal trauma observed on radiographs, not just localized at the crest. The tooth is present in the mouth since childhood, and the surrounding bone mechanics have developed in response to the biomechanical loads. Hence, a tooth is often prepared for any additional forces brought to bear by an attached prosthesis.

The initial reversible signs and symptoms of trauma on natural teeth do not occur with endosteal implants. An absence of soft tissue interface between the implant body and bone results with the greatest magnitude of force localized around the transosteal implant–bone region.[3] The magnitude of stress may cause bone microfractures and mechanical problems with the prosthesis or implant. Instead of reversible signs and symptoms found with teeth, implant bone loss or unsecured restorations most often occur without any warning signs. Implant occlusal sensitivity is uncommon and signifies more advanced complications. The loss of crestal bone around the implant is *not reversible* without surgical intervention, and results in a decreased implant support and increased sulcus pocket depth. As a result, unless the density of bone increases or the amount or duration of force decreases, the condition will progress and even accelerate until implant loss occurs. Elements to decrease crestal bone forces are implemented in occlusal designs presented in this chapter.

Implants are subject to repeated occlusal loads that can lead to microscopic stress fractures, work hardening, and fatigue. The implant components, coping screws, or cement cannot adjust to these conditions and ultimately fracture. The implant needs to perform its service for scores of years, and the long-term complications related to fracture are not yet appreciated. Therefore, forces from occlusion may result in subtle changes that are difficult to discern but may cause more serious long-term problems for survival as a result of bone and/or implant component complications.

Direction of Load to Implant Body

Any occlusal force may be divided into three directions or vectors. The primary direction of the force is greatest in amount or intensity.[3] The primary forces of occlusion should be directed to the long axis of the implant body, not the abutment post. A force along the long axis of the implant body distributes less force to the surrounding crestal bone. Angled abutments are primarily used to improve the path of insertion of the prosthesis. The 30-degree angled abutment loaded in the abutment long axis will transmit greater compressive and tensile stresses to the crest of bone around the implant body compared with the same implant with an angled abutment loaded in the direction of the long axis of the implant body. The greater the angle between the primary force and the implant body, the greater the amount of crestal compressive and tensile stresses with a rigid fixated implant. For example, three-dimensional finite element analysis demonstrates that a vertical load on an implant with 100% bone contact may have compressive stress of 7,000 psi and almost no tensile stress at the bone-implant-crest interface. With a 45 degree load on the same implant design, the compressive stress may increase to 14,000 psi and tensile stress to 4,000 psi on the opposite side. Hence, the compressive stresses are doubled and the tensile stress increase 1,000-fold with a 45 degree load[4] (Fig 32–1). The lateral loads to the implant crestal region further increase when crown height increases or when present on the cantilevered portion of the prosthesis.[3] Therefore, whenever possible, implant bodies should be primarily submitted to the vertical component of the occlusal load. Horizontal or lateral forces magnify the amount of compressive and tensile stress at the transosteal implant crestal site and should be reduced or eliminated, especially when the ratio of crown height to implant length is greater than 1, or present on cantilevered prostheses.

Premature occlusal contacts result with localized loading of the opposing contacting crowns. Because stress is defined as force per area, premature contact provides minimal area to distribute the load, and the amount of stress is dramatically increased. All the occlusal force is applied to one region rather than being shared by several abutments and/or teeth. In addition, the premature contact is most often on an inclined plane,[5] therefore giving a greater horizontal

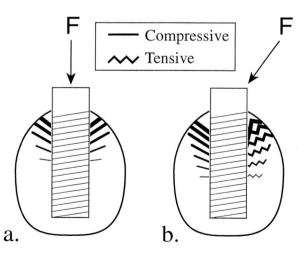

FIG 32–1.
A, axial force results with compressive forces, which are primarily at the transosteal site and rapidly reduced after 5 mm within the bone (for D-1 bone). **B,** angled force results with greater compressive loads on the opposite side and significant tensile forces on the same side as the force.

component to the load and increasing compressive and tensile crestal stresses. Elimination of premature occlusal contacts is especially important with habitual parafunction, as the amount, direction, and duration of the load increase.

Offset loads usually are facial or lingual occlusal contacts, not those in the long axis of the implant body. Occlusal contact rarely is placed over an occlusal access hole for a coping screw, because acrylic rapidly wears and results with no contact. Offset loads therefore are more common when occlusal screws are used in the prosthesis. To avoid esthetic complications for a screw-retained prosthesis, the implant body should be set more lingual, than for a cemented restoration. The offset occlusal load is applied slightly facial to the implant body, and parallel to its long axis. A cement-retained restoration may place the implant directly under the primary occlusal contact. The crown may load the implant body in an axial direction. As a result, fewer offset loads are present on cement-retained prostheses than in screw-retained restorations (Fig 32–2). When offset contacts have an angled force, the distance of the offset contact acts as a moment arm and magnifies the effect of the lateral force. Hence an angled 25 lbf with an offset of 5 mm may result with a 125 lb mm–moment load.

When two or more implants are placed to support a screw-retained restoration, the facial-occlusal contacts over each implant body are similar to the previous scenario for screw-retained implants. However, between the implants, the intermediate marginal ridges and pontics may have more medial primary occlusal contacts, often in the central fossa region instead of the usual mandibular buccal cusp contact. This eliminates the offset loads between the implants, and occlusal loads between the implant bodies are in a more axial direction (Fig 32–3).

FIG 32–2.
A, occlusal load over a cement-retained restoration may load the implant body with axial force.
B, an occlusal access screw hole often is recessed or filled with acrylic, which rapidly wears. Screw-retained restoration often has an offset force toward the facial aspect of the access hole. The distance (*d*) acts as a moment arm with any lateral force and results in a magnified angled load on the implant body.

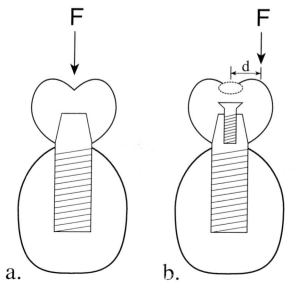

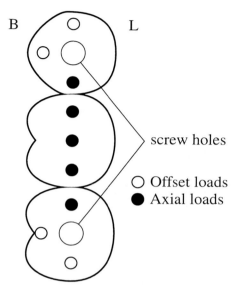

screw holes

○ Offset loads
● Axial loads

FIG 32–3.
Three-unit prosthesis with two screw-retained abutments may place contacts in the central fossa and marginal ridges between the occlusal access holes for more axial loading. Offset loads are buccal, lingual, or lateral to the implant bodies.

Anterior implants with abutments for cement place the implant body under the incisal edge of the prosthesis. Anterior implants with abutments for screw are often placed more lingual, so the access hole is in the cingulum region. Greater offset loads result during lateral excursions, because the incisal edge is more facial. In order to decrease the effect of lateral force during mandibular excursions, natural teeth, when present, receive the greatest load. If this is not possible, more than one implant should distribute the lateral load. The general principles regarding direction of load to the implant body are:

1. Axial loads to the implant body produce less compressive and tensile stress.
2. Horizontal loads produce an increase in both compressive and tensive stress.
3. Premature contacts result with greater stress, often on lateral inclines of cusps.
4. Screw-retained prostheses often have implant bodies more lingual compared to cement-retained restorations, and result with greater offset loads.

Bone Biomechanics

Bone Strength

Bone is strongest under compressive forces, less strong to tensile force, and significantly weakest in shear.[3, 6] Under an axial force, bone has compressive strength of 193 megapascals (MPa), tensile limits of 133 MPa, and shear limits of

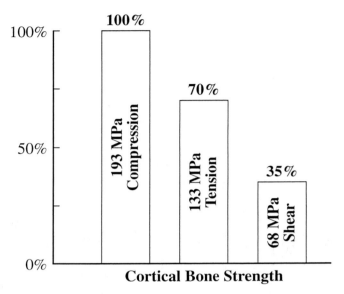

FIG 32–4.
Strength of cortical bone is greatest in compression, 30% weaker in tension, and 65% weaker with shear forces. Therefore occlusal designs should transfer compressive loads.

68 MPa. As a result, occlusal designs aim at reducing tensile force and eliminating shear forces whenever possible (Fig 32–4).

An axial load over the long axis of an implant distributes more compressive stress compared with tensile or shear forces. Any load which is applied at an angle may be separated into normal and shear forces (see Chapter 15). The greater the angle of load to the implant long axis, the greater the compressive, tensile, and shear stresses[3, 4] (Fig 32–5). Therefore, not only is the *amount* of stress increased with an angled load, but the *type* of stress converts to more tensile and shear components. Because bone is stronger in compression, the negative effect of angled loads is enhanced. Because horizontal or lateral loads cause an increase in the amount of tension and shear forces at the crest of the ridge, these loads must be reduced within the occlusal scheme, especially in mechanical systems which increase the force, as cantilevers or crowns with greater crown-implant ratios. A primary vector of compressive force on a unilateral cantilever portion of a fixed partial denture also applies shear and tensile force on the most distant abutment. Therefore it is suggested to establish lighter occlusal contacts on cantilevers.

Direction of Force

The angle of the force to the bone affects the physiologic limit of compressive and tensile strengths of bone. A force applied at a 30 degree angle decreases the

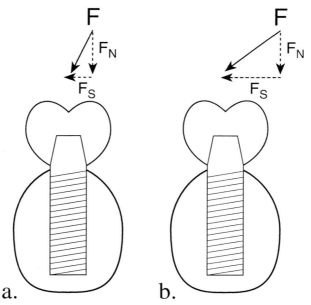

FIG 32–5.
Angled force may be separated in compression, tension (normal forces, F_n), and shear components (F_s). The greater the angle of force the greater the shear component, even though the amount of the force is similar. Therefore the magnitude and direction of the force are important to consider. Occlusal designs should limit the effect of angled loads.

bone strength limits from 193 MPa to 173 MPa under compression and from 133 MPa to 100 MPa with tension. A 60 degree force further reduces the limits to 133 MPa under compression and 60.5 MPa under tension (Table 32–1).

Hence, the angled load increases the amount of stress around the implant body, transforms a *greater* percentage of the force to tensile and shear force, and

TABLE 32–1.
Cortical Bone Strength Related to Angle of Load*

	Strength (MPa)	Direction of Load
Compressive	193.0	Longitudinal
	173.0	30° off axis
	133.0	60° off axis
	133.0	Transverse
Tensile	133.0	Longitudinal
	100.0	30° off axis
	60.5	60° off axis
	51.0	Transverse

*From Cowin SL: *Bone mechanics.* Boca Raton, Fla, CRC Press, 1989.

reduces bone strength in compression and tension. In contrast, the surrounding implant body stress is least and the strength of bone greatest under a load axial to the implant body. All three of these factors mandate the elimination of lateral forces. Axial loading of the implant is especially required when the intensity of force and/or its duration increases (i.e., parafunction). Occlusal designs should include axial loads to implant bodies, and when not possible, should incorporate mechanisms to decrease the negative effect of lateral loads.

Biomechanics

Several features help decrease the effects of horizontal loads responsible for tension and shear on the crest of the ridge. These include the implant diameter[3] and the number of implants supporting the prosthesis and distributing the load. An important parameter in implant prosthesis occlusion is adequate surface area support. Stress is a function of force per area. It is better to err in having too much support, rather than just fall short of necessary requirements. For example, a 25-lb force distributed to two splinted abutments creates less localized stress to the crestal bone than when the same load is applied to one abutment (Fig 32–6). Therefore, whenever lateral force components increase in amount, direction, or duration of application, the number of implants splinted in the region should also increase. Lateral loads frequently occur in the anterior region of the mouth, during mandibular excursions. More splinted implants are therefore placed in this area to reduce and dissipate the resulting crestal stresses.

Wider implants have greater area of bone contact at the crest than narrow implants. As a result, both compressive and tensile forces are reduced with wider implants. On the opposite, narrow root form implants have less surface area and transmit greater stresses at the crest of the ridge[3] (Fig 32–7). Therefore, when narrow implants are used in regions which receive greater forces, additional splinted implants are indicated to compensate for their narrow design and help decrease and distribute the load over a broader region. When forces are increased in intensity, duration, or both (e.g., parafunction), ridge augmentation may be required to place wider implants to compensate for the increased loads. The prosthesis type may also be modified to reduce occlusal loads from a fixed restoration (FP-1 to FP-3) to a removable prosthesis (RP-4). This is most effective when nocturnal parafunction is present and the restoration may be removed to eliminate the condition. In addition, stress-relieving elements may be included in the removable restoration and allow the soft tissue to help dissipate the loads (RP-5 restorations).

The wider the occlusal table, the more frequently offset contacts occur during mastication or parafunction. Wider root form implants offer a broader area for axial occlusal contacts and transmit less forces at the transosteal site under offset loads than narrow plate form or root form implants. The narrower the implant body, the greater the importance of occlusal table width and axial loading the

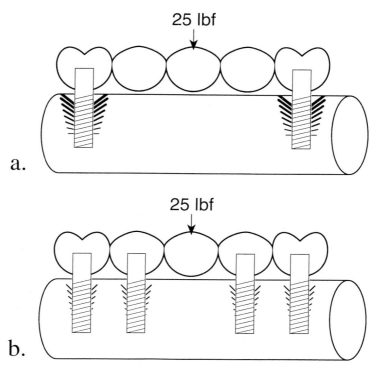

FIG 32–6.
The greater the number of implants supporting a prosthesis, or occlusal force in a segment of the arch the less the stress to each implant transosteal region. **A,** 25 lbf is placed on a fixed prosthesis with two implant abutments. **B,** 25 lbf is placed on a fixed prosthesis with four abutments. There is more crestal stress in **A** than in **B**.

implant body. Therefore the faciolingual dimension of the occlusal table on which contacts are acceptable is directly related to the width of the implant body.

During mastication, the amount of force used to penetrate the food bolus is also related to occlusal table width. For example, less force is required to cut a piece of meat with a sharp knife (narrow occlusal table), than with a dull knife (wider occlusal table). The greater surface area requires greater force to get a similar result. Hence, the wider the occlusal table, the greater force the biologic system uses to penetrate the bolus of food. Therefore, narrow occlusal tables are recommended for use in any unesthetic region of the mouth. Because bone loss occurs at the expence of the facial contour of bone, the occlusal table should be decreased in width from the facial aspect, not from the lingual. This allows the more medial implant to receive a more axial load (Fig 32–8). If the occlusal table cannot be decreased because of esthetics, the opposing arch is decreased from the

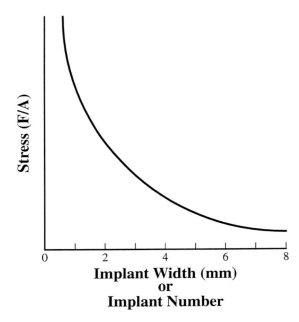

FIG 32–7.
The greater the implant diameter the less stress to the transosteal region. The greater the implant number to support a given load the less the stress to the transosteal region.

facial, and small surface area contacts with greater cusp angle are used to improve masticatory efficiency.

The most common region in which esthetics modify the reduced occlusal table concept is in a maxillary implant reconstruction. The esthetics of the buccal cusps should not be compromised by a reduction in occlusal table width, even when the implant is placed to the lingual aspect of the ridge. The occlusal width remains identical, for ideal esthetics from the buccal cusps. However, narrower occlusal tables are desirable in the mandibular arch to direct occlusal forces over the maxillary implant body. As a result, maxillary implants require the buccal cusps of opposing natural mandibular teeth (or crowns on implants) to be reduced to eliminate the offset load in centric relation occlusion. The maxillary buccal cusp may then be retained for esthetics but the functional occlusal table is reduced. The distal half of the first molar and/or the entire second molar is often in cross-bite to improve the direction of forces, when esthetics are not a concern.

Occlusal Force and Muscles of Mastication

Many occlusal analyses with natural teeth suggest anterior disclusion in excursions.[7–9] The periodontal ligament of natural teeth decreases the amount of crestal load under vertical and horizontal loads[10] compared with rigid fixated implants. The greater cervical diameter of teeth also decrease crestal loads. As a result, natural teeth have a greater stress-relieving element than implants, particularly under lateral forces. If healthy anterior teeth, or natural canines are present, the occlusal scheme uses those teeth to distribute the horizontal load during mandibular excursions.

The stomatognathic system elicits less force when the posterior segments are not in contact. Comparisons of anterior bite force measurements with posterior bite force amounts, and electromyographic studies confirm this result.[11–14] Therefore, whether the anterior section is implant-supported or teeth-supported, the posterior components should be discluded in all lateral excursions when opposing fixed dentitions. The resultant lateral forces are distributed solely to the

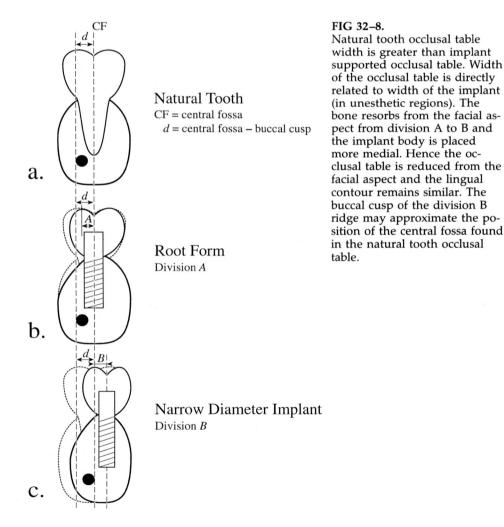

Natural Tooth
CF = central fossa
d = central fossa – buccal cusp

a.

Root Form
Division *A*

b.

Narrow Diameter Implant
Division *B*

c.

FIG 32–8.
Natural tooth occlusal table width is greater than implant supported occlusal table. Width of the occlusal table is directly related to width of the implant (in unesthetic regions). The bone resorbs from the facial aspect from division A to B and the implant body is placed more medial. Hence the occlusal table is reduced from the facial aspect and the lingual contour remains similar. The buccal cusp of the division B ridge may approximate the position of the central fossa found in the natural tooth occlusal table.

anterior segments of the jaws to decrease the quantity of force against the anterior and posterior dentition. In addition, this eliminates completely lateral forces on posterior implants.

Natural Teeth and Implants

There has been controversy regarding whether a rigid fixated implant may remain successful when splinted to natural teeth. Because the implant has no periodontal membrane, concerns center around the potential for the "nonmobile" implant to bear the total load of the prosthesis when joined to the "mobile" natural tooth. The actual mobility of potential natural abutments may influence the treatment more than any other factor. In the implant-tooth-fixed prosthesis, four important components may contribute movement to the system: the implant, bone, tooth, and prosthesis. As demonstrated in Chapter 9, the implant and tooth may be connected, dependent upon all four of these factors.

The concern for the difference in tooth movement and implant movement should not be restricted to situations where these entities are connected. When an implant is placed in a partially edentulous arch, many similar biomechanical elements are present whether the teeth are splinted to the implant or are independent.

The tooth movement ranges from 8 to 28 μ in a vertical direction under a 3 to 5 pound force (lbf), depending upon the size, number, and geometry of the roots and the time elapsed since the last load application.[10, 15–17] Once the initial tooth movement occurs, the secondary tooth movement reflects the property of the surrounding bone and is very similar to the bone-implant movement. The axial movement of an implant ranges from 3 to 5 μm[16] and has little correlation to implant body length.

Because the difference in vertical movement may be as much as 25 μm the initial occlusal contacts should account for this difference, or the implant will be loaded more than the adjacent teeth. Therefore, thin articulating paper is used for the initial occlusal adjustment in centric relation occlusion under a light tapping force. The implant prosthesis should barely contact, and the adjacent teeth should exhibit greater contacts. Only axial occlusal contacts should be present on the implant crown. A heavier centric relation occlusal force is then applied. The contacts should remain axial over the implant body, and may be of similar intensity on the implant crown and the adjacent teeth.

Once the occlusal adjustment is completed in centric relation occlusion, the lateral and protrusive movements may be evaluated. When opposing a fixed dentition, no posterior implants or teeth should contact in any excursive mandibular movement. The horizontal movement of natural anterior teeth ranges from 64 to 108 μm. An implant has a lateral movement which ranges from 12 μm (bucco-lingual in dense bone) to 140 μm in very soft bone (rarely observed in the anterior regions). When a combination of nonsplinted anterior teeth and implants are present in the anterior maxilla or mandible, the forces produced during mandibular lateral excursions should be distributed initially and primarily to the natural teeth. If no anterior teeth are present in the direction of the excursion, two or more splinted implants should distribute the lateral force. Three or more Division A implants may be required for parafunctional forces (bruxism) in each excursive direction.

In summary:

1. Teeth move more in vertical movement (heavier contact than an adjacent or connected implant).
2. Anterior teeth have more horizontal movement (excursions) (initial and heavier contact than an adjacent or connected implant).
3. If only anterior implants, two or more implants should distribute each lateral load (often requires four implants for an edentulous premaxilla); for bruxism, three or more implants are required in each excursion.

Bone Resorption

Once the natural teeth are removed, the bone remodels to the height at or below the lowest level of the lateral cortical plates. Hence, the implant crown is greater than the natural anatomic crown, even in Division A bone. The primary component of the occlusal force is determined before implant placement. In an edentulous ridge with abundant height and width and little resorption, the implant may be placed in a more ideal position for occlusion and aesthetics. A decision is made early in treatment whether an abutment for screw or for cement will be used in the restoration. A cement-retained restoration permits positioning the implant body directly under the primary occlusal contact. An implant is best inserted when it is placed in the middle of the remaining width of bone, or slightly toward the more dense bone of the lingual plate. Facial concavities are avoided, the thinner facial cortical bone is protected, and fewer surgical errors with labial or lingual dehiscence on the implant bodies result with this approach. As a result, whether in the maxilla or the mandible, the implant is placed under the central fossa region of the natural tooth. To load the implant body in an axial direction, the primary occlusal contact should be the central fossa region in division A bone. This permits posterior mandibular natural teeth opposing a maxillary implant to have the mandibular buccal cusp as the primary contact. However, mandibular implants opposing maxillary natural teeth must use the maxillary lingual cusp as the primary contact (Fig 32–9).

The bone continues to resorb from the facial aspect, to further decrease bone width (Division B). In these conditions the implant often is placed under the lingual cusp position relative to the natural tooth in the mandible or maxilla. The implant body should be ideally placed perpendicular to the occlusal plane. In the mandible, the buccal cusp on the implant crown is reduced in height to

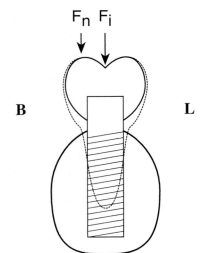

FIG 32–9.
Primary contact on the mandibular posterior natural tooth is the buccal cusp (F_n). This position results with an offset load on an implant placed in the region. The axial implant load (F_i) is in the central fossa region of the original occlusal table for division A bone.

correspond to the original central fossa and the occlusal table is reduced from the facial aspect to permit axial loading of the implant body (Fig 32–10). In the maxilla, the implant crown must retain the offset buccal cusps for esthetics. However, the mandibular occlusal table is modified to permit axial loading of the maxillary implant body, and the maxillary occlusal table may be reduced from the lingual aspect.

In the anterior maxilla, labial concavities may require that the implant be angled away from the labial bone and the abutment toward the facial crown

FIG 32–10.
Division B ridge requires the implant body to be placed in the lingual cusp region of the original natural tooth. The lingual contour of the implant crown may remain the same, but the buccal cusp must be reduced in height and the occlusal table is reduced from the facial region. B = buccal; L = lingual.

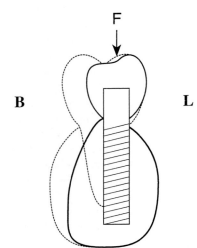

contour. These implant bodies more often are loaded on an angle, and an angled prosthetic abutment is required. Larger diameter implants or more implants are required to reduce crestal bone stress. A ridge augmentation may be necessary prior to implant placement, to improve implant placement and increase the size of the implant diameter, especially in patients with severe bruxism.

In summary, the implant body is placed in the middle of the edentulous crest of bone, which is in the central fossa region or even more lingual. As a result, natural teeth occlusal concepts must be modified so that the primary occlusal contact is axial to the implant body, not the buccal cusp of the mandibular natural tooth.

OCCLUSAL SCHEMES

The goal of an occlusal scheme is to maintain the occlusal load that has been transferred to the implant body within the physiologic limits of each patient. These limits are not the same for all patients and restorations. The forces generated by a patient include parafunction, masticatory dynamics, tongue size, implant arch position, and location and implant arch form (see Chapter 8). The implant dentist can dissipate these force factors by selecting the proper implant size, number, and position, using stress-relieving elements, increasing bone density by progressive loading, and selecting the appropriate occlusal scheme.

The occlusal philosophy for dental implants is highly variable and dependent on several parameters. Implant and natural tooth position, number, size, and design produce a myriad of possible combinations. However, consistent occlusal patterns may be established following the occlusal considerations in this Chapter. The following guidelines are used to restore implant-supported prostheses.

Medial Positioned Lingualized Occlusion

The concepts of medial positioned lingualized occlusion for complete dentures were presented in Chapter 31. Many of these concepts are also indicated for a fixed-implant-supported restoration. When teeth are present, the maxillary edentulous posterior ridge is positioned slightly more facial than the mandibular arch. Once the maxillary teeth are lost, the width of the edentulous ridge resorbs in a medial direction as it evolves: Division A to B, Division B to C, and Division C to D. As a result, in the maxilla the permucosal implant site gradually shifts toward the midline as the ridge resorbs. Subantral augmentation permits endosteal implants even in previous Division D ridges. Therefore the maxillary posterior implant permucosal site even may be lingual to the opposing natural mandibular tooth (Fig 32–11).

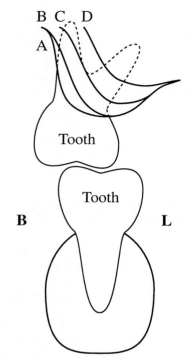

FIG 32–11.
Posterior crest of the maxilla is slightly more lateral than the corresponding mandibular crest. After tooth loss the crest resorbs from the facial aspect (first in width, then in height) and the remaining ridge becomes more medial. *A–D* = bone divisions; *B* = buccal; *L* = lingual.

The maxillary posterior implant most often is positioned under the central fossa region of the natural tooth in Division A bone. The maxillary occlusal table cannot be reduced from the facial aspect because it will affect the esthetics of the restoration and may require a modified ridge lap abutment crown. A maxillary implant opposing a natural mandibular molar may have the lower buccal cusp as primary contact with the central fossa of the maxillary implant crown. The lingual aspect of the maxillary implant crown often is reduced in height and width when the implant is under the maxillary central fossa, to reduce the lingual offset loads in the posterior region (Fig 32–12).

The mandibular posterior implant also is placed under the central fossa region of the natural tooth. When maxillary and mandibular implants oppose each other in the Division A posterior regions, the mandibular buccal cusp may be positioned more medial and of reduced height closer to and over the mandibular implant in the center of the ridge and occlude with the central fossa lingual cusp region of the crowns over the maxillary implant(s), which are reduced in width. This reduces the overall occlusal table in the mandible. If opposing implants cannot load both implant bodies in an axial direction, the weakest implant (in bone density, diameter, length, and so forth) is protected by the axial load at the expense of the more efficient implant regarding these conditions (Fig 32–13).

When the mandibular implant opposes a natural maxillary tooth, the primary contacting cusp becomes the maxillary lingual cusp opposing the mandibular implant crown with the mandibular buccal cusp of decreased height and width over the implant body (Fig 32–14). Hence all contacts are more medial than with natural teeth. The medial positioned lingualized occlusion concept developed by Misch for complete dentures also has direct application for implant fixed prostheses.[18, 19]

Division B maxillary and mandibular implants, which are positioned under the lingual cusp relative to the natural tooth position, require even narrower mandibular occlusal tables, to avoid unwanted occlusal contacts. The primary contact of occlusion on a mandibular implant in Division B bone opposing a natural posterior maxillary tooth is the lingual cusp of the maxillary posterior tooth. The maxillary lingual cusp tip is modified to load the implant body more axially. The buccal cusp of the mandibular implant crown is located over the more medial Division B implant body to dramatically reduce the occlusal table. The medial positioned Division B mandibular implant may even require a single-cusped crown directly over the implant body (Fig 32–15), especially when it is of reduced width as with a plate form implant. The implant in the mandibular

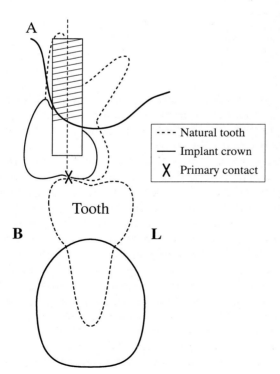

----	Natural tooth
——	Implant crown
X	Primary contact

FIG 32–12.
Maxillary Division *A* bone positions the implant body under the central fossa. In esthetic regions the facial aspect of the maxillary implant crown should remain similar to the natural tooth. This may require a modified ridge lap abutment crown at the cervical region. The lingual contour and cusp may be reduced to reduce offset loads from the opposing natural tooth. *B* = buccal; *L* = lingual.

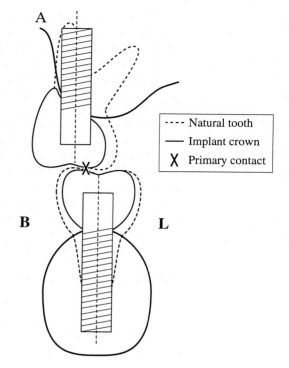

Key
---- Natural tooth
—— Implant crown
X Primary contact

FIG 32–13.
When maxillary and mandibular implants oppose each other in posterior Division *A* bone, each implant is placed under the original central fossa region. The maxillary crown is reduced on the lingual aspect, and the mandibular crown on the facial and lingual aspects, maintaining the same vertical occlusal dimension and reducing the overall occlusal table.

posterior region may on occasion require angulation to avoid the submandibular fossa, and mandates implant placement in a medial angle. As a result, a lingual straight emergence crown profile and/or an angled abutment to limit the extension of the crown toward the tongue is indicated.

A maxillary Division B implant is also often placed under the palatal cusp region. Because the maxillary occlusal table cannot be reduced from the facial for esthetic reasons, the buccal cusp is offset to the facial, but completely out of occlusion in centric relation occlusion and all mandibular excursions. The buccal cusp of the opposing natural tooth is reduced toward the medial aspect and in height, to eliminate any offset load on the maxillary implant. The primary occlusal contact in centric relation occlusion is the maxillary palatal cusp over the implant body and the central fossa region of the mandibular natural tooth.

When Division B position implants are placed in both arches, the maxillary prosthesis is similar to that described in the previous scenario, and the mandibular implant crown is further reduced in width at the expense of the buccal cusp until an axial component of force is realized, at least within 20 degrees. If this is not possible, the weakest implant in bone density, width, or prostheses type (fixed vs. removable) determines the axial load, because it is the most vulnerable arch.

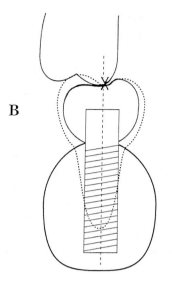

B   L

FIG 32–14.
Mandibular implant in Division A bone is placed under the original central fossa of the natural tooth, which corresponds to the lingual cusp in the maxilla. Hence the buccal cusp is reduced in width, and the height of the buccal implant cusp is similar to that of the natural tooth central fossa. The primary contact is with the maxillary lingual cusp.

In conclusion, the implant body should be loaded in an axial direction. In a Division A maxillary ridge the implant can be placed under the central fossa region of the natural teeth. As a result, the buccal cusp of the natural tooth in the mandibular arch is the dominant cusp. The lingual contour of the maxillary posterior implant crown should be reduced to eliminate offset loads. The position

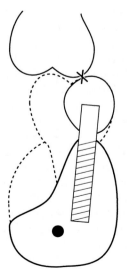

FIG 32–15.
Mandibular posterior Division B bone opposing maxillary natural teeth may require a mandibular single-cusped tooth over the implant body to reduce the offset loads and dramatically reduce the occlusal table. The maxillary lingual cusp may be modified to position the contact more medial.

of the buccal cusp should remain similar to that of the original tooth for proper esthetics and should remain out of occlusion in centric relation and all mandibular excursions.

Once maxillary resorption changes the ridge to Division B, C, or D the maxillary lingual cusp becomes the primary contact, because the implant is located under the lingual cusp. Hence the occlusal contacts are different from the occlusal schemes of a natural tooth, and even may be positioned more medial than the natural lingual cusp tip in the presence of Division C or D bone.

The mandibular arch also resorbs toward the medial position as it changes from Division A to B. In Division A bone, the implant is placed under the central fossa, and in Division B the implant is located under the lingual cusp region of a natural tooth. As a result, mandibular endosteal implants are always positioned more medial than the buccal cusp. All occlusal contacts are more medial than natural mandibular teeth occlusion. Therefore, whether implants are placed in the maxilla or mandible, the occlusion is more medial than most natural occlusal schemes (in which the mandibular buccal cusp is the dominant contact region). The concept of medial positioned lingualized occlusion developed by Misch emphasizes the axial load requirement of an implant occlusion,[18, 19] and may be used for complete dentures supported or opposed by implants and for fixed restorations using implant support.

The Weakest Component

The weakest component philosophy is used when one opposing segment has different factors of force or is more at risk of complications than an opposing area. For example, the occlusal concept in a maxillary completely edentulous area restored with a complete denture opposing an implant-supported restoration in the mandible is determined by the maxilla because it is the weakest area.

The amount of force distributed to a system can be reduced by stress-relieving components that may dramatically reduce impact loads to the implant support. The soft tissue of the traditional completely removable prosthesis opposing an implant prosthesis is displaced more than 2 mm[20] and is an efficient stress reducer. Lateral loads do not result with as great a crestal load to the implants, because the opposing prosthesis is not rigid. As a result, the occlusal concept may be designed to favor the complete removable denture, which is the weakest arch. The most common implant treatment which includes a traditional soft tissue–supported complete denture is a maxillary denture opposing a mandibular implant-supported restoration. The occlusal scheme for this condition raises the posterior plane of occlusion, uses a "medial positioned lingualized occlusion," and bilateral balanced occlusion (see Chapter 31). Whether the mandibular restoration is FP-1, FP-2, FP-3, RP-4, or RP-5, the maxillary denture follows these guidelines.

A bilateral balanced occlusion ideally exhibits contacts in all teeth for all centric and all eccentric occlusal movements. This is a popular occlusal scheme for soft tissue–supported removable prostheses, which improves maxillary denture stability, especially during parafunction. However, the mandibular implant-supported restoration may exert greater force on the premaxilla than a mandibular denture and can cause accelerated bone loss. Therefore, modification of the occlusal scheme aims at protecting the premaxilla under a maxillary denture, by the total elimination of anterior contacts with the mandibular anterior teeth in centric occlusal relation.

The "weakest component" philosophy applies to axial occlusal contacts in the regions of the implant bodies, when cantilevers or offset loaded areas are present. Heavier contacts are applied over the implant bodies to reduce the magnification of the compressive forces from the most distal cantilever and the tensile and shear forces on the most anterior implant abutment. Reduced occlusal forces and absence of lateral contacts in excursions are recommended on posterior cantilevers or anterior offset pontics whenever possible. This reduces the moment forces on the abutments and decreases the amount of crestal bone load on terminal implant abutments. If the implants for both arches cannot be loaded in an axial position, bone density, implant surface area, and prosthesis type determine the area to be protected. The maxillary implants are most likely to be protected with the axial load.

In order to follow the "weaker component" theory, when cantilever pontics are in both arches, they should oppose each other. If maxillary posterior implants cantilever anterior teeth, and mandibular anterior implants cantilever posterior teeth, the occlusal scheme cannot reduce forces on both cantilevers. In this scenario, the weaker component is usually the anterior maxilla, and reduced force in the region would be appropriate. It is better for mandibular cantilever pontics to oppose maxillary implants than the reverse situation.

The "weaker component" occlusal concept also applies to most anterior maxilla implant reconstruction. The implant-restored anterior maxilla is often the weakest section of all other implant reconstructed or natural tooth regions of the mouth. Narrower implants, facial cantilevers, oblique centric contacts, lateral contacts in excursion, D-3 bone density, absence of thick cortical plate at the crest or apex, and the inability to often place central and/or lateral incisor implants are all characteristics of the maxilla which mandate special consideration when establishing the occlusal scheme. Augmentation procedures are indicated for fixed restorations in the maxilla in order to place more and greater diameter implants when greater forces are diagnosed in the implant candidate.

Methods to help reduce force on maxillary anterior implants opposing a fixed dentition or restoration include excursive forces distributed to at least two splinted implants. As a result, anterior implants should be placed in the canine and lateral, or canine and central, or canine and first premolar (in this order of preference) for each anterior quadrant of the arch. Hence the canine is an important position when the anterior teeth are missing. When the canine region cannot be used to place an implant, three implants often are required in the

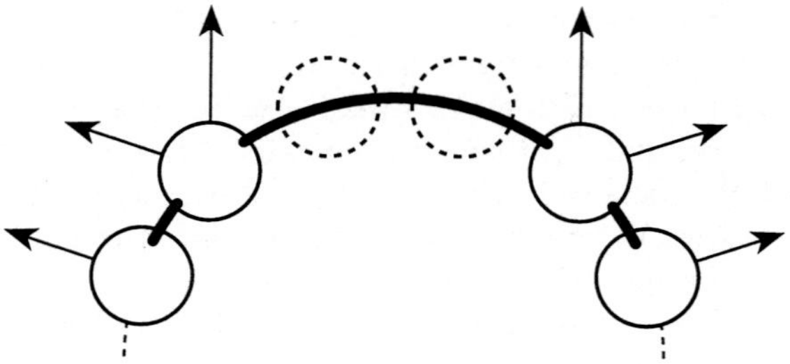

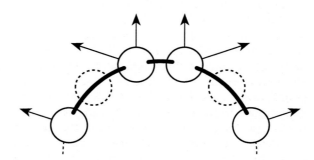

FIG 32–16.
Splinted maxillary implants in the canine and lateral incisor regions allow the lateral incisor implants to support protrusive movement. The right lateral incisor and canine support the right excursive movement, and the left lateral and canine implants support the left excursion. Because more force is generated in a lateral excursion, implants in this arrangement are more ideal.

anterior quadrant of the arch. A first premolar and lateral implant may distribute the working lateral load, and the lateral and a central implant can be used for the protrussive excursion. Hence, a minimum of two anterior implants is most often required in each excursion of a completely edentulous premaxilla, and three implants may be required when there are additional forces (especially with bruxism). Since there are three excursion directions for the mandible, the complete edentulous anterior maxilla often requires four implants. In this usage, one of the implants in a lateral excursion also may be used for the protrussive movement (Figs 32–16 to 32–18).

FIG 32–17.
Splinted maxillary implants in the regions of the central incisors and canines also can disclude lateral forces with two implants. The esthetics of central implant crowns are more difficult than crowns on lateral incisor implants. Lateral excursions include the lateral incisor region more often than the central incisor. Therefore this implant pattern is less ideal.

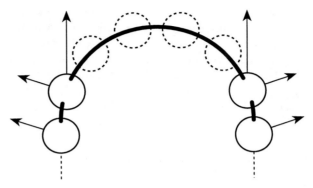

FIG 32–18.
Splinted maxillary implants placed in the canine and first premolar regions are acceptable, but occlusal excursions are difficult to design and have greater force on the implants. Protrusive force on the canines often require altered incisal edge positions for the mandible. Lateral excursions give greater force than the other options because the premolars are in contact. Therefore this pattern is less ideal.

Full Arch Fixed Prostheses (FP-1 to RP-4)

Fixed prostheses or natural teeth opposing FP-1 to RP-4 implant restorations should follow mutually protected occlusal schemes whenever possible. In protrusion, there should be total absence of posterior contact, especially for cantilevered posterior units. The total amount of force in lateral excursions is decreased in absence of posterior contacts.[11–14] This helps reduce the noxious effect of lateral forces on the anterior implants. Two or more implants should share any lateral force. Lateral excursions should occur as far forward as practical, and the canine position should be included.

The posterior component of the restored arch is often independent of the anterior section, especially in the mandible. Mandibular flexures distal to the mental foramen warrant separated sections of the fixed prosthesis.[21–25] In addition, the anterior lateral forces during excursions will not be distributed to the posterior region. As a result, two to four implants support each independent prosthesis, depending on length of span, density of bone, magnitude of force, direction of load, and duration of load. Eight to 10 maxillary implants most often are required for three separated prosthetic units. Posterior implants are more important in the maxilla, to eliminate cantilevers and increase the anterior-posterior implant distance, which further decreases stress to the anterior implants. Six to eight implants to support two or three separate units are suggested in the mandible for a fixed restoration opposing a rigid prosthesis.

The mandible has a torsion movement primarily medial and rotating during opening and clenching.[24, 25] The mandibular bone movement is almost completely limited to the regions posterior to the mental foramen in most individuals. As a result, sufficient numbers of anterior implants with acceptable length and anteroposterior distance may replace the mandibular teeth with a one-piece rigid bilateral posterior cantilever to the first molar region with no consequence related to flexure of the mandible. The posterior cantilevers are the weakest component of the system. Therefore less occlusal contact in the cantilevered regions and no posterior lateral contacts in any lateral excursion are indicated when opposing natural dentition or a fixed restoration.

OCCLUSAL MATERIALS

The materials on the occlusal aspect of the prostheses affect the transmission of force and the maintenance of occlusal schemes. Impact loads give rise to brief episodes of increased force, primarily related to the speed of closure and the dampening effect of the occlusal material (see Chapter 16). Impact loads are affected by the occlusal material, whereas continued forces (for example, with clenching) are affected to a minimum extent. The hardness of a material is related to the stress absorption from impact loads. An all-porcelain occlusal has a hardness of 2.5 times more than natural teeth. Acrylic resin has a Knoop hardness of 17 kg/mm^2, and enamel has a 350 kg/mm^2 hardness.[26] A composite resin may have a hardness of 85% of enamel. Therefore impact loads are reduced with acrylic, increase with composite, increased even more with enamel, and further increased with porcelain. The patient without parafunction may be restored with any occlusal material without risk. The teeth without parafunction occlude less than 30 minutes each day, with less than 30 lbf. However, bruxism increases the duration, speed, and amount of force by 10 times. Therefore the type of occlusal materials can affect the implant-bone interface and components with this condition.

Porcelain, acrylic, and composite fracture with too great a load or even with a decreased load of longer duration, angulation, or frequency. The use of acrylic or composite decreases impact load, but more easily fractures. The compressive strength of acrylic resin is 11,000 psi, compared with 40,000 psi for enamel.[26] Composite resin is three times stronger than acrylic. Material fracture is one of the more common factors that leads to refabrication of a prosthesis. Metal occlusals do not easily fracture, offers good wear resistance, and offers less impact load compared to porcelain.

Progressive bone loading is performed with acrylic transitional prostheses. As the bone matures, the amount of bone in contact with the implant increases, the density of bone increases, and the negative effects of impact loads decrease. It is suggested that patients with parafunction use acrylic transitional restorations for extended periods to improve the bone-implant interface during the progressive loading period. After bone density improves, metal occlusal surfaces should be considered to reduce long-term fracture complications and reduce impact forces compared to porcelain.

Shultz compared the difference of acrylic, gold, and porcelain prostheses related to chewing efficiency in two patients with identical dentures other than the occlusal material. Acrylic was 30% less efficient than porcelain, and gold occlusal surfaces were equal to porcelain surfaces.[27]

OCCLUSAL MAINTENANCE

Wear

The maintenance of an occlusal scheme is related in part to the wear of the material. The definition of wear is the deterioration, change, or loss of a surface caused by use.[28] The factors affecting the amount of wear include magnitude, angle, duration, speed, hardness, and surface finish of the opposing force and surface, together with the lubricant, temperature, and chemical nature of the surrounding environment.[29] The total volume loss of opposing occlusal surfaces are most significant related to occlusal maintenance. A change in occlusal contacts in centric relation occlusion and excursions, vertical relation occlusion, and esthetics are consequence of significant occlusal wear.

A total mean volume loss has been determined for enamel, acrylic, gold, and porcelain opposing each other. Acrylic resin wears 7 to 30 times faster when opposing gold, resin, enamel, or polished porcelain, as compared with gold opposing gold, acrylic, enamel, or porcelain. As a result, designed occlusal contacts are not maintained as well in the long term, and an increase in lateral forces may occur when resin vs. gold is used as the occlusal material.[29] The difference in wear between acrylic and composite resin may be as much as 1.5 mm in cusp height more for acrylic opposing acrylics at 2,000 wear cycles.[30] Therefore the material that decreases impact load more is the material that resists wear least.

Porcelain fused to gold occlusals in esthetic regions opposing gold occlusals in the more nonesthetic areas, or metal occlusals in both arches when parafunction or marginal interarch space is present are the materials most often selected for implant occlusal materials. Acrylic fractures more often when used as a crown and bridge occlusal veneer than does porcelain fused to gold. Porcelain opposing porcelain rarely is used with extreme parafunction because it has the most volume loss and may fracture more often than porcelain opposing metal. A longer progressive bone loading schedule with acrylic occlusals permits porcelain to be used in more esthetic regions. Composite resin teeth are available which wear less than acrylic and are very close to enamel. However, these materials fracture more often than porcelain or gold and are not as color stable as porcelain (Fig 32–19).

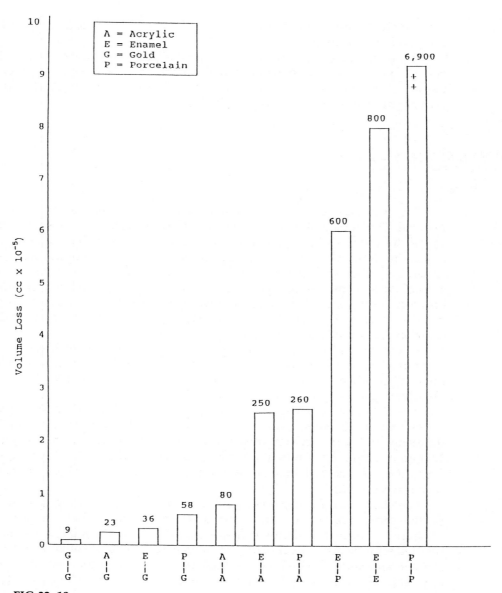

FIG 32–19.
Volume loss of gold, acrylic, enamel, and porcelain opposing each other and in combination. Total volume loss affects occlusal contacts or vertical dimension more than the wearing of one material compared with another.[30] Porcelain to porcelain and porcelain to enamel wear more than any restoring combination. The use of gold, regardless of the opposing combination, always provides the least total volume loss. (Adapted from Mahalick JA, Knap FJ, Weiter EJ: Occlusal wear in prosthodontics, *J Am Dent Assoc* 82:154–159, 1971.)

Material Fracture

Implants, components, and the prosthesis are loaded with a range of magnitude, duration, direction, and frequency. As a consequence, permanent deformation may result, and fatigue fracture and creep are an expected conclusion after years of service. These relate to the factors of force. A long-term view of these complications is not yet appreciated by the majority of the profession. The longevity of dental implants requires the consideration of material, permanent deformation, creep, or fracture. Porcelain fracture is the third most common condition requiring the replacement of a fixed prostheses in natural teeth.[31] The ideal thickness of porcelain to prevent breakage is approximately 2 mm.[32] Unsupported regions of porcelain may occur in porcelain to metal FP-2 or FP-3 prosthesis when the metal superstructure is not properly designed. Many dental laboratories make very thin copings over the implants and teeth, then add porcelain to the final occlusal table. As a result, FP-2 or FP-3 restorations may have more than 6 mm of unsupported porcelain. The incisal edge and occlusal table position of the prosthesis must be clearly planned before the superstructure is fabricated.

Acrylic fracture is a more common complication for fixed FP-3 reconstructions than for complete dentures. Acrylic denture teeth on traditional dentures do not receive the forces demonstrated in implant-supported restorations. In addition, unlike porcelain, acrylic obtains its strength by bulk. The metal superstructure must have mechanical retention regions with proper resistance to forces of occlusion. Posterior acrylic or composite facings often fracture, as inadequate yield and fatigue strengths exist for the bite force obtained in parafunction or on cantilevers for fixed restorations. As a result, porcelain or metal is often selected as the material of choice. Metal occlusals are used in nonesthetic regions, or when parafunction or marginal interarch distance is present. Metal shrinkage is 10 times less than porcelain, which permits a more passive casting, and metal does not fracture or cause wear on the opposing surface as much as porcelain does.

CONCLUSION

The local occlusal considerations in implant dentistry include the transosteal forces, bone biomechanics, basic biomechanics, differences in natural teeth and implants, muscles of mastication and occlusal force, and bone resorption. The incorporation of all these factors lead to an occlusal scheme developed by the author.

Occlusal schemes consider the weakest component, full or partial edentulous arches, and posterior or anterior teeth and/or implants. A medial positioned lingualized occlusion is a consistent approach for implant occlusal schemes.

The material from which the occlusal regions are fabricated may affect implant loading, and also affect implant reaction forces to the opposing arch.

These occlusal materials also affect wear and fracture, which affects the occlusal contacts, vertical occlusal dimension, and esthetics. This chapter blends experience and biological principles for a consistent approach to occlusal considerations.

REFERENCES

1. Glickman I: Inflammation and trauma from occlusion: co-destructive factors in chronic periodontal disease, *J Periodontol* 34:5–10, 1963.
2. Hillam DG: Stresses in the periodontal ligament, *J Periodont Res* 8:51–56, 1973.
3. Bidez MW, Misch CE: Force transfer in implant dentistry: basic concepts and principles, *Oral Implant* 18:264–274, 1992.
4. Misch CE: Three-dimensional finite element analysis of two plate form neck designs (thesis), University of Pittsburgh, 1989.
5. Dawson PE: *Evaluation, diagnosis, and treatment of occlusal problems,* ed 2, St Louis, 1989, CV Mosby.
6. Cowin SC: *Bone mechanics,* Boca Raton, Fla, 1989, CRC Press.
7. Lucia VO: *Modern gnathological concepts,* St Louis, 1961, CV Mosby, p 293.
8. Alexander PC: Analysis of cuspid protected occlusion, *J Prosthet Dent* 13:307–317, 1963.
9. Goldstein GR: The relationship of canine protected occlusion to a periodontal index, *J Prosthet Dent* 41:277–283, 1979.
10. Muhlemann HR, Savdirl S, Rakeitshak KH: Tooth mobility: its cause and significance, *J Periodontol* 36:148–153, 1965.
11. Williamson EH, Lundquist DO: Anterior guidance: its effect on electromyographic activity of the temporal and masseter muscles, *J Prosthet Dent* 49:816–823, 1983.
12. Belser UC, Hannam AG: The influence of working-side occlusal guidance on masticatory muscles and related jaw movement, *J Prosthet Dent* 53:406–413, 1985.
13. Shupe RJ et al: Effects of occlusal guidance on jaw muscle activity, *J Prosthet Dent* 51:811–818, 1984.
14. Manns A, Chan C, Miralles R: Influence of group function and canine guidance on electromyographic activity of elevator muscles, *J Prosthet Dent* 57:494–501, 1987.
15. Muhlemann HR: Tooth mobility: a review of clinical aspects and research findings, *J Periodontol* 38:686, 1967.
16. Sekine H et al: Mobility characteristics and tactile sensitivity of osseointegrated fixture-supporting systems, in van Steenberghe D, editor: *Tissue integration in oral maxillofacial reconstruction,* Amsterdam, 1986, Elsevier, pp 306–332.
17. Parfitt GS: Measurement of the physiologic mobility of individual teeth in an axial direction, *J Dent Res* 39:68, 1960.
18. Misch CE: Classifications and treatment options of the completely edentulous arch in implant dentistry, *Dent Today* 9:26, 30, 1990.
19. Misch CE: *Medial positioned lingualized occlusion in fixed prosthesis* (manual), Dearborn, Mich, Misch Implant Institute, 1989.
20. Lytle RB: Soft tissue displacement beneath removable partial and complete dentures, *J Prosthet Dent* 12:34–43, 1962.

21. Goodkind RJ, Heringlake CB: Mandibular flexure in opening and closure movements, *J Prosthet Dent* 30:134–138, 1973.
22. De Marco TL, Paine S: Mandibular dimensional change, *J Prosthet Dent* 31:482–485, 1974.
23. Fishman BM: The influence of fixed splints on mandibular flexure, *J Prosthet Dent* 35:643–647, 1976.
24. Omar R, Wise MD: Mandibular flexure associated with muscle force applied in the retruded axis position, *J Oral Rehabil* 6:299–321, 1981.
25. Fischman B: The rotational aspect of mandibular flexure, *J Prosthet Dent* 64:483–485, 1990.
26. Leinfelder KF, Lemons JE: *Clinical restoration materials and techniques*, Philadelphia, 1988, Lea and Febiger.
27. Shultz AW: Comfort and chewing efficiency in dentures, *J Prosthet Dent* 65:38–48, 1991.
28. Lipson C, editor: *Wear considerations in design*, Englewood Cliffs, NJ, 1967, Prentice-Hall, pp 1–50.
29. Mahalick JA, Knap FJ, Weiter EJ: Occlusal wear in prosthodontics, *J Am Dent Assoc* 82:154–159, 1971.
30. Von Frauhofer JA, Razaui R, Khan Z: Wear characteristics of high strength denture teeth, *J Prosthet Dent* 60:500–503, 1988.
31. Walton JN, Gardner FM, Agar JR: A survey of crown and fixed partial denture fixtures: Legnth of service and reasons for replacement, *J Prosthet Dent* 56:416–421, 1986.
32. Seghi RR, Daher T, Caputo A: Relative flexural strength of dental restorative ceramics, *Dent Mater* 6:181–184, 1990.

Chapter 33

Maintenance of Dental Implants

Roland M. Meffert

PERIODONTAL ASPECTS OF DENTAL IMPLANTOLOGY

A prerequisite to a successful endosseous dental implant should be obtaining a perimucosal seal of the soft tissue to the implant surface. Failure to achieve or maintain this seal results in the apical migration of the epithelium into the bone-implant interface and possible complete encapsulation of the endosseous or root portion of the implant system.

Perimucosal or Transgingival Area

In the natural dentition, the junctional epithelium provides a seal at the base of the sulcus against the penetration of chemical and bacterial substances. If the seal is disrupted or if the fibers apical to the epithelium are lysed or destroyed, the epithelium migrates rapidly in an apical direction, forming a pocket after cleavage of the soft tissue from the radicular surface. Because there is no cementum or fiber insertion on the surface of an endosseous implant, the perimucosal seal is important. If it is lost, the periodontal pocket extends to the osseous structures.

Is a perimucosal seal possible in the case of an endosseous dental implant? If not, the only barrier to complete epithelial invagination nearing the crestal bone would lie in the tonus of the gingival tissues by means of the circular fibers in the supracrestal soft tissues.[1] Gould et al.[2] reported that epithelial cells attach to the surface of titanium in much the same manner in which the epithelial cells attach to the surface of a natural tooth, that is, a basal lamina and the formation of hemidesmosomes. Schroeder et al.[3] observed that if the post of the implant was situated in a region of immobile, keratinized mucosa, a sign of adhesion of the epithelial cells to the titanium-sprayed surface would be apparent. Wennstrom[4,5] disagrees with Schroeder by maintaining that lack of keratinized gingiva is not necessarily a vulnerable situation, and that a movable mucosa around the neck of the implant, if maintained, will allow for success. To back his premise, Wennstrom cites the presence of attached, keratinized gingiva on 67% (SD 24) and 51% (SD 31) of the buccal and lingual surfaces/jaws in the prospective and retrospective studies by Adell et al.[6] in which 5- to 12-year survival rates of 84% and 93%, are documented for maxilla and mandible, respectively. From these figures, Wennstrom theorizes that keratinized gingiva, though desired, is not essential for maintenance of the perimucosal seal. It is the clinical experience of the author, however, that implant devices, prosthetic devices, and superstructures are quite different from the normal gingival/tooth contours and relationships and that they produce a situation that demands special, detailed instruction and attention in terms of homecare procedures. Add to this the fact that the patients presenting themselves as possible candidates for implant placement are patients with a history of less than optimum homecare in the past, since they are either partially or totally edentulous, and their knowledge of dental hygiene is suspect. Furthermore, from personal experience, the patient with endosseous dental implants is quite wary of effecting vigorous hygiene procedures for fear of causing the restorations to fail by being touched or traumatized with oral hygiene devices.

In the author's experience, keratinized tissue is best acquired by way of soft tissue grafting prior to implant surgery if it is not present in adequate amounts and in the correct location at the time of patient examination and documentation. If an implant (or implants) has already been placed and it is determined that upon reopening that the implant post will be partially or entirely in movable mucosa, the graft can be accomplished during the 3- to 6-month healing period in the mandible and maxillary arch. The least predictable and least satisfactory time for soft tissue grafting is following restorative therapy if approximation of the soft tissue to the implant neck is desired. It is very difficult to impossible to effect any type of junctional epithelium attachment to an implant substrate, be it metallic or nonmetallic in nature.

Jansen[7] disputed the findings of Gould, and reported that hemidesmosome-like contacts were observed only on apatite or polystyrene, never on metallic or carbon surfaces. He felt his results may have differed from those of Gould because of differences in cell population, culture conditions, or treatment of the titanium substrate being used. Irregardless, there is no biological seal or attachment of a predictable nature between the soft tissue and the implant surface, and the adaptation of the soft tissue and the implant surface at the transgingival area is more a result of tonus and close approximation than of any junctional epithelial attachment to the implant surface.

If it is true that junctional epithelial hemidesmosomal attachment is not predictable in a metallic system, can anything be done to retard epithelial invagination? Using a series of laboratory animals, von Recum et al.[8] used collagen and fibronectin to promote fibroblastic proliferation and attachment; the premise was based on the work of Kleinman et al.,[9] which demonstrated that collagen-bound fibronectin provided an excellent substratum for cell attachment in vitro. Von Recum found that the collagen did not enhance attachment; rather, the fibronectin actually retarded healing when applied to an implant surface. He reported that the epithelium in his animals migrated apically at the rate of 2.0 mm weekly and will predictably end up near the osseous crest if the process is not impeded or interrupted. Lowenberg et al.[10] reported good results, however, using a bovine collagen on titanium alloy (Ti6Al4V) to enhance fibroblastic attachment and mitotic activity in a 14-day study in which the demineralized root slice was used as a control. The authors demonstrated that a collagen-coated alloy demonstrated the same attachment results as demineralized root slices. In a direct comparison, no attachment was evidenced on the uncoated alloy.

In another study by the same authors,[11] comparing the attachment of fibroblasts to Ti6Al4V and a zirconium alloy, there was no difference between the materials in terms of fibroblast growth. The study also showed a better attachment to a smooth surface but better orientation of the cells to a porous or rough surface.

Kasten et al.[12] seeded epithelial cells at 75,000 cells/mL onto the surfaces of titanium, titanium alloy, plasma-sprayed titanium, single crystal sapphire, and smooth and rough hydroxylapatites (HA) with and without a collagen coating. When documented at 20 hours, analysis of ten fields or material indicated that human gingival epithelial cells adhered 3 times more frequently to the HA and sapphire surfaces than to metallic or titanium-type implants. In no case was the cell attachment and growth to titanium alloy (7.6 cells/field) plasma-sprayed titanium (7.7 cells/field), or commercially pure titanium (8.6 cells/field) comparable to the sapphire (24.2 cells/field) or the HA (up to 44.1 cells/field). The root control as a comparison averaged 35.3 cells/field in an average of ten fields.

Interestingly enough, the addition of collagen to rough HA did not enhance the activity appreciably, whereas coating the smooth HA surface with collagen increased the surface adherence and growth of epithelial cells from 22.0 cells/field uncoated to 44.1 cells/field coated. This would seem to corroborate the work of Lowenberg relating to a smooth surface being better for cell adherence, but also leading to the conclusion that all surfaces are not the same because the metallic substrates are also smooth in surface texture and they fared poorly in a comparison of epithelial cell growth and adhesion. The effect of collagen coating on cell attachment needs further reevaluation and study.

Laminin has recently been associated with epithelial cell adhesion and prevention of connective tissue growth; it is a potent chemoattractor and, in theory, could prevent epithelial cell migration. Seitz et al.[13] described predictable adhesion to Bioglass when the surface was coated with laminin.

Studies conducted for a 4-month period in dogs[14] demonstrated a cleavage of soft tissue, with deep epithelial invagination when the tissue was approximated to a smooth titanium surface. In the final analysis, if the perimucosal seal breaks down or is not present, a pocket exists and the area is subject to periodontal type disease with resultant osseous defects (Fig 33-1).

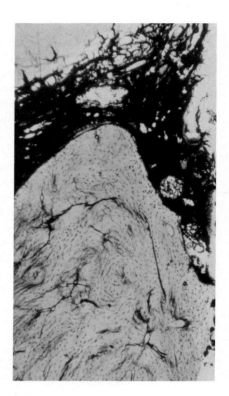

FIG 33–1.
Vertical osseous defect at bone *(left)*–implant *(right)* interface.

To facilitate homecare procedures, the neck of the implant must be smooth and not porous. DePorter et al.[15] placed Ti6Al4V implants in dogs with pore sizes of 50 to 200 μm. These were porous not only in the root portion but also in the transgingival area. The study was terminated prematurely because of severe bone loss and exfoliation of the implant systems. Klawitter et al.[16] placed 44 porous alumina implants in dogs; at a 6-month time frame, only 2 of the 44 implants were still in place. The rest had exfoliated in the face of marked inflammation and bone loss. Hottel and Gibbons[17] reported that a random surface porosity predisposes the implant to develop a thick fibrous capsule, whereas a fully dense implant surface was more liable to effect a perimucosal seal at the interface. All authors came to the same conclusion that a rough surface at the transgingival area was extremely detrimental to tissue health.

Barrier materials are gaining attention in the study of guided tissue regeneration. Substances such as Teflon millipore filters or resorbable collagen materials are placed between the surgical flap and the implant surface to exclude apically proliferating epithelium and gingival connective tissue elements from the substrate surface are gaining attention. The concept defining guided tissue regeneration is to exclude the rapidly regenerative tissues (epithelium or

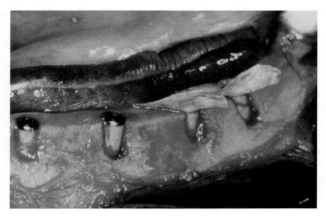

FIG 33–2.
Implants in dog; 3-mm × 5-mm dehiscence defects are shown.

connective tissue) by use of a barrier; this allows for differentiation and migration of pluripotential cells from the periodontal ligament and alveolus into the defect. This would be especially applicable to the dehisced implant surface in which endosseous implant surgical placement may result in facial or lingual osseous dehiscences. Dahlin et al.[18] reported coverage of exposed threads of endosseous implants with new bone in a 6- to 15-week study in rabbits. Zablotsky et al.[19] demonstrated new bone growth over dehisced HA-coated implants in dogs in 4 weeks (Figs 33–2 to 33–4). Both studies utilized the nonresorbable Teflon materials; research utilizing resorbable barrier materials is in progress.

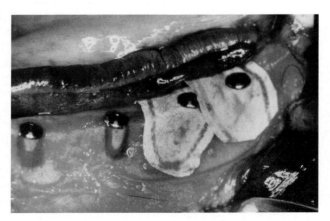

FIG 33–3.
Membrane placed over two test implants; two control implants are to the left of the covered implants.

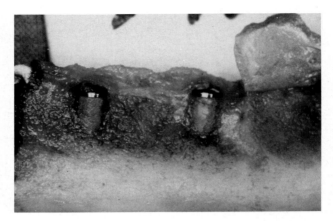

FIG 33–4.
At 1-month healing there is very little growth over the control implants from Figure 33–3 (two at *left*) compared to that protected by membrane *(right)*.

Fibro-Osseous Retention vs. Osseointegration

The two basic means of retention of an endosteal dental implant in function are fibro-osseous retention and osseointegration. According to the American Academy of Implant Dentistry (AAID) Glossary of Terms (1986),[20] the term, fibro-osseous retention is defined as tissue-to-implant contact: interposition of healthy, dense collagenous tissue between the implant and bone. A proponent of the fibro-osseous theory of implant fixation, Weiss[21] defends the presence of collagen fibers at the interface between the implant and bone and interprets it as a peri-implant membrane with an osteogenic effect. He believes that the collagen fibers invest the implant, originating at a trabecula of cancellous bone on one side, weaving around the implant, and reinserting into a trabecula on the other side. When function is applied to the implant, tension is applied to the fiber(s); forces closest to the implant interface cause a compression of the fibers, with a corresponding tension on the fibers placed or inserting into the trabeculae. The difference between the inner aspect (compression) and the outer aspect (tension) of the connective tissue components results in a bioelectric current, and this current (a piezoelectric effect) induces differentiation into connective tissue components associated with bone maintenance. Hence the premise of the fibers being osteogenic.

Weiss[22] speculates that the cylindrical or root form implant now in common use would be invested with a fiber that is too long in which occlusal forces transmitted would be dissipated and the beneficial bioelectric effect not produced. In his theory, fibers around a blade, spiral, or pin-type implant would be short enough for the piezoelectric or osteogenic effect. In other words, connective tissue at the interface of an endosseous implant is a functioning and desirable entity and is directly related to implant design and the length of the fiber more than any other factor in terms of function.

There is no real evidence to suggest, however, that these fibers are functioning in the periodontal ligament mode (from tooth to bone) at the bone-implant interface. Histologic study demonstrates either parallel fiber arrangements to the long axis of the implant (Fig 33–5), fibers with no real functional arrangement, or simply a complete encapsulation. The latter is an obvious failure by anyone's analysis and would never be interpreted as a functioning system. But where does the peri-implant ligament become a pseudoarthrosis? Is it a matter of dimension? This author has never seen a functioning arrangement around an endosseous implant resembling the periodontal ligament (such as horizontal or oblique fiber groups); at this time, the premise, that the peri-implant ligament is osteogenic and exerts a piezoelectric effect is just a hypothesis. This has no direct relation to the success or failure of an implant system unless the width of the connective tissue allows for movement upon manipulation. But we must be careful lest we interpret a histological finding falsely and ascribe powers to it that may not exist.

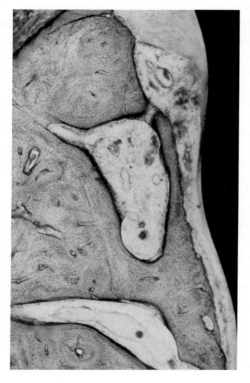

FIG 33–5.
Parallel fiber arrangement in peri-implant space between bone *(left)* and implant *(right)*.

Is there a fibrous tissue interface between titanium implants and bone? Again, the literature is contradictory. Harms and Mausle[23] inserted a series of cylindrical Ti6Al4V implants in the long bones of rats and dogs and described a soft tissue layer after a period of 1 year. Kohler[24] described a fibrous tissue interface of 50 to 250 μm thick around titanium implants in dogs. Cook et al.[25] reported a fibrous layer one to two cell layers thick between implant and bone in porous titanium, textured titanium, and cobalt-chromium-molybdenum alloy implants.

Other authors, however, reported no soft tissue or connective tissue interface between bone and the titanium implant. Linder and Lundskog[26] inserted cylindrical titanium implants in rabbit tibiae, "semi-loaded" them, and found no connective tissue interface. Karagianes[27] inserted porous titanium implants in miniature swine, and described a bony anchorage. Schroeder et al.[28] inserted plasma-sprayed (grit surfaced) porous titanium dental implants in monkey jaws and described a bony anchorage without interposed soft tissue. But the prime proponent of the philosophy that the absence of connective tissue at the bone-implant interface is the key to clinical success in endosseous implantology is Dr. Per-Ingvar Branemark, who coined the term osseointegration and explained it in his text, *Tissue Integrated Prostheses: Osseointegration in Clinical Dentistry.*[29] According to the AAID Glossary of Terms,[20] osseointegration is a contact established between normal and remodeled bone and an implant surface *without* the interposition of nonbone or connective tissue. It must be realized, however, that there is never a 100% bone-implant interface. Johansson and Albrektsson[30] reported a fibrous tissue interface at 1 month following implantation, an average 50% bone-implant contact at 3 months, a 65% bone-implant surface at 6 months, and an average of 85% bone-implant contact 1 year following insertion of a screw-type system in rabbits. Other authors report an average of 25% to 75% osseointegration in the successful case, with the remaining being nonmineralized tissues (vessels, nerves, connective tissue, and so forth). The extreme variance in bone-implant contact can be demonstrated in two figures in which unloaded cylindrical plasma-sprayed implants were placed in dogs for a period of 4 months; both were clinically immobile upon reopening, but neither demonstrated complete investiture of the system with bone (Figs 33–6 and 33–7).

The proponents of the two theories of implant retention and stabilization (fibro-osseous vs. osseointegration) are entirely at odds in their philosophies of tissue maintenance as related to function. According to Weiss,[21] it is the difference between afunction and hypofunction, or between submerging the endosseous portion of the implant for 3 to 6 months (as advocated by Branemark[29]) or protecting it in a hypofunctional mode from the day of insertion until placing it in full function 1 to 2 months after placement (as advocated by Weiss[21]).

Weiss[21] agrees that an afunctional, submerged system will allow for direct bone apposition (osseointegration), but feels that submerging the implant will actually retard healing and that when the implant is placed in full function from an afunctional mode, failure will soon result. Branemark[29] theorizes that the

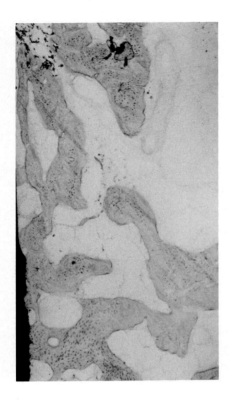

FIG 33–6.
Implant-bone interface, depicting slight bone-to-implant contact. Bone is at *left;* implant, at *right.*

implant must be protected and completely out of function, as he envisions a healing phase of 0 to 12 months in which new bone is formed close to the immobile, resting implant; a remodeling phase of 3 to 18 months when the implant is exposed to masticatory forces; and a steady state after 18 months, in which there is a balance between the forces acting on the implant and the remodeling capacities of the anchoring bone. As documentation to back his premise, the work of Adell et al.[6] is quoted, in which bone loss of 1 to 1.5 mm occurs during the first year (as a result of the surgical trauma) and subsequent marginal bone loss of 0.05 to 0.1 mm occurs annually after the first year (as measured by standardized radiographs).

Exactly, what does happen when an implant is placed in bone? Roberts et al.[31] reports a bridging callus originating within a few millimeters from the implant site and a lattice of woven bone reaching the implant surface in approximately 6 weeks. It is his firm contention that this bridging callus requires complete stability and immobility and has very little load-carrying capability.

The lattice structure of woven bone is filled with well-organized lamellae, and this does not occur to achieve maximum load-carrying capability in the human

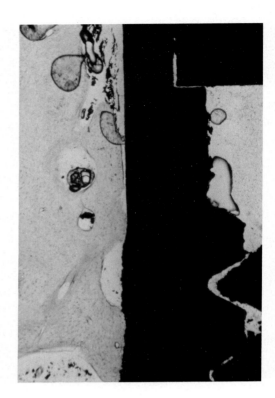

FIG 33–7.
Bone *(left)*–implant *(right)* interface
with denser bone configuration and
more bone-to-implant contact.

being in less than 18 weeks. Furthermore, a maximum compact/composite bone interface is achieved in humans approximately 1 year after implant placement.

So the work of Roberts et al.[31] would seem to correlate very closely with the rationale of Branemark. Maximum load-carrying capability is achieved in 4 to 5 months; Branemark advocates complete immobilization of the system for 3 to 6 months before placing it in function. Conversely, the theory of Weiss,[21] proposing the system be placed in full function in a 1 to 2 months' time frame, long before maximum load-carrying capability is achieved, would be open to question. Early loading before the bridging callus reached the implant site and/or the lattice of woven bone was filled with organized lamellae would certainly be contraindicated if the premise of a peri-implant ligament around the endosseous implant was faulty.

With this in mind, what may cause the formation of a connective tissue interface? In my opinion, the following may account for a lack of osseointegration (absence of connective tissue at bone-implant interface at the light microscopic level).

1. Premature loading of the implant system, earlier than 3 to 6 months.
2. Apical migration of the junctional epithelium into the interface, followed by connective tissue elements (Fig 33–8).
3. Placing the implant with too much pressure. Linkow and Wertman[32] propose that the failure of the endosseous dental implant starts from within and not from the outside and that the system must lie *passively* in the implant site without any pressure. Weiss[21] advocates making the implant site slightly smaller than the implant so it can be tapped into place and that initial retention is gained through a frictional fit.
4. Overheating the bone during site preparation. Bone will resorb if the temperature at the periphery is above 116°F (47°C).[33]
5. Implant not fitting the site exactly. Carlsson et al.[34] created bone-implant gaps of 0 mm, 0.35 mm, and 0.85 mm, respectively, in rabbit tibiae. Those with a gap of 0 mm had direct bone-to-implant contact; a 0.35-mm gap resulted in an average residual gap of 0.22 mm, with few areas of direct contact, and the 0.85-mm gap resulted in no direct

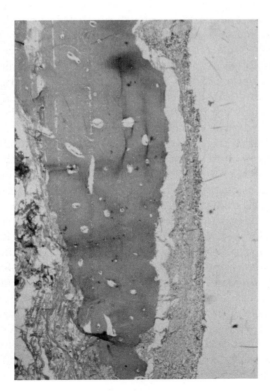

FIG 33–8.
Decalcified section. There is an interface of epithelium and connective tissue between bone *(left)* and implant (removed).

bone-implant contact and an average gap of 0.54 mm, indicating the need for close approximation between bone and implant. Satomi et al.[35] placed threaded screw-type implants in nonthreaded and prethreaded sockets. Six months after insertion, they were examined histologically and histometrically. Implants placed by self-tapping or self-threading healed with direct bony apposition, and those placed in a pre-threaded socket revealed fibrous tissue intervention, again demonstrating the need for close approximation of bone and implant.

Osseointegration vs. Biointegration

As a result of recent research, the terminology used to further define the retention means of dental implants has been altered to osseointegration vs. biointegration. In 1985, dePutter et al.[36] observed that there are two ways of implant anchorage or retention: mechanical and bioactive.

Mechanical retention basically refers to the metallic substrate systems such as titanium or titanium alloy. The retention is based on undercut forms such as vents, slots, dimples, screws, and so forth, and involves direct contact between the dioxide layer on the base metal and bone with no chemical bonding.

Bioactive retention is achieved with bioactive materials such as HA, which bond directly to bone, similar to ankylosis of natural teeth. Bone matrix is deposited on the HA layer as a result of some type of physicochemical interaction between the collagen of bone and the HA crystals of the implant (Denissen et al.[37]). Plasma-spraying and ion-sputter coating are two techniques used to coat metallic implants with HA. Plasma-spraying involves heating the HA by a plasma flame at a temperature of approximately 15,000°C to 20,000°C. The HA is then propelled onto the implant body in an inert environment (usually argon) to a thickness of 50 to 100 μm. Ion-sputter coating is a process by which a thin, dense layer of HA can be coated onto an implant substrate. This technique involves directing an ion beam at a solid-phase HA block, vaporizing it to create a plasma, and then recondensing this plasma on the implant.

Various authors have reported bone formation and maturation occurring at a faster rate and at earlier periods on HA-coated implant than on noncoated implants,[38] a HA-coated system developing an average of 5 to 8 times the mean interfacial strength of an uncoated, grit-surfaced titanium system in 10- to 32-week studies.[39] The HA-coated implants have 66.3% of their surface directly in contact with bone, whereas grit-surfaced titanium implants had only 50.2% of their surface in contact with bone.[40] Davis et al.[41] demonstrated a 75% bone-implant contact when the surface was plasma sprayed, a 49% contact when ion-sputter coating was used, and only a 29% when the Ti6Al4V alloy surface was uncoated—all systems being identical in shape (fluted, threaded), the only difference being coating vs. noncoating. A 12-week study comparing the efficacy of coating blade-type endosseous dental implants with HA vs. leaving them

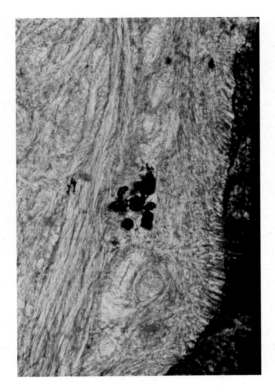

FIG 33–9.
Gingival fibers inserting into layer of osteoid on hydroxylapatite surface.

uncoated demonstrated a 62.62% bone-implant contact with the coated blade in opposition to a 28.22% bone-implant contact when the Ti6Al4V blade was used.[42]

Research in animals has shown that not only is there the possibility of bone growing in a coronal direction on the surface of a material such as HA, but also the possibility of development of a supra-alveolar connective tissue apparatus with new gingival fibers inserting into the osteoid (Fig 33–9). The close interaction between collagen of bone and hydroxylapatite crystals of the implant is demonstrated (Fig 33–10).

Hygiene Protocol and Instrumentation

How is the dental implant maintained? One of the essential questions in the pathogenesis of periodontal disease is the initiation and possible conversion of gingivitis to periodontitis. Or in the case of the endosseous dental implant, what will lead to loss of the perimucosal seal (if present initially) and the change from gingivitis to peri-implantitis?

Increased levels of subgingival spirochetes have been associated with endosseous dental implants (ceramic, ramus frame, blade, and post types made of

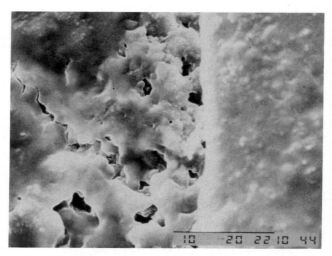

FIG 33–10.
Hydroxylapatite-bone seam (SEM; 5,000×). Bone is at *left;* hydroxylapatite, at *right.*

metal and carbon) considered to be failing because of advanced pocket formation, marked gingival inflammation, and progressive bone loss, while spirochetes have been rarely encountered in subgingival plaque from well-maintained and clinically stable implants.[43] Rams and Link[44] removed plaque samples from the most apical portions of the blade and post-type implant-associated periodontal pockets, and found large numbers of small and medium spirochetes, but no large spirochetes. Oral spirochetes may damage soft tissue or impede soft tissue healing around dental implants by production and release of proteolytic enzymes dissolving fibrin, trypsin-like enzymes disrupting cell-to-cell adhesion, and metabolic end products that are cytotoxic to gingival tissue. Lekholm et al.[45] studied marginal tissues and bacteria associated with healthy, functioning implants. The primary bacteria associated with healthy implants were nonmotile rods and cocci. Mombelli et al.[46] compared clinical and microbiological findings relating to healthy and failing dental implants. Unsuccessful implant sites were characterized by microbiota consisting primarily of gram–negative anaerobic rods. Black-pigmented *Bacteroides* and *Fusobacterium* species were regularly found. Spirochetes and fusiform bacteria were infrequently associated with healthy implant sites. In another study,[47] samples were obtained from 17 patients with 26 failing implants; of the 26 implant samples, *Staphylococcus* spp. was found in eight, *Candida albicans* in nine, gram-negative rods in 10, *Bacteroides intermedius* in three, *Wolinella* spp. in two, *Fusobacterium* spp. in two, *Actinobacillus actinomycetemcomitans* in one, and *Capnocytophaga* spp. in one. Becker et al.,[48] in a clinical and DNA analysis of 36 failing implant sites in 13 patients, found *A. actinomycetemcomitans* in 27% of the sites, *B. intermedius* in 35.4% of the sites, and *Bacteroides gingivalis* in 37.5% of the sites. Wolinsky et al.[49] made a comparison of bacterial adherence to saliva-treated titanium vs. enamel. Initial adherence of *Actinomyces viscosus* to saliva-treated titanium was reduced, while the adherence of *Streptococcus sanguis* was identical in a comparison of titanium and enamel. So even the interaction of bacteria to surface substrate is affected. Even so, most authors and investigators conclude that failing dental implants are associated with bacteria commonly identified as periodontal pathogens.

If bacteria are of significant in the causation of problems identified with the ailing or failing implant, what hygiene techniques, instrumentation, and possibly antimicrobials should be used in maintenance of the dental implant? Thomson-Neal[50] evaluated the in vitro effects of various prophylactic modalities on different implant surfaces such as commercially pure titanium, HA-coated titanium, and the single crystal sapphire (aluminum oxide). The latter was used as the control. It was theorized that because the single crystal sapphire implant was the hardest material used in fabrication of endosseous dental implants, it should be more resistant to changes in surface topography, texture with abrasion, or wear than some of the other materials.

As predicted, the single crystal sapphire was the least affected by any of the modalities employed, with just some surface scratching evidenced. A protocol was directed in terms of application of the modality or instrument on the surface(s), equating it to 15 years of professional service at four visits per year with 8 seconds per surface, or in the case of a polishing agent used by the dental auxiliary at a maintenance visit, polishing for 8 minutes to simulate a 15-year maintenance program.

When the commercially pure titanium, unused and as machined, was viewed at 350× under scanning electron microscopy, its surface was smooth, with only slight machining grooves. Titanium-tipped curettes produced parallel grooves with overlapping strokes (Fig 33–11); stainless-steel curettes produced random grooving, with a marked pitting of the surface (Fig 33–12). The soft titanium surface was pitted in a random fashion with the air abrasive instrument. Ultrasonic scalers and instruments severely abraded the surface and polishing pastes, producing random grooving with corresponding crystals at the end of the grooves. Antimicrobials and hand or motorized toothbrushes produced very little change in surface appearance from the original machined implant with its minute surface irregularities.

The HA-titanium implants were severely altered from the normal, with ultrasonic instruments removing most or all of the HA (Fig 33–13) and the surface topography was changed with the titanium-tipped curette (Fig 33–14). Surface changes were evident in descending order of abrasiveness: ultrasonic instruments, sonic devices, titanium-tipped curettes, interdental brushes, polishing pastes, and antimicrobials.

To summarize Thomson-Neal's study,[50] water and air sonic/ultrasonic units

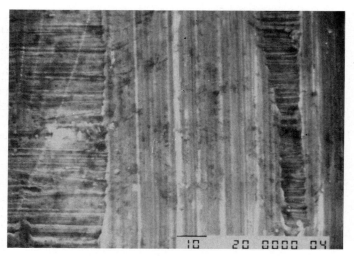

FIG 33–11.
Titanium, treated with titanium-tipped curettes (SEM; 350×).

roughened the surfaces of metal and of single crystal sapphire, a condition that may enhance plaque retention. The same units and modalities removed the HA from the metallic base partially or entirely, a situation that would obviously negate optimum repair and maintenance. It appeared that uni-tufted brushes and antimicrobials were safe, nonabrasive oral hygiene regimens to use on all

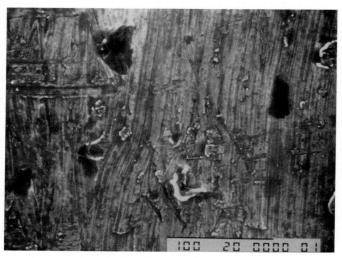

FIG 33–12.
Titanium, treated with stainless-steel curettes (SEM; 350×).

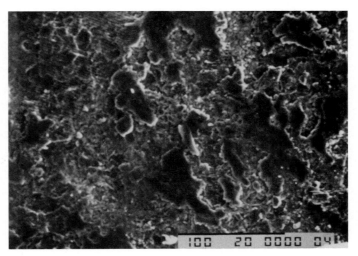

FIG 33–13.
Hydroxylapatite-coated titanium, treated with ultrasonic scaler (SEM; $350\times$).

implant surfaces studied, while the rubber cup polishing with paste was the safest and least abrasive professional modality for use on a regular basis on all implant surfaces. Unpublished studies confirm that plastic curettes produced an insignificant alteration of a titanium implant surface, whereas metal instruments altered the surface at level of significance of $P = 0.001$. In this study,

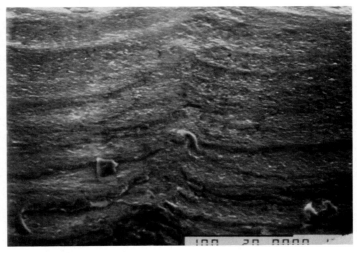

FIG 33–14.
Hydroxylapatite-coated titanium, treated with titanium-tipped curettes (SEM; $350\times$).

titanium-tipped curettes produced a rougher surface than the stainless-steel curette.

Is this surface roughening of any consequence? Commercial firms have marketed plastic instruments for facilitating homecare procedures, but most of these are gross and obviously designed for supragingival instrumentation only. What is obviously needed is the formulation of plastic or Teflon-coated curettes that can effectively treat the subgingival area without changing the surface topography of the implant. Several commercial firms are actively pursuing this goal. Initial studies are quite promising utilizing prototype instruments. It is also advisable to use a plastic disposable probe (available from ProDentec, Batesville, Ark.) to determine the advent and extent of any periodontal or peri-implant problems.

Antimicrobial Treatment

To ensure optimum health around the implant, the following must be accomplished:

1. Plaque must be inhibited
2. Early microbial population on the tooth/implant surfaces must be negated
3. All existing plaque must be eliminated
4. The existing plaque must be altered from pathogenic to nonpathogenic microorganisms.

Antimicrobials effected a minimum alteration of the implant surfaces studied, so an effective means of soft tissue maintenance around the dental implant might be the use of a rinse or mouthwash containing commercially available compounds such as phenolic agents, plant alkaloids, or a prescription containing chlorhexidine gluconate.

Many implant dentists use the chlorhexidine gluconate (Peridex; Procter & Gamble, Cincinnati); approved by the American Dental Association because of its demonstrated substantivity or binding action to the tissues in the oral cavity. It has demonstrated close to 100% bacterial kill of the oral bacteria in a 0.12% concentration even after 5 hours after a 30-second rinse.[51]

Chlorhexidine gluconate is a symmetrical cationic molecule consisting of two 4-chlorphenyl rings and two biguanide groups connected by a central hexamethylene chain. At physiologic pH, it interacts with negative charges on the cell walls of the bacteria and is actually bonded or absorbed to the cell wall. After adherence, the permeability of the cell wall is affected, and leakage of the intracellular components occurs. At high concentrations, precipitation of cytoplasm results. It does not cause lysis of the cells as occurs with penicillin and antiseptics such as hypochlorite but is more related to the extensive intracellular damage.

Follow-up Protocol

To effect optimum home care at the gingival/implant junction, hygiene is most readily accomplished with the use of an interdental brush (Fig 33–15) or a rotary unitufted brush (Rota-Dent; ProDentec) (Fig 33–16). The latter instrument is particularly effective in posterior segments and from the lingual aspect where access is difficult and the superstructure "hides" the implant post from normal oral hygiene procedures. It has been our experience that the patient should be instructed in the use of the instrumentation, area by area, upon insertion of the superstructure. This should be accomplished immediately after placement of the prosthesis and should be part of the treatment protocol.

It is also effective to utilize the antimicrobials with the hand or motorized brushes to achieve maximum contact of the agent with the implant and soft tissue surfaces. Again, the binding action and substantivity of the compound to the soft tissues, tooth, and implant structures will increase the efficacy and longevity of the homecare procedure(s). The patient utilizes the rinse as directed by the manufacturer; chlorhexidine may have the side effect of staining in some individuals so the patient with multiple composite or tooth-colored filling materials is counseled to use a cotton swab, dipped in the antimicrobial, and applied to the site. In our protocol, it is also advisable to dip the hand or motorized brush head in the solution with subsequent application to the implant head and neck. In our maintenance protocol, the patient initiates the rinsing regimen immediately after surgical placement with the one-stage system or upon reopening the implant site in the case of the two-stage system; the combination

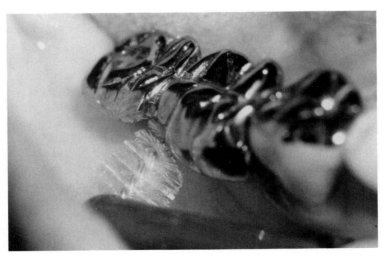

FIG 33–15.
Interdental brush *(bottom)* used to cleanse inter-implant areas.

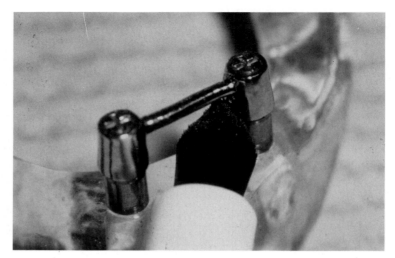

FIG 33–16.
Rotary brush (motorized), used to effect homecare on implant abutments and at soft tissue–implant interface.

rinsing and brushing daily homecare procedures with the antimicrobials begin upon insertion of the prosthesis.

To facilitate homecare procedures, the superstructure must be self-cleansing and completely fixture-borne, with adequate embrasures for hygiene instrument access (Figs 33–17 and 33–18), not one completely unhygienic and lending itself to plaque accumulation, gingival inflammation, and ineffective maintenance (Fig 33–19).

An established maintenance protocol relating to care of the endosseous dental implants might entail a recall visit every 3 months. At this time the effectiveness of hygiene is documented, and the integrity of the fixture or device is verified by inserting an instrument under the prosthesis and gently prying it up, noting any movement of the superstructure. Movement would indicate obvious lack of osseointegration of the implant system, possible failure of the cement bond between superstructure and retainer (in the case of a cemented prosthesis), or screw failure (fracture, loosening) in the case of screwed-in, retrievable super-structure. To complement the 3-month recall visits, a periapical radiograph should be obtained every 6 months to document any changes in osseous topography or the presence of a peri-implant space, denoting a problem or a failing implant. If the prosthesis is retrievable by means of copings or screws, it should be removed every year to ascertain gingival health and implant stability. The appropriate radiographs and hygiene checks can be accomplished at this time.

What happens if crestal bone loss and increased pocket depth are detected at radiographic study and probing (via a plastic-tipped probe) detects and clinical

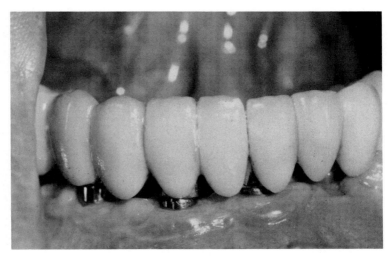

FIG 33–17.
Fixed implant–borne prosthesis with adequate access for homecare procedures.

examination reveals purulence and inflammation? The causes may be multiple: overheating the bone during site preparation; premature loading, resulting in a connective tissue encapsulation; overloading the system, causing microfractures in the bone; trauma to soft or hard tissues during the surgical or restorative phase, and so forth.

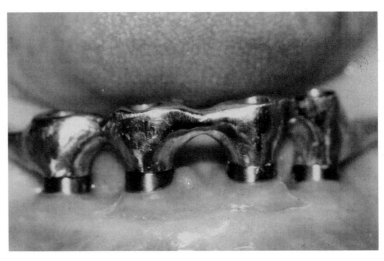

FIG 33–18.
Fixed implant–borne prosthesis with embrasures, access areas for hygiene instrumentation.

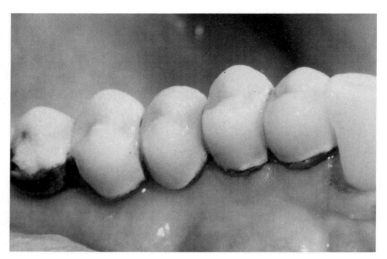

FIG 33–19.
Unhygienic implant-borne fixed appliance with inadequate embrasures (supragingival restorative).

It has been our clinical experience that the endosseous implant may still be "osseointegrated" in terms of lack of clinical mobility, even with severe bone loss patterns. A case in point involves a 61-year-old white woman with two HA-coated implants serving as intermediate and anterior abutments for a fixed partial denture replacing teeth numbers 27 through 31. The implants had been placed in function 2 years prior to the evaluation; she had not reported for maintenance checks but decided to come because the bridge "felt loose." Examination revealed that the screw afixing the superstructure to the distal abutment had backed out and that all the forces were being borne in a torquing, rocking action by the mesial implant abutment. Severe bone loss was noted radiographically; a full-thickness mucoperiosteal flap was reflected, the area had degranulated, and was grafted with HA (Fig 33–20). Radiographs obtained immediately after revealed filling of the defect (Fig 33–21), and 6-month (Fig 33–22) and 18-month (Fig 33–23) radiographs reveal good retention of the grafting material. Tissue health is excellent and the patient is on a strict 3-month maintenance and recall program. This case not only demonstrates the damage caused by lateral, torquing forces on the endosseous dental implant but also the need for the patient to be seen on a strict recall program to preclude severe problems that may not be amenable to any type of therapy.

Repair of the ailing/failing implant can best be accomplished by the alloplastic grafts now commercially available; the purpose of the material is to mechanically obliterate the defect and prevent the ingress of junctional epithelium. In our experience, the surface of the implant should be "detoxified" with either citric acid or chlorhexidine upon exposure and degranulation of the defect, as the surface is obviously contaminated with toxins (enzymes of the anaerobic flora). Guided tissue regeneration with nonresorbable and resorbable materials is being used with great success and will probably be part of future repair protocols.

SUMMARY

Published research reveals the perimucosal seal of the soft tissue to the implant substrate to be tenuous and unpredictable at best; attempts have been made to coat the implant surface with collagen, fibronectin, and laminin in an effort to promote fibroblast and epithelial cell adhesion and mitotic activity. Results have been controversial and require more research. Unpublished studies show that collagen will speed up epithelial cell adhesion and growth on selected implant substrates.

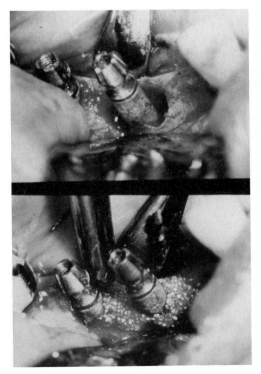

FIG 33–20.
Defect degranulated around implant *(top);* grafted with particulate form of hydroxylapatite *(bottom).*

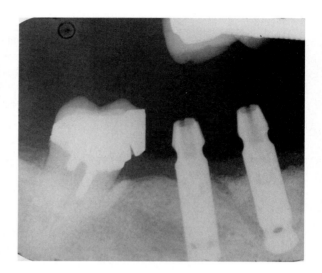

FIG 33–21.
Immediately following grafting
of defect around implant.

If the seal is fragile or nonexistent, soft tissue health is of maximum importance in the maintenance of the dental implant. In the usual case, the tonus of the soft tissue cuff around the implant neck may be accomplished by the gingival circular fibers and prevention of plaque retention and maturation. Furthermore, so as not to disturb this integrity at the interface, subgingival instrumentation must be studiously avoided except in the case of obvious disease patterns and the need for grafting and repair. Unpublished studies show that hand and ultrasonic instrumentation might be detrimental in terms of roughening the implant surface—a situation that would certainly tend toward plaque retention. From present knowledge, the use of antimicrobials and hand or

FIG 33–22.
Six months after grafting of defect around implant.

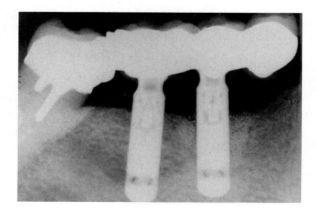

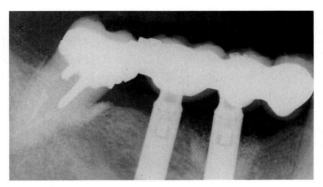

FIG 33–23.
Eighteen months after grafting of defect around implant.

motorized brushes would seem the regimen and instrumentation of choice in maintenance of the dental implant.

The philosophies of fibro-osseous integration vs. osseointegration vs. biointegration are discussed in terms of bioactive and bioinert surfaces. The premise of connective tissue fibers at the bone-implant interface being an osteogenic ligament with bioelectric or piezoelectric properties has not been proved, and the premise that this exists as a viable entity in the endosseous root form implant is suspect. Connective tissue will form at the interface with premature loading, since the work of Roberts[31] shows that bone will not show maximum load-carrying capability before 18 weeks in the human being. Overheating the bone during site preparation will cause bone loss,[33] and it is recommended that speeds of not more than 2,000 rpm with a graded series of drill sizes be used, and that external irrigation would help prevent heating the bone. Other facets such as extraordinary pressure upon placement and the implant not fitting the site will allow for bone loss and/or apical migration of junctional epithelium into the interface. The importance of implant fit to the prepared site has been demonstrated by Carlsson et al.[34] and Satomi et al.[35]

Osseointegration, defined as the absence of connective tissue at the bone-implant interface, is recognized as a histologic finding of bone-implant contact. It is in the range of 25% to 75% in the functioning system and has not been reported at a figure above 85%.[30, 40–42] Biointegration is a different phenomenon, in which bone matrix is deposited on the HA layer as a result of some type of physicochemical interaction between bone collagen and the HA crystals of the implant.[37] This bonding would be similar to ankylosis of the natural tooth.

The design of the superstructure in terms of lack of subgingival extension, open embrasures, and complete accessibility to the implant neck with oral hygiene procedures is of utmost importance in the long-term care of the dental implant.

The patient should be recalled every 3 months for evaluation of the prosthesis and of homecare, with radiographs obtained every 6 months to detect any osseous changes. If the prosthesis is retrievable, it should be removed every year to determine implant stability and gingival integrity, through checking with a plastic-tipped probe.

If bone loss patterns are evident radiographically and/or clinically and the implant is still "integrated" as verified by lack of clinical mobility, grafting materials would seem to be indicated to decrease pocket depths and render the areas more accessible to homecare procedures.

REFERENCES

1. Arnim SS, Hagerman DA: The connective tissue fibers of the marginal gingiva, *J Am Dent Assn* 47:271, 1953.
2. Gould TR, Brunette DM, Westbury L: The attachment mechanism of epithelial cells to titanium in vitro, *J Periodont Res* 16:611–616, 1981.
3. Schroeder A, van der Zypen E, Stich H: The reactions of bone, connective tissue and epithelium to endosteal implants with titanium-sprayed surfaces, *J Oral Maxillofac Surg* 9:15, 1981.
4. Wennstrom J: Keratinized and attached gingiva: regenerative potential and significance for periodontal health (thesis), University of Goteborg, Sweden, 1982.
5. Wennstrom J, Lindhe J: Plaque-induced gingival inflammation in the absence of attached gingiva in dogs, *J Clin Periodontol* 10:266, 1983.
6. Adell R et al: A 15 year study of osseointegrated implants in the treatment of the edentulous jaw, *Int J Oral Surg* 10:387, 1981.
7. Jansen JA: Ultrastructural study of epithelial cell attachment to implant materials, *J Dent Res* 65:5, 1985.
8. von Recum AF, Schreuders PD, Powers DL: Basic healing phenomena around permanent percutaneous implants, International Congress on Tissue Integration, Current Practice Series 29, Amsterdam, 1986, Excerpta Medica, pp 159–169.
9. Kleinman HK, Klebe RJ, Martin GR: Role of collagenous matrices in adhesion and growth of cells, *J Cell Biol* 88:473–485, 1981.
10. Lowenberg BF et al: Attachment, migration and orientation of human gingival fibroblasts to collagen-coated, surface demineralized and nondemineralized dentin in vitro, *J Periodont Res* 65:1106, 1985.
11. Lowenberg BF et al: Migration, attachment and orientation of human gingival fibroblasts to root slices, naked and porous-surfaced titanium alloy discs, and zircalloy-2 discs in vitro, *J Dent Res* 66:1000, 1987.
12. Kasten FH, Soileau K, Meffert RM: Quantitative evaluation of human gingival epithelial cell attachment to implant surfaces in vitro, *Int J Periodont Restor Dent* 10:69–79, 1990.
13. Seitz TL et al: Effect of fibronectin on the adhesion of an established cell line to a surface reactive material, *J Biomed Mater Res* 16:195, 1982.
14. Meffert RM, Block MS, Kent JN: What is osseointegration? *Int J Periodont Restorative Dent* 4:9, 1987.

15. DePorter DA, Friedland B, Watson PA: A clinical and radiographic assessment of a porous-surfaced, titanium alloy dental implant system in dogs, *J Dent Res* 65:1071, 1986.
16. Klawitter JJ, Weinstein AM, Cooke FW: An evaluation of porous-surfaced alumina ceramic implants, *J Dent Res* 56:768, 1977.
17. Hottel TL, Gibbons DF: The effect on change of surface microstructure of carbon oral implants on gingival structures, *J Oral Maxillofac Surg* 40:647, 1982.
18. Dahlin C et al: Generation of new bone around titanium implants using a membrane technique: an experimental study in rabbits, *Int J Oral Maxillofac Implants*, 4:19–25, 1989.
19. Zablotsky M, Meffert RM, Caudill R, et al: Histological and clinical comparisons of guided tissue regeneration on dehisced hydroxylapatite-coated and titanium endosseous implant surfaces: A pilot study, *Int J Oral Maxillofac Implants* 6:295–303, 1991.
20. American Academy of Implant Dentistry Glossary of Terms, *Oral Implant* 12:284, 1986.
21. Weiss CM: A comparative analysis of fibro-osteal and osteal integration and other variables that affect long term bone maintenance around dental implants, *J Oral Implant* 13:467, 1987.
22. Weiss CM: Tissue integration of dental endosseous implants: description and comparative analysis of fibro-osseous and osseointegration systems, *J Oral Implant* 12:169, 1986.
23. Harms J, Mausle E: Biokompatibilitat von implanten in der orthopadie, *Hefte Unfalheilkd.* 144:1, 1980.
24. Kohler S: Untersuchungen der grenzflachen zwischen implantat and knocken mit dem electronenstrahlmikdranalysator (EMSA), *Zahn Mund Kiederheilkd* 69:4, 1981.
25. Cook SD et al: Interface mechanics and histology of titanium and hydroxylapatite-coated titanium for dental implant applications, *Int J Oral Maxillofac Implants* 2:1, 15, 1987.
26. Linder L, Lindskog J: Incorporation of stainless steel, titanium and vitallium in bone, *Injury* 6:277, 1975.
27. Karagianes MT: Development and evaluation of porous-surfaced dental implants in miniature swine, *J Dent Res* 55:85, 1976.
28. Schroeder A, Pohler O, Sutter F: Gewebsreaktion auf ein Titan-hohlzylinder implantat mit titan-sprizoberflachhe, *Schweiz., Mschr., Zahnheilk.* 86:713, 1976.
29. Branemark P-I, Zarb G, Albrektsson T: *Tissue integrated prostheses: osseointegration in clinical dentistry,* Chicago, 1985, Quintessence, pp 11–77, 129–145.
30. Johansson C, Albrektsson T: Integration of screw implants in the rabbit: a 1-year follow-up of removal torque of titanium implants, *Int J Oral Maxillofac Surg* 2:69, 1987.
31. Roberts WE et al: Bone physiology and metabolism, *J Calif Dent Assoc* 54:32–39, 1987.
32. Linkow LI, Wertman E: Re-entry implants and their procedures, *J Oral Implant* 12:590–626, 1986.
33. Eriksson RA, Albrektsson T: The effect of heat on bone regeneration, *J Oral Maxillofac Surg* 42:701–711, 1984.
34. Carlsson L et al: Implant fixation improved by close fit, *Acta Orthop Scand* 59:272, 1988.

35. Satomi K et al: Bone-implant interface structures after nontapping and tapping insertion of screw-type titanium alloy endosseous implants, *J Prosthet Dent* 59:339, 1988.

36. dePutter C, deLange GL, deGroot K: Permucosal oral implants of dense hydroxylapatite: fixation in alveolar bone, International Congress on Tissue Integration in Oral and Maxillofacial Reconstruction, May 1985; Current Practice Series 29. Amsterdam, Excerpta Medica, 1986, pp 389–394.

37. Denissen HW, Veldhuis AAH, van der Hooff A: Hydroxylapatite titanium implants, International Congress on Tissue Integration in Oral and Maxillofacial Reconstruction, May 1985; Excerpta Medica, Current Practice Series 29, 1986, pp 372–389.

38. Block MS, Kent JN, Kay JF: Evaluation of hydroxylapatite-coated titanium dental implants in dogs, *J Oral Maxillofac Surg* 45:601, 1987.

39. Cook SD et al: Interface mechanics and histology of titanium and hydroxylapatite-coated titanium for dental implant applications, *Int J Oral Maxillofac Implants* 2:1, 15, 1987.

40. Block M et al: Loaded HA-coated and grit titanium implants in dogs (abstract), *J Dent Res* 67:178, 1989.

41. Davis TS et al: A histologic comparison of the bone-implant interface utilizing the Integral(TM) and three surface variations of the Micro-Vent(TM) implant, submitted for publication.

42. Dickerson AC et al: Titanium vs. hydroxylapatite-coated blade implants, submitted for publication.

43. Rams T et al: The subgingival microbial flora associated with human dental implants, *J Prosthet Dent* 51:529, 1984.

44. Rams T, Link C Jr: Microbiology of failing dental implants in humans: electron microscopic observations, *J Oral Implant* 11:93, 1983.

45. Lekholm U et al: The condition of soft tissue at tooth and fixture abutments supporting fixed bridges: a microbiological and histological study, *J Clin Periodontol* 13:558, 1986.

46. Mombelli A et al: The microbiota associated with successful or failing osseointegrated titanium implants, *Oral Microbiol Immunol* 2:145, 1987.

47. Alcoforado GAP et al: Microbiology of failing osseointegrated dental implants, abstract, ASM Annual meeting, New Orleans, 1989.

48. Becker W et al: Clinical and microbiologic findings that may contribute to dental implant failure, *Int J Oral Maxillofac Implants* 5:31–38, 1990.

49. Wolinsky LE, Camargo PM, Erard JC: A study of in vitro attachment of *Streptococcus sanguis* and *Actinomyces viscosus* to saliva-treated titanium, *Int J Oral Maxillofac Implants* 4:27–31, 1989.

50. Thomson-Neal D et al: A SEM evaluation of various prophylactic modalities on different implants, *Int J Perio Rest Dent* 4; 1989.

51. Briner WW et al: Effect of chlorhexidine gluconate mouthrinse on plaque bacteria, *J Periodont Res* 16(suppl):44–52, 1986.

Index